Stahl's Essential Psychopharmacology

Neuroscientific Basis and Practical Application

Fourth Edition

Stephen M. Stahl
Adjunct Professor of Psychiatry, University of California at San Diego, CA, USA;
Honorary Visiting Senior Fellow in Psychiatry, University of Cambridge, Cambridge, UK

with illustrations by
Nancy Muntner

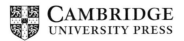
CAMBRIDGE
UNIVERSITY PRESS

CAMBRIDGE
UNIVERSITY PRESS

University Printing House, Cambridge CB2 8BS, United Kingdom

Published in the United States of America by Cambridge University Press, New York

Cambridge University Press is part of the University of Cambridge.

It furthers the University's mission by disseminating knowledge in the pursuit of education, learning and research at the highest international levels of excellence.

www.cambridge.org
Information on this title: www.cambridge.org/9781107025981

First edition published 1996
Second edition published 2000
Third edition published 2008
Fourth edition published 2013
Reprinted 2013

Printed in Spain by Grafos SA, Arte Sobre Papel, Barcelona

A catalog record for this publication is available from the British Library

Library of Congress Cataloging in Publication data

Stahl, S. M.
   Stahl's essential psychopharmacology : neuroscientific basis and practical
application / Stephen M. Stahl ; with illustrations by Nancy Muntner. – 4th ed.
      p. ; cm.
   Essential psychopharmacology
   Includes bibliographical references and index.
   ISBN 978-1-107-02598-1 (Hardback) – ISBN 978-1-107-68646-5 (Paperback)
   I. Title.   II. Title: Essential psychopharmacology.
   [DNLM: 1. Mental Disorders–drug therapy.   2. Central Nervous System–
drug effects.   3. Psychotropic Drugs–pharmacology.   WM 402]
   616.89′18–dc23
                                                                       2012036791

ISBN 978-1-107-02598-1 Hardback
ISBN 978-1-107-68646-5 Paperback

In memory of Daniel X. Freedman, mentor, colleague, and scientific father

To Cindy, Jennifer, and Victoria

Contents

Preface to the fourth edition

For this fourth edition of *Stahl's Essential Psychopharmacology* you will notice there is a new look and feel. With a new layout, displayed over two columns, and an increased page size we have eliminated redundancies across chapters, have added significant new material, and yet have decreased the overall size of the book.

Highlights of what has been added or changed since the 3rd edition include:

- Integrating much of the basic neurosciences into the clinical chapters, thus reducing the number of introductory chapters solely covering basic neurosciences.
- Major revision of the psychosis chapter, including much more detailed coverage of the neurocircuitry of schizophrenia, the role of glutamate, genomics, and neuroimaging.
- One of the most extensively revised chapters is on antipsychotics, which now has:
  - new discussion and illustrations on how the current atypical antipsychotics act upon serotonin, dopamine, and glutamate circuitry
  - new discussion of the roles of neurotransmitter receptors in the mechanisms of actions of some but not all atypical antipsychotics
    - $5HT_7$ receptors
    - $5HT_{2C}$ receptors
    - α_1-adrenergic receptors
  - completely revamped visuals for displaying the relative binding properties of 17 individual antipsychotics agents, based upon log binding data made qualitative and visual with novel graphics
  - reorganization of the known atypical antipsychotics as
    - the "pines" (peens)
    - the "dones"
    - two "pips"
    - and a "rip"
- inclusion of several new antipsychotics
  - iloperidone (Fanapt)
  - asenapine (Saphris)
  - lurasidone (Latuda)
- extensive coverage of switching from one antipsychotic to another
- new ideas about using high dosing and polypharmacy for treatment resistance and violence
- new antipsychotics in the pipeline
  - brexpiprazole
  - cariprazine
  - selective glycine reuptake inhibitors (SGRIs, e.g., bitopertin [RG1678], Org25935, SSR103800)
- The mood chapter has expanded coverage of stress, neurocircuitry, and genetics.
- The antidepressant and mood stabilizer chapters have:
  - new discussion and illustrations on circadian rhythms
  - discussion of the roles of neurotransmitter receptors in the mechanisms of actions of some antidepressants
    - melatonin receptors
    - $5HT_{1A}$ receptors
    - $5HT_{2C}$ receptors
    - $5HT_3$ receptors
    - $5HT_7$ receptors
    - NMDA glutamate receptors
  - inclusion of several new antidepressants
    - agomelatine (Valdoxan)
    - vilazodone (Viibryd)

- vortioxetine (LuAA21004)
- ketamine (rapid onset for treatment resistance)
- The anxiety chapter provides new coverage of the concepts of fear conditioning, fear extinction, and reconsolidation, with OCD moved to the impulsivity chapter.
- The pain chapter updates neuropathic pain states.
- The sleep/wake chapter provides expanded coverage of melatonin and new discussion of orexin pathways and orexin receptors, as well as new drugs targeting orexin receptors as antagonists, such as:
  - suvorexant/MK-6096
  - almorexant
  - SB-649868
- The ADHD chapter includes new discussion on how norepinephrine and dopamine tune pyramidal neurons in prefrontal cortex, and expanded discussion on new treatments such as:
  - guanfacine ER (Intuniv)
  - lisdexamfetamine (Vyvanse)
- The dementia chapter has been extensively revamped to emphasize the new diagnostic criteria for Alzheimer's disease, and the integration of biomarkers into diagnostic schemes including:
  - Alzheimer's diagnostics
    - CSF Aβ and tau levels
    - amyloid PET scans, FDG-PET scans, structural MRI scans
  - multiple new drugs in the pipeline targeting amyloid plaques, tangles, and tau
    - vaccines/immunotherapy (e.g., bapineuzumab, solenezumab, crenezumab), intravenous immunoglobulin
    - γ-secretase inhibitors (GSIs, e.g., semagacestat)
    - β-secretase inhibitors (e.g., LY2886721, SCH 1381252, CTS21666, others)
- The impulsivity–compulsivity and addiction chapter is another of the most extensively revised chapters in this fourth edition, significantly expanding the drug abuse chapter of the third edition to include now a large number of related "impulsive–compulsive" disorders that hypothetically share the same brain circuitry:

- neurocircuitry of impulsivity and reward involving the ventral striatum
- neurocircuitry of compulsivity and habits including drug addiction and behavioral addiction involving the dorsal striatum
- "bottom-up" striatal drives and "top-down" inhibitory controls from the prefrontal cortex
- update on the neurobiology and available treatments for the drug addictions (stimulants, nicotine, alcohol, opioids, hallucinogens, and others)
- behavioral addictions
  - major new section on obesity, eating disorders, and food addiction, including the role of hypothalamic circuits and new treatments for obesity
  - lorcaserin (Belviq)
  - phentermine/topiramate ER (Qsymia)
  - bupropion/naltrexone (Contrave)
  - zonisamide/naltrexone
  - obsessive–compulsive and spectrum disorders
  - gambling, impulsive violence, mania, ADHD and many others

One of the major themes emphasized in this new edition is the notion of **symptom endophenotypes**, or dimensions of psychopathology that cut across numerous syndromes. This is seen perhaps most dramatically in the organization of numerous disorders of impulsivity/compulsivity, where impulsivity and/ or compulsivity are present in many psychiatric conditions and thus "travel" trans-diagnostically without respecting the DSM (*Diagnostic and Statistical Manual*) of the American Psychiatric Association or the ICD (*International Classification of Diseases*). This is the future of psychiatry – the matching of symptom endophenotypes to hypothetically malfunctioning brain circuits, regulated by genes, the environment, and neurotransmitters. Hypothetically, inefficiency of information processing in these brain circuits creates symptom expression in various psychiatric disorders that can be changed with psychopharmacologic agents. Even the DSM recognizes this concept and calls it Research Domain Criteria (or RDoC). Thus, impulsivity and compulsivity can be seen as domains of psychopathology; other domains include mood, cognition, anxiety, motivation, and many more. Each chapter in this fourth edition discusses "symptoms and circuits" and how to exploit domains of psychopathology both to become a neurobiologically empowered psychopharmacologist, and to select and combine treatments for individual patients in psychopharmacology practice.

What has not changed in this new edition is the **didactic style** of the first three editions. This text attempts to present the fundamentals of psychopharmacology in **simplified and readily readable form**. We emphasize current formulations of disease mechanisms and also drug mechanisms. As in previous editions, the text is not extensively referenced to original papers, but rather to textbooks and reviews and a few selected original papers, with only a limited reading list for each chapter, but preparing the reader to consult more sophisticated textbooks as well as the professional literature.

The organization of information continues to apply the principles of **programmed learning** for the reader, namely repetition and interaction, which has been shown to enhance retention. Therefore, it is suggested that novices first approach this text by going through it from beginning to end, reviewing only the color graphics and the legends for those graphics. Virtually everything covered in the text is also covered in the graphics and icons. Once having gone through all the color graphics in these chapters, it is recommended that the reader then go back to the beginning of the book, and read the entire text, reviewing the graphics at the same time. After the text has been read, the entire book can be rapidly reviewed again merely by referring to the various color graphics in the book. This mechanism of using the materials will create a certain amount of programmed learning by incorporating the elements of repetition, as well as interaction with visual learning through graphics. Hopefully, the visual concepts learned via graphics will reinforce abstract concepts learned from the written text, especially for those of you who are primarily "visual learners" (i.e., those who retain information better from visualizing concepts than from reading about them). For those of you who are already familiar with psychopharmacology, this book should provide easy reading from beginning to end. Going back and forth between the text and the graphics should provide interaction. Following review of the complete text, it should be simple to review the entire book by going through the graphics once again.

Expansion of *Essential Psychopharmacology* books

This fourth edition of *Essential Psychopharmacology* is the flagship, but not the entire fleet, as the *Essential Psychopharmacology* series has expanded now to an entire suite of products for the interested reader. For those of you interested in specific prescribing information, there are now three prescriber's guides:

- for psychotropic drugs, *Stahl's Essential Psychopharmacology: the Prescriber's Guide*
- for neurology drugs, *Essential Neuropharmacology: the Prescriber's Guide*
- for pain drugs: *Essential Pain Pharmacology: the Prescriber's Guide*

For those interested in how the textbook and prescriber's guides get applied in clinical practice there is a book covering 40 cases from my own clinical practice:

- *Case Studies: Stahl's Essential Psychopharmacology*

For teachers and students wanting to assess objectively their state of expertise, to pursue maintenance of certification credits for board recertification in psychiatry in the US, and for background on instructional design and how to teach there are two books:

- *Stahl's Self-Assessment Examination in Psychiatry: Multiple Choice Questions for Clinicians*
- *Best Practices in Medical Teaching*

For those interested in expanded visual coverage of specialty topics in psychopharmacology, there is the *Stahl's Illustrated* series:

- *Antidepressants*
- *Antipsychotics: Treating Psychosis, Mania and Depression*, 2nd edition
- *Anxiety, Stress, and PTSD*
- *Attention Deficit Hyperactivity Disorder*
- *Chronic Pain and Fibromyalgia*
- *Mood Stabilizers*
- *Substance Use and Impulsive Disorders*

Finally, there is an ever-growing edited series of subspecialty topics:

- *Next Generation Antidepressants*
- *Essential Evidence-Based Psychopharmacology*, 2nd edition
- *Essential CNS Drug Development*

Essential Psychopharmacology Online

Now, you also have the option of accessing all these books plus additional features online by going to *Essential Psychopharmacology Online* at **www.stahlonline. org**. We are proud to announce the continuing update of this new website which allows you to search online within the entire *Essential Psychopharmacology* suite of products. With publication of the fourth edition, two new features will become available on the website:

- downloadable slides of all the figures in the book
- narrated animations of several figures in the textbook, hyperlinked to the online version of the book, playable with a click

In addition, **www.stahlonline.org** is now linked to:

- our new journal *CNS Spectrums* (**www.journals. cambridge.org/CNS**), of which I am the new editor-in-chief, and which is now the official journal of the Neuroscience Education Institute (NEI), free online to NEI members. This journal now features readable and illustrated reviews of current topics in psychiatry, mental health, neurology, and the neurosciences as well as psychopharmacology
- the NEI website, **www.neiglobal.com**:

- for CME credits for reading the books and the journal, and for completing numerous additional programs both online and live
- for access to the live course and playback encore features from the annual NEI Psychopharmacology Congress
- for access to the NEI Master Psychopharmacology Program, an online fellowship with certification

- plans for expansion to a Cambridge University Health Partners co-accredited online Masterclass and Certificate in Psychopharmacology, based upon live programs held on campus in Cambridge and taught by University of Cambridge faculty, including myself, having joined the faculty there as an Honorary Visiting Senior Fellow

Hopefully the reader can appreciate that this is an incredibly exciting time for the fields of neuroscience and mental health, creating fascinating opportunities for clinicians to utilize current therapeutics and to anticipate future medications that are likely to transform the field of psychopharmacology. Best wishes for your first step on this fascinating journey.

Stephen M. Stahl, MD, PhD

CME information

Release/expiration dates

Release date: February 1, 2013

CME credit expiration date: January 31, 2016 (*if this date has passed, please contact NEI for updated information*)

Target audience

This activity has been developed for prescribers specializing in psychiatry. There are no prerequisites. All other healthcare providers who are interested in psychopharmacology are welcome for advanced study, especially primary care physicians, nurse practitioners, psychologists, and pharmacists.

Statement of need

Psychiatric illnesses have a neurobiological basis and are primarily treated by pharmacological agents; understanding each of these, as well as the relationship between them, is essential in order to select appropriate treatment for a patient. The field of psychopharmacology has experienced incredible growth; it has also experienced a major paradigm shift from a limited focus on neurotransmitters and receptors to an emphasis as well upon brain circuits, neuroimaging, genetics, and signal transduction cascades.

The following unmet needs and professional practice gaps regarding mental health were revealed following a critical analysis of activity feedback, expert faculty assessment, literature review, and through new medical knowledge:

- Mental disorders are highly prevalent and carry substantial burden that can be alleviated through treatment; unfortunately, many patients with mental disorders do not receive treatment or receive suboptimal treatment.
- There is a documented gap between evidence-based practice guidelines and actual care in clinical practice for patients with mental illnesses.
- This gap is due at least in part to lack of clinician confidence and knowledge in terms of appropriate usage of the therapeutic tools available to them.

To help address clinician performance gaps with respect to diagnosis and treatment of mental health disorders, quality improvement efforts need to provide education regarding (1) the fundamentals of neurobiology as it relates to the most recent research regarding the neurobiology of mental illnesses; (2) the mechanisms of action of treatment options for mental illnesses and the relationship to the pathophysiology of the disease states; and (3) new therapeutic tools and research that are likely to affect clinical practice.

Learning objectives

After completing this activity, participants should be better able to

- apply fundamental principles of neurobiology to the assessment of psychiatric disease states
- differentiate the neurobiological targets for psychotropic medications
- link the relationship of psychotropic drug mechanism of action to the pathophysiology of disease states
- identify novel research and treatment approaches that are expected to affect clinical practice

Accreditation and credit designation statements

The Neuroscience Education Institute (NEI) is accredited by the Accreditation Council for Continuing Medical Education (ACCME) to provide continuing medical education for physicians.

The Neuroscience Education Institute designates this enduring material for a maximum of 67 *AMA PRA Category 1 Credits*™. Physicians should claim only the credit commensurate with the extent of their participation in the activity.

Nurses: for all of your CE requirements for recertification, the ANCC will accept *AMA PRA Category 1 Credits*™ from organizations accredited by the ACCME.

Physician assistants: the NCCPA accepts *AMA PRA Category 1 Credits*™ from organizations accredited by the AMA (providers accredited by the ACCME).

A certificate of participation for completing this activity will also be available.

Activity instructions

This CME activity is in the form of a printed monograph and incorporates instructional design to enhance your retention of the information and pharmacological concepts that are being presented. You are advised to go through the figures in this activity from beginning to end, followed by the text, and then complete the posttests and evaluations. The estimated time for completion of this activity is 67 hours.

Instructions for CME credit

Certificates of CME credit or participation are available for each topical section of the book (total of 12 sections). To receive a section-specific certificate of CME credit or participation, please complete the relevant posttest and evaluation, available only online at **www.neiglobal.com/CME** (under "Book"). If a passing score of 70% or more is attained (required to receive credit), you can immediately print your certificate. There is a fee for each post test (varies per section), which is waived for NEI members. If you have questions, please call 888–535–5600, or email customerservice@neiglobal.com.

NEI disclosure policy

It is the policy of the Neuroscience Education Institute to ensure balance, independence, objectivity, and scientific rigor in all its educational activities. Therefore, all individuals in a position to influence or control content development are required by NEI to disclose any financial relationships or apparent conflicts of interest. Although potential conflicts of interest are identified and resolved prior to the activity, it remains for the audience to determine whether outside interests reflect a possible bias in either the exposition or the conclusions presented.

These materials have been peer-reviewed to ensure the scientific accuracy and medical relevance of information presented and its independence from commercial bias. The Neuroscience Education Institute takes responsibility for the content, quality, and scientific integrity of this CME activity.

Individual disclosure statements

Author
Stephen M. Stahl, MD, PhD
Adjunct Professor, Department of Psychiatry, University of California, San Diego School of Medicine

Honorary Visiting Senior Fellow, University of Cambridge, UK

Grant/research: AstraZeneca, CeNeRx Bio-Pharma, Forest, Genomind, Lilly, Merck, Neuronetics, Pamlab, Pfizer, Roche, Sunovion, Servier, Shire, Torrent, Trovis

Consultant/advisor: Abbott, ACADIA, AstraZeneca, AVANIR, BioMarin, Bristol-Myers Squibb, CeNeRx, Forest, Genomind, GlaxoSmithKline, Johnson & Johnson, Lilly, Lundbeck, Merck, Mylan (f/k/a Dey), Neuronetics, Novartis, Noven, Ono Pharma, Orexigen, Otsuka America, Pamlab, Pfizer, RCT LOGIC, Rexahn, Roche, Servier, Shire, Sunovion, Trius, Trovis, Valeant

Speakers bureau: Arbor Scientia, AstraZeneca, Forest, Johnson & Johnson, Lilly, Merck, Pfizer, Servier, Sunovion

Board member: Genomind

Content editors
Meghan Grady
Director, Content Development, Neuroscience Education Institute, Carlsbad, CA

No financial relationships to disclose

Debbi Ann Morrissette, PhD
Adjunct Professor, Biological Sciences, California State University, San Marcos

Medical Writer, Neuroscience Education Institute, Carlsbad, CA

No financial relationships to disclose

Peer reviewers
Steve S. Simring, MD
Clinical Associate Professor, Department of Psychiatry, Columbia University College of Physicians and Surgeons, New York State Psychiatric Institute, New York City

No financial relationships to disclose

Electa Stern, PharmD
Clinical Supervisor, Pharmacy Services, Sharp Grossmont Hospital, La Mesa, CA

No financial relationships to disclose

Ronnie G. Swift, MD

Professor and Associate Chairman, Department of Psychiatry and Behavioral Sciences, New York Medical College, Valhalla

Professor of Clinical Public Health, School of Public Health, New York; New York Medical College, Valhalla

Chief of Psychiatry and Associate Medical Director, Metropolitan Hospital Center, New York City

No financial relationships to disclose

Mark Williams, MD

Assistant Professor, Department of Psychiatry and Psychology, Mayo Clinic, Rochester, MN

No financial relationships to disclose

Design staff

Nancy Muntner

Director, Medical Illustrations, Neuroscience Education Institute, Carlsbad, CA

No financial relationships to disclose

Disclosed financial relationships with conflicts of interest have been reviewed by the Neuroscience Education Institute CME Advisory Board Chair and resolved. All faculty and planning committee members have attested that their financial relationships, if any, do not affect their ability to present well-balanced, evidence-based content for this activity.

Disclosure of off-label use

This educational activity may include discussion of unlabeled and/or investigational uses of agents that are not currently labeled for such use by the FDA. Please consult the product prescribing information for full disclosure of labeled uses.

Disclaimer

Participants have an implied responsibility to use the newly acquired information from this activity to enhance patient outcomes and their own professional development. The information presented in this educational activity is not meant to serve as a guideline for patient management. Any procedures, medications, or other courses of diagnosis or treatment discussed or suggested in this educational activity should not be used by clinicians without evaluation of their patients' conditions and possible contraindications or dangers in use, review of any applicable manufacturer's product information, and comparison with recommendations of other authorities. Primary references and full prescribing information should be consulted.

Cultural and linguistic competency

A variety of resources addressing cultural and linguistic competency can be found at http://cdn.neiglobal.com/content/cme/regulations/ca_ab_1195_handout_non-ca_2008.pdf.

Sponsor

This activity is sponsored by the Neuroscience Education Institute.

Support

This activity is supported solely by the sponsor, Neuroscience Education Institute.

Chemical neurotransmission

Modern psychopharmacology is largely the story of chemical neurotransmission. To understand the actions of drugs on the brain, to grasp the impact of diseases upon the central nervous system, and to interpret the behavioral consequences of psychiatric medicines, one must be fluent in the language and principles of chemical neurotransmission. The importance of this fact cannot be overstated for the student of psychopharmacology. This chapter forms the foundation for the entire book, and the roadmap for one's journey through one of the most exciting topics in science today, namely the neuroscience of how disorders and drugs act upon the central nervous system.

Anatomical versus chemical basis of neurotransmission

What is neurotransmission? Neurotransmission can be described in many ways: anatomically, chemically, electrically. The *anatomical* basis of neurotransmission is neurons (Figures 1-1 through 1-3) and the connections between them, called synapses (Figure 1-4), sometimes also called the *anatomically addressed* nervous system, a complex of "hard-wired" synaptic connections between neurons, not unlike millions of telephone wires within thousands upon thousands of cables. The anatomically addressed brain is thus a complex wiring diagram, ferrying electrical impulses to wherever the "wire" is plugged in (i.e., at a synapse). Synapses can form on many parts of a neuron, not just the dendrites as axodendritic synapses, but also on the soma as axosomatic synapses, and even at the beginning and at the end of axons (axoaxonic synapses) (Figure 1-2). Such synapses are said to be "asymmetric" since communication is structurally designed to be in one direction; that is, anterograde from the axon of the first neuron to the dendrite, soma, or axon of the second neuron (Figures 1-2 and 1-3). This means that there are presynaptic elements that differ from postsynaptic elements (Figure 1-4). Specifically, neurotransmitter is packaged in the presynaptic nerve terminal like ammunition in a loaded gun, and then fired at the postsynaptic neuron to target its receptors.

Neurons are the cells of chemical communication in the brain. Human brains are comprised of tens of billions of neurons, and each is linked to thousands of other neurons. Thus, the brain has trillions of specialized connections known as synapses. Neurons

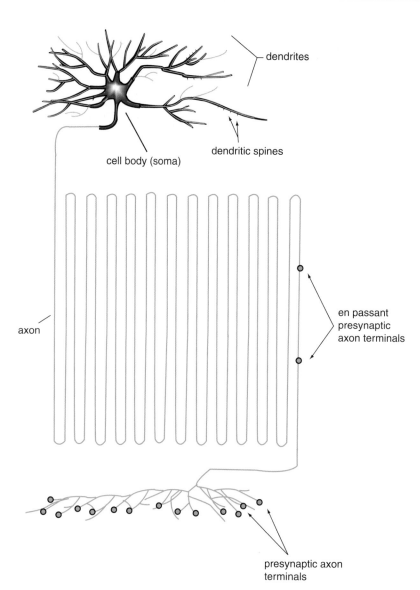

Figure 1-1. **General structure of a neuron.** This is an artist's conception of the generic structure of a neuron. All neurons have a cell body known as the soma, which is the command center of the nerve and contains the nucleus of the cell. All neurons are also set up structurally to both send and receive information. Neurons send information via an axon that forms presynaptic terminals as the axon passes by (en passant) or as the axon ends.

have many sizes, lengths, and shapes that determine their functions. Localization within the brain also determines function. When neurons malfunction, behavioral symptoms may occur. When drugs alter neuronal function, behavioral symptoms may be relieved, worsened, or produced.

General structure of a neuron. Although this textbook will often portray neurons with a generic structure (such as that shown in Figures 1-1 through 1-3), the truth is that many neurons have unique structures depending upon where in the brain they are located and what their function is. All neurons have a cell body known as the soma, and are set up structurally to receive information from other neurons through dendrites, sometimes via spines on the dendrites and often through an elaborately branching "tree" of dendrites (Figure 1-2). Neurons are also set up structurally to send information to other neurons via an axon that forms presynaptic terminals as the axon passes by (en passant, Figure 1-1) or as the axon ends (presynaptic axon terminals, Figures 1-1 through 1-4).

Neurotransmission has an *anatomical* infrastructure, but it is fundamentally a very elegant *chemical* operation. Complementary to the anatomically addressed nervous system is the *chemically addressed* nervous system, which forms the *chemical* basis of neurotransmission: namely, how chemical signals

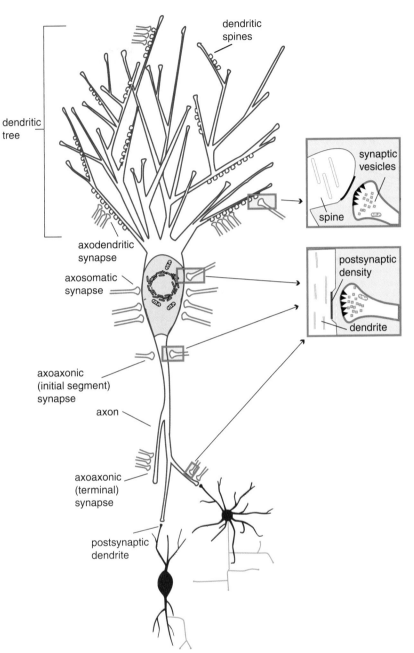

Figure 1-2. Axodendritic, axosomatic, and axoaxonic connections. After neurons migrate, they form synapses. As shown in this figure, synaptic connections can form not just between the axon and dendrites of two neurons (axodendritic) but also between the axon and the soma (axosomatic) or the axons of the two neurons (axoaxonic). Communication is anterograde from the axon of the first neuron to the dendrite, soma, or axon of the second neuron.

are coded, decoded, transduced, and sent along the way. Understanding the principles of chemical neurotransmission is a fundamental requirement for grasping how psychopharmacologic agents work, because they target key molecules involved in neurotransmission. Drug targeting of specific chemical sites that influence neurotransmission is discussed in Chapters 2 and 3.

Understanding the chemically addressed nervous system is also a prerequisite for becoming a "neurobiologically informed" clinician: that is, being able to translate exciting new findings on brain circuitry, functional neuroimaging, and genetics into clinical practice, and potentially improving the manner in which psychiatric disorders and their symptoms are diagnosed and treated. The chemistry of neurotransmission in specific

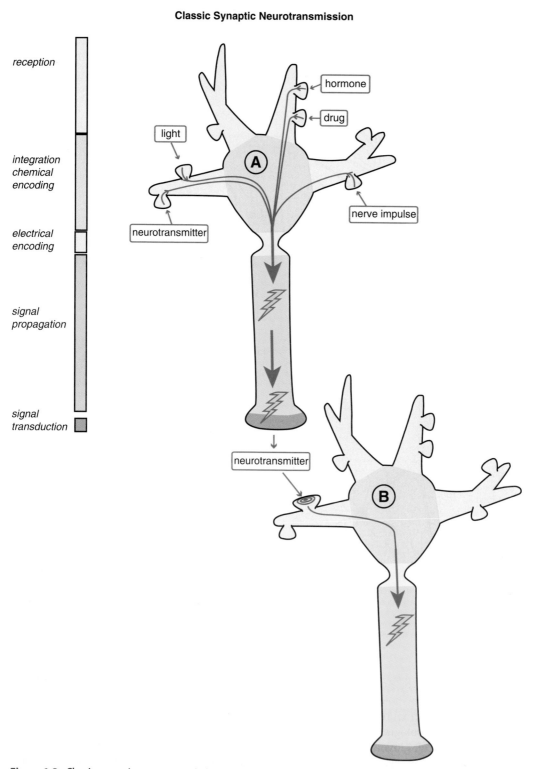

Figure 1-3. Classic synaptic neurotransmission. In classic synaptic neurotransmission, stimulation of a presynaptic neuron (e.g., by neurotransmitters, light, drugs, hormones, nerve impulses) causes electrical impulses to be sent to its axon terminal. These electrical impulses are then converted into chemical messengers and released to stimulate the receptors of a postsynaptic neuron. Thus, although communication *within* a neuron can be electrical, communication *between* neurons is chemical.

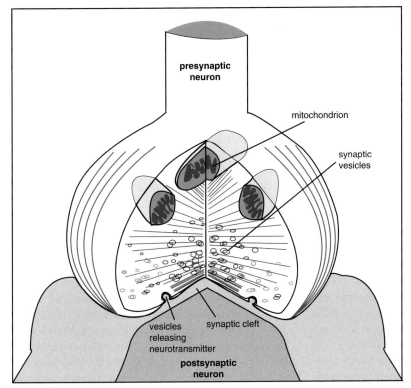

Figure 1-4. Enlarged synapse. The synapse is enlarged conceptually here to show the specialized structures that enable chemical neurotransmission to occur. Specifically, a presynaptic neuron sends its axon terminal to form a synapse with a postsynaptic neuron. Energy for neurotransmission from the presynaptic neuron is provided by mitochondria there. Chemical neurotransmitters are stored in small vesicles, ready for release upon firing of the presynaptic neuron. The synaptic cleft is the gap between the presynaptic neuron and the postsynaptic neuron; it contains proteins and scaffolding and molecular forms of "synaptic glue" to reinforce the connection between the neurons. Receptors are present on both sides of this cleft and are key elements of chemical neurotransmission.

brain regions and how these principles are applied to various specific psychiatric disorders and treated with various specific psychotropic drugs are discussed throughout the rest of the book.

Principles of chemical neurotransmission

Neurotransmitters

There are more than a dozen known or suspected neurotransmitters in the brain. For psychopharmacologists, it is particularly important to know the six key neurotransmitter systems targeted by psychotropic drugs:

- serotonin
- norepinephrine
- dopamine
- acetylcholine
- glutamate
- GABA (γ-aminobutyric acid)

Each is discussed in detail in the clinical chapters related to the specific drugs that target them. Other neurotransmitters that are also important neurotransmitters and neuromodulators, such as histamine and various neuropeptides and hormones, are mentioned in brief throughout the relevant clinical chapters in this textbook.

Some neurotransmitters are very similar to drugs and have been called "God's pharmacopeia." For example, it is well known that the brain makes its own morphine (i.e., β-endorphin) and its own marijuana (i.e., anandamide). The brain may even make its own antidepressants, anxiolytics, and hallucinogens. Drugs often mimic the brain's natural neurotransmitters, and some drugs have been discovered prior to the natural neurotransmitter. Thus, morphine was used in clinical practice before the discovery of β-endorphin; marijuana was smoked before the discovery of cannabinoid receptors and anandamide; the benzodiazepines Valium (diazepam) and Xanax (alprazolam) were prescribed before the discovery of benzodiazepine receptors; and the antidepressants Elavil (amitriptyline) and Prozac (fluoxetine) entered clinical practice before molecular clarification of the serotonin transporter site. This underscores the point that the great majority of drugs that act in the central nervous system act upon the process of neurotransmission. Indeed, this apparently occurs at times in a manner that can mimic the actions of the brain itself, when the brain uses its own chemicals.

Input to any neuron can involve many different neurotransmitters coming from many different neuronal circuits. Understanding these inputs to neurons within functioning circuits can provide a rational basis for selecting and combining therapeutic agents. This theme is discussed extensively in each chapter on the various psychiatric disorders. The idea is that for the modern psychopharmacologist to influence abnormal neurotransmission in patients with psychiatric disorders, it may be necessary to target neurons in specific circuits. Since these networks of neurons send and receive information via a variety of neurotransmitters, it may therefore be not only rational but necessary to use multiple drugs with multiple neurotransmitter actions for patients with psychiatric disorders, especially if single agents with single neurotransmitter mechanisms are not effective in relieving symptoms.

Neurotransmission: classic, retrograde, and volume

Classic neurotransmission begins with an electrical process by which neurons send electrical impulses from one part of the cell to another part of the same cell via their axons (see neuron A in Figure 1-3). However, these electrical impulses do not jump directly to other neurons. Classic neurotransmission between neurons involves one neuron hurling a chemical messenger, or neurotransmitter, at the receptors of a second neuron (see the synapse between neuron A and neuron B in Figure 1-3). This happens frequently but not exclusively at the sites of synaptic connections. In the human brain, a hundred billion neurons each make thousands of synapses with other neurons for an estimated trillion chemically neurotransmitting synapses.

Communication *between* all these neurons at synapses is chemical, not electrical. That is, an electrical impulse in the first neuron is converted to a chemical signal at the synapse between it and a second

neuron, in a process known as excitation–secretion coupling, the first stage of chemical neurotransmission. This occurs predominantly but not exclusively in one direction, from the *presynaptic* axon terminal to a second *postsynaptic* neuron (Figures 1-2 and 1-3). Finally, neurotransmission continues in the second neuron either by converting the chemical information from the first neuron back into an electrical impulse in the second neuron, or, perhaps more elegantly, by the chemical information from the first neuron triggering a cascade of further chemical messages within the second neuron to change that neuron's molecular and genetic functioning (Figure 1-3).

An interesting twist to chemical neurotransmission is the discovery that postsynaptic neurons can also "talk back" to their presynaptic neurons. They can do this via *retrograde neurotransmission* from the second neuron to the first at the synapse between them (Figure 1-5, right panel). Chemicals produced specifically as retrograde neurotransmitters at some synapses include the endocannabinoids (EC, also known as "endogenous marijuana"), which are synthesized in the postsynaptic neuron. They are then released and diffuse to presynaptic cannabinoid receptors such as the CB1 or cannabinoid 1 receptor (Figure 1-5, right panel). Another retrograde neurotransmitter is the gaseous neurotransmitter NO, or nitric oxide, which is synthesized postsynaptically and then diffuses out of the postsynaptic membrane and into the presynaptic membrane to interact with cyclic guanosine monophosphate (cGMP)-sensitive targets there (Figure 1-5, right panel). A third group of retrograde neurotransmitter are neurotrophic factors such as NGF (nerve growth factor), which is released from postsynaptic sites and then diffuses to the presynaptic neuron, where it is taken up into vesicles and transported all the way back to the cell nucleus via retrograde transport systems to interact with the genome there (Figure 1-5, right panel). What these retrograde neurotransmitters have to say to the presynaptic neuron and how this modifies or regulates the communication between pre- and postsynaptic neuron are subjects of intense active investigation.

In addition to "reverse" or retrograde neurotransmission at synapses, some neurotransmission does not need a synapse at all! Neurotransmission without a synapse is called *volume neurotransmission*, or nonsynaptic diffusion neurotransmission (examples are shown in Figures 1-6 through 1-8). Chemical messengers sent by one neuron to another can spill over to

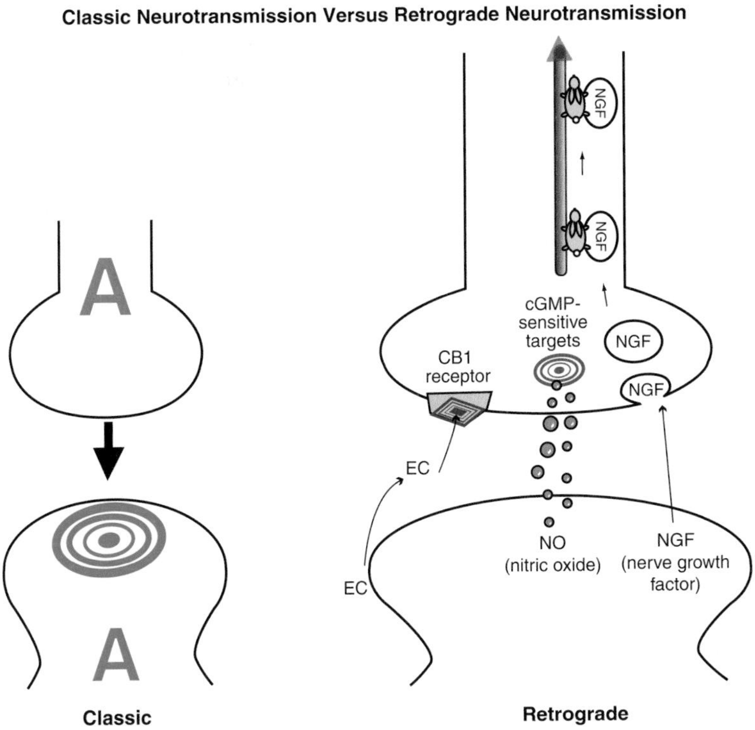

Classic Neurotransmission Versus Retrograde Neurotransmission

Classic

Retrograde

Figure 1-5. Retrograde neurotransmission. Not all neurotransmission is classic or anterograde or from top to bottom – namely, presynaptic to postsynaptic (left). Postsynaptic neurons may also communicate with presynaptic neurons from the bottom to the top via retrograde neurotransmission, from postsynaptic neuron to presynaptic neuron (right). Some neurotransmitters produced specifically as retrograde neurotransmitters at some synapses include the endocannabinoids (ECs, or "endogenous marijuana"), which are synthesized in the postsynaptic neuron, released, and diffuse to presynaptic cannabinoid receptors such as the cannabinoid 1 receptor (CB1); the gaseous neurotransmitter nitric oxide (NO), which is synthesized postsynaptically and then diffuses both out of the postsynaptic membrane and into the presynaptic membrane to interact with cyclic guanosine monophosphate (cGMP)-sensitive targets there; and neurotrophic factors such as nerve growth factor (NGF), which is released from postsynaptic sites and diffuses to the presynaptic neuron, where it is taken up into vesicles and transported all the way back to the cell nucleus via retrograde transport systems to interact with the genome there.

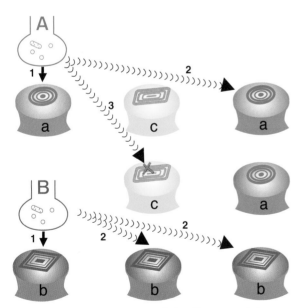

Figure 1-6. Volume neurotransmission. Neurotransmission can also occur without a synapse; this is called volume neurotransmission or nonsynaptic diffusion. In this figure, two anatomically addressed synapses (neurons A and B) are shown communicating with their corresponding postsynaptic receptors (a and b, arrows 1). However, there are also receptors for neurotransmitter A, neurotransmitter B, and neurotransmitter C,

sites distant to the synapse by diffusion (Figure 1-6). Thus, neurotransmission can occur at any compatible receptor within the diffusion radius of the neurotransmitter, not unlike modern communication with cellular telephones, which function within the transmitting radius of a given cell tower (Figure 1-6). This concept is part of the chemically addressed nervous system, and here neurotransmission occurs in chemical "puffs" (Figures 1-6 through 1-8). The brain is thus not only a collection of wires, but also a sophisticated "chemical soup." The chemically addressed

which are distant from the synaptic connections of the anatomically addressed nervous system. If neurotransmitter A or B can diffuse away from its synapse before it is destroyed, it will be able to interact with other matching receptor sites distant from its own synapse (arrows 2). If neurotransmitter A or B encounters a different receptor not capable of recognizing it (receptor c), it will not interact with that receptor even if it diffuses there (arrow 3). Thus, a chemical messenger sent by one neuron to another can spill over by diffusion to sites distant from its own synapse. Neurotransmission can occur at a compatible receptor within the diffusion radius of the matched neurotransmitter. This is analogous to modern communication with cellular telephones, which function within the transmitting radius of a given cell. This concept is called the chemically addressed nervous system, in which neurotransmission occurs in chemical "puffs." The brain is thus not only a collection of wires but also a sophisticated "chemical soup."

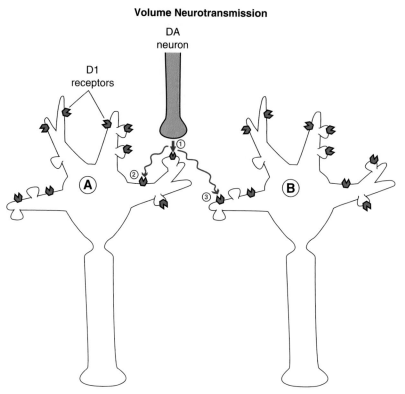

Volume Neurotransmission

Synaptic neurotransmission at 1 and diffusion to 2 and 3

Figure 1-7. Volume neurotransmission: dopamine. An example of volume neurotransmission would be that of dopamine in the prefrontal cortex. Since there are few dopamine reuptake pumps in the prefrontal cortex, dopamine is available to diffuse to nearby receptor sites. Thus, dopamine released from a synapse (arrow 1) targeting postsynaptic neuron A is free to diffuse further in the absence of a reuptake pump and can reach dopamine receptors on that same neuron but outside of the synapse from which it was released, on neighboring dendrites (arrow 2). Shown here is dopamine also reaching extrasynaptic receptors on a neighboring neuron (arrow 3).

nervous system is particularly important in mediating the actions of drugs that act at various neurotransmitter receptors, since such drugs will act wherever there are relevant receptors, and not just where such receptors are innervated with synapses by the anatomically addressed nervous system. Modifying volume neurotransmission may indeed be a major way in which several psychotropic drugs work in the brain.

A good example of volume neurotransmission is dopamine action in the prefrontal cortex. Here there are very few dopamine reuptake transport pumps (dopamine transporters or DATs) to terminate the action of dopamine released in the prefrontal cortex during neurotransmission. This is much different from other brain areas, such as the striatum, where dopamine reuptake pumps are present in abundance. Thus, when dopamine neurotransmission occurs at a synapse in the prefrontal cortex, dopamine is free to spill over from that synapse and diffuse to neighboring dopamine receptors to stimulate them, even though there is no synapse at these "spillover" sites (Figure 1-7).

Another important example of volume neurotransmission is at the sites of autoreceptors on monoamine neurons (Figure 1-8). At the somatodendritic end of the neuron (top of the neurons in Figure 1-8) are autoreceptors that inhibit the release of neurotransmitter from the axonal end of the neuron (bottom of the neurons in Figure 1-8). Although some recurrent axon collaterals and other monoamine neurons may directly innervate somatodendritic receptors, these so-called somatodendritic autoreceptors also receive neurotransmitter from dendritic release (Figure 1-8, middle and right panels). There is no synapse here, just neurotransmitter leaked from the neuron upon its own receptors. The nature of a neuron's regulation by its somatodendritic autoreceptors is a subject of intense interest, and is theoretically linked to the mechanism of action of many antidepressants, as will be explained in Chapter 7. The take-home point here is that not all chemical neurotransmission occurs at synapses.

Excitation–secretion coupling

An electrical impulse in the first – or presynaptic – neuron is converted into a chemical signal at the synapse by a process known as *excitation–secretion*

○ autoreceptor
◉ synaptic vesicles
◗ dendritic monoamine

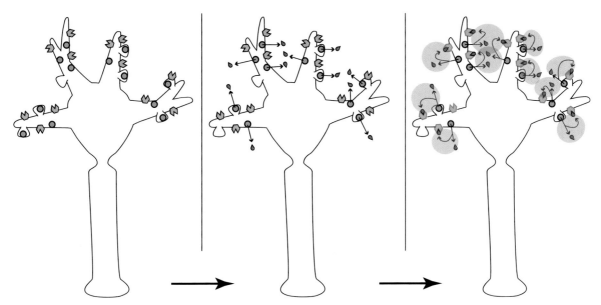

Figure 1-8. Volume neurotransmission: monoamine autoreceptors. Another example of volume neurotransmission could involve autoreceptors on monoamine neurons. Autoreceptors located on the dendrites and soma of a neuron (at the top of the neuron in the left panel) normally inhibit release of neurotransmitter from the axon of that neuron (at the bottom of the neuron in the left panel), and thus inhibit impulse flow through that neuron from top to bottom. Monoamines released from the dendrites of this neuron (at the top of the neuron in the middle panel), then bind to these autoreceptors (at the top of the neuron in the right panel) and would inhibit neuronal impulse flow in that neuron (from the bottom of the neuron in the right panel). This action occurs due to volume neurotransmission and despite the absence of synaptic neurotransmission in the somatodendritic areas of these neurons.

coupling. Once an electrical impulse invades the presynaptic axon terminal, it causes the release of chemical neurotransmitter stored there (Figures 1-3 and 1-4). Electrical impulses open ion channels – both *voltage-sensitive sodium channels* (VSSCs) and *voltage-sensitive calcium channels* (VSCCs) – by changing the ionic charge across neuronal membranes. As sodium flows into the presynaptic nerve through sodium channels in the axon membrane, the electrical charge of the action potential moves along the axon until it reaches the presynaptic nerve terminal, where it also opens calcium channels. As calcium flows into the presynaptic nerve terminal, it causes synaptic vesicles anchored to the inner membrane to spill their chemical contents into the synapse. The way is paved for chemical communication by previous synthesis of neurotransmitter and storage of neurotransmitter in the first neuron's presynaptic axon terminal.

Excitation–secretion coupling is thus the way that the neuron transduces an electrical stimulus into a chemical event. This happens very quickly once the electrical impulse enters the presynaptic neuron. It is also possible for the neuron to transduce a chemical message from a presynaptic neuron back into an electrical chemical message in the postsynaptic neuron by opening ion channels linked to neurotransmitters there. This also happens very quickly when chemical neurotransmitters open ion channels that change the flow of charge into the neuron, and ultimately, action potentials in the postsynaptic neuron. Thus, the process of neurotransmission is constantly transducing chemical signals into electrical signals, and electrical signals back into chemical signals.

Signal transduction cascades
Overview

Neurotransmission can be seen as part of a much larger process than just the communication of a presynaptic axon with a postsynaptic neuron at the

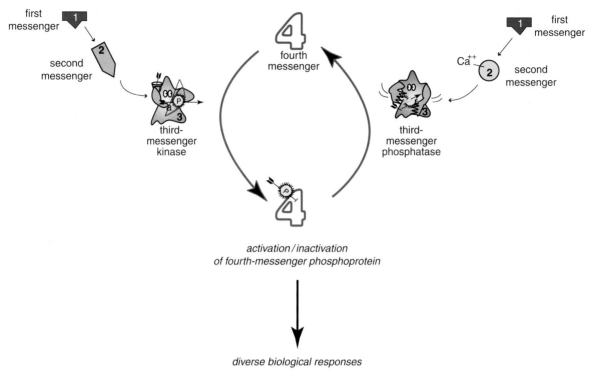

first messenger 1

second messenger 2

third-messenger kinase

fourth messenger 4

Ca++

first messenger 1

second messenger 2

third-messenger phosphatase

activation/inactivation of fourth-messenger phosphoprotein

diverse biological responses

Figure 1-9. Signal transduction cascade. The cascade of events that occurs following stimulation of a postsynaptic receptor is known as signal transduction. Signal transduction cascades can activate third-messenger enzymes known as kinases, which add phosphate groups to proteins to create phosphoproteins (on the left). Other signal transduction cascades can activate third-messenger enzymes known as phosphatases, which remove phosphates from phosphoproteins (on the right). The balance between kinase and phosphatase activity, signaled by the balance between the two neurotransmitters that activate each of them, determines the degree of downstream chemical activity that gets translated into diverse biological responses, such as gene expression and synaptogenesis.

synapse between them. That is, neurotransmission can also be seen as communication from the genome of the presynaptic neuron (neuron A in Figure 1-3) to the genome of the postsynaptic neuron (neuron B in Figure 1-3), and then back from the genome of the postsynaptic neuron to the genome of the presynaptic neuron via retrograde neurotransmission (right panel in Figure 1-5). Such a process involves long strings of chemical messages within both presynaptic and postsynaptic neurons, called signal transduction cascades.

Signal transduction cascades triggered by chemical neurotransmission thus involve numerous molecules, starting with neurotransmitter first messenger, and proceeding to second, third, fourth, and more messengers (Figures 1-9 through 1-30). The initial events occur in less than a second, but the long-term consequences are mediated by downstream messengers that take hours to days to activate, yet can last for many days or even for the lifetime of a synapse or neuron (Figure 1-10). Signal

transduction cascades are somewhat akin to a molecular "pony express" with specialized molecules acting as a sequence of riders, handing on the message to the next specialized molecule, until the message has reached a functional destination, such as gene expression or activation of otherwise "sleeping" and inactive molecules (see for example, Figures 1-9 through 1-19).

An overview of such a molecular "pony express," from first-messenger neurotransmitter through several "molecular riders" to the production of diverse biological responses, is shown in Figure 1-9. Specifically, a first-messenger neurotransmitter on the left activates the production of a chemical second messenger that in turn activates a third messenger, namely an enzyme known as a kinase that adds phosphate groups to fourth-messenger proteins to create phosphoproteins (Figure 1-9, left). Another signal transduction cascade is shown on the right with a first-messenger neurotransmitter opening an ion channel that allows calcium to enter the neuron and

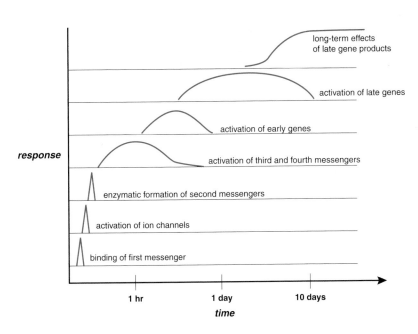

Time Course of Signal Transduction

long-term effects of late gene products

activation of late genes

activation of early genes

response

activation of third and fourth messengers

enzymatic formation of second messengers

activation of ion channels

binding of first messenger

1 hr   1 day   10 days

time

Figure 1-10. Time course of signal transduction. The time course of signal transduction is shown here. The process begins with binding of a first messenger (bottom), which leads to activation of ion channels or enzymatic formation of second messengers. This, in turn, can cause activation of third and fourth messengers, which are often phosphoproteins. If genes are subsequently activated, this leads to the synthesis of new proteins, which can alter the neuron's functions. Once initiated, the functional changes due to protein activation or new protein synthesis can last for at least many days and possibly much longer. Thus, the ultimate effects of signal transduction cascades triggered by chemical neurotransmission are not only delayed but also long-lasting.

act as the second messenger for this cascade system (Figure 1-9, right). Calcium then activates a different third messenger, namely an enzyme known as a phosphatase that removes phosphate groups from fourth-messenger phosphoproteins and thus reverses the actions of the third messenger on the left. The balance between kinase and phosphatase activity, signaled by the balance between the two neurotransmitters that activate each of them, determines the degree of downstream chemical activity that gets translated into active fourth messengers able to trigger diverse biological responses, such as gene expression and synaptogenesis (Figure 1-9). Each molecular site within the transduction cascade of chemical and electrical messages is a potential location for a malfunction associated with a mental illness; it is also a potential target for a psychotropic drug. Thus, the various elements of multiple signal transduction cascades play very important roles in psychopharmacology.

Four of the most important signal transduction cascades in the brain are shown in Figure 1-11. These include G-protein-linked systems, ion-channel-linked systems, hormone-linked systems, and neurotrophin-linked systems. There are many chemical messengers for each of these four critical signal transduction cascades; the G-protein-linked and the ion-channel-linked cascades are triggered by neurotransmitters (Figure 1-11). Many of the psychotropic drugs used in clinical practice today target one of these two signal transduction cascades. Drugs that target the G-protein-linked system are discussed in Chapter 2; drugs that target the ion-channel-linked system are discussed in Chapter 3.

Forming a second messenger

Each of the four signal transduction cascades (Figure 1-11) passes its message from an extracellular first messenger to an intracellular second messenger. In the case of G-protein-linked systems, the second messenger is a chemical, but in the case of an ion-channel-linked system, the second messenger can be an ion such as calcium (Figure 1-11). For some hormone-linked systems, a second messenger is formed when the hormone finds its receptor in the cytoplasm and binds to it to form a hormone–nuclear receptor complex (Figure 1-11). For neurotrophins, a complex set of various second messengers exist (Figure 1-11), including proteins that are kinase enzymes with an alphabet soup of complicated names.

The transduction of an extracellular first neurotransmitter from the presynaptic neuron into an intracellular second messenger in the postsynaptic neuron is known in detail for some second-messenger

11

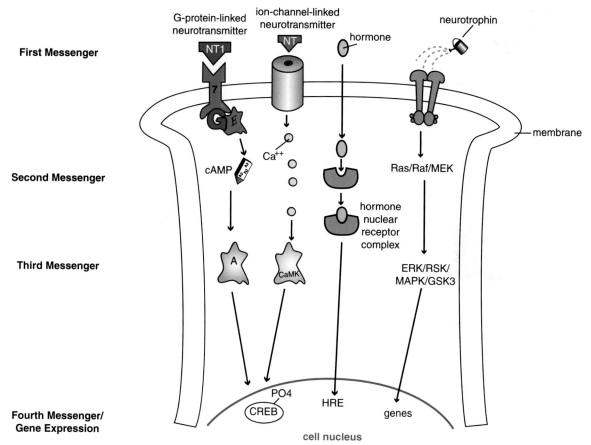

First Messenger

Second Messenger

Third Messenger

**Fourth Messenger/
Gene Expression**

Figure 1-11. Different signal transduction cascades. Four of the most important signal transduction cascades in the brain are shown here. These include G-protein-linked systems, ion-channel-linked systems, hormone-linked systems, and neurotrophin-linked systems. Each begins with a different first messenger binding to a unique receptor, leading to activation of very different downstream second, third, and subsequent chemical messengers. Having many different signal transduction cascades allows neurons to respond in amazingly diverse biological ways to a whole array of chemical messaging systems. Neurotransmitters (NT) activate both the G-protein-linked system and the ion-channel-linked system on the left, and both of these systems activate genes in the cell nucleus by phosphorylating a protein there called cAMP response element-binding protein (CREB). The G-protein-linked system works through a cascade involving cAMP (cyclic adenosine monophosphate) and protein kinase A, whereas the ion-channel-linked system works through calcium and its ability to activate a different kinase called calcium/calmodulin-dependent protein kinase (CaMK). Certain hormones, such as estrogen and other steroids, can enter the neuron, find their receptors in the cytoplasm, and bind them to form a hormone–nuclear receptor complex. This complex can then enter the cell nucleus to interact with hormone response elements (HRE) there to trigger activation of specific genes. Finally, the neurotrophin system on the far right activates a series of kinase enzymes, with a confusing alphabet soup of names, to trigger gene expression, which may control such functions as synaptogenesis and neuronal survival. Ras is a G protein, Raf is a kinase, and the other elements in this cascade are proteins as well (MEK stands for mitogen-activated protein kinase/extracellular-signal-regulated kinase; ERK stands for extracellular-signal-regulated kinase itself; RSK is ribosomal S6 kinase; MAPK is MAP kinase itself, and GSK-3 is glycogen synthase kinase 3).

systems, such as those that are linked to G proteins (Figures 1-12 through 1-15). There are four key elements to this second-messenger system:

- the first-messenger neurotransmitter;
- a receptor for the neurotransmitter that belongs to the receptor superfamily in which all have the structure of seven transmembrane regions (designated by the number 7 on the receptor in Figures 1-12 through 1-15);

- a G protein capable of binding both to certain conformations of the neurotransmitter receptor (7) and to an enzyme system (E) that can synthesize the second messenger;
- and finally the enzyme system itself for the second messenger.

The first step is the neurotransmitter binding to its receptor (Figure 1-13). This changes the conformation of the receptor so it can now fit with the G protein, as

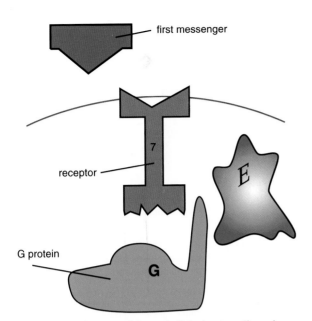

Figure 1-12. Elements of G-protein-linked system. Shown here are the four elements of a G-protein-linked second-messenger system. The first element is the neurotransmitter itself, sometimes also referred to as the first messenger. The second element is the G-protein-linked neurotransmitter receptor, which is a protein with seven transmembrane regions. The third element, a G protein, is a connecting protein. The fourth element of the second-messenger system is an enzyme (E), which can synthesize a second messenger when activated.

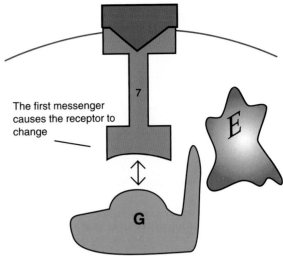

G protein can now bind to the receptor

Figure 1-13. First messenger. In this figure, the neurotransmitter has docked into its receptor. The first messenger does its job by transforming the conformation of the receptor so that the receptor can bind to the G protein, indicated here by the receptor turning the same color as the neurotransmitter and changing its shape at the bottom in order to make it capable of binding to the G protein.

indicated by the receptor (7) turning green and its shape changing at the bottom. Next comes the binding of the G protein to this new conformation of the receptor–neurotransmitter complex (Figure 1-14). The two receptors cooperate with each other: namely, the neurotransmitter receptor itself and the G protein, which can be thought of as another type of receptor associated with the inner membrane of the cell. This cooperation is indicated in Figure 1-14 by the G protein turning green and its conformation changing on the right so it is now capable of binding to an enzyme (E) that synthesizes the second messenger. Finally, the enzyme, in this case adenylate cyclase, binds to the G protein and synthesizes cAMP (cyclic adenosine monophosphate), which serves as second messenger (Figure 1-15). This is indicated in Figure 1-15 by the enzyme turning green and generating cAMP (the icon with number 2 on it).

Beyond the second messenger to phosphoprotein messengers

Recent research has begun to clarify the complex molecular links between the second messenger and its ultimate effects upon cellular functions. These links are specifically the third, fourth, and subsequent chemical messengers in the signal transduction cascades shown in Figures 1-9, 1-11, and 1-16 through 1-30. Each of the four classes of signal transduction cascades shown in Figure 1-11 not only begins with a different first messenger binding to a unique receptor, but also leads to activation of very different downstream second, third, and subsequent chemical messengers. Having many different signal transduction cascades allows neurons to respond in amazingly diverse biological ways to a whole array of chemical messaging systems.

What is the ultimate target of signal transduction? There are two major targets of signal transduction: phosphoproteins and genes. Many of the intermediate targets along the way to the gene are phosphoproteins, such as the fourth-messenger phosphoproteins shown in Figures 1-18 and 1-19 that lie dormant in the neuron until signal transduction wakes them up and they can spring into action.

The actions shown in Figure 1-9 on fourth-messenger phosphoproteins as targets of signal transduction can be seen in more detail in Figures 1-16 through 1-19. Thus, one signal transduction pathway can activate a third-messenger kinase through second-messenger cAMP (Figure 1-16), whereas another signal transduction pathway can activate a third-messenger phosphatase through second-messenger calcium

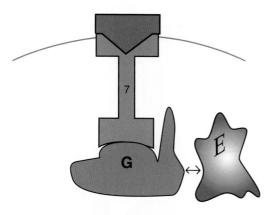

Once bound to the receptor, the G protein changes shape so it can bind to an enzyme capable of synthesizing a second messenger.

Figure 1-14. G protein. The next stage in producing a second messenger is for the transformed neurotransmitter receptor to bind to the G protein, depicted here by the G protein turning the same color as the neurotransmitter and its receptor. Binding of the binary neurotransmitter receptor complex to the G protein causes yet another conformational change, this time in the G protein, represented here as a change in the shape of the right-hand side of the G protein. This prepares the G protein to bind to the enzyme capable of synthesizing the second messenger.

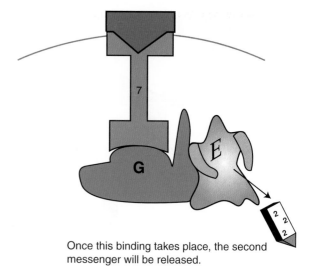

Once this binding takes place, the second messenger will be released.

Figure 1-15. Second messenger. The final step in formation of the second messenger is for the ternary complex neurotransmitter–receptor–G protein to bind to a messenger-synthesizing enzyme, depicted here by the enzyme turning the same color as the ternary complex. Once the enzyme binds to this ternary complex, it becomes activated and capable of synthesizing the second messenger. Thus, it is the cooperation of all four elements, wrapped together as a quaternary complex, that leads to the production of the second messenger. Information from the first messenger thus passes to the second messenger through use of receptor–G protein–enzyme intermediaries.

Activating a Third-Messenger Kinase through Cyclic AMP

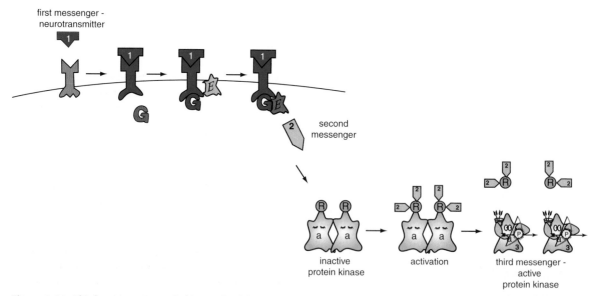

Figure 1-16. Third-messenger protein kinase. This figure illustrates activation of a third-messenger protein kinase through the second-messenger cAMP. Neurotransmitters begin the process of activating genes by producing a second messenger (cAMP), as shown in Figures 1-12 through 1-15. Some second messengers activate intracellular enzymes known as protein kinases. This enzyme is shown here as inactive when it is paired with another copy of the enzyme plus two regulatory units (R). In this case, two copies of the second messenger interact with the regulatory units, dissociating them from the protein kinase dimer. This dissociation activates each protein kinase, readying this enzyme to phosphorylate other proteins.

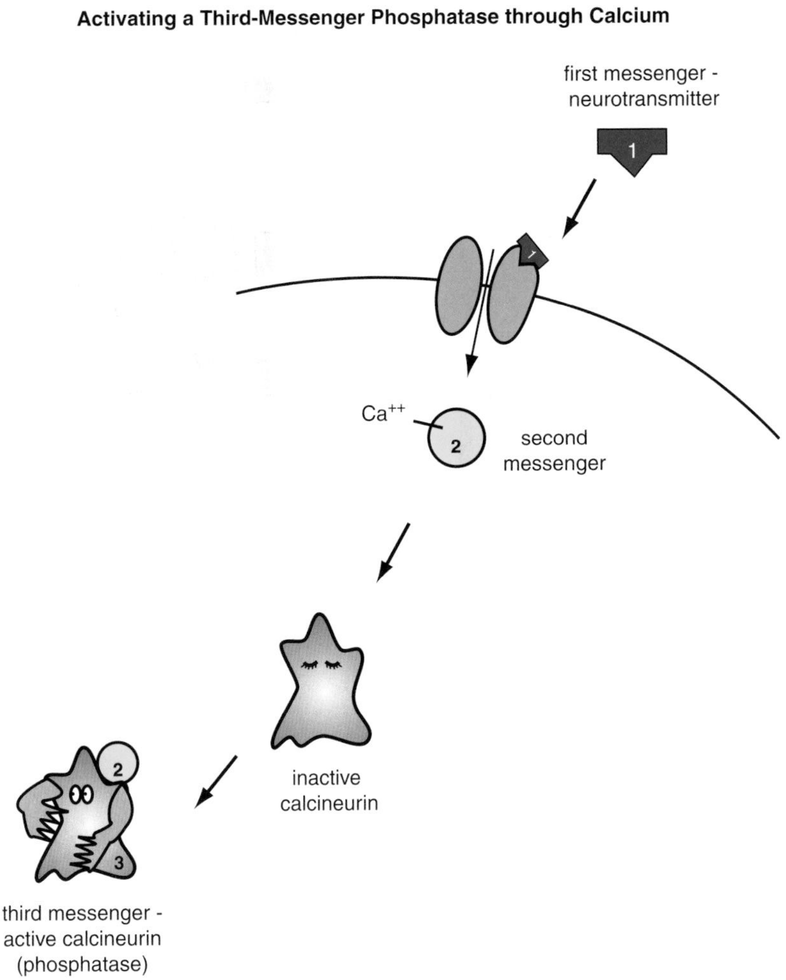

Activating a Third-Messenger Phosphatase through Calcium

first messenger -
neurotransmitter

Ca^{++}

second
messenger

inactive
calcineurin

third messenger -
active calcineurin
(phosphatase)

Figure 1-17. Third-messenger phosphatase. This figure illustrates activation of a third-messenger phosphatase through the second-messenger calcium. Shown here is calcium binding to an inactive phosphatase known as calcineurin, thereby activating it and thus readying it to remove phosphates from fourth-messenger phosphoproteins.

(Figure 1-17). In the case of kinase activation, two copies of the second messenger target each regulatory unit of dormant or "sleeping" protein kinase (Figure 1-16). When some protein kinases are inactive, they exist in dimers (two copies of the enzyme) while binding to a regulatory unit, thus rendering them in a conformation that is not active. In this example, when two copies of cAMP bind to each regulatory unit, the regulatory unit dissociates from the enzyme, the dimer dissociates into two copies of the enzyme, and the protein kinase is now activated, shown with bow and arrow ready to shoot phosphate groups into unsuspecting fourth-messenger phosphoproteins (Figure 1-16).

Meanwhile, the nemesis of protein kinase is also forming, namely a protein phosphatase (Figure 1-17). Another first messenger is opening an ion channel here, allowing second-messenger calcium to enter, which activates the phosphatase enzyme calcineurin.

In the presence of calcium, calcineurin becomes activated, shown with scissor fingers ready to rip phosphate groups off fourth-messenger phosphoproteins (Figure 1-17).

The clash between kinase and phosphatase can be seen by comparing what happens in Figures 1-18 and 1-19. In Figure 1-18, third-messenger kinase is putting phosphates onto various fourth-messenger phosphoproteins such as ligand-gated ion channels, voltage-gated ion channels, and enzymes. In Figure 1-19, third-messenger phosphatase is taking those phosphates off. Sometimes phosphorylation activates a dormant phosphoprotein; for other phosphoproteins, dephosphorylation can be activating. Activation of fourth-messenger phosphoproteins can change the synthesis of neurotransmitters, alter neurotransmitter release, change the conductance of ions, and generally maintain the chemical neurotransmission apparatus in

Third-Messenger Kinase put Phosphates on Critical Proteins

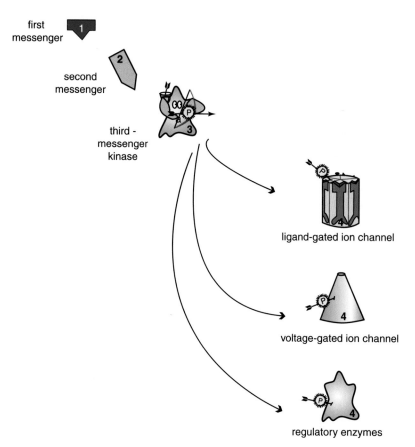

first
messenger

second
messenger

third -
messenger
kinase

ligand-gated ion channel

voltage-gated ion channel

regulatory enzymes

Figure 1-18. Third-messenger kinase puts phosphates on critical proteins. Here the activation of a third-messenger kinase adds phosphates to a variety of phosphoproteins, such as ligand-gated ion channels, voltage-gated ion channels, and various regulatory enzymes. Adding a phosphate group to some phosphoproteins activates them; for other proteins, this inactivates them.

either a state of readiness or dormancy. The balance between phosphorylation and dephosphorylation of fourth-messenger kinases and phosphatases plays a vital role in regulating many molecules critical to the chemical neurotransmission process.

Beyond the second messenger to a phosphoprotein cascade triggering gene expression

The ultimate cellular function that neurotransmission often seeks to modify is gene expression, either turning a gene on or turning a gene off. All four signal transduction cascades shown in Figure 1-11 end with the last molecule influencing gene transcription. Both cascades triggered by neurotransmitters are shown acting upon the CREB system, which is responsive to phosphorylation of its regulatory units (Figure 1-11 on the left). CREB is cAMP response

element-binding protein, a transcription factor in the cell nucleus capable of activating expression of genes, especially a type of gene known as immediate genes or immediate early genes. When G-protein-linked receptors activate protein kinase A, this activated enzyme can translocate or move into the cell nucleus and stick a phosphate group on CREB, thus activating this transcription factor and causing the nearby gene to become activated. This leads to gene expression, first as RNA and then as the protein coded by the gene.

Interestingly, it is also possible for ion-channel-linked receptors that enhance intracellular second-messenger calcium levels to activate CREB by phosphorylating it. A protein known as calmodulin, which interacts with calcium, can lead to activation of certain kinases called calcium/calmodulin-dependent protein kinases (Figure 1-11). This is an entirely different enzyme than the phosphatase shown in Figures 1-9, 1-17 and 1-19. Here, a kinase and not a phosphatase is activated. When activated, this kinase can translocate into the

Third-Messenger Phosphatases Undo what Kinases Create - Take Phosphates Off Critical Proteins

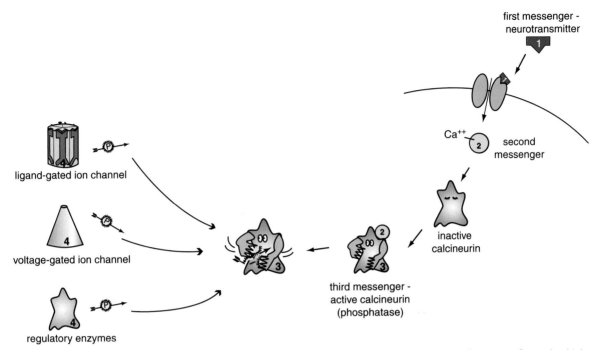

Figure 1-19. Third-messenger phosphatase removes phosphates from critical proteins. In contrast to the previous figure, the third messenger here is a phosphatase; this enzyme removes phosphate groups from phosphoproteins such as ligand-gated ion channels, voltage-gated ion channels, and various regulatory enzymes. Removing a phosphate group from some phosphoproteins activates them; for others, it inactivates them.

cell nucleus and, just like the kinase activated by the G-protein system, add a phosphate group to CREB and activate this transcription factor so that gene expression is triggered.

It is important to bear in mind that calcium is thus able to activate both kinases and phosphatases. There is a very rich and sometimes confusing array of kinases and phosphatases, and the net result of calcium action is dependent upon what substrates are activated, because different phosphatases and kinases target very different substrates. Thus, it is important to keep in mind the specific signal transduction cascade under discussion, and the specific phosphoproteins acting as messengers in the cascade, in order to understand the net effect of various signal transduction cascades. In the case illustrated in Figure 1-11, the G-protein system and the ion-channel system are working together to produce more activated kinases and thus more activation of CREB. However, in Figures 1-9, and 1-16 through 1-19, they are working in opposition.

Genes are also the ultimate target of the hormone signal transduction cascade in Figure 1-11. Some

hormones, such as estrogen, thyroid, and cortisol, act at cytoplasmic receptors, bind them, and produce a hormone–nuclear receptor complex that translocates to the cell nucleus, finds elements in the gene that it can influence (called hormone response elements, or HREs), and then acts as a transcription factor to trigger activation of nearby genes (Figure 1-11).

Finally, a very complicated signal transduction system with terrible-sounding names for their downstream signal cascade messengers is activated by neurotrophins and related molecules. Activating this system by first-messenger neurotrophins leads to activation of enzymes that are mostly kinases, one kinase activating another until finally one of them phosphorylates a transcription factor in the cell nucleus and starts transcribing genes (Figure 1-11). Ras is a G protein that activates a cascade of kinases with confusing names. For those who are good sports with an interest in the specifics, this cascade starts with Ras activating Raf, which phosphorylates and activates MEK (MAP kinase/ERK kinase, or mitogen-activated protein kinase/extracellular-signal-regulated kinase kinase), which activates ERK

17

(extracellular signal-regulated kinase itself), RSK (ribosomal S6 kinase), MAPK (MAP kinase itself), or GSK-3 (glycogen synthase kinase), leading ultimately to changes in gene expression. Confused? It is actually not important to know the names, but to remember the take-away point that neurotrophins trigger an important signal transduction pathway that activates kinase enzyme after kinase enzyme, ultimately changing gene expression. This is worth knowing, because this signal transduction pathway may be responsible for the expression of genes that regulate many critical functions of the neuron, such as synaptogensis and cell survival, as well as the plastic changes that are necessary for learning, memory, and even disease expression in various brain circuits. Both drugs and the environment target gene expression in ways that are just beginning to be understood, including how such actions contribute to the cause of mental illnesses and to the mechanism of action of effective treatments for mental illnesses.

In the meantime, it is mostly important to realize that a very wide variety of genes are targeted by all four of these signal transduction pathways. These range from the genes that make synthetic enzymes for neurotransmitters, to growth factors, cytoskeleton proteins, cellular adhesion proteins, ion channels, receptors, and the intracellular signaling proteins themselves, among many others. When genes are expressed by any of the signal transduction pathways shown in Figure 1-11, this can lead to making more or fewer copies of any of these proteins. Synthesis of such proteins is obviously a critical aspect of the neuron performing its many and varied functions. Numerous diverse biological actions are effected within neurons that alter behaviors in individuals due to gene expression that is triggered by the four major signal transduction cascades. These functions include synaptogensis, strengthening of a synapse, neurogenesis, apoptosis, increasing or decreasing the efficiency of information processing in cortical circuits, to behavioral responses such as learning, memory, antidepressant responses to antidepressant administration, symptom reduction by psychotherapy, and possibly even the production of a mental illness.

How neurotransmission triggers gene expression

How does the gene express the protein it codes? The discussion above has shown how the molecular "pony express" of signal transduction has a message encoded with chemical information from the neurotransmitter–receptor complex that is passed along from molecular rider to molecular rider until the message is delivered to the appropriate phosphoprotein mailbox (Figures 1-9 and 1-16 through 1-19) or DNA mailbox in the postsynaptic neuron's genome (Figures 1-11 and 1-20 through 1-30). Since the most powerful way for a neuron to alter its function is to change which genes are being turned on or off, it is important to understand the molecular mechanisms by which neurotransmission regulates gene expression.

How many potential genes can neurotransmission target? It is estimated that the human genome contains approximately *20 000 to 30 000 genes* located within *3 million base pairs* of DNA on 23 chromosomes. Incredibly, however, genes only occupy a few percent of this DNA. The other 97% used to be called "junk" DNA since it does not code proteins, but it is now known that these sections of DNA are critical for regulating whether or not a gene is expressed or is silent. It is not just the number of genes we have, it is whether, when, how often, and under what circumstances they are expressed that seems to be the important factor in regulating neuronal function. These same factors of gene expression are now thought to also underlie the actions of psychopharmacologic drugs and the mechanisms of psychiatric disorders within the central nervous system.

Molecular mechanism of gene expression

Chemical neurotransmission converts receptor occupancy by a neurotransmitter into the creation of third, fourth, and subsequent messengers that eventually activate transcription factors that turn on genes (Figures 1-20 through 1-30). Most genes have two regions, a *coding region* and a *regulatory region* with enhancers and promoters of gene transcription (Figure 1-20). The coding region is the direct template for making its corresponding RNA. This DNA can be transcribed into its RNA with the help of an enzyme called *RNA polymerase*. However, RNA polymerase must be activated or it won't work.

Luckily, the regulatory region of the gene can make this happen. It has an *enhancer element* and a *promoter element* (Figure 1-20), which can initiate gene expression with the help of transcription factors (Figure 1-21). Transcription factors themselves can be activated when they are phosphorylated, which allows them to bind to the regulatory region of the gene (Figure 1-21). This in turn activates RNA polymerase and off we go, with the coding part of the gene *transcribing* itself into its mRNA (Figure 1-22). Once

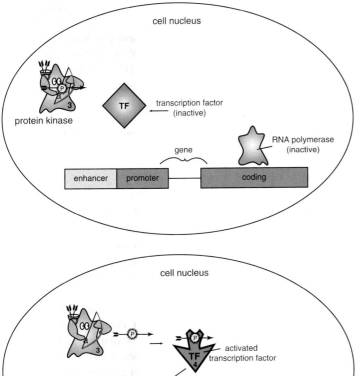

Figure 1-20. Activation of a gene, part 1: gene is off. The elements of gene activation shown here include the enzyme protein kinase; a transcription factor, a type of protein that can activate a gene; RNA polymerase, the enzyme that synthesizes RNA from DNA when the gene is transcribed; the regulatory regions of DNA, such as enhancer and promoter areas; and finally the gene itself. This particular gene is off because the transcription factor has not yet been activated. The DNA for this gene contains both a regulatory region and a coding region. The regulatory region has both an enhancer element and a promoter element, which can initiate gene expression when they interact with activated transcription factors. The coding region is directly transcribed into its corresponding RNA once the gene is activated.

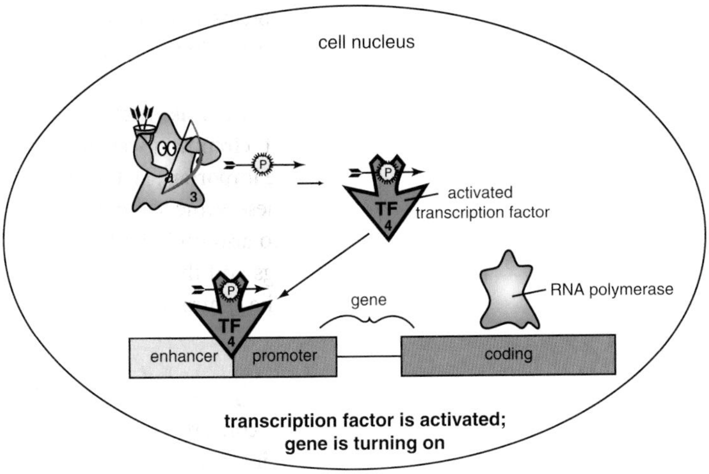

Figure 1-21. Activation of a gene, part 2: gene turns on. The transcription factor is now activated because it has been phosphorylated by protein kinase, allowing it to bind to the regulatory region of the gene.

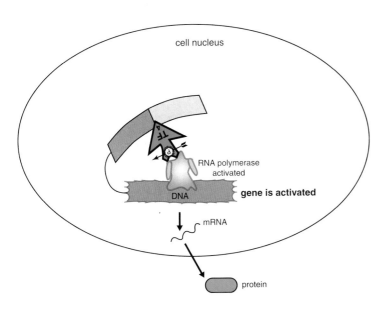

Figure 1-22. Activation of a gene, part 3: gene product. The gene itself is now activated because the transcription factor has bound to the regulatory region of the gene, in turn activating the enzyme RNA polymerase. The gene is transcribed into messenger RNA (mRNA), which in turn is translated into its corresponding protein. This protein is thus the product of activation of this particular gene.

Third-Messenger Activating a Transcription Factor for an Early Gene

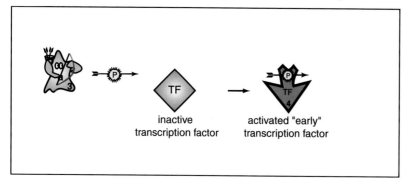

inactive
transcription factor

activated "early"
transcription factor

Figure 1-23. Immediate early gene. Some genes are known as immediate early genes. Shown here is a third-messenger protein kinase enzyme activating a transcription factor, or fourth messenger, capable of activating, in turn, an early gene.

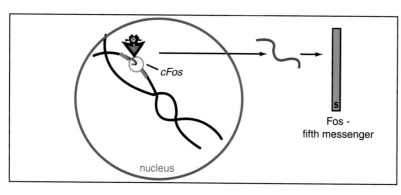

cFos

nucleus

Fos -
fifth messenger

Figure 1-24. Early genes activate late genes, part 1. In the top panel, a transcription factor is activating the immediate early gene *cFos* and producing the protein product Fos. While the *cFos* gene is being activated, another immediate early gene, *cJun*, is being simultaneously activated and producing its protein, Jun, as shown in the bottom panel. Fos and Jun can be thought of as fifth messengers.

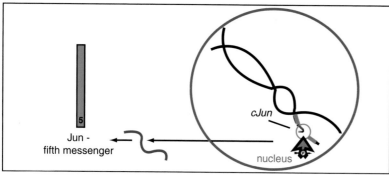

Jun -
fifth messenger

cJun

nucleus

transcribed, of course, the RNA goes on to *translate* itself into the corresponding protein (Figure 1-22).

Some genes are known as immediate early genes (Figure 1-23). They have weird names such as *cJun* and *cFos* (Figures 1-24 and 1-25) and belong to a family called "leucine zippers" (Figure 1-25). These immediate early genes function as rapid responders to the neurotransmitter's input, like the special ops troops sent into combat quickly and ahead of the full army. Such rapid-deployment forces of immediate early genes are thus the first to

respond to the neurotransmission signal by making the proteins they encode. In this example, it is Jun and Fos proteins coming from *cJun* and *cFos* genes (Figure 1-24). These are nuclear proteins; that is, they live and work in the nucleus. They get started within 15 minutes of receiving a neurotransmission but last for only a half hour to an hour (Figure 1-10).

When Jun and Fos team up, they form a leucine zipper type of transcription factor (Figure 1-25), which in turn activates many kinds of later-onset genes

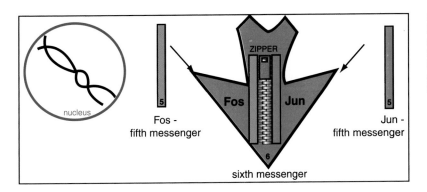

Figure 1-25. Early genes activate late genes, part 2. Once Fos and Jun proteins are synthesized, they can collaborate as partners and produce a Fos-Jun combination protein, which now acts as a sixth-messenger transcription factor for late genes.

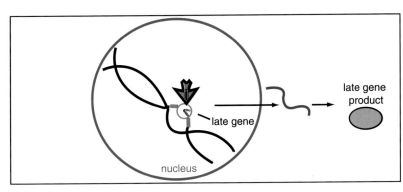

Figure 1-26. Early genes activate late genes, part 3. The Fos-Jun transcription factor belongs to a family of proteins called leucine zippers. The leucine zipper transcription factor formed by the products of the activated early genes *cFos* and *cJun* now returns to the genome and finds another gene. Since this gene is being activated later than the others, it is called a late gene. Thus, early genes activate late genes when the products of early genes are themselves transcription factors. The product of the late gene can be any protein the neuron needs, such as an enzyme, a transport factor, or a growth factor.

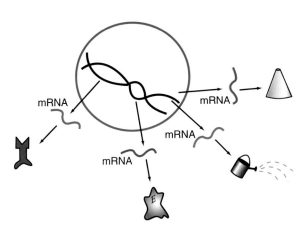

Figure 1-27. Examples of late gene activation. A receptor, an enzyme, a neurotrophic growth factor, and an ion channel are all being expressed owing to activation of their respective genes. Such gene products go on to modify neuronal function for many hours or days.

(Figures 1-26, 1-27, 1-29). Thus, Jun and Fos serve to wake up the much larger army of inactive genes. Which individual "late" soldier genes are so drafted to active gene duty depends upon a number of factors, not the least of which is which neurotransmitter is sending the message, how frequently it is sending the message, and

whether it is working in concert or in opposition with other neurotransmitters talking to other parts of the same neuron at the same time. When Jun and Fos partner together to form a leucine zipper type of transcription factor, this can lead to the activation of genes to make anything you can think of, from enzymes to receptors to structural proteins (Figure 1-27).

In summary, one can trace the events from neurotransmitting first messenger through gene transcription (Figures 1-9, 1-11, 1-28, 1-29). Once the second-messenger cAMP is formed from its first-messenger neurotransmitter (Figure 1-28), it can interact with a protein kinase third messenger. cAMP binds to the inactive or sleeping version of this enzyme, wakes it up, and thereby activates protein kinase. Once awakened, the protein kinase third messenger's job is to activate transcription factors by phosphorylating them (Figure 1-28). It does this by traveling straight to the cell nucleus and finding a sleeping transcription factor. By sticking a phosphate onto the transcription factor, protein kinase is able to "wake up" that transcription factor and form a fourth messenger (Figure 1-28). Once a transcription factor is aroused, it will bind to genes and cause protein

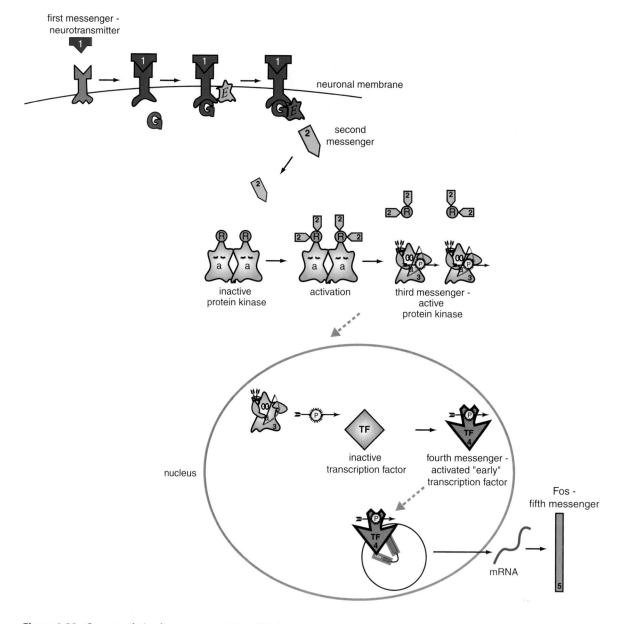

first messenger -
neurotransmitter

neuronal membrane

second
messenger

inactive
protein kinase

activation

third messenger -
active
protein kinase

nucleus

inactive
transcription factor

fourth messenger -
activated "early"
transcription factor

Fos -
fifth messenger

mRNA

Figure 1-28. Gene regulation by neurotransmitters. This figure summarizes gene regulation by neurotransmitters, from first-messenger extracellular neurotransmitter to intracellular second messenger, to third-messenger protein kinase, to fourth-messenger transcription factor, to fifth-messenger protein, which is the gene product of an early gene.

synthesis; in this case, the product of an immediate early gene, which functions as a fifth messenger. Two such gene products bind together to form yet another activated transcription factor, and this is the sixth messenger (Figure 1-29). Finally, the sixth messenger causes the expression of a late gene product, which could be thought of as a seventh-messenger protein product of the activated gene. This late gene product

then mediates some biological response important to the functioning of the neuron.

Of course, neurotransmitter-induced molecular cascades into the cell nucleus lead to changes not only in the synthesis of its own receptors but also in that of many other important postsynaptic proteins, including enzymes and receptors for other neurotransmitters. If such changes in genetic expression lead to changes

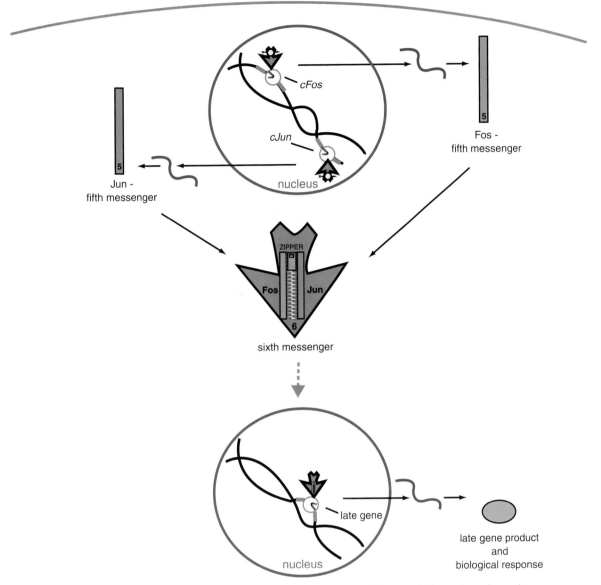

Figure 1-29. Activating a late gene. This figure summarizes the process of activating a late gene. At the top, immediate early genes *cFos* and *cJun* are expressed and their fifth-messenger protein products Fos and Jun are formed. Next, a transcription factor, namely a leucine zipper, is created by the cooperation of Fos and Jun together, combining to form the sixth messenger. Finally, this transcription factor goes on to activate a late gene, resulting in the expression of its own gene product and the biological response triggered by that late gene product.

in connections and in the functions that these connections perform, it is easy to understand how genes can *modify behavior*. The details of nerve functioning – and thus the behavior derived from this nerve functioning – are controlled by genes and the products they produce. Since mental processes and the behaviors they cause come from the connections between neurons in the brain, genes therefore exert significant control over behavior. But can behavior modify genes? Learning as well as experiences from the environment can indeed alter which genes are expressed and thus can give rise to changes in neuronal connections. In this way, human experiences, education, and even psychotherapy may change the expression of genes that alter the distribution and "strength" of specific synaptic connections. This in turn may produce long-term changes in behavior caused by the original experience and mediated by the genetic changes triggered by that original experience.

Thus, genes modify behavior and behavior modifies genes. Genes do not directly regulate neuronal functioning. Rather, they directly regulate the proteins that create neuronal functioning. Changes in function have to wait until the changes in protein synthesis occur and the events they cause start to happen.

Epigenetics

Genetics is the DNA code for what a cell can transcribe into specific types of RNA or translate into specific proteins. However, just because there are over 20 000 genes in the human genome, it does not mean that every gene is expressed, even in the brain. Epigenetics is a parallel system that determines whether any given gene is actually made into its specific RNA and protein, or if it is instead ignored or silenced. If the genome is a lexicon of all protein "words," then the epigenome is a "story" resulting from arranging the "words" into a coherent tale. The genomic lexicon of all potential proteins is the same in every one of the 10+ billion neurons in the brain, and indeed is the same in all of the 200+ types of cells in the body. So, the plot of how a normal neuron becomes a malfunctioning neuron in a psychiatric disorder, as well as how a neuron becomes a neuron instead of a liver cell, is the selection of which specific genes are expressed or silenced. In addition, malfunctioning neurons are impacted by inherited genes that have abnormal nucleotide sequences, which if expressed contribute to mental disorders. Thus, the story of the brain depends not only on which genes are inherited but also on whether any abnormal genes are expressed or even whether normal genes are expressed when they should be silent or silenced when they should be expressed. Neurotransmission, genes themselves, drugs, and the environment all regulate which genes are expressed or silenced, and thus all affect whether the story of the brain is a compelling narrative such as learning and memory, a regrettable tragedy such as drug abuse, stress reactions, and psychiatric disorders, or therapeutic improvement of a psychiatric disorder by medications or psychotherapy.

What are the molecular mechanisms of epigenetics?

Epigenetic mechanisms turn genes on and off by modifying the structure of chromatin in the cell nucleus (Figure 1-30). The character of a cell is fundamentally determined by its chromatin, a substance composed of nucleosomes (Figure 1-30). Nucleosomes are an octet of proteins called histones around which DNA is wrapped (Figure 1-30). Epigenetic control over whether a gene is read (i.e., expressed) or is not read (i.e., silenced), is achieved by modifying the structure of chromatin. Chemical modifications that can do this include not only methylation, but also acetylation, phosphorylation, and other processes that are regulated by neurotransmission, drugs, and the environment (Figure 1-30). For example, when DNA or histones are methylated, this compacts the chromatin and acts to close off access of molecular transcription factors to the promoter regions of DNA, with the consequence that the gene in this region is silenced, and not expressed, so no RNA or protein is manufactured (Figure 1-30). Silenced DNA means molecular features that are not part of a given cell's personality.

Histones are methylated by enzymes called histone methyl-transferases, and this is reversed by enzymes called histone demethylases (Figure 1-30). Methylation of histones can silence genes, whereas demethylation of histones can activate genes. DNA can also be methylated, and this also silences genes. Demethylation of DNA reverses this. Methylation of DNA is regulated by DNA methyl-transferase (DNMT) enzymes, and demethylation of DNA by DNA demethylase enzymes (Figure 1-30). There are many forms of methyl-transferase enzymes, and they all tag their substrates with methyl groups donated from L-methylfolate via S-adenosyl-methionine (SAMe) (Figure 1-30). When neurotransmission, drugs, or the environment affect methylation, this regulates whether genes are epigenetically silenced or expressed.

Methylation of DNA can eventually lead to deacetylation of histones as well, by activating enzymes called histone deacetylases (HDACs). Deacetylation of histones also has a silencing action on gene expression (Figure 1-30). Methylation and deacetylation compress chromatin, as though a molecular gate has been closed. This prevents transcription factors from accessing the promoter regions that activate genes; thus, the genes are silenced and not transcribed into RNA or translated into proteins (Figure 1-30). On the other hand, demethylation and acetylation do just the opposite: they decompress chromatin as though a molecular gate has been opened, and thus transcription factors can get to the promoter regions of genes and activate them (Figure 1-30). Activated genes thus become part of the molecular personality of a given cell.

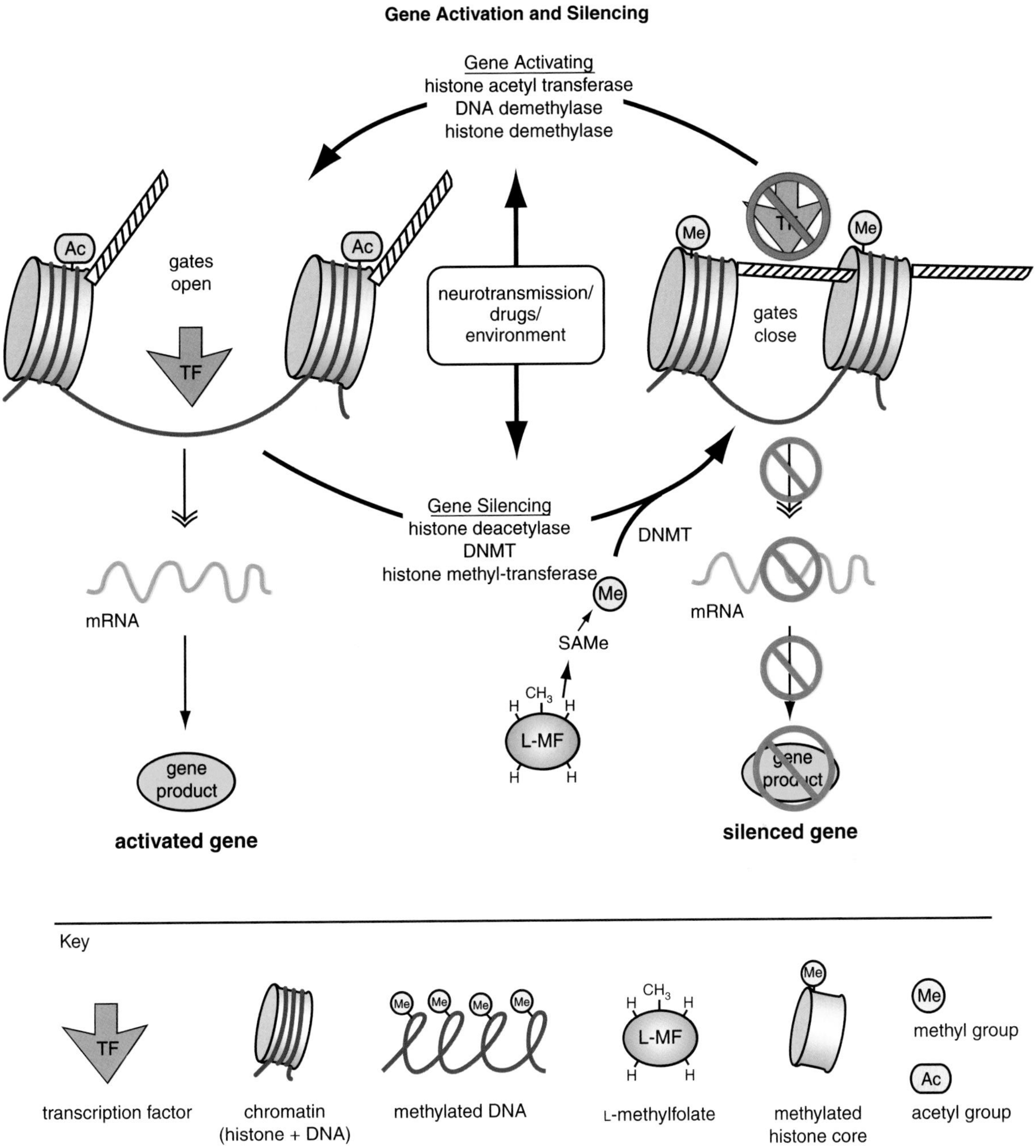

Figure 1-30. Gene activation and silencing. Molecular gates are opened by acetylation and/or demethylation of histones, allowing transcription factors access to genes, thus activating them. Molecular gates are closed by deacetylation and/or methylation provided by the methyl donor SAMe derived from L-methylfolate. This prevents access of transcription factors to genes, thus silencing them. Ac, acetyl; Me, methyl; DNMT, DNA methyl-transferase; TF, transcription factor; SAMe, S-adenosyl-methionine; L-MF, L-methylfolate.

How epigenetics maintains or changes the status quo

Some enzymes try to maintain the status quo of a cell, such as DNMT1 (DNA methyl-transferase 1), which maintains the methylation of specific areas of DNA and keeps various genes quiet for a lifetime. That is, this process keeps a neuron a neuron and a liver cell a liver cell, including when a cell divides into another one. Presumably, methylation is maintained at genes that one cell does not need, even though another cell type might.

It used to be thought that, once a cell differentiated, the epigenetic pattern of gene activation and gene silencing remained stable for the lifetime of that cell. Now, however, it is known that there are various circumstances in which epigenetics may change in mature, differentiated neurons. Although the initial epigenetic pattern of a neuron is indeed set during neurodevelopment to give each neuron its own lifelong "personality," it now appears that the storyline of some neurons is that they respond to their narrative experiences throughout life with a changing character arc, thus causing de novo alterations in their epigenome. Depending upon what happens to a neuron (such as child abuse, adult stress, dietary deficiencies, productive new encounters, psychotherapy, drugs of abuse, or psychotropic therapeutic medications), it now seems that previously silenced genes can become activated and/or previously active genes can become silenced (Figure 1-30). When this happens, both favorable and unfavorable developments can occur in the character of neurons. Favorable epigenetic mechanisms may be triggered in order for one to learn (e.g., spatial memory formation) or to experience the therapeutic actions of psychopharmacologic agents. On the other hand, unfavorable epigenetic mechanisms may be triggered in order for one to become addicted to drugs of abuse or to experience various forms of "abnormal learning," such as when one develops fear conditioning, an anxiety disorder, or a chronic pain condition.

How these epigenetic mechanisms arrive at the scene of the crime remains a compelling neurobiological and psychiatric mystery. Nevertheless, a legion of scientific detectives is working on these cases and is beginning to show how epigenetic mechanisms are mediators of psychiatric disorders. There is also the possibility that epigenetic mechanisms can be harnessed to treat addictions, extinguish fear, and prevent the development of chronic pain states. It may even be possible to prevent disease progression of psychiatric disorders such as schizophrenia by identifying high-risk individuals before the "plot thickens" and the disorder is irreversibly established and relentlessly marches on to an unwanted destiny.

One of the mechanisms for changing the status quo of epigenomic patterns in a mature cell is via de novo DNA methylation by a type of DNMT enzyme known as DNMT2 or DNMT3 (Figure 1-30). These enzymes target neuronal genes for silencing that were previously active in a mature neuron. Of course, deacetylation of histones near previously active genes would do the same thing, namely silence them, and this is mediated by the enzymes called histone deacetylases (HDACs). In reverse, demethylation or acetylation both activate genes that were previously silent. The real question is, how does a neuron know which genes among its thousands to silence or activate in response to the environment, including stress, drugs, and diet? How might this go wrong when a psychiatric disorder develops? This part of the story remains a twisted mystery, but some very interesting detective work has already been done by various investigators who hope to understand how some neuronal stories evolve into psychiatric tragedies. These investigations may set the stage for rewriting the narrative of various psychiatric disorders by therapeutically altering the epigenetics of key neuronal characters so that the story has a happy ending.

Summary

The reader should now appreciate that chemical neurotransmission is the foundation of psychopharmacology. There are many neurotransmitters, and all neurons receive input from a multitude of neurotransmitters in classic presynaptic to postsynaptic asymmetrical neurotransmission. Presynaptic to postsynaptic neurotransmissions at the brain's trillion synapses are key to chemical neurotransmission, but some neurotransmission is retrograde from postsynaptic neuron to presynaptic neuron, and other types of neurotransmission, such as volume neurotransmission, do not require a synapse at all.

The reader should also have an appreciation for elegant if complex molecular cascades precipitated by a neurotransmitter, with molecule-by-molecule transfer of the transmitted message inside the neuron receiving that message, eventually altering the biochemical machinery of that cell in order to act upon the message that was sent to it. Thus, the function of chemical neurotransmission is not so much to have a presynaptic neurotransmitter communicate with its postsynaptic receptors, but to have a *presynaptic genome converse with a postsynaptic genome*: DNA to DNA, presynaptic "command center" to postsynaptic "command center" and back.

The message of chemical neurotransmission is transferred via three sequential "molecular pony express" routes: (1) a presynaptic neurotransmitter synthesis route from presynaptic genome to the synthesis and packaging of neurotransmitter and supporting enzymes and receptors; (2) a postsynaptic route from receptor occupancy through second messengers all the way to the genome, which turns on postsynaptic genes; and (3) another postsynaptic route starting from the newly expressed postsynaptic genes transferring information as a molecular cascade of biochemical consequences throughout the postsynaptic neuron.

It should now be clear that neurotransmission does not end when a neurotransmitter binds to a receptor, or even when ion flows have been altered or second messengers have been created. Events such as these all start and end within milliseconds to seconds following release of presynaptic neurotransmitter. The ultimate goal of neurotransmission is to alter the biochemical activities of the postsynaptic target neuron in a profound and enduring manner. Since the postsynaptic DNA has to wait until molecular pony express messengers make their way from the postsynaptic receptors, often located on dendrites, to phosphoproteins within the neuron, or to transcription factors and genes in the postsynaptic neuron's cell nucleus, it can take a while

for neurotransmission to begin influencing the postsynaptic target neuron's biochemical processes. The time it takes from receptor occupancy by neurotransmitter to gene expression is usually hours. Furthermore, since the last messenger triggered by neurotransmission – called a transcription factor – only initiates the very beginning of gene action, it takes even longer for the gene activation to be fully implemented via the series of biochemical events it triggers. These biochemical events can begin many hours to days after the neurotransmission occurred, and can last days or weeks once they are put in motion.

Thus, a brief puff of chemical neurotransmission from a presynaptic neuron can trigger a profound postsynaptic reaction that takes hours to days to develop and that can last days to weeks or even a lifetime. Every conceivable component of this entire process of chemical neurotransmission is a candidate for modification by drugs. Most psychotropic drugs act upon the processes that control chemical neurotransmission at the level of the neurotransmitters themselves, their enzymes, and especially their receptors. Future psychotropic drugs will undoubtedly act directly upon the biochemical cascades, particularly upon those elements that control the expression of pre- and postsynaptic genes. Also, mental and neurological illnesses are known or suspected to affect these same aspects of chemical neurotransmission. The neuron is dynamically modifying its synaptic connections throughout its life, in response to learning, life experiences, genetic programming, epigenetic changes, drugs, and diseases, with chemical neurotransmission being the key aspect underlying the regulation of all these important processes.

Chapter

2

Transporters, receptors, and enzymes as targets of psychopharmacological drug action

Psychotropic drugs have many mechanisms of action, but they all target specific molecular sites that have profound effects upon neurotransmission. It is thus necessary to understand the anatomical infrastructure and chemical substrates of neurotransmission (Chapter 1) in order to grasp how psychotropic drugs work. Although there are over 100 essential psychotropic drugs utilized in clinical practice today (see *Stahl's Essential Psychopharmacology: the Prescriber's Guide*), there are only a few sites of action for all these therapeutic agents (Figure 2-1). Specifically, about a third of psychotropic drugs target one of the transporters for a neurotransmitter; another third target receptors coupled to G proteins; and perhaps only 10% target enzymes. All three of these sites of action will be discussed in this chapter. The balance of psychotropic drugs target various types of ion channels, which will be discussed in Chapter 3. Thus, mastering how just a few molecular sites regulate neurotransmission allows the psychopharmacologist to understand the theories about the mechanisms of action of virtually all psychopharmacological agents.

Neurotransmitter transporters as targets of drug action
Classification and structure

Neuronal membranes normally serve to keep the internal milieu of the neuron constant by acting as barriers to the intrusion of outside molecules and to the leakage of internal molecules. However, selective permeability of the membrane is required to allow discharge as well as uptake of specific molecules, to respond to the needs of cellular functioning. Good examples of this are neurotransmitters, which are released from neurons during neurotransmission and, in many cases, are also transported back into presynaptic neurons as a recapture mechanism following their release. This recapture – or reuptake – is done in order for neurotransmitter to be reused in a subsequent neurotransmission. Also, once inside the neuron, most neurotransmitters are transported again into synaptic vesicles for storage, protection from metabolism, and immediate use during a volley of future neurotransmission.

The Five Molecular Targets of Psychotropic Drugs

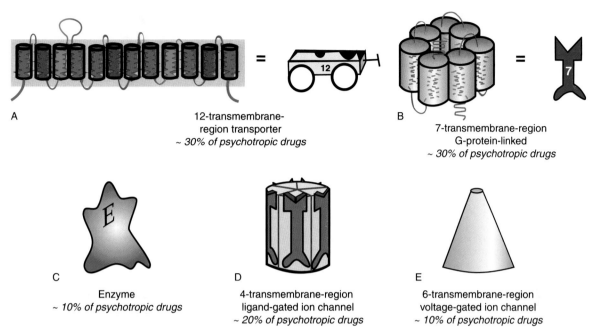

A

12-transmembrane-
region transporter
~ 30% of psychotropic drugs

B

7-transmembrane-region
G-protein-linked
~ 30% of psychotropic drugs

C

Enzyme
~ 10% of psychotropic drugs

D

4-transmembrane-region
ligand-gated ion channel
~ 20% of psychotropic drugs

E

6-transmembrane-region
voltage-gated ion channel
~ 10% of psychotropic drugs

Figure 2-1. The molecular targets of psychotropic drugs. There are only a few major sites of action for the wide expanse of psychotropic drugs utilized in clinical practice. Approximately one-third of psychotropic drugs target one of the twelve-transmembrane-region transporters for a neurotransmitter (A), while another third target seven-transmembrane-region receptors coupled to G proteins (B). The sites of action for the remaining third of psychotropic drugs include enzymes (C), four-transmembrane-region ligand-gated ion channels (D), and six-transmembrane-region voltage-sensitive ion channels (E).

Both types of neurotransmitter transport – presynaptic reuptake as well as vesicular storage – utilize a molecular transporter belonging to a "superfamily" of twelve-transmembrane-region proteins (Figures 2-1A and 2-2). That is, neurotransmitter transporters have in common the structure of going in and out of the membrane 12 times (Figure 2-1A). These transporters are a type of receptor that binds to the neurotransmitter prior to transporting that neurotransmitter across the membrane.

Recently, details of the structures of neurotransmitter transporters have been determined; this has led to a proposed subclassification of neurotransmitter transporters. That is, there are two major subclasses of *plasma membrane transporters* for neurotransmitters. Some of these transporters are presynaptic and others are on glial membranes. The first subclass consists of sodium/chloride-coupled transporters, called the solute carrier SLC6 gene family, and includes transporters for the mono-amines serotonin, norepinephrine, and dopamine (Table 2-1 and Figure 2-2A) as well as for the neurotransmitter GABA (gamma-aminobutyric acid) and

the amino acid glycine (Table 2-2 and Figure 2-2A). The second subclass consists of high-affinity glutamate transporters, also called the solute carrier SLC1 gene family (Table 2-2 and Figure 2-2A).

In addition, there are three subclasses of *intracellular synaptic vesicle transporters* for neurotransmitters. The SLC18 gene family comprises the vesicular monoamine transporters (VMATs) for serotonin, norepinephrine, dopamine, and histamine and the vesicular acetylcholine transporter (VAChT). The SLC32 gene family consists of the vesicular inhibitory amino acid transporters (VIAATs). Finally, the SLC17 gene family consists of the vesicular glutamate transporters, such as VGluT1–3 (Table 2-3 and Figure 2-2B).

Monoamine transporters (SLC6 gene family) as targets of psychotropic drugs

Reuptake mechanisms for monoamines utilize unique presynaptic transporters (Figure 2-2A) but the same vesicular transporter in all three monoamine neurons (histamine neurons also use the same vesicular

Table 2-1 Presynaptic monoamine transporters

Transporter	Common abbreviation	Gene family	Endogenous substrate	False substrate
Serotonin transporter	SERT	SLC6	Serotonin	Ecstasy (MDMA)
Norepinephrine transporter	NET	SLC6	Norepinephrine	Dopamine Epinephrine Amphetamine
Dopamine transporter	DAT	SLC6	Dopamine	Norepinephrine Epinephrine Amphetamine

MDMA, 3,4-methylenedioxymethamphetamine

Table 2-2 Neuronal and glial GABA and amino acid transporters

Transporter	Common abbreviation	Gene family	Endogenous substrate
GABA transporter 1 (neuronal and glial)	GAT1	SLC6	GABA
GABA transporter 2 (neuronal and glial)	GAT2	SLC6	GABA β-alanine
GABA transporter 3 (mostly glial)	GAT3	SLC6	GABA β-alanine
GABA transporter 4, also called betaine transporter (neuronal and glial)	GAT4 BGT1	SLC6	GABA betaine
Glycine transporter 1 (mostly glial)	GlyT1	SLC6	Glycine
Glycine transporter 2 (neuronal)	GlyT2	SLC6	Glycine
Excitatory amino acid transporters 1–5	EAAT1–5	SLC1	L-glutamate L-aspartate

transporter) (Figure 2-2B). That is, the unique presynaptic transporter for serotonin is known as SERT, for norepinephrine is known as NET, and for dopamine is known as DAT (Table 2-1 and Figure 2-2A). All three of these monoamines are then transported into synaptic vesicles of their respective neurons by the same vesicular transporter, known as VMAT2 (vesicular monoamine transporter 2) (Figure 2-2B and Table 2-3).

Although the three presynaptic transporters – SERT, NET, and DAT – are unique in their amino acid sequences and binding affinities for monoamines, each presynaptic monoamine transporter nevertheless has appreciable affinity for amines other than the one matched to its own neuron (Table 2-1). Thus, if other transportable neurotransmitters or drugs are in the vicinity of a given monoamine transporter, they may also be transported into the presynaptic neuron by hitchhiking a ride on certain transporters that can carry them into the neuron.

For example, the norepinephrine transporter (NET) has high affinity for the transport of dopamine as well as for norepinephrine, the dopamine transporter (DAT) has high affinity for the transport of amphetamines as well as for dopamine, and the serotonin transporter (SERT) has high affinity for the transport of "ecstasy" (the drug of abuse MDMA or 3,4-methylenedioxymethamphetamine) as well as for serotonin (Table 2-1).

How are neurotransmitters transported? Monoamines are not passively shuttled into the presynaptic neuron, because it requires energy to concentrate monoamines into a presynaptic neuron. That energy is provided by transporters in the SLC6 gene family coupling the "downhill" transport of sodium (down a concentration gradient) with the "uphill" transport of the monoamine (up a concentration gradient) (Figure 2-2A). Thus, the monoamine transporters are really sodium-dependent cotransporters; in most cases, this involves the additional cotransport of chloride, and in some cases the countertransport of

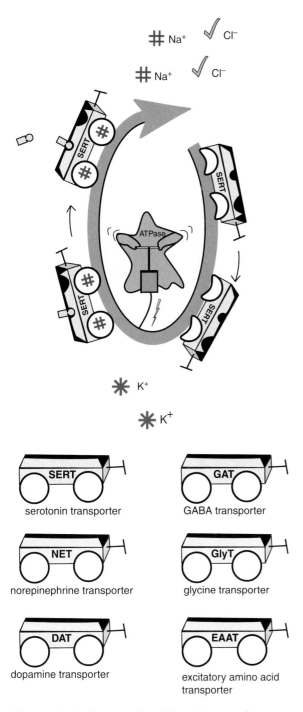

potassium. All of this is made possible by coupling monoamine transport to the activity of sodium-potassium ATPase (adenosine triphosphatase), an enzyme sometimes called the "sodium pump" that creates the downhill gradient for sodium by continuously pumping sodium out of the neuron (Figure 2-2A).

The structure of a monoamine transporter from the SLC6 family has recently been proposed to have binding sites not only for the monoamine, but also for two sodium ions (Figure 2-2A). In addition, these transporters may exist as dimers, or two copies working together with each other, but the manner in which they cooperate is not yet well understood and is not shown in the figures. There are other sites on this transporter – not well defined – for drugs such as antidepressants, which bind to the transporter and inhibit reuptake of monoamines but do not bind to the substrate site and are not transported into the neuron (thus they are *allosteric*, meaning "other site").

In the absence of sodium, there is low affinity of the monoamine transporter for its monoamine substrate, and thus binding of neither sodium nor monoamine. An example of this is shown for the serotonin transporter SERT in Figure 2-2A, where some of the transport "wagons" have flat tires, indicating no binding of sodium as well as absence of binding of serotonin to its substrate binding site, since the transporter has low affinity for serotonin in the absence of sodium. The allosteric site for antidepressant binding is also empty (the front seat in Figure 2-2A). However, in the presence of sodium ions, the tires are "inflated" by sodium binding and serotonin can also bind to its substrate site on SERT. The situation is now primed for serotonin transport back into the serotonergic neuron, along with cotransport of sodium and chloride down the gradient and into the neuron and countertransport of potassium out of the neuron (Figure 2-2A). But if a drug binds to an inhibitory allosteric site on SERT, this reduces the affinity of the serotonin transporter SERT for its substrate serotonin, and serotonin binding is prevented.

Figure 2-2A. Sodium-potassium ATPase. Transport of many neurotransmitters into the presynaptic neuron is not passive, but rather requires energy. This energy is supplied by sodium-potassium ATPase (adenosine triphosphatase), an enzyme that is also sometimes referred to as the sodium pump. Sodium-potassium ATPase continuously pumps sodium out of the neuron, creating a downhill gradient. The "downhill" transport of sodium is coupled to the "uphill" transport of the neurotransmitter. In many cases this also involves cotransport of chloride and in some cases countertransport of potassium. Examples of neurotransmitter transporters include the serotonin transporter (SERT), the norepinephrine transporter (NET), the dopamine transporter (DAT), the GABA transporter (GAT), the glycine transporter (GlyT), and the excitatory amino acid transporter (EAAT).

Table 2-3 Vesicular neurotransmitter transporters

Transporter	Common abbreviation	Gene family	Endogenous substrate
Vesicular monoamine transporters 1 and 2	VMAT1 VMAT2	SLC18	Serotonin Norepinephrine Dopamine
Vesicular acetylcholine transporter	VAChT	SLC18	Acetylcholine
Vesicular inhibitory amino acid transporter	VIAAT	SLC32	GABA
Vesicular glutamate transporters 1–3	VGluT1–3	SLC17	Glutamate

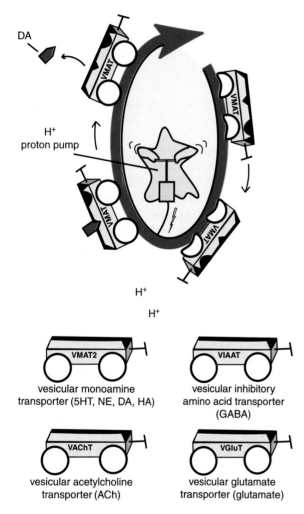

vesicular monoamine transporter (5HT, NE, DA, HA)

vesicular inhibitory amino acid transporter (GABA)

vesicular acetylcholine transporter (ACh)

vesicular glutamate transporter (glutamate)

Figure 2-2B. Vesicular transporters. Vesicular transporters package neurotransmitters into synaptic vesicles through the use of a proton ATPase, or proton pump. The proton pump utilizes energy to pump positively charged protons continuously out of the synaptic vesicle. Neurotransmitter can then be transported into the synaptic vesicle, keeping the charge inside the vesicle constant. Examples of vesicular transporters include the vesicular monoamine transporter (VMAT2), which transports serotonin, norepinephrine, dopamine, and histamine; the vesicular acetylcholine transporter (VAChT), which transports acetylcholine; the vesicular inhibitory amino acid transporter (VIAAT), which transports GABA; and the vesicular glutamate transporter (VGluT), which transports glutamate.

Why does this matter? Blocking the presynaptic monoamine transporter has a huge impact on neurotransmission at any synapse that utilizes that neurotransmitter. The normal recapture of neurotransmitter by the presynaptic neurotransmitter transporter in Figure 2-2A keeps the levels of this neurotransmitter from accumulating in the synapse. Normally, following release from the presynaptic neuron, neurotransmitters only have time for a brief dance on their synaptic receptors, and the party is soon over because the monoamines climb back into the presynaptic neuron on their transporters (Figure 2-2A). If one wants to enhance normal synaptic activity of these neurotransmitters, or restore their diminished synaptic activity, this can be accomplished by blocking these transporters. Although this might not seem to be a very dramatic thing, the fact is that this alteration in chemical neurotransmission – namely the enhancement of synaptic monoamine action – is thought to underlie the clinical effects of all the agents that block monoamine transporters, including most known antidepressants and stimulants. Specifically, many antidepressants enhance serotonin, norepinephrine, or both, due to actions on SERT and/or NET. Some antidepressants act on DAT, as do stimulants. Also, recall that many antidepressants that block monoamine transporters are also effective anxiolytics, reduce neuropathic pain, and have additional therapeutic actions as well. Thus, it may come as no surprise that drugs that block monoamine transporters are among the most frequently prescribed psychotropic drugs. In fact, about a third of the currently prescribed essential psychotropic drugs act by targeting one or more of the three monoamine transporters.

Other neurotransmitter transporters (SLC6 and SLC1 gene families) as targets of psychotropic drugs

In addition to the three transporters for monoamines discussed in detail above, there are several other transporters for various different neurotransmitters or their precursors. Although this includes a dozen additional transporters, there is only one psychotropic drug used clinically that is known to bind to any of these transporters. Thus, there is a presynaptic transporter for choline, the precursor to the neurotransmitter acetylcholine, but no known drugs target this transporter. There are also several transporters for the ubiquitous inhibitory neurotransmitter GABA, known as GAT1–4 (Table 2-2). Although debate continues about the exact localization of these subtypes at presynaptic neurons, neighboring glia, or even postsynaptic neurons, it is clear that a key presynaptic transporter of GABA is the GAT1 transporter, which is selectively blocked by the anticonvulsant tiagabine, thereby increasing synaptic GABA concentrations. In addition to anticonvulsant actions, this increase in synaptic GABA may have therapeutic actions in anxiety, sleep disorders, and pain. No other inhibitors of this transporter are available for clinical use.

Finally, there are multiple transporters for two amino acid neurotransmitters, glycine and glutamate (Table 2-2). There are no drugs utilized in clinical practice that are known to block glycine transporters, although new agents are in clinical trials for treating schizophrenia. The glycine transporters, along with the choline and GABA transporters, are all members of the same family to which the monoamine transporters belong and have a similar structure (Figure 2-2A, Tables 2-1 and 2-2). However, the glutamate transporters belong to a unique family, SLC1, and have a unique structure and somewhat different functions compared to those transporters of the SLC6 family (Table 2-2).

Specifically, there are several transporters for glutamate, known as excitatory amino acid transporters 1–5, or EAAT1–5 (Table 2-2). The exact localization of these various transporters at presynaptic neurons, postsynaptic neurons, or glia is still under investigation, but the uptake of glutamate into glia is well known to be a key system for recapturing glutamate for reuse once it has been released. Transport into glia results in conversion of glutamate into glutamine, and then glutamine enters the presynaptic neuron for reconversion back into glutamate. No drugs utilized in clinical practice are known to block glutamate transporters.

One difference between transport of neurotransmitters by the SLC6 gene family and transport of glutamate by the SLC1 gene family is that glutamate does not seem to cotransport chloride with sodium when it also cotransports glutamate. Also, glutamate transport is almost always characterized by the countertransport of potassium, whereas this is not always the case with SLC6 gene family transporters. Glutamate transporters may work together as trimers rather than dimers, as the SLC6 transporters seem to do. The functional significance of these differences remains obscure, but may become more apparent if clinically useful psychopharmacologic agents that target glutamate transporters are discovered. Since it may often be desirable to diminish rather than enhance glutamate neurotransmission, the future utility of glutamate transporters as therapeutic targets is also unclear.

Where are the transporters for histamine and neuropeptides?

It is an interesting observation that apparently not all neurotransmitters are regulated by reuptake transporters. The central neurotransmitter histamine apparently does not have a presynaptic transporter (although it is transported into synaptic vesicles by VMAT2, the same transporter used by the monoamines – see Figure 2-2B). Histamine's inactivation is thus thought to be entirely enzymatic. The same can be said for neuropeptides, since reuptake pumps and presynaptic transporters have not been found for them, and are thus thought to be lacking for this class of neurotransmitter. Inactivation of neuropeptides is apparently by diffusion, sequestration, and enzymatic destruction, but not by presynaptic transport. It is always possible that a transporter will be discovered in the future for some of these neurotransmitters, but at the present time there are no known presynaptic transporters for either histamine or neuropeptides.

Vesicular transporters: subtypes and function

Vesicular transporters for the monoamines (VMATs) are members of the SLC18 gene family and have already been discussed above. They are shown in

Figure 2-2B and listed in Table 2-3, as is the vesicular transporter for acetylcholine – also a member of the SLC18 gene family but known as VAChT. The GABA vesicular transporter is a member of the SLC32 gene family and is called VIAAT (vesicular inhibitory amino acid transporter; Figure 2-2B and Table 2-3). Finally, vesicular transporters for glutamate, called vGluT1–3 (vesicular glutamate transporters 1, 2, and 3) are members of the SLC17 gene family – and are also shown in Figure 2-2B and listed in Table 2-3. The SV2A transporter is a novel twelve-transmembrane-region synaptic vesicle transporter of uncertain mechanism and with unclear substrates; it is localized within the synaptic vesicle membrane and binds the anticonvulsant levetiracetam, perhaps interfering with neurotransmitter release and thereby reducing seizures.

How do neurotransmitters get inside synaptic vesicles? In the case of vesicular transporters, storage of neurotransmitters is facilitated by a proton ATPase, known as the "proton pump," that utilizes energy to pump positively charged protons continuously out of the synaptic vesicle (Figure 2-2B). The neurotransmitters can then be concentrated against a gradient by substituting their own positive charge inside the vesicle for the positive charge of the proton being pumped out. Thus, neurotransmitters are not so much transported as "antiported" – i.e., they go in while the protons are actively transported out, keeping charge inside the vesicle constant. This concept is shown in Figure 2-2B for the VMAT transporting dopamine in exchange for protons. Contrast this with Figure 2-2A, where a monoamine transporter on the presynaptic membrane is cotransporting a monoamine along with sodium and chloride, but with the help of a sodium-potassium ATPase (sodium pump) rather than a proton pump.

Vesicular transporters (SLC18 gene family) as targets of psychotropic drugs

Vesicular transporters for acetylcholine (SLC18 gene family), GABA (SLC32 gene family), and glutamate (SLC17 gene family) are not known to be targeted by any drug utilized by humans. However, vesicular transporters for monoamines in the SLC18 gene family, or VMATs, particularly those in dopamine and norepinephrine neurons, are potently targeted by several drugs including amphetamine, tetrabenazine, and reserpine.

Amphetamine thus has two targets: monoamine transporters as well as VMATs. In contrast, other stimulants such as methylphenidate and cocaine target only the monoamine transporters, and in much the same manner as described for antidepressants (see Chapter 7).

G-protein-linked receptors
Structure and function

Another major target of psychotropic drugs is the class of receptors linked to G proteins. These receptors all have the structure of seven transmembrane regions, meaning that they span the membrane seven times (Figure 2-1). Each of the transmembrane regions clusters around a central core that contains a binding site for a neurotransmitter. Drugs can interact at this neurotransmitter binding site or at other sites (allosteric sites) on the receptor. This can lead to a wide range of modifications of receptor actions due to mimicking or blocking, partially or fully, the neurotransmitter function that normally occurs at this receptor. These drug actions can thus change downstream molecular events such as which phosphoproteins are activated or inactivated and therefore which enzymes, receptors, or ion channels are modified by neurotransmission. Such drug actions can also change which genes are expressed, and thus which proteins are synthesized and which functions are amplified, from synaptogenesis, to receptor and enzyme synthesis, to communication with downstream neurons innervated by the neuron with the G-protein-linked receptor.

These actions on neurotransmission by G-protein-linked receptors are described in detail in Chapter 1 on signal transduction and chemical neurotransmission. The reader should have a good command of the function of G-protein-linked receptors and their role in signal transduction from specific neurotransmitters, as described in Chapter 1, in order to understand how drugs acting at G-protein-linked receptors modify the signal transduction that arises from these receptors. This is important to understand because such drug-induced modifications in signal transduction from G-protein-linked receptors can have profound actions on psychiatric symptoms. In fact, the single most common action of psychotropic drugs utilized in clinical practice is to modify the actions of G-protein-linked receptors, resulting in either therapeutic actions or side effects. Here we will describe how various drugs stimulate or block these receptors, and throughout the textbook we will show how specific drugs acting at specific G-protein-linked receptors have specific actions on specific psychiatric disorders.

G-protein-linked receptors as targets of psychotropic drugs

G-protein-linked receptors are a large superfamily of receptors that interact with many neurotransmitters and with many psychotropic drugs (Figure 2-1B). There are numerous ways to subtype these receptors, but pharmacologic subtypes are perhaps the most important to understand for clinicians who wish to target specific receptors with psychotropic drugs utilized in clinical practice. That is, the natural neurotransmitter interacts at all of its receptor subtypes, but many drugs are more selective than the neurotransmitter itself for certain receptor subtypes and thus define a pharmacologic subtype of receptor at which they specifically interact. This is not unlike the concept of the neurotransmitter being a master key that opens all the doors, and a drug that interacts at pharmacologically specific receptor subtypes functioning as a specific key opening only one door. Here we will develop the concept that drugs have many different ways of interacting at pharmacologic subtypes of G-protein-linked receptors, which occur across an agonist spectrum (Figure 2-3).

No agonist

An important concept for the agonist spectrum is that the absence of agonist does not necessarily mean that nothing is happening with signal transduction at G-protein-linked receptors. Agonists are thought to produce a conformational change in G-protein-linked receptors that leads to full receptor activation, and thus full signal transduction. In the absence of agonist, this same conformational change may still be occurring at some receptor systems, but only at very low frequency. This is referred to as *constitutive activity*, which may be present especially in receptor systems and brain areas where there is a high density of receptors. Thus, when something occurs at very low frequency but among a high number of receptors, it can still produce detectable signal transduction output. This is represented as a small – but not absent – amount of signal transduction in Figure 2-4.

Agonists

An agonist produces a conformational change in the G-protein-linked receptor that turns on the synthesis of second messenger to the greatest extent possible (i.e., the action of a *full agonist*). The full agonist is generally represented by the naturally occurring neurotransmitter itself, although some drugs can also act in as full a manner as the natural neurotransmitter. What this means from the perspective of chemical neurotransmission is that the full array of downstream signal transduction is triggered by a full

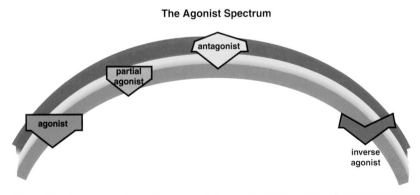

The Agonist Spectrum

Figure 2-3. Agonist spectrum. Shown here is the agonist spectrum. Naturally occurring neurotransmitters stimulate receptors and are thus agonists. Some drugs also stimulate receptors and are therefore agonists as well. It is possible for drugs to stimulate receptors to a lesser degree than the natural neurotransmitter; these are called partial agonists or stabilizers. It is a common misconception that antagonists are the opposite of agonists because they block the actions of agonists. However, although antagonists prevent the actions of agonists, they have no activity of their own in the absence of the agonist. For this reason, antagonists are sometimes called "silent." Inverse agonists, on the other hand, do have opposite actions compared to agonists. That is, they not only block agonists but can also reduce activity below the baseline level when no agonist is present. Thus, the agonist spectrum reaches from full agonists to partial agonists through to "silent" antagonists and finally inverse agonists.

No Agonist: Constitutive Activity

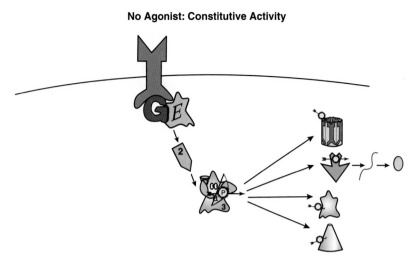

Figure 2-4. Constitutive activity. The absence of agonist does not mean that there is no activity related to G-protein-linked receptors. Rather, in the absence of agonist, the receptor's conformation is such that it leads to a low level of activity, or constitutive activity. Thus, signal transduction still occurs, but at a low frequency. Whether this constitutive activity leads to detectable signal transduction is affected by the receptor density in that brain region.

agonist (Figure 2-5). Thus, downstream proteins are maximally phosphorylated, and genes are maximally impacted. Loss of the agonist actions of a neurotransmitter at G-protein-linked receptors, due to deficient neurotransmission of any cause, would lead to the loss of this rich downstream chemical tour de force. Thus, agonists that restore this natural action would be potentially useful in states where reduced signal transduction leads to undesirable symptoms.

There are two major ways to stimulate G-protein-linked receptors with full agonist action. First, several drugs *directly* bind to the neurotransmitter site and produce the same array of signal transduction effects as a full agonist (Table 2-4). These are direct-acting agonists. Second, many drugs can *indirectly* act to boost the levels of the natural full agonist neurotransmitter (Table 2-5). This happens when neurotransmitter inactivation mechanisms are blocked. The most prominent examples of indirect full agonist actions have already been discussed above, namely inhibition of the monoamine transporters SERT, NET, and DAT and the GABA transporter GAT1. Another way to accomplish indirect full agonist action is to block the enzymatic destruction of neurotransmitters (Table 2-5). Two examples of this are inhibition of the enzymes monoamine oxidase (MAO) and acetylcholinesterase.

Antagonists

On the other hand, it is also possible that full agonist action can be too much of a good thing and that maximal activation of the signal transduction cascade is not always desirable, as in states of overstimulation

by neurotransmitters. In such cases, blocking the action of the natural neurotransmitter agonist may be desirable. This is the property of an antagonist. Antagonists produce a conformational change in the G-protein-linked receptor that causes no change in signal transduction – including no change in whatever amount of any constitutive activity that may have been present in the absence of agonist (compare Figure 2-4 with Figure 2-6). Thus, true antagonists are "neutral" and, since they have no actions of their own, are also called "silent."

There are many more examples in clinical practice of important antagonists of G-protein-linked receptors than there are of direct-acting full agonists (Table 2-4). Antagonists are well known both as the mediators of therapeutic actions in psychiatric disorders and as the cause of undesirable side effects (Table 2-4). Some of these may prove to be inverse agonists (see below), but most antagonists utilized in clinical practice are characterized simply as "antagonists."

Antagonists block the actions of everything in the agonist spectrum (Figure 2-3). In the presence of an agonist, an antagonist will block the actions of that agonist but does nothing itself (Figure 2-6). The antagonist simply returns the receptor conformation back to the same state as exists when no agonist is present (Figure 2-4). Interestingly, an antagonist will also block the actions of a partial agonist. Partial agonists are thought to produce a conformational change in the G-protein-linked receptor that is intermediate between a full agonist and the baseline conformation of the receptor in the absence of

Full Agonist: Maximum Signal Transduction

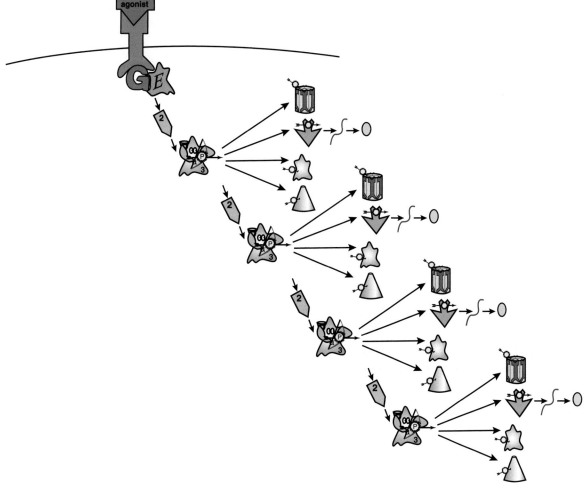

Figure 2-5. Full agonist: maximum signal transduction. When a full agonist binds to G-protein-linked receptors, it causes conformational changes that lead to maximum signal transduction. Thus, all the downstream effects of signal transduction, such as phosphorylation of proteins and gene activation, are maximized.

agonist (Figures 2-7 and 2-8). An antagonist reverses the action of a partial agonist by returning the G-protein-linked receptor to the same conformation (Figure 2-6) as exists when no agonist is present (Figure 2-4). Finally, an antagonist reverses an inverse agonist. Inverse agonists are thought to produce a conformational state of the receptor that totally inactivates it and even removes the baseline constitutive activity (Figure 2-9). An antagonist reverses this back to the baseline state that allows constitutive activity (Figure 2-6), the same as exists for the receptor in the absence of the neurotransmitter agonist (Figure 2-4).

By themselves, therefore, it is easy to see that true antagonists have no activity, and why they are sometimes referred to as "silent." Silent antagonists return the entire spectrum of drug-induced conformational changes in the G-protein-linked receptor (Figures 2-3 and 2-10) to the same place (Figure 2-6) – i.e., the conformation that exists in the absence of agonist (Figure 2-4).

Partial agonists

It is possible to produce signal transduction that is something more than an antagonist yet something less than a full agonist. Turning down the gain a bit

Table 2-4 Key G-protein-linked receptors directly targeted by psychotropic drugs

Neurotransmitter	G-protein receptor and pharmacologic subtype directly targeted	Pharmacologic action	Drug class	Therapeutic action
Dopamine	D_2	Antagonist or partial agonist	Conventional antipsychotic; atypical antipsychotic	Antipsychotic; antimanic
Serotonin	$5HT_{2A}$	Antagonist or inverse agonist	Atypical antipsychotic	Reduced motor side effects; possible mood stabilizing and antidepressant actions in bipolar disorder
			Antidepressant, hypnotic	Improve mood and insomnia
	$5HT_{1A}$ $5HT_{1B/D}$ $5HT_{2C}$ $5HT_6$ $5HT_7$	Antagonist or partial agonist	Atypical antipsychotic	Unknown secondary receptor actions, possibly contributing to efficacy and tolerability
	$5HT_{1A}$	Partial agonist	Anxiolytic	Anxiolytic; booster of antidepressant action
Norepinephrine	$Alpha_2$	Antagonist Agonist	Antidepressant Antihypertensive	Antidepressant Cognition and behavioral disturbance in attention deficit hyperactivity disorder
	$Alpha_1$	Antagonist	Many antipsychotics and antidepressants	Side effects of orthostatic hypotension and possibly sedation
GABA	$GABA_B$	Agonist	Gamma hydroxybutyrate/sodium oxybate	Cataplexy, sleepiness in narcolepsy; possible enhanced slow-wave sleep and pain reduction
Melatonin	MT_1 MT_2	Agonist Agonist	Hypnotic Hypnotic	Improve insomnia Improve insomnia
Histamine	H_1	Antagonist	Many antipsychotics and antidepressants; some anxiolytics	Therapeutic effect for anxiety and insomnia; side effect of sedation and weight gain
Acetylcholine	M_1	Antagonist	Many antipsychotics and antidepressants	Side effects of memory disturbance, sedation, dry mouth, blurred vision, constipation, urinary retention
	M_3/M_5	Antagonist	Some atypical antipsychotics	May contribute to metabolic dysregulation (dyslipidemia and diabetes)

Table 2-5 Key G-protein-linked receptors indirectly targeted by psychotropic drugs

Neurotransmitter	G-protein receptor and pharmacologic subtype indirectly targeted	Pharmacologic action	Drug class	Therapeutic action
Dopamine	D_1 and D_2 (possibly D_3, D_4)	Agonist via increasing dopamine itself at all dopamine receptors	Stimulant (actions at dopamine and/or synaptic vesicle transporters DAT and VMAT2)	Improvement of attention deficit hyperactivity disorder (ADHD)
			Antidepressant (actions at dopamine and/or norepinephrine transporters DAT and/or NET)	Antidepressant; ADHD
			MAO inhibitor (reducing dopamine metabolism)	Antidepressant
Serotonin	$5HT_{1A}$ (presynaptic somadendritic autoreceptors)	Agonist via increasing serotonin itself at all serotonin receptors	Antidepressant (actions at serotonin transporters SERT)	Antidepressant; anxiolytic
	$5HT_{2A}$ postsynaptic receptors; possibly $5HT_{1A}$, $5HT_{2C}$, $5HT_6$, $5HT_7$ postsynaptic receptors			
			MAO inhibitor (reducing serotonin metabolism)	Antidepressant
Norepinephrine	$Beta_2$ postsynaptic; possibly $alpha_2$ presynaptic and postsynaptic	Agonist via increasing norepinephrine itself at all norepinephrine receptors	Antidepressant; neuropathic pain (actions at norepinephrine transporter NET)	Antidepressant; improve ADHD; for chronic pain (when combined with SERT inhibition)
			MAO inhibitor (reducing norepinephrine metabolism)	Antidepressant
GABA	$GABA_A$ and $GABA_B$	Agonist via increasing GABA itself at all GABA receptors	Anticonvulsant (actions at the GABA GAT1 transporter)	Anticonvulsant; possibly anxiolytic, for chronic pain, for slow-wave sleep
Acetylcholine	M_1 (possibly M_2–M_5)	Agonist via increasing acetylcholine itself at all acetylcholine receptors	Acetylcholinesterase inhibitor (reducing acetylcholine metabolism)	Slowing progression in Alzheimer's disease

DAT, dopamine transporter; MAO, monoamine oxidase; NET, norepinephrine transporter; SERT, serotonin transporter; VMAT, vesicular monoamine transporter.

**"Silent" Antagonist: Back to Baseline,
Constitutive Activity Only, Same as No Agonist**

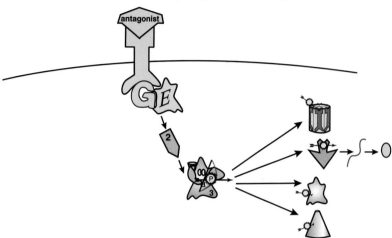

Figure 2-6. "Silent" antagonist. An antagonist blocks agonists (both full and partial) from binding to G-protein-linked receptors, thus preventing agonists from causing maximum signal transduction and instead changing the receptor's conformation back to the same state as exists when no agonist is present. Antagonists also reverse the effects of inverse agonists, again by blocking the inverse agonists from binding and then returning the receptor conformation to the baseline state. Antagonists do not have any impact on signal transduction in the absence of an agonist.

from full agonist actions, but not all the way to zero, is the property of a partial agonist (Figure 2-7). This action can also be seen as turning up the gain a bit from silent antagonist actions, but not all the way to a full agonist. Depending upon how close this partial agonist is to a full agonist or to a silent antagonist on the agonist spectrum will determine the impact of a partial agonist on downstream signal transduction events.

The amount of "partiality" that is desired between agonist and antagonist – that is, where a partial agonist should sit on the agonist spectrum – is a matter of debate as well as trial and error. The ideal therapeutic agent may have signal transduction through G-protein-linked receptors that is not too "hot," yet not too "cold," but "just right," sometimes called the "Goldilocks" solution. Such an ideal state may vary from one clinical situation to another, depending upon the balance between full agonism and silent antagonism that is desired.

In cases where there is unstable neurotransmission throughout the brain, such as when pyramidal neurons in the prefrontal cortex are out of "tune," it may be desirable to find a state of signal transduction that stabilizes G-protein-linked receptor output somewhere between too much and too little downstream action. For this reason, partial agonists are also called "stabilizers," since they have the theoretical capacity to find a stable solution between the extremes of too much full agonist action and no agonist action at all (Figure 2-7).

Since partial agonists exert an effect less than that of a full agonist, they are also sometimes called "weak," with the implication that partial agonism means partial clinical efficacy. That is certainly possible in some cases, but it is more sophisticated to understand the potential stabilizing and "tuning" actions of this class of therapeutic agents, and not to use terms that imply clinical actions for the entire class of drugs that may only apply to some individual agents. A few partial agonists are utilized in clinical practice (Table 2-4) and more are in clinical development.

Light and dark as an analogy for partial agonists

It was originally conceived that a neurotransmitter could only act at receptors like a light switch, turning things on when the neurotransmitter is present and turning things off when the neurotransmitter is absent. We now know that many receptors, including the G-protein-linked receptor family, can function rather more like a rheostat. That is, a full agonist will turn the lights all the way on (Figure 2-8A), but a partial agonist will only turn the light on partially (Figure 2-8B). If neither full agonist nor partial agonist is present, the room is dark (Figure 2-8C).

Each partial agonist has its own set point engineered into the molecule, such that it cannot turn the lights on brighter even with a higher dose. No matter how much partial agonist is given, only a certain degree of brightness will result. A series of partial agonists will differ one from the other in the degree

Partial Agonist: Partially Enhanced Signal Transduction

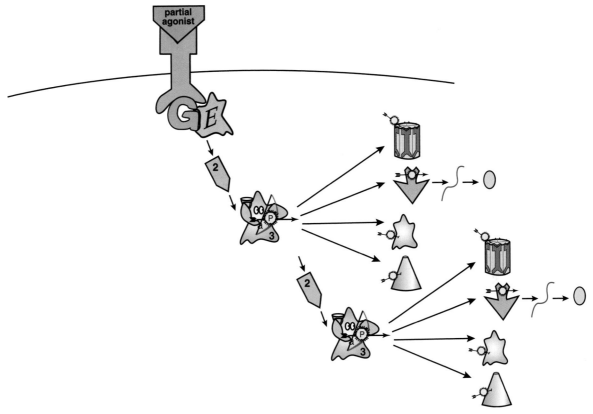

Figure 2-7. Partial agonist. Partial agonists stimulate G-protein-linked receptors to enhance signal transduction but do not lead to maximum signal transduction the way full agonists do. Thus, in the absence of a full agonist, partial agonists increase signal transduction. However, in the presence of a full agonist, the partial agonist will actually turn down the strength of various downstream signals. For this reason, partial agonists are sometimes referred to as stabilizers.

FULL AGONIST --
light is at its brightest

PARTIAL AGONIST --
light is dimmed but still shining

NO AGONIST --
light is off

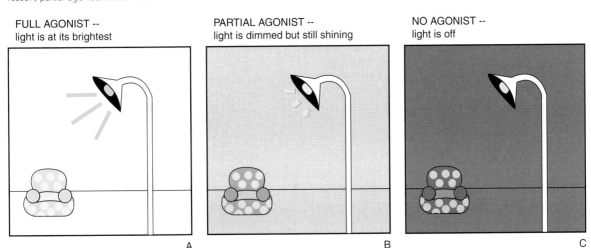

A   B   C

Figure 2-8. Agonist spectrum: rheostat. A useful analogy for the agonist spectrum is a light controlled by a rheostat. The light will be brightest after a full agonist turns the light switch fully on (A). A partial agonist will also act as a net agonist and turn the light on, but only partially, according to the level preset in the partial agonist's rheostat (B). If the light is already on, a partial agonist will "dim" the lights, thus acting as a net antagonist. When no full or partial agonist is present, the situation is analogous to the light being switched off (C).

of partiality, so that theoretically all degrees of brightness can be covered within the range from "off" to "on," but each partial agonist has its own unique degree of brightness associated with it.

What is so interesting about partial agonists is that they can appear as a net agonist, or as a net antagonist, depending upon the amount of naturally occurring full agonist neurotransmitter that is present. Thus, when a full agonist neurotransmitter is absent, a partial agonist will be a net agonist. That is, from the resting state, a partial agonist initiates somewhat of an increase in the signal transduction cascade from the G-protein-linked second-messenger system. However, when full agonist neurotransmitter is present, the same partial agonist will become a net antagonist. That is, it will decrease the level of full signal output to a lesser level, but not to zero. Thus, a partial agonist can simultaneously *boost* deficient neurotransmitter activity yet *block* excessive neurotransmitter activity, another reason that partial agonists are called stabilizers.

Returning to the light-switch analogy, a room will be dark when agonist is missing and the light switch is off (Figure 2-8C). A room will be brightly lit when it is full of natural full agonist and the light switch is fully on (Figure 2-8A). Adding partial agonist to the dark room where there is no natural full agonist neurotransmitter will turn the lights up, but only as far as the partial agonist works on the rheostat (Figure 2-8B). Relative to the dark room as a starting point, a partial agonist acts therefore as a net agonist. On the other hand, adding a partial agonist to the fully lit room will have the effect of turning the lights down to the intermediate level of lower brightness on the rheostat (Figure 2-8B). This is a net antagonistic effect relative to the fully lit room. Thus, after adding partial agonist to the dark room and to the brightly lit room, both rooms will be equally light. The degree of brightness is that of being partially turned on, as dictated by the properties of the partial agonist. However, in the dark room, the partial agonist has acted as a net agonist, whereas in the brightly lit room, the partial agonist has acted as a net antagonist.

An agonist and an antagonist in the same molecule is quite a new dimension to therapeutics. This concept has led to proposals that partial agonists could treat not only states that are theoretically deficient in full agonist, but also those that have a theoretical excess of full agonist. A partial agonist may even be able to treat simultaneously states that are mixtures of both excess and deficiency in neurotransmitter activity.

Inverse Agonist: Beyond Antagonism; Even the Constitutive Activity is Blocked

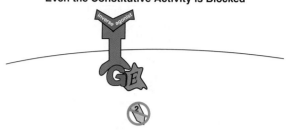

Figure 2-9. Inverse agonist. Inverse agonists produce conformational change in the G-protein-linked receptor that renders it inactive. This leads to reduced signal transduction as compared not only to that associated with agonists but also to that associated with antagonists or the absence of an agonist. The impact of an inverse agonist is dependent on the receptor density in that brain region. That is, if the receptor density is so low that constitutive activity does not lead to detectable signal transduction, then reducing the constitutive activity would not have any appreciable effect.

Inverse agonists

Inverse agonists are more than simple antagonists, and are neither neutral nor silent. These agents have an action that is thought to produce a conformational change in the G-protein-linked receptor that stabilizes it in a totally inactive form (Figure 2-9). Thus, this conformation produces a functional reduction in signal transduction (Figure 2-9) that is even less than that produced when there is either no agonist present (Figure 2-4) or a silent antagonist present (Figure 2-6). The result of an inverse agonist is to shut down even the constitutive activity of the G-protein-linked receptor system. Of course, if a given receptor system has no constitutive activity, perhaps in cases when receptors are present in low density, then there will be no reduction in activity and the inverse agonist will look like an antagonist.

In many ways, therefore, inverse agonists do the *opposite* of agonists. If an agonist increases signal transduction from baseline, an inverse agonist decreases it, even below baseline levels. In contrast to agonists and antagonists, therefore, an *inverse agonist* neither increases signal transduction like an agonist (Figure 2-5) nor merely blocks the agonist from increasing signal transduction like an antagonist (Figure 2-6); rather, an inverse agonist binds the receptor in a fashion so as to provoke an action opposite to that of the agonist, namely causing the receptor to *decrease* its baseline signal transduction level (Figure 2-9). It is unclear from a clinical point of view what the relevant differences are between an inverse agonist and a silent antagonist. In fact, some drugs that have long been considered to be silent antagonists may turn out in some areas of the brain to be

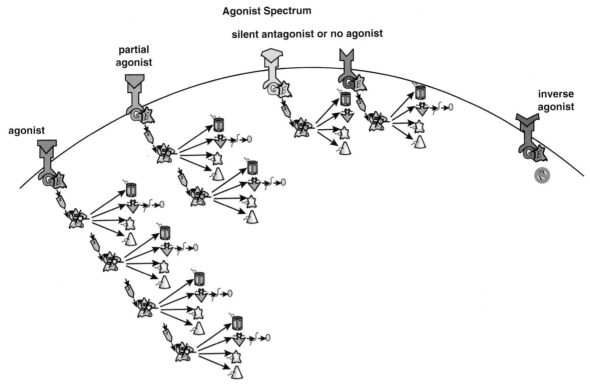

Figure 2-10. Agonist spectrum. This figure summarizes the implications of the agonist spectrum. Full agonists cause maximum signal transduction, while partial agonists increase signal transduction compared to no agonist but decrease it compared to full agonist. Antagonists allow constitutive activity and thus, in the absence of an agonist, have no effects themselves; in the presence of an agonist, antagonists lead to reduced signal transduction. Inverse agonists are the functional opposites of agonists and actually reduce signal transduction beyond that produced in the absence of an agonist.

inverse agonists. Thus, the concept of an inverse agonist as clinically distinguishable from a silent antagonist remains to be proven. In the meantime, inverse agonists remain an interesting pharmacological concept.

In summary, G-protein-linked receptors act along an agonist spectrum, and drugs have been described that can produce conformational changes in these receptors to create any state from full agonist, to partial agonist, to silent antagonist, to inverse agonist (Figure 2-10). When one considers signal transduction along this spectrum (Figure 2-10), it is easy to understand why agents at each point along the agonist spectrum differ so much from each other, and why their clinical actions are so different.

Enzymes as targets of psychotropic drugs

Enzymes are involved in multiple aspects of chemical neurotransmission, as discussed extensively in Chapter 1 on signal transduction. Every enzyme is the theoretical target for a drug acting as an enzyme inhibitor. However, in practice, only a minority of currently known drugs

utilized in the clinical practice of psychopharmacology are enzyme inhibitors.

Enzyme activity is the conversion of one molecule into another, namely a substrate into a product (Figure 2-11). The substrates for each enzyme are unique and selective, as are the products. A substrate (Figure 2-11A) comes to the enzyme to bind at the enzyme's active site (Figure 2-11B), and departs as a changed molecular entity called the product (Figure 2-11C). The inhibitors of an enzyme are also unique and selective for one enzyme compared to another. In the presence of an enzyme inhibitor, the enzyme cannot bind to its substrates. The binding of inhibitors can be either irreversible (Figure 2-12) or reversible (Figure 2-13).

When an irreversible inhibitor binds to the enzyme, it cannot be displaced by the substrate; thus, that inhibitor binds irreversibly (Figure 2-12). This is depicted as binding with chains (Figure 2-12A) that cannot be cut with scissors by the substrate (Figure 2-12B). The irreversible type of enzyme inhibitor is sometimes called a

After a Substrate Binds to an Enzyme, it is Turned Into a Product Which is Then Released From the Enzyme.

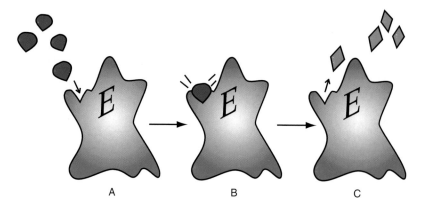

A   B   C

Figure 2-11. Enzyme activity. Enzyme activity is the conversion of one molecule into another. Thus, a substrate is said to be turned into a product by enzymatic modification of the substrate molecule. The enzyme has an active site at which the substrate can bind specifically (A). The substrate then finds the active site of the enzyme and binds to it (B), so that a molecular transformation can occur, changing the substrate into the product (C).

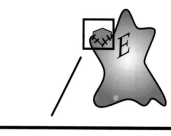

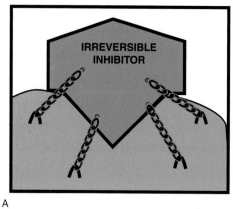

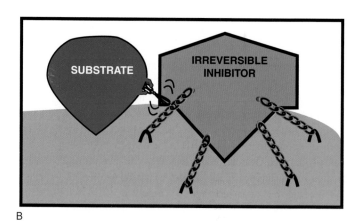

A   B

Figure 2-12. Irreversible enzyme inhibitors. Some drugs are inhibitors of enzymes. Shown here is an irreversible inhibitor of an enzyme, depicted as binding to the enzyme with chains (A). A competing substrate cannot remove an irreversible inhibitor from the enzyme, depicted as scissors unsuccessfully attempting to cut the chains off the inhibitor (B). The binding is locked so permanently that such irreversible enzyme inhibition is sometimes called the work of a "suicide inhibitor," since the enzyme essentially commits suicide by binding to the irreversible inhibitor. Enzyme activity cannot be restored unless another molecule of enzyme is synthesized by the cell's DNA.

"suicide inhibitor" because it covalently and irreversibly binds to the enzyme protein, permanently inhibiting it and therefore essentially "killing" it by making the enzyme nonfunctional forever (Figure 2-12). Enzyme activity in this case is only restored when new enzyme molecules are synthesized.

However, in the case of reversible enzyme inhibitors, an enzyme's substrate is able to compete with

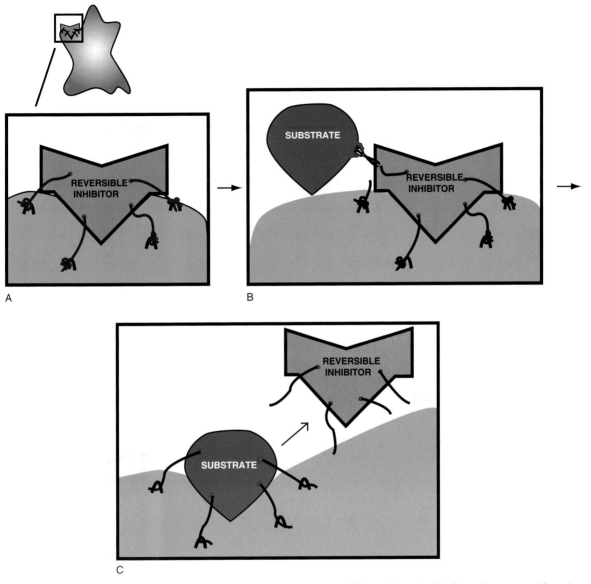

Figure 2-13. Reversible enzyme inhibitors. Other drugs are reversible enzyme inhibitors, depicted as binding to the enzyme with a string (A). A reversible inhibitor can be challenged by a competing substrate for the same enzyme. In the case of a reversible inhibitor, the molecular properties of the substrate are such that it can get rid of the reversible inhibitor, depicted as scissors cutting the string that binds the reversible inhibitor to the enzyme (B). The consequence of a substrate competing successfully for reversal of enzyme inhibition is that the substrate displaces the inhibitor and shoves it off (C). Because the substrate has this capability, the inhibition is said to be reversible.

that reversible inhibitor for binding to the enzyme, and shove it off the enzyme (Figure 2-13). Whether the substrate or the inhibitor "wins" or predominates depends upon which one has the greater affinity for the enzyme and/or is present in the greater concentration. Such binding is called "reversible." Reversible enzyme inhibition is depicted as binding with strings (Figure 2-13A), such that the substrate can cut them with scissors (Figure 2-13B) and displace the enzyme inhibitor, then bind the enzyme itself with its own strings (Figure 2-13C).

These concepts can be applied potentially to any enzyme system. Several enzymes are involved in neurotransmission, including in the synthesis and destruction of neurotransmitters as well as in signal transduction. Only three enzymes are known to be targeted by

GSK-3 (Glycogen Synthetase Kinase): Possible Target for Lithium and Other Mood Stabilizers

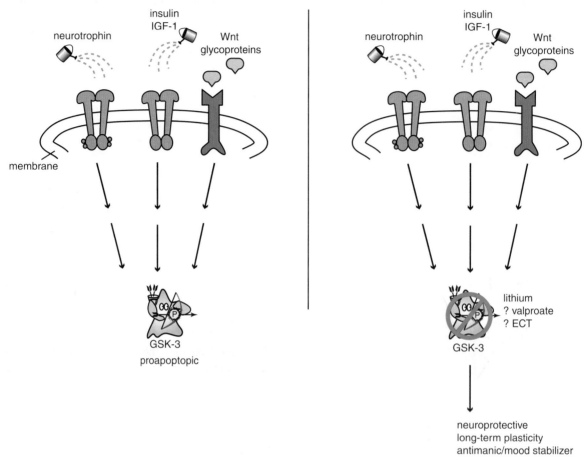

Figure 2-14. Receptor tyrosine kinases. Receptor tyrosine kinases are potential targets for novel psychotropic drugs. Left: Some neurotrophins, growth factors, and other signaling pathways act through a downstream phosphoprotein, an enzyme called GSK-3 (glycogen synthase kinase), to promote cell death (proapoptotic actions). Right: Lithium and possibly some other mood stabilizers may inhibit this enzyme, which could lead to neuroprotective actions and long-term plasticity as well as possibly contribute to mood-stabilizing actions.

psychotropic drugs currently used in clinical practice, namely monoamine oxidase (MAO), acetylcholinesterase, and glycogen synthase kinase (GSK). MAO inhibitors are discussed in more detail in Chapter 7 on antidepressants, and acetylcholinesterase inhibitors are discussed in more detail in Chapter 13 on cognition. Lithium may target an important enzyme in the signal transduction pathway of neurotrophic factors (Figure 2-14). That is, some neurotrophins, growth factors, and other signaling pathways act through a specific downstream phosphoprotein, an enzyme called GSK-3, to promote cell death (proapoptotic actions). Lithium has the capacity to inhibit this enzyme (Figure 2-14). It is possible that

inhibition of this enzyme is physiologically relevant, because this action could lead to neuroprotective actions and long-term plasticity and may contribute to the antimanic and mood-stabilizing actions known to be associated with lithium. The development of novel GSK-3 inhibitors is in progress.

Cytochrome P450 drug metabolizing enzymes as targets of psychotropic drugs

Pharmacokinetic actions are mediated through the hepatic and gut drug metabolizing system known as the cytochrome P450 (CYP) enzyme system. **Pharmacokinetics** is the study of how the body acts upon drugs, especially to absorb, distribute, metabolize, and excrete them. The CYP enzymes and the pharmacokinetic actions they represent must be contrasted with the **pharmacodynamic** actions of drugs, the latter being the major emphasis of this book. Pharmacodynamic actions account for the therapeutic effects and side effects of drugs. However, many psychotropic drugs also target the CYP drug metabolizing enzymes, and a brief overview of these enzymes and their interactions with psychotropic drugs is in order.

CYP enzymes follow the same principles of enzymes transforming substrates into products as illustrated in Figures 2-11 through 2-13. Figure 2-15 depicts the concept of a psychotropic drug being absorbed through the gut wall on the left and then sent to the big blue enzyme in the liver to be

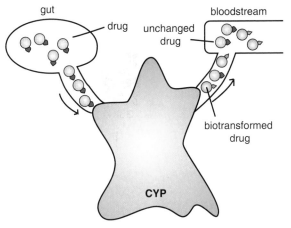

Figure 2-15. Cytochrome P450. The cytochrome P450 (CYP) enzyme system mediates how the body metabolizes many drugs, including antipsychotics. The CYP enzyme in the gut wall or liver converts the drug into a biotransformed product in the bloodstream. After passing through the gut wall and liver (left), the drug will exist partly as unchanged drug and partly as biotransformed drug (right).

biotransformed so that the drug can be sent back into the bloodstream to be excreted from the body via the kidney. Specifically, CYP enzymes in the gut wall or liver convert the drug substrate into a biotransformed product in the bloodstream. After passing through the gut wall and liver, the drug will exist partially as unchanged drug and partially as biotransformed product in the bloodstream (Figure 2-15).

There are several known CYP systems. Five of the most important enzymes for antidepressant drug metabolism are shown in Figure 2-16. There are over 30 known CYP enzymes, and probably many more awaiting discovery and classification. Not all individuals have all the same CYP enzymes. In such cases, their enzymes are said to be polymorphic. For example, about 5–10% of Caucasians are poor metabolizers via the enzyme CYP 2D6, and approximately 20% of Asians may have reduced activity of another CYP enzyme, 2C19. Such individuals with genetically low enzyme activity must metabolize drugs by alternative routes that may not be as efficient as the traditional routes; thus, these patients often have elevated drug levels in their bloodstreams and in their brains compared to individuals with normal enzyme activity. Other individuals may inherit a CYP enzyme that is extensively active compared to normal enzyme activity, and thus have lower drug levels compared to patients with normal enzyme activity. The genes for these CYP enzymes can now be measured and can be used to predict which patients might need to have up or down dosage adjustments of certain drugs for best results.

CYP 1A2

One important CYP enzyme is 1A2. Several antipsychotics and antidepressants are substrates for 1A2, as are caffeine and theophylline (Figure 2-17). An inhibitor

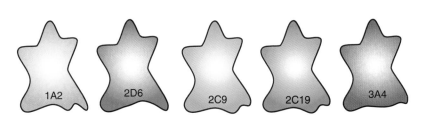

Figure 2-16. Five CYP enzymes. There are many cytochrome P450 (CYP) systems; these are classified according to family, subtype, and gene product. Five of the most important are shown here: CYP 1A2, 2D6, 2C9, 2C19, and 3A4.

1 = family
A = subtype
1 = gene product

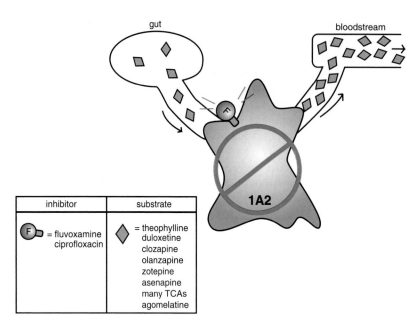

Figure 2-17. Consequences of CYP 1A2 inhibition. Numerous drugs (theophylline, duloxetine, clozapine, olanzapine, zotepine, asenapine, certain tricyclic antidepressants (TCAs), and agomelatine) are substrates for CYP 1A2. Thus, in the presence of a CYP 1A2 inhibitor (fluvoxamine, ciprofloxacin) their levels will rise. In many cases, this means that the dose of the substrate must often be lowered in order to avoid side effects.

inhibitor	substrate
= fluvoxamine ciprofloxacin	= theophylline duloxetine clozapine olanzapine zotepine asenapine many TCAs agomelatine

of 1A2 is the antidepressant fluvoxamine (Figure 2-17). This means that when substrates of 1A2, such as olanzapine, clozapine, zotepine, asenapine, duloxetine, or theophylline, are given concomitantly with an inhibitor of 1A2, such as fluvoxamine, the blood and brain levels of 1A2 substrates could rise (Figure 2-17). Although this may not be particularly clinically important for olanzapine or asenapine (possibly causing slightly increased sedation), it could potentially raise plasma levels sufficiently in the case of clozapine, zotepine, duloxetine, or theophylline to increase side effects, including possibly increasing the risk of seizures. Thus, the dose of clozapine or zotepine (or olanzapine and asenapine, as well as duloxetine) may need to be lowered when administered with fluvoxamine, or an antidepressant other than fluvoxamine may need to be chosen.

1A2 can also be induced, or increased in activity, by smoking. When patients smoke, any substrate of 1A2 may have its blood and brain levels fall and require more dosage. Also, patients stabilized on an antipsychotic dose who start smoking may relapse if the drug levels fall too low. Cigarette smokers may require higher doses of 1A2 substrates than nonsmokers (Figure 2-18).

CYP 2D6

Another CYP enzyme of importance to many psychotropic drugs is 2D6. Many antipsychotics and some antidepressants are substrates for 2D6, and several

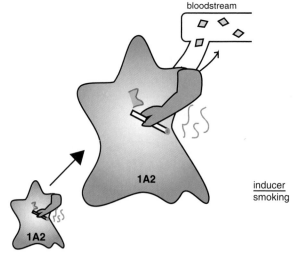

Figure 2-18. CYP 1A2 and smoking. Cigarette smoking, quite common among patients with schizophrenia, can induce the enzyme CYP 1A2 and lower the concentration of drugs metabolized by this enzyme, such as olanzapine, clozapine, zotepine, and others. Smokers may also require higher doses of these drugs than nonsmokers.

antidepressants are also inhibitors of this enzyme (Figure 2-19). This enzyme converts two drugs, risperidone and venlafaxine, into active drugs (i.e., paliperidone and desvenlafaxine, respectively) rather than inactive metabolites. Giving a substrate of 2D6 to a patient who is either a genetically poor metabolizer of this enzyme or who is taking an inhibitor of

No Hydroxylation

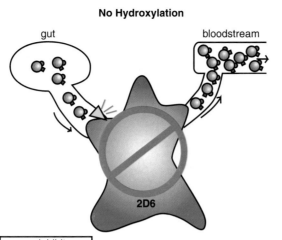

some substrates	some inhibitors
= TCA	= paroxetine
thioridazine	fluoxetine
codeine	duloxetine
some beta blockers	bupropion
atomoxetine	quinidine
venlafaxine	ritonavir
duloxetine	asenapine
paroxetine	
risperidone	
clozapine	
olanzapine	
aripiprazole	
iloperidone	

Figure 2-19. Consequences of CYP 2D6 inhibition. If a tricyclic antidepressant (a substrate for CYP 2D6) is given concomitantly with an agent that is an inhibitor of CYP 2D6 (e.g., paroxetine, fluoxetine), this will cause the levels of the tricyclic antidepressant to increase, which can be toxic. Therefore either monitoring of tricyclic plasma concentration with dose reduction or avoidance of this combination is required. Many other psychotropic medications are also substrates for CYP 2D6 and may therefore have increased blood levels when given with a CYP 2D6 inhibitor.

2D6 can raise the blood and brain levels of the substrate. This can be especially important for patients taking the 2D6 substrates tricyclic antidepressants, atomoxetine, thioridazine, iloperidone, and codeine, for example, so dose adjustments or using an alternative drug may be necessary for maximum safety and efficacy. Asenapine is an inhibitor of 2D6 and can raise the levels of drugs that are substrates of 2D6.

CYP 3A4

This enzyme metabolizes several psychotropic drugs as well as several of the HMG-CoA reductase inhibitors (statins) for treating high cholesterol (Figure 2-20). Several psychotropic drugs are weak inhibitors of this enzyme, including the antidepressants fluvoxamine, nefazodone, and the active metabolite of fluoxetine, norfluoxetine (Figure 2-20). Several nonpsychotropic drugs are powerful inhibitors of 3A4, including ketoconazole (antifungal), protease inhibitors (for AIDS/HIV), and erythromycin (antibiotic) (Figure 2-20). For the substrates of 3A4, co-administration of a 3A4 inhibitor may require dosage reduction of the substrate. Specifically, combining a 3A4 inhibitor with the 3A4 substrate pimozide can result in elevated plasma pimozide levels, with consequent QTc prolongation and dangerous cardiac arrhythmias. Combining a 3A4 inhibitor with alprazolam or triazolam can cause significant sedation due to elevated plasma drug levels of these latter agents. Combining a 3A4 inhibitor with certain cholesterol-lowering drugs that are 3A4 substrates (e.g., simvastatin, atorvastatin, lovastatin, or cerevastatin, but not pravastatin or fluvastatin) can increase the risk of muscle damage and rhabdomyolysis from elevated plasma levels of these statins.

There are also some drugs that can induce 3A4, including carbamazepine, rifampin, and some reverse transcriptase inhibitors for HIV/AIDS (Figure 2-21). Since carbamazepine is a mood stabilizer frequently mixed with atypical antipsychotics, it is possible that carbamazepine added to the regimen of a patient previously stabilized on clozapine, quetiapine, ziprasidone, sertindole, aripiprazole, iloperidone, lurasidone, or zotepine could reduce the blood and brain

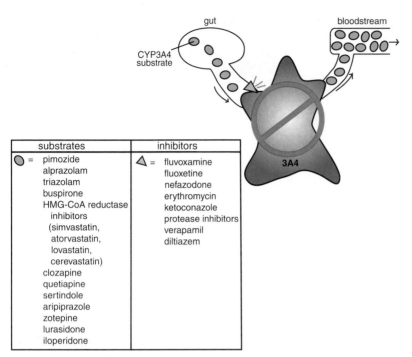

Figure 2-20. Substrates and inhibitors for CYP 3A4. The antipsychotic pimozide, the benzodiazepines alprazolam and triazolam, the anxiolytic buspirone, HMG-CoA reductase inhibitors (statins), and multiple antipsychotics are all substrates for CYP 3A4. Fluvoxamine, fluoxetine, and nefazodone are moderate CYP 3A4 inhibitors, as are some nonpsychotropic agents.

substrates	inhibitors
◉ = pimozide	△ = fluvoxamine
alprazolam	fluoxetine
triazolam	nefazodone
buspirone	erythromycin
HMG-CoA reductase	ketoconazole
inhibitors	protease inhibitors
(simvastatin,	verapamil
atorvastatin,	diltiazem
lovastatin,	
cerevastatin)	
clozapine	
quetiapine	
sertindole	
aripiprazole	
zotepine	
lurasidone	
iloperidone	

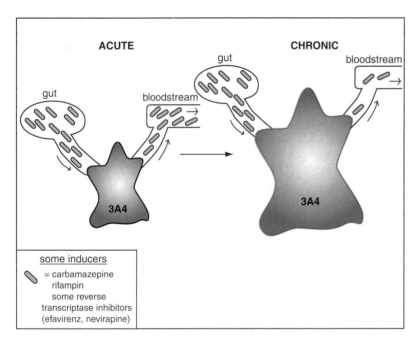

Figure 2-21. CYP 3A4 induced by carbamazepine. The enzyme CYP 3A4 can be induced by the anticonvulsant and mood stabilizer carbamazepine, as well as by rifampin and some reverse transcriptase inhibitors. This would lead to increased metabolism of substrates for 3A4 (e.g., clozapine, quetiapine, ziprasidone, sertindole, aripiprazole, and zotepine) and may therefore require higher doses of these agents when given concomitantly with carbamazepine.

levels of these agents, requiring their doses to be increased. On the other hand, if carbamazepine is stopped in a patient receiving one of these atypical antipsychotics, their doses may need to be reduced, because the autoinduction of 3A4 by carbamazepine will reverse over time.

Drug interactions mediated by CYP enzymes are constantly being discovered, and the active clinician who combines drugs must be alert to these, and thus be continually updated on what drug interactions are important. Here we present only the general concepts of drug interactions at CYP enzyme systems, but the specifics should be found in a comprehensive and up-to-date reference source (such as *Stahl's Essential Psychopharmacology: the Prescriber's Guide*, a companion to this textbook) before prescribing.

Summary

About a third of psychotropic drugs in clinical practice bind to a neurotransmitter transporter, and another third of psychotropic drugs bind to G-protein-linked receptors. These two molecular sites of action, their impact upon neurotransmission, and various specific drugs that act at these sites have all been reviewed in this chapter.

Specifically, there are two subclasses of plasma membrane transporters for neurotransmitters and three subclasses of intracellular synaptic vesicular transporters for neurotransmitters. The monoamine transporters (SERT for serotonin, NET for norepinephrine, and DAT for dopamine) are key targets for most of the known antidepressants. In addition, stimulants target DAT. The vesicular transporter for all three of these monoamines is known as VMAT2 (vesicular monoamine transporter 2) and is also a target of the stimulant amphetamine.

G-protein receptors are the most common targets of psychotropic drugs, and their actions can lead to both therapeutic and side effects. Drug actions at these receptors occur in a spectrum, from full agonist actions, to partial agonist actions, to antagonism, and even to inverse agonism. Natural neurotransmitters are full agonists, as are some drugs used in clinical practice. However, most drugs that act directly on G-protein-linked receptors act as antagonists. A few act as partial agonists, and some as inverse agonists. Each drug interacting at a G-protein-linked receptor causes a conformational change in that receptor that defines where on the agonist spectrum it will act. Thus, a full agonist produces a conformational change that turns on signal transduction and second-messenger formation to the maximum extent. One novel concept is that of a partial agonist, which acts somewhat like an agonist, but to a lesser extent. An antagonist causes a conformational change that stabilizes the receptor in the baseline state and thus is "silent." In the presence of agonists or partial agonists, an antagonist causes the receptor to return to this baseline state as well, and thus reverses their actions. A novel receptor action is that of an inverse agonist that leads to a conformation of the receptor that stops all activity, even baseline actions. Understanding the agonist spectrum can lead to prediction of downstream consequences on signal transduction, including clinical actions.

Chapter 3

Ion channels as targets of psychopharmacological drug action

Many important psychopharmacological drugs target ion channels. The roles of ion channels as important regulators of synaptic neurotransmission were covered in Chapter 1. Here we discuss how targeting these molecular sites causes alterations in synaptic neurotransmission that are linked in turn to the therapeutic actions of various psychotropic drugs. Specifically, we cover ligand-gated ion channels and voltage-sensitive ion channels as targets of psychopharmacological drug action.

Ligand-gated ion channels as targets of psychopharmacological drug action
Ligand-gated ion channels, ionotropic receptors, and ion-channel-linked receptors: different terms for the same receptor/ion-channel complex

Ions normally cannot penetrate membranes because of their charge. In order to selectively control access of ions into and out of neurons, their membranes are decorated with all sorts of ion channels. The most important ion channels in psychopharmacology regulate calcium, sodium, chloride, and potassium. Many

can be modified by various drugs, and this will be discussed throughout this chapter.

There are two major classes of ion channels, and each class has several names. One class of ion channels is opened by neurotransmitters and goes by the names *ligand-gated ion channels*, *ionotropic receptors*, and *ion-channel-linked receptors*. These channels and their associated receptors will be discussed next. The other major class of ion channel is opened by the charge or voltage across the membrane and is called either a *voltage-sensitive* or a *voltage-gated* ion channel; these will be discussed later in this chapter.

Ion channels that are opened and closed by actions of neurotransmitter ligands at receptors acting as gatekeepers are shown conceptually in Figure 3-1. When a neurotransmitter binds to a gatekeeper receptor on an ion channel, that neurotransmitter causes a conformational change in the receptor that opens the ion channel (Figure 3-1A). A neurotransmitter, drug, or hormone that binds to a receptor is sometimes called a *ligand* (literally, "tying"). Thus, ion channels linked to receptors that regulate their opening and closing are often called *ligand-gated ion channels*. Since these ion channels are also receptors, they are sometimes also called *ionotropic receptors* or *ion-channel-linked receptors*.

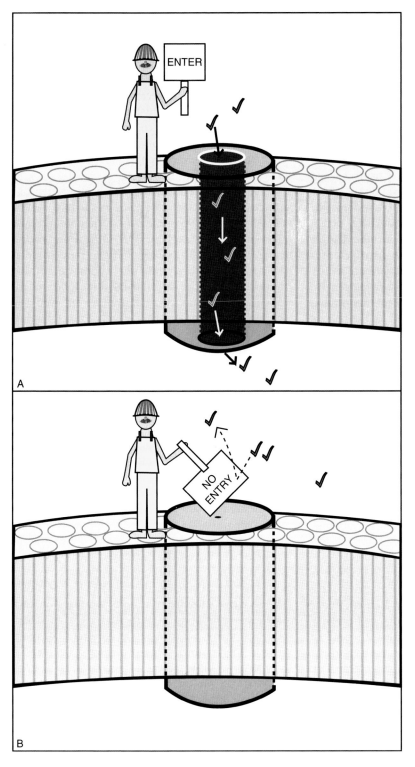

Figure 3-1. Ligand-gated ion channel gatekeeper. This schematic shows a ligand-gated ion channel. In panel A, a receptor is serving as a molecular gatekeeper that acts on instruction from neurotransmission to open the channel and allow ions to travel into the cell. In panel B, the gatekeeper is keeping the channel closed so that ions cannot get into the cell. Ligand-gated ion channels are a type of receptor that forms an ion channel and are thus also called ion-channel-linked receptors or ionotropic receptors.

These terms will be used interchangeably with ligand-gated ion channels here.

Numerous drugs act at many sites around such receptor/ion-channel complexes, leading to a wide variety of modifications of receptor/ion-channel actions. These modifications not only immediately alter the flow of ions through the channels, but with a delay can also change the downstream events that result from transduction of the signal that begins at these receptors. The downstream actions have been extensively discussed in Chapter 1 and include both activation and inactivation of phosphoproteins, shifting the activity of enzymes, the sensitivity of receptors, and the conductivity of ion channels. Other downstream actions include changes in gene expression and thus changes in which proteins are synthesized and which functions are amplified. Such functions can range from synaptogenesis, to receptor and enzyme synthesis, to communication with downstream neurons innervated by the neuron with the ionotropic receptor, and many more. The reader should have a good command of the function of signal transduction pathways described in Chapter 1 in order to understand how drugs acting at ligand-gated ion channels modify the signal transduction that arises from these receptors.

Drug-induced modifications in signal transduction from ionotropic (sometimes called ionotrophic) receptors can have profound actions on psychiatric symptoms. About a fifth of psychotropic drugs currently utilized in clinical practice, including many drugs for the treatment of anxiety and insomnia such as the benzodiazepines, are known to act at these receptors. Because ionotropic receptors immediately change the flow of ions, drugs that act on these receptors can have an almost immediate effect, which is why many anxiolytics and hypnotics that act at these receptors may have immediate clinical onset. This is in contrast to the actions of many drugs at G-protein-linked receptors described in Chapter 2, some of which have clinical effects – such as antidepressant actions – that may occur with a delay necessitated by awaiting initiation of changes in cellular functions activated through the signal transduction cascade. Here we will describe how various drugs stimulate or block various molecular sites around the receptor/ion-channel complex. Throughout the textbook we will show how specific drugs acting at specific ionotropic receptors have specific actions on specific psychiatric disorders.

Ligand-gated ion channels: structure and function

Are ligand-gated ion channels receptors or ion channels? The answer is "yes" – ligand-gated ion channels are a type of receptor and they also form an ion channel. That is why they are called not only a channel (ligand-gated ion channel) but also a receptor (ionotropic receptor or ion-channel-linked receptor). These terms try to capture the dual function of these ion channels/receptors.

Ligand-gated ion channels comprise several long strings of amino acids assembled as subunits around an ion channel. Decorating these subunits are also multiple binding sites for everything from neurotransmitters to ions to drugs. That is, these complex proteins have several sites where some ions travel through a channel and others also bind to the channel; where one neurotransmitter or even two cotransmitters act at separate and distinct binding sites; where numerous allosteric modulators – i.e., natural substances or drugs that bind to a site different than where the neurotransmitter binds – increase or decrease the sensitivity of channel opening.

Pentameric subtypes

Many ligand-gated ion channels are assembled from five protein subunits; that is why they are called pentameric. The subunits for pentameric subtypes of ligand-gated ion channels each have four transmembrane regions (Figure 3-2A). These membrane proteins go in and out of the membrane four times (Figure 3-2A). When five copies of these subunits are selected (Figure 3-2B), they come together in space to form a fully functional pentameric receptor with the ion channel in the middle (Figure 3-2C). The receptor sites are in various locations on each of the subunits; some binding sites are in the channel, but many are present at different locations outside the channel. This pentameric structure is typical for $GABA_A$ receptors, nicotinic cholinergic receptors, serotonin $5HT_3$ receptors, and glycine receptors (Table 3-1). Drugs that act directly on pentameric ligand-gated ion channels are listed in Table 3-2.

If this structure were not complicated enough, pentameric ionotropic receptors actually have many different subtypes. Subtypes of pentameric ionotropic receptors are defined based upon which forms of each

Table 3-1 Pentameric ligand-gated ion channels

4 transmembrane regions 5 subunits	
Neurotransmitter	**Receptor subtype**
Acetylcholine	Nicotinic receptors (e.g., α_7-nicotinic receptors; $\alpha_4\beta_2$-nicotinic receptors)
GABA	$GABA_A$ receptors (e.g., α_1 subunits)
Glycine	Strychnine-sensitive glycine receptors
Serotonin	$5HT_3$ receptors

of the five subunits are chosen for assembly into a fully constituted receptor. That is, there are several subtypes for each of the four transmembrane subunits, making it possible to piece together several different constellations of fully constituted receptors. Although the natural neurotransmitter binds to every subtype of ionotropic receptor, some drugs used in clinical practice, and many more in clinical trials, are able to bind selectively to one or more of these subtypes, but not to others. This may have functional and clinical consequences. Specific receptor subtypes and the specific drugs that bind to them selectively are discussed in chapters that cover their specific clinical use.

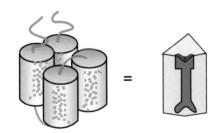

A

Figure 3-2. Ligand-gated ion channel structure. The four transmembrane regions of a single subunit of a pentameric ligand-gated ion channel form a cluster, as shown in panel A. An icon for this subunit is shown on the right in panel A. Five copies of the subunits come together in space (panel B) to form a functional ion channel in the middle (panel C). Pentameric ligand-gated ion channels have receptor binding sites located on all five subunits, both inside and outside the channel.

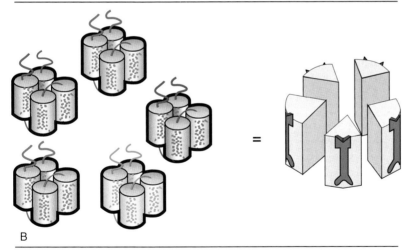

B

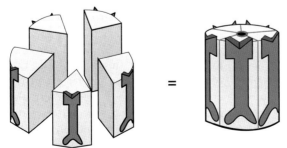

C

Table 3-2 Key ligand-gated ion channels directly targeted by psychotropic drugs

Neurotransmitter	Ligand-gated ion-channel receptor subtype directly targeted	Pharmacologic action	Drug class	Therapeutic action
Acetylcholine	$\alpha_4\beta_2$-nicotinic receptors	Partial agonist	Nicotinic receptor partial agonist (NRPA) (varenicline)	Smoking cessation
GABA	GABA$_A$ benzodiazepine receptors	Full agonist	Benzodiazepines	Anxiolytic
	GABA$_A$ non-benzodiazepine PAM sites	Full agonist	"Z drugs"/hypnotics (zolpidem, zaleplon, zopiclone, eszopiclone)	Improve insomnia
Glutamate	NMDA NAM channel sites/ Mg^{++} sites	Antagonist	NMDA glutamate antagonist (memantine)	Slowing progression in Alzheimer's disease
	NMDA open channel sites	Antagonist	PCP (phencyclidine) Ketamine	Hallucinogen anesthetic
Serotonin	5HT$_3$	Antagonist	Antidepressant (mirtazapine)	Unknown; reduce nausea
	5HT$_3$	Antagonist	Antiemetic	Reduce chemotherapy-induced emesis

PAM, positive allosteric modulator; NAM, negative allosteric modulator; NMDA, *N*-methyl-D-aspartate; Mg, magnesium.

Tetrameric subtypes

Ionotropic glutamate receptors have a different structure from the pentameric ionotropic receptors just discussed. The ligand-gated ion channels for glutamate comprise subunits that have three full transmembrane regions and a fourth re-entrant loop (Figure 3-3A), rather than four full transmembrane regions as shown in Figure 3-2A. When four copies of these subunits are selected (Figure 3-3B), they come together in space to form a fully functional ion channel in the middle with the four re-entrant loops lining the ion channel (Figure 3-3C). Thus, tetrameric subtypes of ion channels (Figure 3-3) are analogous to pentameric subtypes of ion channels (Figure 3-2), but have just four subunits rather than five. Receptor sites are in various locations on each of the subunits; some binding sites are in the channel, but many are present at different locations outside the channel.

This tetrameric structure is typical of the ionotropic glutamate receptors known as AMPA (α-amino-3-hydroxy-5-methyl-4-isoxazole-propionic acid) and NMDA (*N*-methyl-D-aspartate) subtypes (Table 3-3). Drugs that act directly at tetrameric ionotropic

glutamate receptors are listed in Table 3-2. Receptor subtypes for glutamate according to the selective agonist acting at that receptor, as well as the specific molecular subunits that comprise that subtype, are listed in Table 3-3. Subtype-selective drugs for ionotropic glutamate receptors are under investigation but not currently used in clinical practice.

The agonist spectrum

The concept of an agonist spectrum for G-protein-linked receptors, discussed extensively in Chapter 2, can also be applied to ligand-gated ion channels (Figure 3-4). Thus, **full agonists** change the conformation of the receptor to open the ion channel the maximal amount and frequency allowed by that binding site (Figure 3-5). This then triggers the maximal amount of downstream signal transduction possible to be mediated by this binding site. The ion channel can open to an even greater extent (i.e., more frequently) than with a full agonist alone, but this requires the help of a second receptor site, that of a positive allosteric modulator, or PAM, as will be shown later.

Table 3-3 Tetrameric ligand-gated ion channels

3 transmembrane regions and one re-entrant loop 4 subunits	
Neurotransmitter	**Receptor subtype**
Glutamate	AMPA (e.g., GluR1–4 subunits)
	KAINATE (e.g., GluR5–7, KA1–2 subunits)
	NMDA (e.g., NMDAR1, NMDAR2A–D, NMDAR3A subunits)

AMPA, α-amino-3-hydroxy-5-methyl-4-isoxazole-propionic acid; NMDA, N-methyl-D-aspartate.

Antagonists stabilize the receptor in the resting state, which is the same as the state of the receptor in the absence of agonist (Figure 3-6). Since there is no difference between the presence and absence of the antagonist, the antagonist is said to be neutral or silent. The resting state is not a fully closed ion channel, so there is some degree of ion flow through the channel even in the absence of agonist (Figure 3-6A) and even in the presence of antagonist (Figure 3-6B). This is due to occasional and infrequent opening of the channel even when an agonist is not present and even when an antagonist is present. This is called constitutive activity and is also discussed in Chapter 2 for G-protein-linked receptors. Antagonists

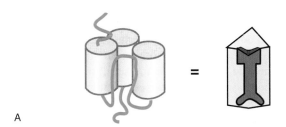

A

Figure 3-3. Tetrameric ligand-gated ion channel structure. A single subunit of a tetrameric ligand-gated ion channel is shown to form a cluster in panel A, with an icon for this subunit shown on the right in panel A. Four copies of these subunits come together in space (panel B) to form a functional ion channel in the middle (panel C). Tetrameric ligand-gated ion channels have receptor binding sites located on all four subunits, both inside and outside the channel.

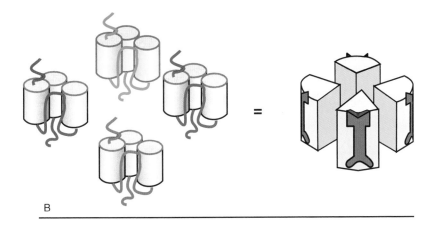

B

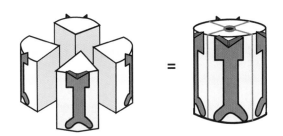

C

The Agonist Spectrum

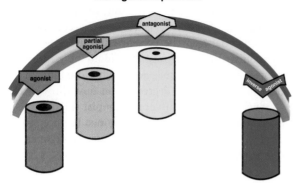

Figure 3-4. Agonist spectrum. The agonist spectrum and its corresponding effects on the ion channel are shown here. This spectrum ranges from agonists (on the far left), which open the channel the maximal amount and frequency allowed by that binding site, through antagonists (middle of the spectrum), which retain the resting state with infrequent opening of the channel, to inverse agonists (on the far right), which put the ion channel into a closed and inactive state. Between agonists and antagonists are partial agonists, which increase the degree and frequency of ion-channel opening as compared to the resting state, but not as much as a full agonist. Antagonists can block anything in the agonist spectrum, returning the ion channel to the resting state in each instance.

of ion-channel-linked receptors reverse the action of agonists (Figure 3-7) and bring the receptor conformation back to the resting baseline state, but do not block any constitutive activity.

Partial agonists produce a change in receptor conformation such that the ion channel opens to a greater extent and more frequently than in its resting state but less than in the presence of a full agonist (Figures 3-8 and 3-9). An antagonist reverses a partial agonist, just as it reverses a full agonist, returning the receptor to its resting state (Figure 3-10). Partial agonists thus produce ion flow and downstream signal transduction that is something more than the resting state in the absence of agonist, yet something less than a full agonist. Just as is the case for G-protein-linked receptors, how close this partial agonist is to a full agonist or to a silent antagonist on the agonist spectrum will determine the impact of a partial agonist on downstream signal transduction events.

The ideal therapeutic agent in some cases may need to have ion flow and signal transduction that is not too hot, yet not too cold, but just right, called the "Goldilocks" solution in Chapter 2, a concept that can apply here to ligand-gated ion channels as well. Such

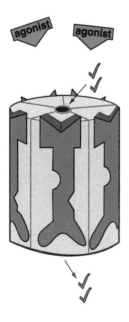

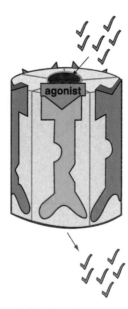

Figure 3-5. Actions of an agonist. In panel A, the ion channel is in its resting state, during which the channel opens infrequently (constitutive activity). In panel B, the agonist occupies its binding site on the ligand-gated ion channel, increasing the frequency at which the channel opens. This is represented as the red agonist turning the receptor red and opening the ion channel.

channel in its resting state in the absence of agonist

A

agonist binds to the receptor and the channel is more frequently open

B

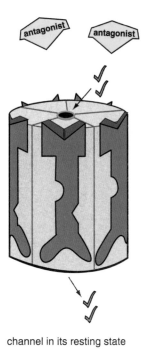

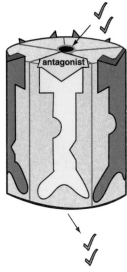

channel in its resting state

antagonist binds to the receptor, not affecting
the frequency of opening of the channel
compared to the resting
state of no agonist

A

B

Figure 3-6. Antagonists acting alone. In panel A, the ion channel is in its resting state, during which the channel opens infrequently. In panel B, the antagonist occupies the binding site normally occupied by the agonist on the ligand-gated ion channel. However, there is no consequence to this, and the ion channel does not affect the degree or frequency of opening of the channel compared to the resting state. This is represented as the yellow antagonist docking into the binding site and turning the receptor yellow but not affecting the state of the ion channel.

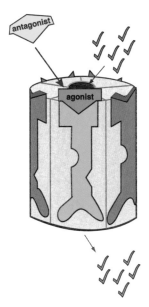

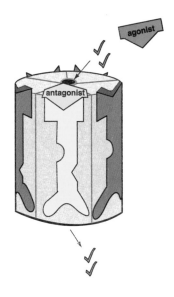

the agonist causes the channel to become
open more frequently

the antagonist takes over and puts
the channel back into the resting state

A

B

Figure 3-7. Antagonist acting in presence of agonist. In panel A, the ion channel is bound by an agonist, which causes it to open at a greater frequency than in the resting state. This is represented as the red agonist turning the receptor red and opening the ion channel as it docks into its binding site. In panel B, the yellow antagonist prevails and shoves the red agonist off the binding site, reversing the agonist's actions and restoring the resting state. Thus, the ion channel has returned to its status before the agonist acted.

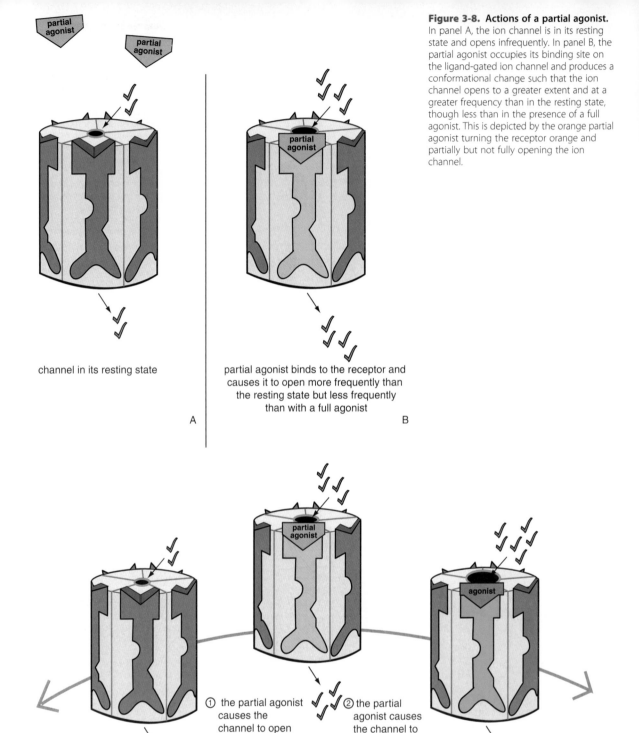

Figure 3-8. Actions of a partial agonist. In panel A, the ion channel is in its resting state and opens infrequently. In panel B, the partial agonist occupies its binding site on the ligand-gated ion channel and produces a conformational change such that the ion channel opens to a greater extent and at a greater frequency than in the resting state, though less than in the presence of a full agonist. This is depicted by the orange partial agonist turning the receptor orange and partially but not fully opening the ion channel.

channel in its resting state

partial agonist binds to the receptor and causes it to open more frequently than the resting state but less frequently than with a full agonist

A

B

① the partial agonist causes the channel to open more frequently; in this case the partial agonist is having a net agonist action

② the partial agonist causes the channel to open less frequently; in this case the partial agonist is having a net antagonist action

channel in its resting state

the full agonist opens the channel maximally and frequently

Figure 3-9. Net effect of partial agonist. Partial agonists act either as net agonists or as net antagonists, depending on the amount of agonist present. When full agonist is absent (on the far left), a partial agonist causes the channel to open more frequently as compared to the resting state and thus has a net agonist action (moving from left to right). However, in the presence of a full agonist (on the far right), a partial agonist decreases the frequency of channel opening in comparison to the full agonist and thus acts as a net antagonist (moving from right to left).

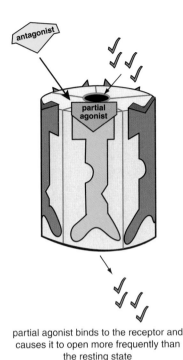

partial agonist binds to the receptor and
causes it to open more frequently than
the resting state

A

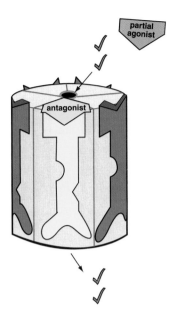

the antagonist causes the channel
to return to baseline

B

Figure 3-10. Antagonist acting in presence of partial agonist. In panel A, a partial agonist occupies its binding site and causes the ion channel to open more frequently than in the resting state. This is represented as the orange partial agonist docking to its binding site, turning the receptor orange, and partially opening the ion channel. In panel B, the yellow antagonist prevails and shoves the orange partial agonist off the binding site, reversing the partial agonist's actions. Thus the ion channel is returned to its resting state.

an ideal state may vary from one clinical situation to another, depending upon the balance between full agonism and silent antagonism that is desired. In cases where there is unstable neurotransmission throughout the brain, finding such a balance may stabilize receptor output somewhere between too much and too little downstream action. For this reason, partial agonists are also called "*stabilizers*," since they have the theoretical capacity to find the stable solution between the extremes of too much full agonist action and no agonist action at all (Figure 3-9).

Just as is the case for G-protein-linked receptors, partial agonists at ligand-gated ion channels can appear as net agonists, or as net antagonists, depending upon the amount of naturally occurring full agonist neurotransmitter that is present. Thus, when a full agonist neurotransmitter is absent, a partial agonist will be a net agonist (Figure 3-9). That is, from the resting state, a partial agonist initiates somewhat of an increase in the ion flow and downstream signal transduction cascade from the ion-channel-linked receptor. However, when full agonist neurotransmitter is present, the same partial agonist will become a net antagonist (Figure 3-9): it will decrease the

level of full signal output to a lesser level, but not to zero. Thus, a partial agonist can simultaneously *boost* deficient neurotransmitter activity yet *block* excessive neurotransmitter activity, another reason that partial agonists are called stabilizers. An agonist and an antagonist in the same molecule acting at ligand-gated ion channels is quite an interesting new dimension to therapeutics. This concept has led to proposals that partial agonists could treat not only states that are theoretically deficient in full agonist, but also states that are theoretically in excess of full agonist. As mentioned in the discussion of G-protein-linked receptors in Chapter 2, a partial agonist at ligand-gated ion channels could also theoretically treat states that are mixtures of both excessive and deficient neurotransmitter activity. Partial agonists at ligand-gated ion channels are just beginning to enter use in clinical practice (Table 3-2), and several more are in clinical development.

Inverse agonists at ligand-gated ion channels are different from simple antagonists, and are neither neutral nor silent. Inverse agonists are explained in Chapter 2 in relation to G-protein-linked receptors. Inverse agonists at ligand-gated ion channels are thought to produce

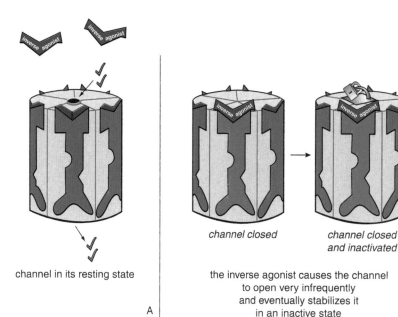

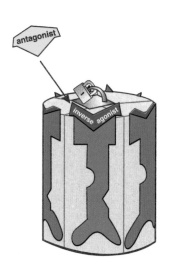

Figure 3-11. Actions of an inverse agonist. In panel A, the ion channel is in its resting state and opens infrequently. In panel B, the inverse agonist occupies the binding site on the ligand-gated ion channel and causes it to close. This is the opposite of what an agonist does and is represented by the purple inverse agonist turning the receptor purple and closing the ion channel. Eventually, the inverse agonist stabilizes the ion channel in an inactive state, represented by the padlock on the channel itself.

channel closed

channel closed and inactivated

channel in its resting state

the inverse agonist causes the channel to open very infrequently and eventually stabilizes it in an inactive state

A

B

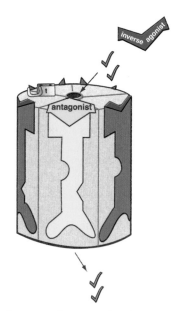

Figure 3-12. Antagonist acting in presence of inverse agonist. In panel A, the ion channel has been stabilized in an inactive form by the inverse agonist occupying its binding site on the ligand-gated ion channel. This is represented as the purple inverse agonist turning the receptor purple and closing and padlocking the ion channel. In panel B, the yellow antagonist prevails and shoves the purple inverse agonist off the binding site, returning the ion channel to its resting state. In this way, the antagonist's effects on an inverse agonist's actions are similar to its effects on an agonist's actions; namely, it returns the ion channel to its resting state. However, in the presence of an inverse agonist, the antagonist increases the frequency of channel opening, whereas in the presence of an agonist, the antagonist decreases the frequency of channel opening. Thus an antagonist can reverse the actions of either an agonist or an inverse agonist despite the fact that it does nothing on its own.

the inverse agonist causes the channel to stabilize in an inactive form

the antagonist returns the channel to the resting state

A

B

a conformational change in these receptors that first closes the channel and then stabilizes it in an inactive form (Figure 3-11). Thus, this inactive conformation (Figure 3-11B) produces a functional reduction in ion flow and in consequent signal transduction compared to the resting state (Figure 3-11A) that is even less than that produced when there is either no agonist present or when a silent antagonist is present. Antagonists reverse

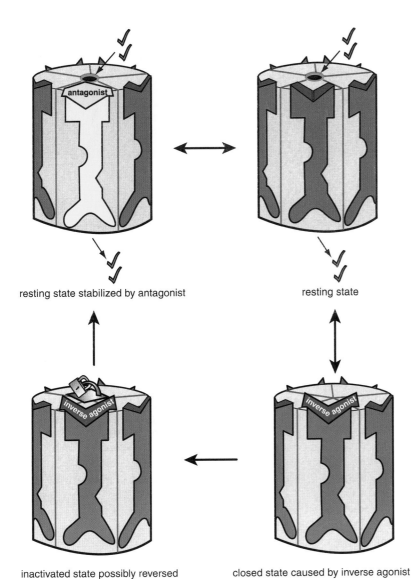

resting state stabilized by antagonist

resting state

inactivated state possibly reversed immediately by an antagonist

closed state caused by inverse agonist

Figure 3-13. Inverse agonist actions reversed by antagonist. Antagonists cause conformational change in ligand-gated ion channels that stabilizes the receptors in the resting state (top left), the same state they are in when no agonist or inverse agonist is present (top right). Inverse agonists cause conformational change that closes the ion channel (bottom right). When an inverse agonist is bound over time, it may eventually stabilize the ion channel in an inactive conformation (bottom left). This stabilized conformation of an inactive ion channel can be quickly reversed by an antagonist, which restabilizes it in the resting state (top left).

this inactive state caused by inverse agonists, returning the channel to the resting state (Figure 3-12).

In many ways, therefore, an inverse agonist does the *opposite* of an agonist. If an agonist increases signal transduction from baseline, an inverse agonist decreases it, even below baseline levels. Also, in contrast to antagonists, which stabilize the resting state, inverse agonists stabilize an inactivated state (Figures 3-11 and 3-13). It is not yet clear if the inactivated state of the inverse agonist can be distinguished clinically from the resting state of the silent antagonist at ionotropic receptors. In the

meantime, inverse agonists remain an interesting pharmacological concept.

In summary, ion-channel-linked receptors act along an agonist spectrum, and drugs have been described that can produce conformational changes in these receptors to create any state from full agonist, to partial agonist, to silent antagonist, to inverse agonist (Figure 3-4). When one considers signal transduction along this spectrum, it is easy to understand why agents at each point along the agonist spectrum differ so much from each other, and why their clinical actions are so different.

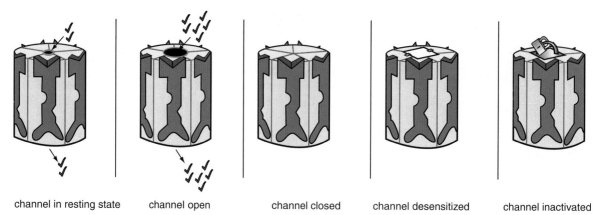

channel in resting state   channel open   channel closed   channel desensitized   channel inactivated

Figure 3-14. Five states of ligand-gated ion channels. Summarized here are five well-known states of ligand-gated ion channels. In the resting state, ligand-gated ion channels open infrequently, with consequent constitutive activity that may or may not lead to detectable signal transduction. In the open state, ligand-gated ion channels open to allow ion conductance through the channel, leading to signal transduction. In the closed state, ligand-gated ion channels are closed, allowing no ion flow to occur and thus reducing signal transduction to even less than is produced in the resting state. Channel desensitization is an adaptive state in which the receptor stops responding to agonist even if it is still bound. Channel inactivation is a state in which a closed ion channel over time becomes stabilized in an inactive conformation.

Different states of ligand-gated ion channels

There are even more states of ligand-gated ion channels than those determined by the agonist spectrum discussed above and shown in Figures 3-4 through 3-13. The states discussed so far are those that occur predominantly with acute administration of agents that work across the agonist spectrum. These range from the maximal opening of the ion channel caused by a full agonist to the maximal closing of the ion channel caused by an inverse agonist. Such changes in conformation caused by the acute action of agents across this spectrum are subject to change over time, because these receptors have the capacity to adapt, particularly when there is chronic or excessive exposure to such agents.

We have already discussed the resting state, the open state, and the closed state shown in Figure 3-14. The best-known adaptive states are those of desensitization and inactivation, also shown in Figure 3-14. We have also briefly discussed inactivation as a state that can be caused by acute administration of an inverse agonist, beginning with a rapid conformational change in the ion channel that first closes it, but over time stabilizes the channel in an inactive conformation that can be relatively quickly reversed by an antagonist, which then restabilizes the ion channel in the resting state (Figures 3-11 through 3-13).

Desensitization is yet another state of the ligand-gated ion channel shown in Figure 3-14. Ion-channel-linked receptor desensitization can be caused by prolonged exposure to agonists, and may be a way for receptors to protect themselves from overstimulation. An agonist acting at a ligand-gated ion channel first induces a change in receptor conformation that opens the channel, but the continuous presence of the agonist over time leads to another conformational change where the receptor essentially stops responding to the agonist even though the agonist is still present. This receptor is then considered to be desensitized (Figures 3-14 and 3-15). This state of desensitization can at first be reversed relatively quickly by removal of the agonist (Figure 3-15). However, if the agonist stays much longer, on the order of hours, then the receptor converts from a state of simple desensitization to one of inactivation (Figure 3-15). This state does not reverse simply upon removal of the agonist, since it also takes hours in the absence of agonist to revert to the resting state where the receptor is again sensitive to new exposure to agonist (Figure 3-15).

The state of inactivation may be best characterized for nicotinic cholinergic receptors, ligand-gated ion channels that are normally responsive to the endogenous neurotransmitter acetylcholine. Acetylcholine is quickly hydrolyzed by an abundance of the enzyme acetylcholinesterase, so it rarely gets the chance to desensitize and inactivate its nicotinic receptors. However, the drug nicotine is not hydrolyzed by acetylcholinesterase, and is famous for stimulating nicotinic cholinergic receptors so profoundly and so

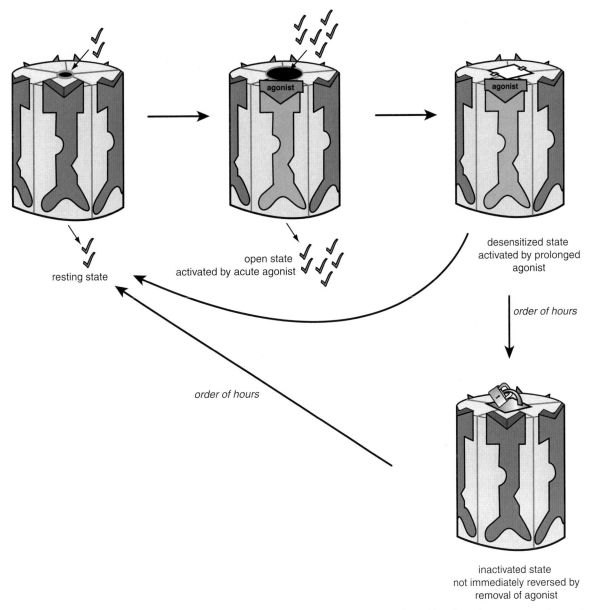

Figure 3-15. Opening, desensitizing, and inactivating by agonists. Agonists cause ligand-gated ion channels to open more frequently, increasing ion conductance in comparison to the resting state. Prolonged exposure to agonists can cause a ligand-gated ion channel to enter a desensitized state in which it no longer responds to the agonist even if it is still bound. Prompt removal of the agonist can reverse this state fairly quickly. However, if the agonist stays longer, it can cause a conformational change that leads to inactivation of the ion channel. This state is not immediately reversed when the agonist is removed.

enduringly that the receptors are not only rapidly desensitized, but enduringly inactivated, requiring hours in the absence of agonist to get back to the resting state. These transitions among various receptor states induced by agonists are shown in Figure 3-15. Desensitization of nicotinic receptors is discussed in further detail in Chapter 14.

Allosteric modulation: PAMs and NAMs

Ligand-gated ion channels are regulated by more than the neurotransmitter(s) that bind to them. That is, there are other molecules that are not neurotransmitters but that can bind to the receptor/ion-channel complex at different sites from where

Positive Allosteric Modulation (PAM)

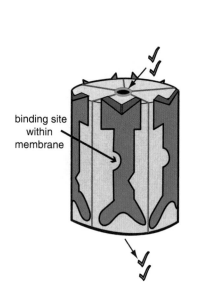
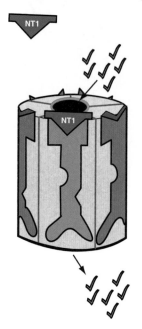
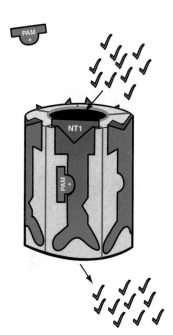

binding site within membrane

When a neurotransmitter binds to receptors making up an ion channel, the channel opens more frequently. However, when BOTH the neurotransmitter and a positive allosteric modulator (PAM) are bound to the receptor, the channel opens much more frequently, allowing more ions into the cell.

Figure 3-16. Positive allosteric modulators (PAMs). Allosteric modulators are ligands that bind to sites other than the neurotransmitter site on an ion-channel-linked receptor. Allosteric modulators have no activity of their own but rather enhance (positive allosteric modulators, or PAMs) or block (negative allosteric modulators, or NAMs) the actions of neurotransmitters. When a PAM binds to its site while an agonist is also bound, the channel opens more frequently than when only the agonist is bound, therefore allowing more ions into the cell.

neurotransmitter(s) bind. These sites are called *allosteric* (literally, "other site") and ligands that bind there are called allosteric modulators. These ligands are modulators rather than neurotransmitters because they have little or no activity on their own in the absence of the neurotransmitter. Allosteric modulators thus only work in the presence of the neurotransmitter.

There are two forms of allosteric modulators – those that boost what the neurotransmitter does and are thus called positive allosteric modulators (PAMs), and those that block what the neurotransmitter does and are thus called negative allosteric modulators (NAMs).

Specifically, when PAMs or NAMs bind to their allosteric sites while the neurotransmitter is *not* binding to its site, the PAM and the NAM do nothing. However, when a PAM binds to its allosteric site while the neurotransmitter is sitting at its site, the PAM causes conformational changes in the ligand-gated ion channel that

open the channel even further and more frequently than happens with a full agonist by itself (Figure 3-16). That is why the PAM is called "positive." Good examples of PAMs are benzodiazepines. These ligands boost the action of GABA at $GABA_A$ types of ligand-gated chloride ion channels. GABA binding to $GABA_A$ sites increases chloride ion flux by opening the ion channel, and benzodiazepines acting as agonists at benzodiazepine receptors elsewhere on the $GABA_A$ receptor complex cause the effect of GABA to be amplified in terms of chloride ion flux by opening the ion channel to a greater degree or more frequently. Clinically, this is exhibited as anxiolytic, hypnotic, anticonvulsant, amnestic, and muscle relaxant actions. In this example, benzodiazepines are acting as full agonists at the PAM site.

On the other hand, when a NAM binds to its allosteric site while the neurotransmitter resides at its agonist binding site, the NAM causes conformational

Negative Allosteric Modulation (NAM)

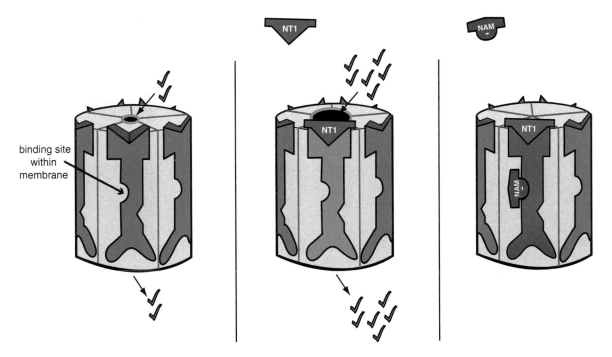

When a neurotransmitter binds to receptors making up an ion channel, the channel opens more frequently. However, when BOTH the neurotransmitter and a negative allosteric modulator (NAM) are bound to the receptor, the channel opens much less frequently, allowing fewer ions into the cell.

Figure 3-17. Negative allosteric modulators (NAMs). Allosteric modulators are ligands that bind to sites other than the neurotransmitter site on an ion-channel-linked receptor. Allosteric modulators have no activity of their own but rather enhance (positive allosteric modulators, or PAMs) or block (negative allosteric modulators, or NAMs) the actions of neurotransmitters. When a NAM binds to its site while an agonist is also bound, the channel opens less frequently than when only the agonist is bound, therefore allowing fewer ions into the cell.

changes in the ligand-gated ion channel that block or reduce the actions that normally occur when the neurotransmitter acts alone (Figure 3-17). That is why the NAM is called "negative." One example of a NAM is a benzodiazepine inverse agonist. Although these are only experimental, as expected, they have the opposite actions of benzodiazepine full agonists and thus diminish chloride conductance through the ion channel so much that they cause panic attacks, seizures, and some improvement in memory – the opposite clinical effects of a benzodiazepine full agonist. Thus, the same allosteric site can have either NAM or PAM actions, depending upon whether the ligand is a full agonist or an inverse agonist. NAMs for NMDA receptors include phencyclidine (PCP, also called "angel dust") and its structurally related anesthetic agent ketamine. These agents bind to a site in the calcium channel, but can get into the channel to block it only when the channel is open. When either PCP or ketamine bind to their NAM site, they prevent glutamate/glycine cotransmission from opening the channel.

Voltage-sensitive ion channels as targets of psychopharmacological drug action
Structure and function

Not all ion channels are regulated by neurotransmitter ligands. Indeed, critical aspects of nerve conduction, action potentials, and neurotransmitter release are all mediated by another class of ion channels known as *voltage-sensitive* or *voltage-gated*; they are so called because their opening and closing are

Ionic Components of an Action Potential

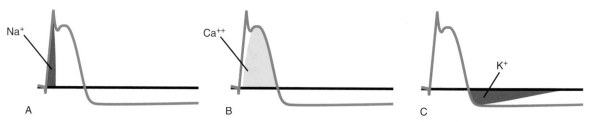

Figure 3-18. Ionic components of an action potential. The ionic components of an action potential are shown graphically here. First, voltage-sensitive sodium channels (VSSCs) open to allow an influx of "downhill" sodium into the negatively charged internal milieu of the neuron (A). The change of voltage potential caused by the influx of sodium triggers voltage-sensitive calcium channels (VSCCs) to open and allow calcium influx (B). Finally, after the action potential is gone, potassium enters the cell while sodium is pumped out, restoring the neuron's baseline internal electrical milieu (C).

regulated by the ionic charge or voltage potential across the membrane in which they reside. An electrical impulse in a neuron, also known as the action potential, is triggered by summation of the various neurochemical and electrical events of neurotransmission. These are discussed extensively in Chapter 1, which covers the chemical basis of neurotransmission and signal transduction.

The ionic components of an action potential are shown in Figure 3-18. The first phase is sodium rushing "downhill" into the sodium-deficient, negatively charged internal milieu of the neuron (Figure 3-18A). This is made possible when voltage-gated sodium channels open the gates and let the sodium in. A few milliseconds later, the calcium channels get the same idea, with their voltage-gated ion channels opened by the change in voltage potential caused by the sodium rushing in (Figure 3-18B). Finally, after the action potential is gone, during recovery of the neuron's baseline internal electrical milieu, potassium makes its way back into the cell through potassium channels while sodium is again pumped out (Figure 3-18C). It is now known or suspected that several psychotropic drugs work on voltage-sensitive sodium channels (VSSCs) and voltage-sensitive calcium channels (VSCCs). These classes of ion channels will be discussed here. Potassium channels are less well known to be targeted by psychotropic drugs and will thus not be emphasized.

VSSCs (voltage-sensitive sodium channels)

Many dimensions of ion-channel structure are similar for VSSCs and VSCCs. Both have a "pore" that is the channel itself, allowing ions to travel from one side of the membrane to the other. However,

voltage-gated ion channels have a more complicated structure than just a hole or pore in the membrane. These channels are long strings of amino acids, comprising subunits, and four different subunits are connected to form the critical pore, known as an α subunit. In addition, other proteins are associated with the four subunits, and these appear to have regulatory functions.

Let us now build a voltage-sensitive ion channel from scratch and describe the known functions for each part of the proteins that make up these channels. The subunit of a pore-forming protein has six transmembrane segments (Figure 3-19). Transmembrane segment 4 can detect the difference in charge across the membrane and is thus the most electrically sensitive part of the voltage-sensitive channel. Transmembrane segment 4 thus functions like a voltmeter, and when it detects a change in ion charge across the membrane, it can alert the rest of the protein and begin conformational changes of the ion channel to either open it or close it. This same general structure exists for both VSSCs (Figure 3-19A) and VSCCs (Figure 3-19B), but the exact amino acid sequences of the protein subunits are obviously different for VSSCs compared to VSCCs.

Each subunit of a voltage-sensitive ion channel has an extracellular amino acid loop between transmembrane segments 5 and 6 (Figure 3-19). This section of amino acids serves as an "ionic filter" and is located in a position so that it can cover the outside opening of the pore. This is illustrated as a colander configured molecularly to allow only sodium ions to filter through the sodium channel on the left and only calcium channels to filter through the calcium channel on the right (Figure 3-19).

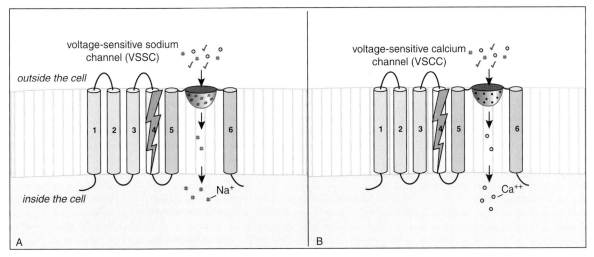

Figure 3-19. Ionic filter of voltage-sensitive sodium and calcium channels. The extracellular loop between transmembrane segments 5 and 6 of an α pore unit acts as an ionic filter (illustrated here as a colander). In the α pore unit of a voltage-sensitive sodium channel, the ionic filter allows only sodium ions to enter the cell (A). In the α pore unit of a voltage-sensitive calcium channel, the ionic filter allows only calcium ions to enter the cell (B).

Four copies of the sodium-channel version of this protein are strung together to form one complete ion-channel pore of a VSSC (Figure 3-20A). The cytoplasmic loops of amino acids that tie these four subunits together are sites that regulate various functions of the sodium channel. For example, on the connector loop between the third and fourth subunits of a VSSC, there are amino acids that act as a "plug" to close the channel. Like a ball on an amino acid chain, this "pore inactivator" stops up the channel on the inner membrane surface of the pore (Figure 3-20A and B). This is a physical blocking of the hole in the pore, and reminiscent of an old-fashioned bathtub plug stopping up the drain in a bathtub. The pore-forming unit of the VSSC is also shown as an icon in Figure 3-20B with a hole in the middle of the pore, and a pore inactivator ready to plug the hole from the inside.

Many figures in textbooks represent voltage-gated ion channels with the outside of the cell on the top of a figure; this is the way the ion channel is shown in Figure 3-20A and B. Here, we also show what the channel looks like when the inside of the cell is at the top of the figure, since throughout this book these channels will often be shown on presynaptic membranes where the inside of the neuron is up and the outside of the neuron, namely its synapse, is down, like the orientation represented in Figure 3-20C. In either case, the sodium is kept out of the neuron when the channel is closed or inactivated and the direction of sodium flow is into the neuron when the channel is open, activated, and the pore is not plugged up with the pore-inactivating amino acid loops.

Voltage-sensitive sodium channels may have one or more regulatory proteins, some of which are called β units, located in the transmembrane area and flanking the α pore-forming unit (Figure 3-20C). The function of these β subunits is not clearly established, but they may modify the actions of the α unit and thereby indirectly influence the opening and closing of the channel. It is possible that β units may be phosphoproteins and that their state of phosphorylation or dephosphorylation could regulate how much influence they exert on ion-channel regulation. Indeed, the α unit itself may also be a phosphoprotein, with the possibility that its own phosphorylation state could be regulated by signal transduction cascades and thus increase or decrease the sensitivity of the ion channel to changes in the ionic environment. This is discussed in Chapter 1 as part of the signal transduction cascade, and ion channels in some cases may act as third, fourth, or subsequent messengers triggered by neurotransmission. Both β subunits and the α subunit itself may have various sites where various psychotropic drugs act, especially anticonvulsants, some of which are also useful as mood stabilizers or as treatments for chronic pain. Specific drugs will be discussed in further detail in the chapters on mood stabilizers (Chapter 8) and pain (Chapter 10).

Four Subunits Combine to Form the Alpha Pore Subunit, or Channel, for Sodium of a VSSC (Voltage-Sensitive Sodium Channel)

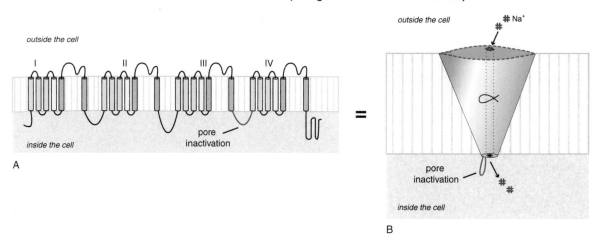

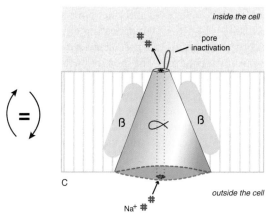

Figure 3-20. Alpha pore of voltage-sensitive sodium channel. The α pore of a voltage-sensitive sodium channel comprises four subunits (A). Amino acids in the intracellular loop between the third and fourth subunits act as a pore inactivator, "plugging" the channel. An iconic version of the α unit is shown here, with the extracellular portion on top (B) and with the intracellular portion on top (C).

Three different states of a VSSC are shown in Figure 3-21. The channel can be open and active, a state allowing maximum ion flow through the α unit (Figure 3-21A). When a sodium channel needs to stop ion flow, it has two states that can do this. One state acts very quickly to flip the pore inactivator into place, stopping ion flow so fast that the channel has not yet even closed (Figure 3-21B). Another state of inactivation actually closes the channel with conformational changes in the ion channel's shape (Figure 3-21C). The pore inactivation mechanism may be for fast inactivation, and the channel closing mechanism

may be for a more stable state of inactivation, but it is not entirely clear.

There are many subtypes of sodium channels, but the details of how they are differentiated from each other by location in the brain, functions, and drug actions are only beginning to be clarified. For the psychopharmacologist, what is now of interest is the fact that various sodium channels may be the sites of action of several anticonvulsants, some of which have mood-stabilizing and pain-reducing properties. Most currently available anticonvulsants probably have multiple sites of action, including multiple sites of

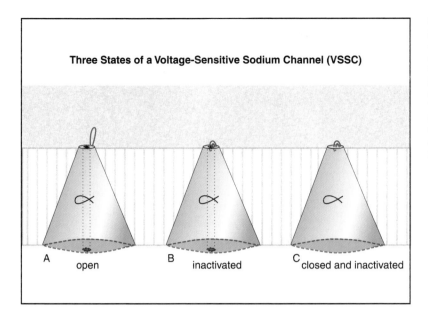

Three States of a Voltage-Sensitive Sodium Channel (VSSC)

A   open

B   inactivated

C   closed and inactivated

Figure 3-21. States of a voltage-sensitive sodium channel. VSSCs can be in the open state, in which the ion channel is open and active and ions flow through the α unit (left). They may also be in an inactivated state, in which the channel is not yet closed but has been "plugged" by the pore inactivator, preventing ion flow (middle). Finally, conformational changes in the ion channel can cause it to close, the third state (right).

action at multiple types of ion channels. The specific actions of specific drugs will be discussed in the chapters that cover specific disorders.

VSCCs (voltage-sensitive calcium channels)

Many aspects of VSCCs and VSSCs are similar – not just their names. Like their sodium-channel cousins, the voltage-sensitive calcium channels also have subunits with six transmembrane segments, with segment 4 a voltmeter and with the extracellular amino acids connecting segments 5 and 6 acting as an ionic filter – only this time as a colander allowing calcium to come into the cell, not sodium (Figure 3-19B). Obviously, the exact sequence of amino acids differs between a sodium channel and a calcium channel, but they have a very similar overall organization and structure.

Just like voltage-gated sodium channels, VSCCs also string together four of their subunits to form a pore, in this case called an α_1 unit (Figure 3-22). The connecting string of amino acids also has functional activities that can regulate calcium-channel functioning, but in this case the functions are different from those for sodium channels. That is, there is no pore inactivator working as a plug for the VSCC, as was described above for the VSSC; instead, the amino acids connecting the second and third subunits of the voltage-sensitive calcium channel work as a "snare" to hook up with synaptic vesicles and regulate

the release of neurotransmitter into the synapse during synaptic neurotransmission (Figures 3-22A and 3-23). The orientation of the calcium channel in Figure 3-22B is with the outside of the cell at the top of the page, and this is switched in Figure 3-22C so that the inside of the cell is now at the top of the page, so the reader can see how these channels might look in various configurations in space. In all cases, the direction of ion flow is from outside the cell to the inside when that channel opens to allow ion flow to occur.

Several proteins flank the α_1 pore-forming unit of a VSCC, called γ, β, and $\alpha_2\delta$. Shown in Figure 3-22C are γ units that span the membrane, cytoplasmic β units, and a curious protein called $\alpha_2\delta$, because it has two parts: a δ part that is transmembrane, and an α_2 part that is extracellular (Figure 3-22C). The functions of all these proteins associated with the α_1 pore-forming unit of a voltage-sensitive calcium channel are just beginning to be understood, but already it is known that the $\alpha_2\delta$ protein is the target of certain psychotropic drugs, such as the anticonvulsants pregabalin and gabapentin, and that this $\alpha_2\delta$ protein may be involved in regulating conformational changes of the ion channel to change the way the ion channel opens and closes.

As would be expected, there are several subtypes of VSCCs (Table 3-4). The vast array of voltage-sensitive calcium channels indicates that the term "calcium channel" is much too general, and in fact

Four Subunits Combine to Form the Alpha-1 Pore Subunit, or Channel, for Calcium of a VSCC (Voltage-Sensitive Calcium Channel)

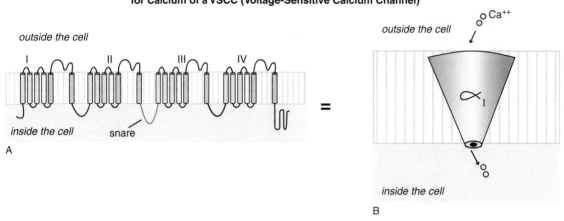

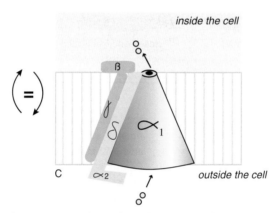

Figure 3-22. Alpha-1 pore of voltage-sensitive calcium channel. The α pore of a voltage-sensitive calcium channel, termed an α_1 unit, comprises four subunits (A). Amino acids in the cytoplasmic loop between the second and third subunits act as a snare to connect with synaptic vesicles, thereby controlling neurotransmitter release (A). An iconic version of the α_1 unit is also shown here, with the extracellular portion on top (B) and with the intracellular portion on top (C).

Opening a Presynaptic Voltage-Sensitive N or P/Q Calcium Channel: Triggers Neurotransmitter Release

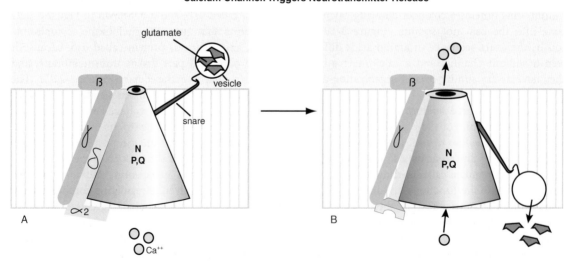

Figure 3-23. N and P/Q voltage-sensitive calcium channels. The voltage-sensitive calcium channels that are most relevant to psychopharmacology are termed N and P/Q channels. These ion channels are presynaptic and involved in the regulation of neurotransmitter release. The intracellular amino acids linking the second and third subunits of the α_1 unit form a snare that hooks onto synaptic vesicles (A). When a nerve impulse arrives, the snare "fires," leading to neurotransmitter release (B).

Table 3-4 Subtypes of voltage-sensitive calcium channels (VSCCs)

Type	Pore-forming subunit	Location	Function
L	Ca_V 1.2, 1.3	Cell bodies, dendrites	Gene expression, synaptic integration
N	Ca_V 2.2	*Nerve terminals* Dendrites, cell bodies	*Transmitter release* Synaptic integration
P/Q	Ca_V 2.1	*Nerve terminals* Dendrites, cell bodies	*Transmitter release* Synaptic integration
R	Ca_V 2.3	*Nerve terminals* Cell bodies, dendrites	*Transmitter release* Repetitive firing, synaptic integration
T	Ca_V 3.1, 3.2, 3.3	Cell bodies, dendrites	Pacemaking, repetitive firing, synaptic integration

can be confusing. For example, calcium channels associated with the ligand-gated ion channels discussed in the previous section, especially those associated with glutamate and nicotinic cholinergic ionotropic receptors, are members of an entirely different class of ion channels from the voltage-sensitive calcium channels under discussion here. As we have mentioned, calcium channels associated with this previously discussed class of ion channels are called ligand-gated ion channels, ionotropic receptors, or ion-channel-linked receptors, to distinguish them from VSCCs.

The specific subtypes of VSCCs of most interest to psychopharmacology are those that are presynaptic, that regulate neurotransmitter release, and that are targeted by certain psychotropic drugs. This subtype designation of VSCCs is shown in Table 3-4, and such channels are known as N or P/Q channels.

Another well-known subtype of VSCC is the L channel. This channel exists not only in the central nervous system, where its functions are still being clarified, but also on vascular smooth muscle, where it regulates blood pressure and where a group of drugs known as dihydropyridine "calcium channel blockers" interact as therapeutic antihypertensives to lower blood pressure. R and T channels are also of interest, and some anticonvulsants and psychotropic drugs may also interact there, but the exact roles of these channels are still being clarified.

Presynaptic N and P/Q VSCCs have a specialized role in regulating neurotransmitter release because they are linked by molecular "snares" to synaptic vesicles (Figure 3-23). That is, these channels are literally hooked to synaptic vesicles. Some experts think of this as a cocked gun – loaded with neurotransmitters packed in a synaptic vesicle bullet (Figure 3-23A) ready

to be fired at the postsynaptic neuron as soon as a nerve impulse arrives (Figure 3-23B). Some of the structural details of the molecular links – namely, with snare proteins – that connect the N and P/Q VSCCs with the synaptic vesicle are shown in Figure 3-24. If a drug interferes with the ability of the channel to open and let in calcium, the synaptic vesicle stays tethered to the voltage-gated calcium channel. Neurotransmission can thus be prevented, which may be desirable in states of excessive neurotransmission, such as pain, seizures, mania, or anxiety. This may explain the action of certain anticonvulsants.

Indeed, it is neurotransmitter release that is the *raison d'être* for presynaptic voltage-sensitive N and P/Q channels. When a nerve impulse invades the presynaptic area, this causes the charge across the membrane to change, in turn opening the VSCC, allowing calcium to enter; this makes the synaptic vesicle dock into and merge with the presynaptic membrane, spewing its neurotransmitter contents into the synapse to effect neurotransmission (Figures 3-25 and 3-26). This conversion of an electrical impulse into a chemical message is triggered by calcium and sometimes called excitation–secretion coupling.

Anticonvulsants are thought to act at various VSSCs and VSCCs and will be discussed in further detail in the relevant clinical chapters. Many of these anticonvulsants have several uses in psychopharmacology, from chronic pain to migraine, from bipolar mania to bipolar depression to bipolar maintenance, and possibly as anxiolytics and sleep aids. These specific applications and more details about hypothetical mechanisms of action are explored in depth in the clinical chapters dealing with the various psychiatric disorders.

Docking of Synaptic Vesicle with Presynaptic Membrane, VSCC (Voltage-Sensitive Calcium Channel), and Snare Proteins

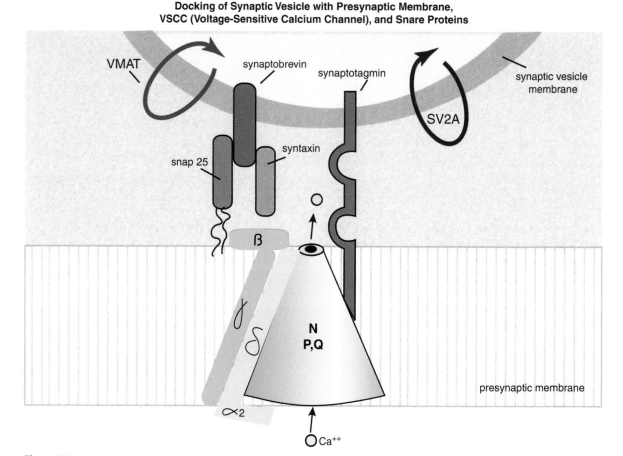

Figure 3-24. Snare proteins. Proteins that link the voltage-sensitive calcium channel to the synaptic vesicle, called snare proteins, are shown here; they include SNAP 25, synaptobrevin, syntaxin, and synaptotagmin. A VMAT (vesicular monoamine transporter) is shown on the left. Another transporter, SV2A, is shown on the right. The mechanism of this transporter is not yet clear, but the anticonvulsant levetiracetam is known to bind to this site.

Ion channels and neurotransmission

Although the various subtypes of ligand-gated and voltage-gated ion channels are presented separately, the reality is that they work cooperatively during neurotransmission. When the actions of all these ion channels are well orchestrated, brain communication becomes a magical mix of electrical and chemical messages made possible by ion channels. The coordinated acts of ion channels during neurotransmission are illustrated in Figures 3-25 and 3-26.

The initiation of chemical neurotransmission by a neuron's ability to integrate all of its inputs and then translate them into an electrical impulse is presented in Chapter 1. We now show how ion channels are involved in this process. After a neuron receives and integrates its inputs from other neurons, it then encodes them into an action potential, and that nerve impulse is next sent along the axon via voltage-sensitive sodium channels that line the axon (Figure 3-25).

The action potential could be described as lighting a fuse, with the fuse burning from the initial segment of the axon to the axon terminal. Movement of the burning edge of the fuse is carried out by a sequence of VSSCs that open one after the other, allowing sodium to pass into the neuron and then carrying the electrical impulse along to the next VSSC in line (Figure 3-25). When the electrical impulse reaches the axon terminal, it meets voltage-sensitive calcium channels in the presynaptic neuronal membrane, already loaded with synaptic vesicles and ready to fire (see axon terminal of neuron A in Figure 3-25).

Summary: From Presynaptic to Postsynaptic Signal Propagation

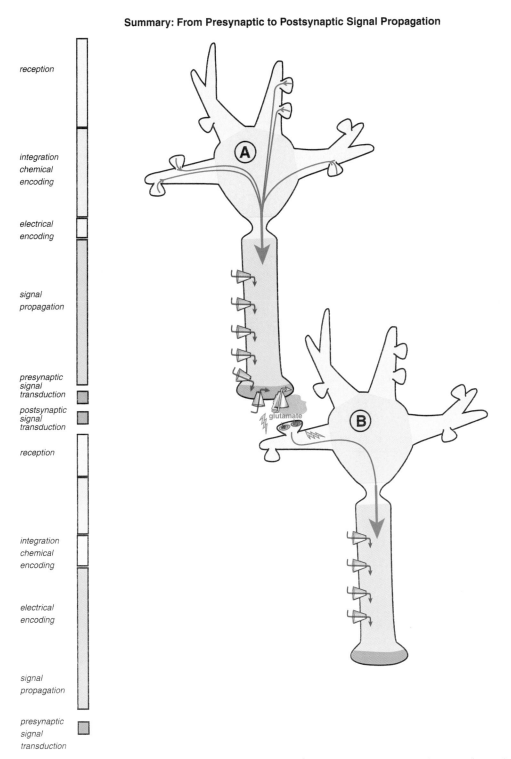

Figure 3-25. Signal propagation. Summary of signal propagation from presynaptic to postsynaptic neuron. A nerve impulse is generated in neuron A, and the action potential is sent along the axon via voltage-sensitive sodium channels until it reaches voltage-sensitive calcium channels linked to synaptic vesicles full of neurotransmitters in the axon terminal. Opening of the voltage-sensitive calcium channel and consequent calcium influx causes neurotransmitter release into the synapse. Arrival of neurotransmitter at postsynaptic receptors on the dendrite of neuron B triggers depolarization of the membrane in that neuron and, consequently, postsynaptic signal propagation.

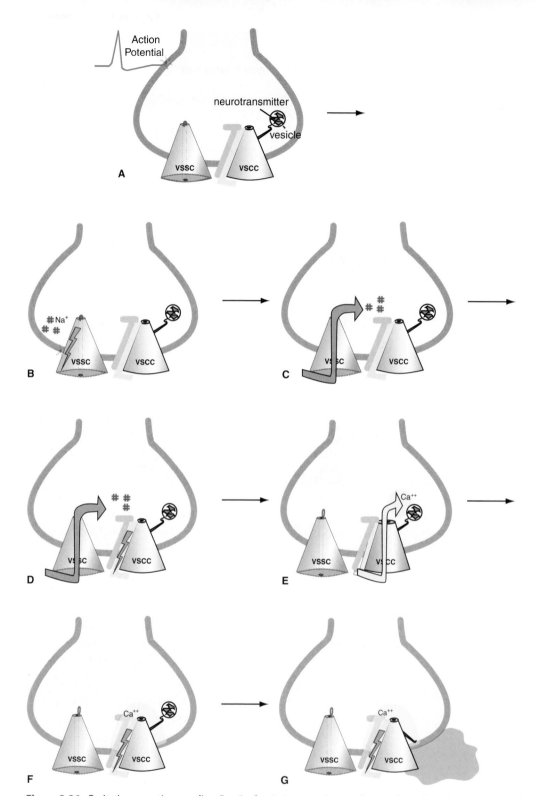

Figure 3-26. Excitation–secretion coupling. Details of excitation–secretion coupling are shown here. An action potential is encoded by the neuron and sent to the axon terminal via voltage-sensitive sodium channels along the axon (A). The sodium released by those channels triggers a voltage-sensitive sodium channel at the axon terminal to open (B), allowing sodium influx into the presynaptic neuron (C). Sodium influx changes the electrical charge of the voltage-sensitive calcium channel (D), causing it to open and allow calcium influx (E). As the intraneuronal concentration of calcium increases (F), the synaptic vesicle is caused to dock and merge with the presynaptic membrane, leading to neurotransmitter release (G).

When the electrical impulse is detected by the voltmeter in the voltage-sensitive calcium channel, it opens the calcium channel, allowing calcium to enter, and bang! – the neurotransmitter is released in a cloud of synaptic chemicals from the presynaptic axon terminal via excitation–secretion coupling (see axon terminal of neuron A in Figure 3-25 and enlarged illustrations of this in Figure 3-26). Details of this process of excitation–secretion coupling are shown in Figure 3-26, beginning with the action potential about to invade the presynaptic terminal and with a closed VSSC sitting next to a closed but poised VSCC snared to its synaptic vesicle (Figure 3-26A). As the nerve impulse arrives in the axon terminal, it first hits the VSSC as a wave of positive sodium charges delivered by the openings of upstream sodium channels, which are detected by the sodium channel's voltmeter (Figure 3-26B). This opens the last sodium channel shown, allowing sodium to enter (Figure 3-26C). The consequence of this sodium entry is to change the electrical charge near the calcium channel; this is then detected by the VSCC's voltmeter (Figure 3-26D). Next, the calcium channel opens (Figure 3-26E). At this point, chemical neurotransmission has now been irreversibly triggered, and the translation of an electrical message into a chemical message has begun. Calcium entry from the VSCC now increases the local concentrations of this ion in the vicinity of the VSCC, the synaptic vesicle, and the neurotransmitter release machinery (Figure 3-26F). This causes the synaptic vesicle to dock into the inside of the presynaptic membrane, then merge with it, spewing its neurotransmitter contents out of the membrane and into the synapse (Figure 3-26G). This amazing process occurs almost instantaneously and simultaneously from many VSCCs releasing neurotransmitter from many synaptic vesicles.

By now, only about half of the sequential phenomena of chemical neurotransmission have been described. The other half occur on the other side of the synapse. That is, reception of the released neurotransmitter now occurs in neuron B (Figure 3-25), which can set up another nerve impulse in neuron B. This whole process – from the generation of a nerve impulse and its propagation along neuron A to its nerve terminal, then sending chemical neurotransmission to neuron B, and finally propagating this second nerve impulse along neuron B – is summarized in Figure 3-25. Voltage-sensitive sodium channels in presynaptic neuron A propagate the impulse there, and then voltage-sensitive calcium channels in presynaptic neuron A release the neurotransmitter glutamate. Ligand-gated ion channels on dendrites in postsynaptic neuron B next receive this chemical input, and translate this chemical message back into a nerve impulse propagated in neuron B by voltage-sensitive sodium channels in that neuron. Also, ligand-gated ion channels in postsynaptic neuron B translate the glutamate chemical signal into another type of electrical phenomenon called long-term potentiation, to cause changes in the function of neuron B.

Summary

Ion channels are key targets of many psychotropic drugs. This is not surprising, because these targets are key regulators of chemical neurotransmission and the signal transduction cascade.

There are two major classes of ion channels: ligand-gated ion channels and voltage-sensitive ion channels. The opening of ligand-gated ion channels is regulated by neurotransmitters, whereas the opening of voltage-sensitive ion channels is regulated by the charge across the membrane in which they reside.

Ligand-gated ion channels are both ion channels and receptors. They are also commonly called ionotropic receptors as well as ion-channel-linked receptors. One subclass of ligand-gated ion channels has a pentameric structure and includes $GABA_A$, nicotinic cholinergic, serotonin 3, and glycine receptors. The other subclass of ligand-gated ion channels has a tetrameric structure, and includes many glutamate receptors, including the AMPA, kainate, and NMDA subtypes.

Ligands act at ligand-gated ion channels across an agonist spectrum, from full agonist, to partial agonist, to antagonist, to inverse agonist. Ligand-gated ion channels can be regulated not only by neurotransmitters acting as agonists, but also by molecules interacting at other sites on the receptor, either boosting the action of neurotransmitter agonists as positive allosteric modulators (PAMs), or diminishing the action of neurotransmitter agonists as negative allosteric modulators (NAMs). In addition, these receptors exist in several states, from open, to resting, to closed, to inactivated, to desensitized.

The second major class of ion channels is called either voltage-sensitive or voltage-gated, since they are opened and closed by the voltage charge across the membrane. The major channels from this class that are of interest to psychopharmacologists are the voltage-sensitive sodium channels (VSSCs) and the voltage-sensitive calcium channels (VSCCs). Numerous anticonvulsants bind to various sites on these channels and may exert their anticonvulsant actions by this mechanism, as well as their actions as mood stabilizers, treatments for chronic pain, anxiolytics, and sleep medications.

Psychosis and schizophrenia

Psychosis is a difficult term to define and is frequently misused, not only in the media but unfortunately among mental health professionals as well. Stigma and fear surround the concept of psychosis, and sometimes the pejorative term "crazy" is used for psychosis. This chapter is not intended to list the diagnostic criteria for all the different mental disorders in which psychosis is either a defining feature or an associated feature. The reader is referred to standard reference sources such as the DSM (*Diagnostic and Statistical Manual*) of the American Psychiatric Association and the ICD (*International Classification of Diseases*) for that information. Although schizophrenia is emphasized here, we will approach psychosis as a syndrome associated with a variety of illnesses that are all targets for antipsychotic drug treatment.

Symptom dimensions in schizophrenia
Clinical description of psychosis

Psychosis is a syndrome – that is, a mixture of symptoms – that can be associated with many different psychiatric disorders, but is not a specific disorder itself in diagnostic schemes such as the DSM or ICD. At a minimum, psychosis means delusions and hallucinations. It generally also includes symptoms such as disorganized speech, disorganized behavior, and gross distortions of reality.

Therefore, psychosis can be considered to be a set of symptoms in which a person's mental capacity, affective response, and capacity to recognize reality, communicate, and relate to others is impaired. Psychotic disorders have psychotic symptoms as their defining features; there are other disorders in which psychotic symptoms may be present, but are not necessary for the diagnosis.

Those **disorders that require the presence of psychosis** as a *defining* feature of the diagnosis include schizophrenia, substance-induced (i.e., drug-induced) psychotic disorders, schizophreniform disorder, schizoaffective disorder, delusional disorder, brief psychotic disorder, and psychotic disorder due to a general medical condition (Table 4-1). **Disorders that may or may not have psychotic symptoms** as *associated* features include mania and depression as well as several cognitive disorders such as Alzheimer's dementia (Table 4-2).

Psychosis itself can be paranoid, disorganized/excited, or depressive. Perceptual distortions and motor disturbances can be associated with any type of psychosis. *Perceptual distortions* include being distressed by hallucinatory voices; hearing voices that accuse, blame, or threaten punishment; seeing visions;

Table 4-1 Disorders in which psychosis is a defining feature

Schizophrenia

Substance-induced (i.e., drug-induced) psychotic disorders

Schizophreniform disorder

Schizoaffective disorder

Delusional disorder

Brief psychotic disorder

Psychotic disorder due to a general medical condition

Table 4-2 Disorders in which psychosis is an associated feature

Mania

Depression

Cognitive disorders

Alzheimer's dementia

reporting hallucinations of touch, taste or odor; or reporting that familiar things and people seem changed. *Motor disturbances* are peculiar, rigid postures; overt signs of tension; inappropriate grins or giggles; peculiar repetitive gestures; talking, muttering, or mumbling to oneself; or glancing around as if hearing voices.

In **paranoid psychosis**, the patient has paranoid projections, hostile belligerence and grandiose expansiveness. *Paranoid projection* includes preoccupation with delusional beliefs; believing that people are talking about oneself; believing one is being persecuted or being conspired against; and believing people or external forces control one's actions. *Hostile belligerence* is verbal expression of feelings of hostility; expressing an attitude of disdain; manifesting a hostile, sullen attitude; manifesting irritability and grouchiness; tending to blame others for problems; expressing feelings of resentment; complaining and finding fault; as well as expressing suspicion of people. *Grandiose expansiveness* is exhibiting an attitude of superiority; hearing voices that praise and extol; believing one has unusual powers or is a well-known personality, or that one has a divine mission.

In a **disorganized/excited psychosis** there is conceptual disorganization, disorientation, and excitement. *Conceptual disorganization* can be characterized by giving answers that are irrelevant or incoherent, drifting off the subject, using neologisms, or repeating certain words or phrases. *Disorientation* is not knowing where one is, the season of the year, the calendar year, or one's own age. *Excitement* is expressing feelings without restraint; manifesting speech that is hurried; exhibiting an elevated mood; an attitude of superiority;

dramatizing oneself or one's symptoms; manifesting loud and boisterous speech; exhibiting overactivity or restlessness; and exhibiting excess of speech.

Depressive psychosis is characterized by psychomotor retardation, apathy, and anxious self-punishment and blame. *Psychomotor retardation* and *apathy* are manifested by slowed speech; indifference to one's future; fixed facial expression; slowed movements; deficiencies in recent memory; blocking in speech; apathy toward oneself or one's problems; slovenly appearance; low or whispered speech; and failure to answer questions. *Anxious self-punishment and blame* is the tendency to blame or condemn oneself; anxiety about specific matters; apprehensiveness regarding vague future events; an attitude of self-deprecation, manifesting as a depressed mood; expressing feelings of guilt and remorse; preoccupation with suicidal thoughts, unwanted ideas, and specific fears; and feeling unworthy or sinful.

This discussion of clusters of psychotic symptoms does not constitute diagnostic criteria for any psychotic disorder. It is given merely as a description of several types of symptoms in psychosis to give the reader an overview of the nature of behavioral disturbances associated with the various psychotic illnesses.

Schizophrenia is more than a psychosis

Although schizophrenia is the commonest and best-known psychotic illness, it is not synonymous with psychosis, but is just one of many causes of psychosis. Schizophrenia affects 1% of the population, and in the US there are over 300 000 acute schizophrenic episodes annually. Between 25% and 50% of schizophrenia patients attempt suicide, and 10% eventually succeed, contributing to a mortality rate eight times greater than that of the general population. Life expectancy of a patient with schizophrenia may be 20–30 years shorter than the general population, not only due to suicide, but in particular due to premature cardiovascular disease. Accelerated mortality from premature cardiovascular disease in patients with schizophrenia is caused not only by genetic and lifestyle factors, such as smoking, unhealthy diet, and lack of exercise leading to obesity and diabetes, but also – sorrily – from treatment with some antipsychotic drugs which themselves cause an increased incidence of obesity and diabetes, and thus increase cardiac risk. In the US, over 20% of all social security benefits are used for the care of patients with schizophrenia. The direct and indirect costs of schizophrenia in the US alone are estimated to be in the tens of billions of dollars every year.

Schizophrenia by definition is a disturbance that must last for six months or longer, including at least one month of delusions, hallucinations, disorganized speech, grossly disorganized or catatonic behavior, or negative symptoms. **Positive symptoms** are listed in Table 4-3 and shown in Figure 4-1. These symptoms

Table 4-3 Positive symptoms of psychosis and schizophrenia

Delusions

Hallucinations

Distortions or exaggerations in language and communication

Disorganized speech

Disorganized behavior

Catatonic behavior

Agitation

of schizophrenia are often emphasized, since they can be dramatic, can erupt suddenly when a patient decompensates into a psychotic episode (often called a psychotic "break," as in break from reality), and are the symptoms most effectively treated by antipsychotic medications. *Delusions* are one type of positive symptom, and these usually involve a misinterpretation of perceptions or experiences. The most common content of a delusion in schizophrenia is persecutory, but it may include a variety of other themes including referential (i.e., erroneously thinking that something refers to oneself), somatic, religious, or grandiose. *Hallucinations* are also a type of positive symptom (Table 4-3) and may occur in any sensory modality (e.g., auditory, visual, olfactory, gustatory, and tactile), but auditory hallucinations are by far the most common and characteristic hallucinations in schizophrenia. Positive symptoms generally reflect an *excess* of normal functions, and in addition to delusions and hallucinations may also include distortions or exaggerations in language and communication (disorganized speech), as well as in behavioral monitoring (grossly disorganized or catatonic or agitated behavior). Positive symptoms are well known because they are dramatic, are often the cause of bringing a patient to the attention of medical professionals and law enforcement, and are the major target of antipsychotic drug treatments.

Negative symptoms are listed in Tables 4-4 and 4-5 and shown in Figure 4-1. Classically, there are at

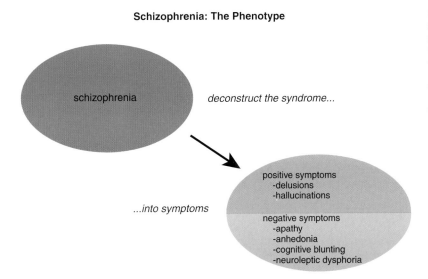

Schizophrenia: The Phenotype

schizophrenia

deconstruct the syndrome...

...into symptoms

positive symptoms
-delusions
-hallucinations

negative symptoms
-apathy
-anhedonia
-cognitive blunting
-neuroleptic dysphoria

Figure 4-1. Positive and negative symptoms of schizophrenia. The syndrome of schizophrenia consists of a mixture of symptoms that are commonly divided into two major categories, positive and negative. Positive symptoms, such as delusions and hallucinations, reflect the development of the symptoms of psychosis; they can be dramatic and may reflect loss of touch with reality. Negative symptoms reflect the loss of normal functions and feelings, such as losing interest in things and not being able to experience pleasure.

least five types of negative symptoms all starting with the letter A (Table 4-5):

- *alogia* – dysfunction of communication; restrictions in the fluency and productivity of thought and speech
- *affective blunting or flattening* – restrictions in the range and intensity of emotional expression
- *asociality* – reduced social drive and interaction
- *anhedonia* – reduced ability to experience pleasure
- *avolition* – reduced desire, motivation or persistence; restrictions in the initiation of goal-directed behavior

Table 4-4 Negative symptoms of schizophrenia

Blunted affect

Emotional withdrawal

Poor rapport

Passivity

Apathetic social withdrawal

Difficulty in abstract thinking

Lack of spontaneity

Stereotyped thinking

Alogia: restrictions in fluency and productivity of thought and speech

Avolition: restrictions in initiation of goal-directed behavior

Anhedonia: lack of pleasure

Attentional impairment

Negative symptoms in schizophrenia, such as blunted affect, emotional withdrawal, poor rapport, passivity and apathetic social withdrawal, difficulty in abstract thinking, stereotyped thinking and lack of spontaneity, commonly are considered a reduction in normal functions and are associated with long periods of hospitalization and poor social functioning. Although this reduction in normal functioning may not be as dramatic as positive symptoms, it is interesting to note that negative symptoms of schizophrenia determine whether a patient ultimately functions well or has a poor outcome. Certainly, patients will have disruptions in their ability to interact with others when their positive symptoms are out of control, but their degree of negative symptoms will largely determine whether patients with schizophrenia can live independently, maintain stable social relationships, or re-enter the workplace.

Although formal rating scales can be used to measure negative symptoms in research studies, in clinical practice it may be more practical to identify and monitor negative symptoms quickly by observation alone (Figure 4-2) or by some simple questioning (Figure 4-3). Negative symptoms are not just part of the syndrome of schizophrenia – they can also be part of a "prodrome" that begins with subsyndromal symptoms that do not meet the diagnostic criteria of schizophrenia and occur before the onset of the full syndrome of schizophrenia. Prodromal negative symptoms are important to detect and monitor over time in high-risk patients so that treatment can be initiated at the first signs of psychosis. Negative

Table 4-5 What are negative symptoms?

Domain	Descriptive Term	Translation
Dysfunction of communication	Alogia	Poverty of speech; e.g., talks little, uses few words
Dysfunction of affect	Affective blunting	Reduced range of emotions (perception, experience and expression); e.g., feels numb or empty inside, recalls few emotional experiences, good or bad
Dysfunction of socialization	Asociality	Reduced social drive and interaction; e.g., little sexual interest, few friends, little interest in spending time with (or little time spent with) friends
Dysfunction of capacity for pleasure	Anhedonia	Reduced ability to experience pleasure; e.g., finds previous hobbies or interests unpleasurable
Dysfunction of motivation	Avolition	Reduced desire, motivation, persistence; e.g., reduced ability to undertake and complete everyday tasks; may have poor personal hygiene

Key Negative Symptoms Identified Solely on Observation

Reduced speech: Patient has restricted speech quantity, uses few words and nonverbal responses. May also have impoverished content of speech, when words convey little meaning*

A

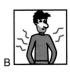

Poor grooming: Patient has poor grooming and hygiene, clothes are dirty or stained, or subject has an odor*

B

Limited eye contact: Patient rarely makes eye contact with the interviewer*

C

*symptoms are described for patients at the more severe end of the spectrum

Figure 4-2. Negative symptoms identified by observation. Some negative symptoms of schizophrenia – such as reduced speech, poor grooming, and limited eye contact – can be identified solely by observing the patient.

Key Negative Symptoms Identified With Some Questioning

Reduced emotional responsiveness: Patient exhibits few emotions or changes in facial expression, and when questioned can recall few occasions of emotional experience*

A

Reduced interest: Reduced interests and hobbies, little or nothing stimulates interest, limited life goals and inability to proceed with them*

B

Reduced social drive: Patient has reduced desire to initiate social contacts and may have few or no friends or close relationships*

C

*symptoms are described for patients at the more severe end of the spectrum

Figure 4-3. Negative symptoms identified by questioning. Other negative symptoms of schizophrenia can be identified by simple questioning. For example, brief questioning can reveal the degree of emotional responsiveness, interest level in hobbies or pursuing life goals, and desire to initiate and maintain social contacts.

symptoms can also persist between psychotic episodes once schizophrenia has begun, and reduce social and occupational functioning in the absence of positive symptoms.

Current antipsychotic drug treatments are limited in their ability to treat negative symptoms, but psychosocial interventions along with antipsychotics can be helpful in reducing negative symptoms. There is even the possibility that instituting treatment for negative symptoms during the prodromal phase of schizophrenia may delay or prevent the onset of the illness, but this is still a matter of current research.

Beyond positive and negative symptoms of schizophrenia

Although not recognized formally as part of the diagnostic criteria for schizophrenia, numerous studies subcategorize the symptoms of this illness into five dimensions: not just positive and negative symptoms, but also cognitive symptoms, aggressive symptoms, and affective symptoms (Figure 4-4). This is perhaps a more sophisticated, if complicated, manner of describing the symptoms of schizophrenia.

Aggressive symptoms such as assaultiveness, verbally abusive behaviors, and frank violence can

Match Each Symptom to Hypothetically Malfunctioning Brain Circuits

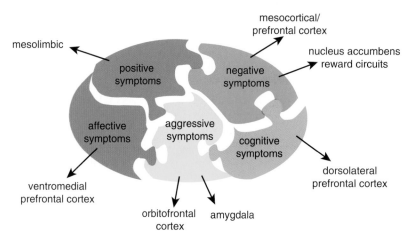

Figure 4-4. Localization of symptom domains. The different symptom domains of schizophrenia are hypothesized to be regulated by unique brain regions. Positive symptoms of schizophrenia are hypothetically modulated by malfunctioning mesolimbic circuits, while negative symptoms are hypothetically linked to malfunctioning mesocortical circuits and may also involve mesolimbic regions such as the nucleus accumbens, which is part of the brain's reward circuitry and thus plays a role in motivation. The nucleus accumbens may also be involved in the increased rate of substance use and abuse seen in patients with schizophrenia. Affective symptoms are associated with the ventromedial prefrontal cortex, while aggressive symptoms (related to impulse control) are associated with abnormal information processing in the orbitofrontal cortex and amygdala. Cognitive symptoms are associated with problematic information processing in the dorsolateral prefrontal cortex. Although there is overlap in function among different brain regions, understanding which brain regions may be predominantly involved in specific symptoms can aid in customization of treatment to the particular symptom profile of each individual patient with schizophrenia.

occur with positive symptoms such as delusions and hallucinations, and be confused with positive symptoms. Behavioral interventions may be particularly helpful to prevent violence linked to poor impulsivity by reducing provocations from the environment. Certain antipsychotic drugs such as clozapine, or very high doses of standard antipsychotic drugs, or occasionally the use of two antipsychotic drugs simultaneously, may also be useful for aggressive symptoms and violence in some patients.

It can also be difficult to separate the symptoms of formal cognitive dysfunction from the symptoms of affective dysfunction and from negative symptoms, but research is attempting to localize the specific areas of brain dysfunction for each symptom domain in schizophrenia in the hope of developing better treatments for the often-neglected negative, cognitive, and affective symptoms of schizophrenia. In particular, neuropsychological assessment batteries are being developed to quantify cognitive symptoms, in order to detect cognitive improvement after treatment with a number of novel psychotropic drugs currently being

tested. Cognitive symptoms of schizophrenia are impaired attention and impaired information processing manifested as impaired verbal fluency (ability to produce spontaneous speech), problems with serial learning (of a list of items or a sequence of events), and impairment in vigilance for executive functioning (problems with sustaining and focusing attention, concentrating, prioritizing, and modulating behavior based upon social cues).

Important cognitive symptoms of schizophrenia are listed in Table 4-6. These do not include symptoms of dementia and memory disturbance more characteristic of Alzheimer's disease, but cognitive symptoms of schizophrenia emphasize "executive dysfunction," which includes problems representing and maintaining goals, allocating attentional resources, evaluating and monitoring performance, and utilizing these skills to solve problems. Cognitive symptoms of schizophrenia are important to recognize and monitor because they are the single strongest correlate of real-world functioning, even stronger than negative symptoms.

Table 4-6 Cognitive symptoms of schizophrenia

Problems representing and maintaining goals

Problems allocating attentional resources

Problems focusing attention

Problems sustaining attention

Problems evaluating functions

Problems monitoring performance

Problems prioritizing

Problems modulating behavior based upon social cues

Problems with serial learning

Impaired verbal fluency

Difficulty with problem solving

Symptoms of schizophrenia are not necessarily unique to schizophrenia

It is important to recognize that several illnesses other than schizophrenia can share some of the same five symptom dimensions as described here for schizophrenia and shown in Figure 4-4. Thus, disorders in addition to schizophrenia that can have *positive symptoms* include bipolar disorder, schizoaffective disorder, psychotic depression, Alzheimer's disease and other organic dementias, childhood psychotic illnesses, drug-induced psychoses, and others. *Negative symptoms* can also occur in other disorders and can also overlap with cognitive and affective symptoms that occur in these other disorders. However, as a primary deficit state, negative symptoms are fairly unique to schizophrenia. Schizophrenia is certainly not the only disorder with *cognitive symptoms*. Autism, post-stroke (vascular or multi-infarct) dementia, Alzheimer's disease, and many other organic dementias (Parkinsonian/Lewy body dementia, frontotemporal/Pick's dementia, etc.) can also be associated with cognitive dysfunctions similar to those seen in schizophrenia.

Affective symptoms are frequently associated with schizophrenia but this does not necessarily mean that they fulfill the diagnostic criteria for a comorbid anxiety or affective disorder. Nevertheless, depressed mood, anxious mood, guilt, tension, irritability, and worry frequently accompany schizophrenia. These various symptoms are also prominent features of major depressive disorder, psychotic depression,

bipolar disorder, schizoaffective disorder, organic dementias, childhood psychotic disorders, and treatment-resistant cases of depression, bipolar disorder, and schizophrenia, among others. Finally, *aggressive and hostile symptoms* occur in numerous other disorders, especially those with problems of impulse control. Symptoms include overt hostility, such as verbal or physical abusiveness or assault, self-injurious behaviors including suicide, and arson or other property damage. Other types of impulsiveness such as sexual acting out are also in this category of aggressive and hostile symptoms. These same symptoms are frequently associated with bipolar disorder, childhood psychosis, borderline personality disorder, antisocial personality disorder, drug abuse, Alzheimer's and other dementias, attention deficit hyperactivity disorder, conduct disorders in children, and many others.

Brain circuits and symptom dimensions in schizophrenia

The various symptoms of schizophrenia are hypothesized to be localized in unique brain regions (Figure 4-4). Specifically, the positive symptoms of schizophrenia have long been hypothesized to be localized to malfunctioning mesolimbic circuits, especially involving the nucleus accumbens. The nucleus accumbens is considered to be part of the brain's reward circuitry, so it is not surprising that problems with reward and motivation in schizophrenia, symptoms that can overlap with negative symptoms and lead to smoking, drug and alcohol abuse, may be linked to this brain area as well. The prefrontal cortex is considered to be a key node in the nexus of malfunctioning cerebral circuitry responsible for each of the remaining symptoms of schizophrenia: specifically, the mesocortical and ventromedial prefrontal cortex with negative symptoms and affective symptoms, the dorsolateral prefrontal cortex with cognitive symptoms, and the orbitofrontal cortex and its connections to amygdala with aggressive, impulsive symptoms (Figure 4-4).

This model is obviously oversimplified and reductionistic, because every brain area has several functions, and every function is certainly distributed to more than one brain area. Nevertheless, allocating specific symptom dimensions to unique brain areas not only assists research studies, but has both heuristic and clinical value. Specifically, every patient has unique symptoms, and unique responses to medication. In order to optimize and individualize treatment, it can be useful to consider which specific symptoms any given patient is expressing, and therefore which areas of that particular patient's brain are hypothetically malfunctioning (Figure 4-4). Each brain area has unique neurotransmitters, receptors, enzymes, and genes that regulate it, with some overlap, but also with some unique regional differences, and knowing this can assist the clinician in choosing medications and in monitoring the effectiveness of treatment.

Neurotransmitters and circuits in schizophrenia

Dopamine

The leading hypothesis for schizophrenia is based upon the neurotransmitter dopamine. To understand the potential role of dopamine in schizophrenia, it is first important to review how dopamine is synthesized, metabolized, and regulated; and the role of dopamine receptors and the localization of key dopamine pathways in the brain.

Dopaminergic neurons

Dopaminergic neurons utilize the neurotransmitter dopamine (DA), which is synthesized in dopaminergic nerve terminals from the amino acid tyrosine after it is taken up into the neuron from the extracellular space and bloodstream by a tyrosine pump, or transporter (Figure 4-5). Tyrosine is converted into DA first by the rate-limiting enzyme tyrosine hydroxylase (TOH) and then by the enzyme DOPA decarboxylase (DDC) (Figure 4-5). DA is then taken up into synaptic vesicles by a vesicular monoamine transporter (VMAT2) and stored there until it is used during neurotransmission.

The DA neuron has a presynaptic transporter (reuptake pump) called DAT, which is unique for DA and which terminates DA's synaptic action by whisking it out of the synapse back into the presynaptic nerve terminal; there it can be re-stored in synaptic vesicles for subsequent reuse in another neurotransmission (Figure 4-6). DATs are not present in high density at the axon terminals of all DA neurons. For example, in prefrontal cortex, DATs are relatively sparse and DA is inactivated by other mechanisms. Excess DA that

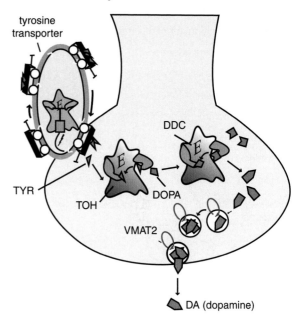

Dopamine is Produced

Figure 4-5. Dopamine synthesis. Tyrosine (TYR), a precursor to dopamine, is taken up into dopamine nerve terminals via a tyrosine transporter and converted into DOPA by the enzyme tyrosine hydroxylase (TOH). DOPA is then converted into dopamine (DA) by the enzyme DOPA decarboxylase (DDC). After synthesis, dopamine is packaged into synaptic vesicles via the vesicular monoamine transporter (VMAT2) and stored there until its release into the synapse during neurotransmission.

escapes storage in synaptic vesicles can be destroyed within the neuron by the enzymes monoamine oxidase (MAO)-A or MAO-B, or outside the neuron by the enzyme catechol-*O*-methyl-transferase (COMT) (Figure 4-6). DA that diffuses away from synapses can also be transported by norepinephrine transporters (NETs) as a "false" substrate, and DA action will be terminated in this manner.

Receptors for dopamine also regulate dopaminergic neurotransmission (Figure 4-7). The DA transporter DAT and the vesicular transporter VMAT2 are both types of receptors. A plethora of additional dopamine receptors exist, including at least five pharmacological subtypes and several more molecular isoforms. Perhaps the most extensively investigated dopamine receptor is the dopamine 2 (D_2) receptor, as it is stimulated by dopamine agonists for the treatment of Parkinson's disease, and blocked by dopamine antagonist antipsychotics for the treatment of schizophrenia. As will be discussed in greater detail in Chapter 5 on antipsychotic drugs, dopamine 1, 2, 3,

Dopamine's Action is Terminated

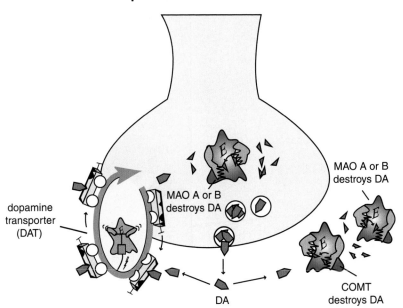

dopamine transporter (DAT)

MAO A or B destroys DA

MAO A or B destroys DA

COMT destroys DA

DA

Figure 4-6. Dopamine's action is terminated. Dopamine's action can be terminated through multiple mechanisms. Dopamine can be transported out of the synaptic cleft and back into the presynaptic neuron via the dopamine transporter (DAT), where it may be repackaged for future use. Alternatively, dopamine may be broken down extracellularly via the enzyme catechol-O-methyl-transferase (COMT). Other enzymes that break down dopamine are monoamine oxidase A (MAO-A) and monoamine oxidase B (MAO-B), which are present in mitochondria within the presynaptic neuron and in other cells such as glia.

Dopamine Receptors

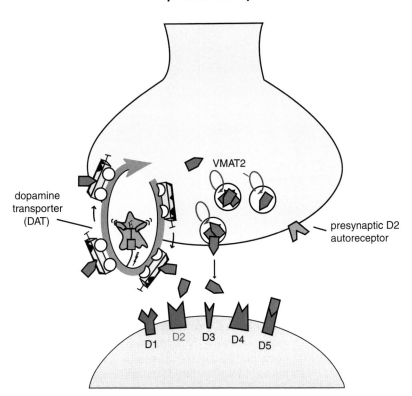

dopamine transporter (DAT)

VMAT2

presynaptic D2 autoreceptor

D1 D2 D3 D4 D5

Figure 4-7. Dopamine receptors. Shown here are receptors for dopamine that regulate its neurotransmission. The dopamine transporter (DAT) exists presynaptically and is responsible for clearing excess dopamine out of the synapse. The vesicular monoamine transporter (VMAT2) takes dopamine up into synaptic vesicles for future neurotransmission. There is also a presynaptic dopamine D_2 autoreceptor, which regulates release of dopamine from the presynaptic neuron. In addition, there are several postsynaptic receptors. These include D_1, D_2, D_3, D_4, and D_5 receptors. The functions of the D_2 receptors are best understood, because this is the primary binding site for virtually all antipsychotic agents as well as for dopamine agonists used to treat Parkinson's disease.

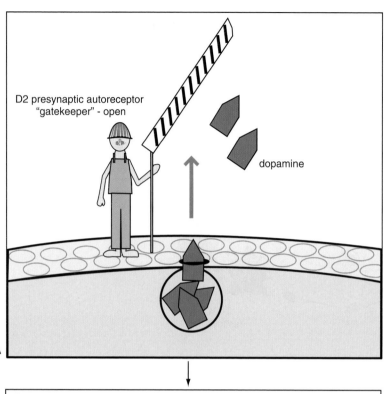

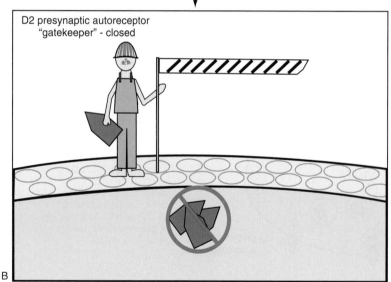

Figure 4-8. Presynaptic dopamine 2 (D₂) autoreceptors. Presynaptic D₂ autoreceptors are "gatekeepers" for dopamine. That is, when these gatekeeping receptors are not bound by dopamine (no dopamine in the gatekeeper's hand), they open a molecular gate, allowing dopamine release (A). However, when dopamine binds to the gatekeeping receptors (now the gatekeeper has dopamine in his hand), they close the molecular gate and prevent dopamine from being released (B).

and 4 receptors are all blocked by some atypical antipsychotic drugs, but it is not clear to what extent dopamine 1, 3, or 4 receptors contribute to the clinical properties of these drugs.

Dopamine 2 receptors can be presynaptic, where they function as autoreceptors (Figure 4-7).

Presynaptic D₂ receptors thus act as "gatekeepers," either allowing DA release when they are not occupied by DA (Figure 4-8A) or inhibiting DA release when DA builds up in the synapse and occupies these gatekeeping presynaptic autoreceptors (Figure 4-8B). Such receptors are located either on

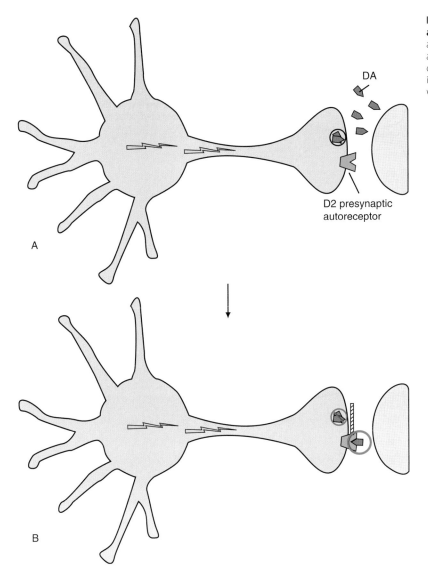

Figure 4-9. Presynaptic dopamine-2 autoreceptors. Presynaptic D_2 autoreceptors can be located on the axon terminal, as shown here. When dopamine builds up in the synapse (A), it is available to bind to the autoreceptor, which then inhibits dopamine release (B).

DA

D2 presynaptic autoreceptor

A

B

the axon terminal (Figure 4-9) or on the other end of the neuron in the somatodendritic area (Figure 4-10). In both cases, occupancy of these D_2 receptors provides negative feedback input, or a braking action upon the release of dopamine from the presynaptic neuron.

Key dopamine pathways in the brain

The five dopamine pathways in the brain are shown in Figure 4-11. They include the mesolimbic dopamine pathway, the mesocortical dopamine pathway, the nigrostriatal dopamine pathway, the tuberoinfundibular dopamine pathway, and a fifth pathway that innervates the thalamus.

The dopamine hypothesis of schizophrenia: the mesolimbic dopamine pathway and positive symptoms of schizophrenia

The *mesolimbic dopamine pathway* projects from dopaminergic cell bodies in the ventral tegmental area of the brainstem to axon terminals in one of the limbic areas of the brain, namely the nucleus accumbens in the ventral striatum (Figure 4-11). This pathway is thought to have an important role in several emotional behaviors, including the positive symptoms of psychosis, such as delusions and hallucinations (Figure 4-12). The mesolimbic dopamine pathway also is important for motivation, pleasure, and reward.

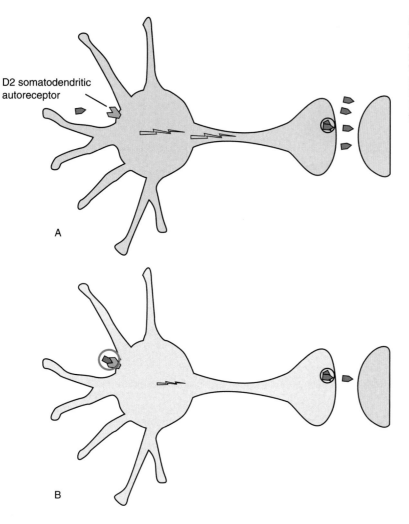

D2 somatodendritic
autoreceptor

A

B

Figure 4-10. Somatodendritic dopamine-2 autoreceptors. D_2 autoreceptors can also be located in the somatodendritic area, as shown here (A). When dopamine binds to the receptor here, it shuts off neuronal impulse flow in the dopamine neuron (see loss of lightning bolts in the neuron in B), and this stops further dopamine release.

For more than 40 years, it has been observed that diseases or drugs that increase dopamine will enhance or produce positive psychotic symptoms, whereas drugs that decrease dopamine will decrease or stop positive symptoms. For example, stimulant drugs such as amphetamine and cocaine release dopamine, and if given repetitively can cause a paranoid psychosis virtually indistinguishable from the positive symptoms of schizophrenia. Stimulant drugs are discussed in detail in subsequent chapters on treatment of attention deficit hyperactivity disorder, and on drug abuse.

All known antipsychotic drugs capable of treating positive psychotic symptoms are blockers of the dopamine D_2 receptor. Antipsychotic drugs are discussed in Chapter 5. These observations have been formulated into a theory of psychosis sometimes referred to as the "dopamine hypothesis of schizophrenia."

Perhaps a more precise modern designation is the "mesolimbic dopamine hypothesis of positive symptoms of schizophrenia," since it is believed that it is hyperactivity specifically in this particular dopamine pathway that mediates the positive symptoms of psychosis (Figure 4-13). Hyperactivity of the mesolimbic dopamine pathway hypothetically accounts for positive psychotic symptoms whether those symptoms are part of the illness of schizophrenia, or of drug-induced psychosis, or whether they are positive psychotic symptoms accompanying mania, depression, or dementia. Hyperactivity of mesolimbic dopamine neurons may also play a role in aggressive and hostile symptoms in schizophrenia and related illnesses, especially if serotonergic control of dopamine is aberrant in patients who lack impulse control. Although it is not known what causes this mesolimbic

Dopamine Pathways and Key Brain Regions

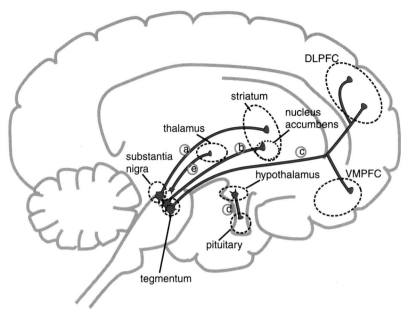

Figure 4-11. Five dopamine pathways in the brain. The neuroanatomy of dopamine neuronal pathways in the brain can explain the symptoms of schizophrenia as well as the therapeutic effects and side effects of antipsychotic drugs. (a) The **nigrostriatal dopamine pathway**, which projects from the substantia nigra to the basal ganglia or striatum, is part of the extrapyramidal nervous system and controls motor function and movement. (b) The **mesolimbic dopamine pathway** projects from the midbrain ventral tegmental area to the nucleus accumbens, a part of the limbic system of the brain thought to be involved in many behaviors such as pleasurable sensations, the powerful euphoria of drugs of abuse, as well as delusions and hallucinations of psychosis. (c) A pathway related to the mesolimbic dopamine pathway is the **mesocortical dopamine pathway**. It also projects from the midbrain ventral tegmental area but sends its axons to areas of the prefrontal cortex, where they may have a role in mediating cognitive symptoms (dorsolateral prefrontal cortex, DLPFC) and affective symptoms (ventromedial prefrontal cortex, VMPFC) of schizophrenia. (d) The fourth dopamine pathway of interest, the **tuberoinfundibular dopamine pathway**, projects from the hypothalamus to the anterior pituitary gland and controls prolactin secretion. (e) The fifth dopamine pathway arises from multiple sites, including the periaqueductal gray, ventral mesencephalon, hypothalamic nuclei, and lateral parabrachial nucleus, and it projects to the thalamus. Its function is not currently well known.

Mesolimbic Pathway

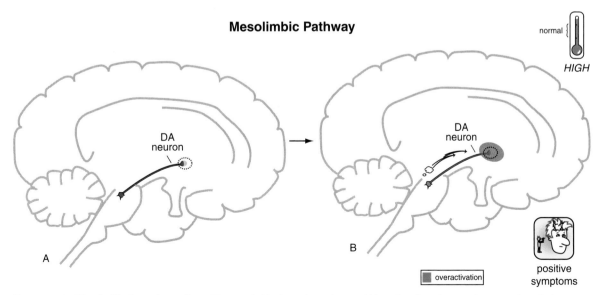

Figure 4-12. Mesolimbic dopamine pathway. The mesolimbic dopamine pathway, which projects from the ventral tegmental area in the brainstem to the nucleus accumbens in the ventral striatum (A), is involved in regulation of emotional behaviors and is believed to be the predominant pathway regulating positive symptoms of psychosis. Specifically, hyperactivity of this pathway is believed to account for delusions and hallucinations (B).

The Mesolimbic Dopamine Hypothesis of Positive Symptoms of Schizophrenia

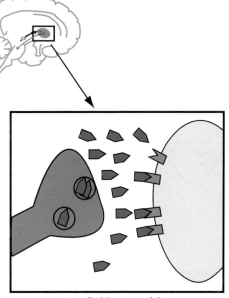

mesolimbic overactivity =
positive symptoms of schizophrenia

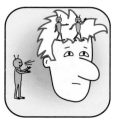

positive symptoms

Figure 4-13. Mesolimbic dopamine hypothesis. Hyperactivity of dopamine neurons in the mesolimbic dopamine pathway theoretically mediates the positive symptoms of psychosis such as delusions and hallucinations. This pathway is also involved in pleasure, reward, and reinforcing behavior, and many drugs of abuse interact here.

dopamine hyperactivity, current theories now state that it is the downstream consequence of dysfunction in prefrontal cortex and hippocampal glutamate activity, as will be discussed below.

The mesocortical dopamine pathway and cognitive, negative, and affective symptoms of schizophrenia

Another pathway also arising from cell bodies in the ventral tegmental area, but projecting to areas of the prefrontal cortex, is known as the *mesocortical dopamine pathway* (Figures 4-14 and 4-15). Branches of this pathway into the dorsolateral prefrontal cortex are hypothesized to regulate cognition and executive functions (Figure 4-14), whereas branches of this pathway into the ventromedial parts of the prefrontal cortex are hypothesized to regulate emotions and affect (Figure 4-15). The exact role of the mesocortical dopamine pathway in mediating symptoms of schizophrenia is still a matter of debate, but many researchers believe that cognitive and some negative symptoms of schizophrenia may be due to a *deficit* of dopamine activity in mesocortical projections to dorsolateral prefrontal cortex (Figure 4-14), whereas affective and other negative symptoms of schizophrenia may be due to a *deficit* of dopamine activity in mesocortical projections to ventromedial prefrontal cortex (Figure 4-15).

The behavioral deficit state suggested by negative symptoms certainly implies underactivity or lack of proper functioning of mesocortical dopamine projections that may be the consequence of neurodevelopmental abnormalities in the NMDA (*N*-methyl-D-aspartate) glutamate system, described in the next section. Whatever the cause, a corollary to the original DA hypothesis of schizophrenia now incorporates theories for the cognitive, negative, and affective symptoms, and might be more precisely designated as the "mesocortical dopamine hypothesis of cognitive, negative, and affective symptoms of schizophrenia," since it is believed that it is underactivity specifically in mesocortical projections to prefrontal cortex that mediate the cognitive, negative, and affective symptoms of schizophrenia (Figure 4-16).

Theoretically, increasing dopamine in the mesocortical dopamine pathway might improve negative, cognitive, and affective symptoms of schizophrenia. However, since there is hypothetically an excess of dopamine elsewhere in the brain – within the mesolimbic dopamine pathway – any further increase of dopamine in that pathway would actually worsen positive symptoms. Thus, this state of affairs for dopamine activity in the brain of patients with schizophrenia poses a therapeutic dilemma: how do you

Mesocortical Pathway to DLPFC

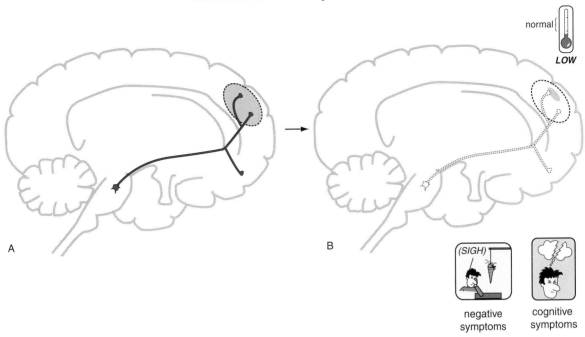

Figure 4-14. Mesocortical pathway to dorsolateral prefrontal cortex. Another major dopaminergic pathway is the mesocortical dopamine pathway, which projects from the ventral tegmental area to the prefrontal cortex (A). Projections specifically to the dorsolateral prefrontal cortex (DLPFC) are believed to be involved in the negative and cognitive symptoms of schizophrenia. In this case, expression of these symptoms is thought to be associated with hypoactivity of this pathway (B).

Mesocortical Pathway to VMPFC

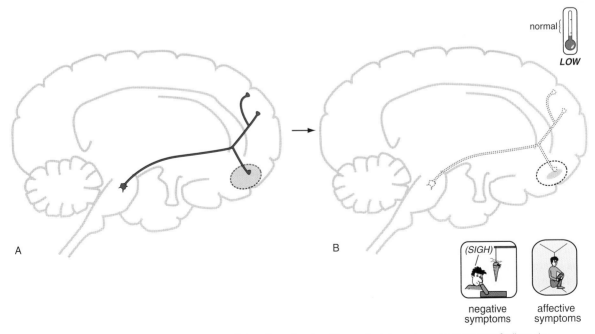

Figure 4-15. Mesocortical pathway to ventromedial prefrontal cortex. Mesocortical dopamine projections specifically to the ventromedial prefrontal cortex (VMPFC) are believed to mediate negative and affective symptoms associated with schizophrenia (A). These symptoms are believed to arise from hypoactivity in this pathway (B).

The Mesocortical Dopamine Hypothesis of Cognitive, Negative, and Affective Symptoms of Schizophrenia

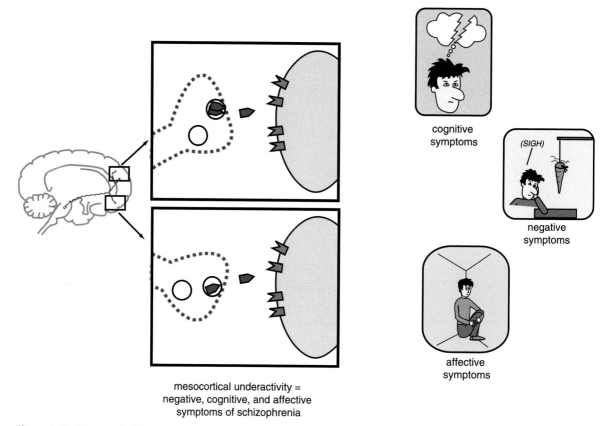

cognitive symptoms

negative symptoms

affective symptoms

mesocortical underactivity =
negative, cognitive, and affective
symptoms of schizophrenia

Figure 4-16. Mesocortical dopamine hypothesis of negative, cognitive, and affective symptoms of schizophrenia. Hypoactivity of dopamine neurons in the mesocortical dopamine pathway theoretically mediates the cognitive, negative, and affective symptoms of schizophrenia.

increase dopamine in the mesocortical pathway while simultaneously decreasing dopamine activity in the mesolimbic dopamine pathway? The extent to which atypical antipsychotics have provided a solution to this therapeutic dilemma will be discussed in Chapter 5.

Mesolimbic dopamine pathway, reward and negative symptoms

When a patient with schizophrenia loses motivation and interest, and has anhedonia and lack of pleasure, such symptoms could also implicate a deficient functioning of the mesolimbic dopamine pathway, not just deficient functioning in the mesocortical dopamine pathway. This idea is supported by observations that treating patients with antipsychotics, particularly the conventional antipsychotics, can produce a worsening of negative symptoms and a state of "neurolepsis" that looks very much like negative symptoms of schizophrenia. Since the prefrontal cortex does not have a high density of D_2 receptors, this implicates possible deficient functioning within the mesolimbic dopamine system causing inadequate reward mechanisms, exhibited as behaviors such as anhedonia and drug abuse, as well as negative symptoms, exhibited as lack of rewarding social interactions, and lack of general motivation and interest. Perhaps the much higher incidence of substance abuse in schizophrenia than in healthy adults, especially of nicotine but also of stimulants and other substances of abuse, could be partially explained as an attempt to boost the function of defective mesolimbic dopaminergic pleasure centers, perhaps at the cost of activating positive symptoms.

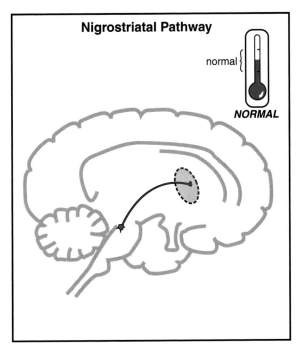

Figure 4-17. Nigrostriatal dopamine pathway. The nigrostriatal dopamine pathway projects from the substantia nigra to the basal ganglia or striatum. It is part of the extrapyramidal nervous system and plays a key role in regulating movements. When dopamine is deficient, it can cause parkinsonism with tremor, rigidity, and akinesia/bradykinesia. When DA is in excess, it can cause hyperkinetic movements such as tics and dyskinesias. In untreated schizophrenia, activation of this pathway is believed to be "normal."

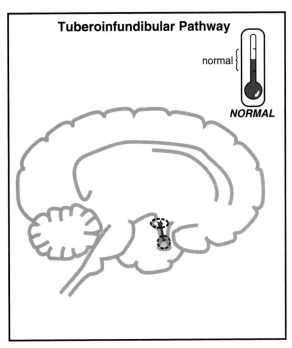

Figure 4-18. Tuberoinfundibular dopamine pathway. The tuberoinfundibular dopamine pathway from the hypothalamus to the anterior pituitary regulates prolactin secretion into the circulation. Dopamine inhibits prolactin secretion. In untreated schizophrenia, activation of this pathway is believed to be "normal."

Nigrostriatal dopamine pathway

Another key dopamine pathway in the brain is the nigrostriatal dopamine pathway, which projects from dopaminergic cell bodies in the brainstem substantia nigra via axons terminating in the basal ganglia or striatum (Figure 4-17). The nigrostriatal dopamine pathway is a part of the extrapyramidal nervous system, and controls motor movements. Deficiencies in dopamine in this pathway cause movement disorders including Parkinson's disease, characterized by rigidity, akinesia/bradykinesia (i.e., lack of movement or slowing of movement), and tremor. Dopamine deficiency in the basal ganglia also can produce akathisia (a type of restlessness), and dystonia (twisting movements especially of the face and neck). These movement disorders can be replicated by drugs that block D_2 receptors in this pathway, and this will be discussed briefly in Chapter 5.

Hyperactivity of dopamine in the nigrostriatal pathway is thought to underlie various hyperkinetic movement disorders such as chorea, dyskinesias, and

tics. Chronic blockade of D_2 receptors in this pathway may result in a hyperkinetic movement disorder known as neuroleptic-induced tardive dyskinesia. This will also be discussed briefly in Chapter 5. In schizophrenia, the nigrostriatal pathway in untreated patients may be relatively preserved (Figure 4-17).

Tuberoinfundibular dopamine pathway

The dopamine neurons that project from hypothalamus to anterior pituitary are part of the tuberoinfundibular dopamine pathway (Figure 4-18). Normally, these neurons are active and *inhibit* prolactin release. In the postpartum state, however, the activity of these dopamine neurons is decreased. Prolactin levels can therefore rise during breastfeeding so that lactation will occur. If the functioning of tuberoinfundibular dopamine neurons is disrupted by lesions or drugs, prolactin levels can also rise. Elevated prolactin levels are associated with galactorrhea (breast secretions), amenorrhea (loss of ovulation and menstrual periods), and possibly other problems such as sexual dysfunction. Such problems can occur after treatment with many antipsychotic drugs that block

D_2 receptors, and will be discussed further in Chapter 5. In untreated schizophrenia, the function of the tuberoinfundibular pathway may be relatively preserved (Figure 4-18).

Thalamic dopamine pathway

Recently, a dopamine pathway that innervates the thalamus in primates has been described. It arises from multiple sites, including the periaqueductal gray matter, the ventral mesencephalon, various hypothalamic nuclei, and the lateral parabrachial nucleus (Figure 4-11). Its function is still under investigation, but it may be involved in sleep and arousal mechanisms by gating information passing through the thalamus to the cortex and other brain areas. There is no evidence at this point for abnormal functioning of this dopamine pathway in schizophrenia.

Glutamate

In recent years, the neurotransmitter glutamate has attained a key theoretical role in the hypothesized pathophysiology of schizophrenia, as well as in a number of other psychiatric disorders, including depression. It is also now a key target of novel psychopharmacologic agents for future treatments of schizophrenia and depression. In order to understand theories about glutamate in schizophrenia and other psychiatric disorders, how the malfunctioning of glutamate systems impacts dopamine systems in schizophrenia, and how glutamate systems might become important targets of new therapeutic drugs for schizophrenia, it is necessary to review the regulation of glutamate neurotransmission. Glutamate is the major excitatory neurotransmitter in the central nervous system and sometimes considered to be the "master switch" of the brain, since it can excite and turn on virtually all CNS neurons. The synthesis, metabolism, receptor regulation, and key pathways of glutamate are therefore critical to the functioning of the brain and will be reviewed here.

Glutamate synthesis

Glutamate or glutamic acid is a neurotransmitter which is an amino acid. Its predominant use is not as a neurotransmitter, but as an amino acid building block for protein biosynthesis. When used as a neurotransmitter, it is synthesized from glutamine in glia, which also assist in the recycling and regeneration of more glutamate following glutamate

release during neurotransmission. When glutamate is released from synaptic vesicles stored within glutamate neurons, it interacts with receptors in the synapse and is then taken up into neighboring glia by a reuptake pump known as an excitatory amino acid transporter (EAAT) (Figure 4-19A). The presynaptic glutamate neuron and the postsynaptic site of glutamate neurotransmission may also have EAATs (not shown in the figures), but these EAATs do not appear to play as important a role in glutamate recycling and regeneration as the EAATs in glia (Figure 4-19A).

After reuptake into glia, glutamate is converted into glutamine inside the glia by an enzyme known as glutamine synthetase (arrow 3 in Figure 4-19B). It is possible that glutamate is not simply reused, but rather converted into glutamine, to keep it in a pool for neurotransmitter use, rather than being lost into the pool for protein synthesis. Glutamine is released from glia by reverse transport out of them by a pump or transporter known as a specific neutral amino acid transporter, (SNAT, arrow 4 in Figure 4-19C). Glutamine may also be transported out of glia by a second transporter known as a glial alanine-serine-cysteine transporter or ASC-T (not shown). When glial SNATs and ASC-Ts operate in the inward direction, they transport glutamine and other amino acids into glia. Here, they are reversed so that glutamine can get out of the glia and hop a ride into a neuron via a different type of neuronal SNAT, operating inwardly in a reuptake manner (arrow 5 in Figure 4-19C).

Once inside the neuron, glutamine is converted back into glutamate for use as a neurotransmitter by an enzyme in mitochondria called glutaminase (arrow 6 in Figure 4-19D). Glutamate is then transported into synaptic vesicles via a vesicular glutamate transporter (vGluT, arrow 7 in Figure 4-19D) where it is stored for subsequent release during neurotransmission. Once it is released, glutamate's actions are stopped not by enzymatic breakdown, as in other neurotransmitter systems, but by removal by EAATs on neurons or glia, and the whole cycle is started again (Figures 4-19A through D).

Synthesis of glutamate cotransmitters glycine and D-serine

Glutamate systems are curious in that one of the key receptors for glutamate requires a cotransmitter in addition to glutamate in order to function.

Glutamate is Recycled and Regenerated: Part 1

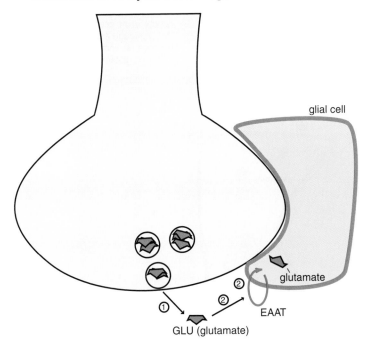

Figure 4-19A. Glutamate is recycled and regenerated, part 1. After release of glutamate from the presynaptic neuron (1), it is taken up into glial cells via the EAAT, or excitatory amino acid transporter (2).

Glutamate is Recycled and Regenerated: Part 2

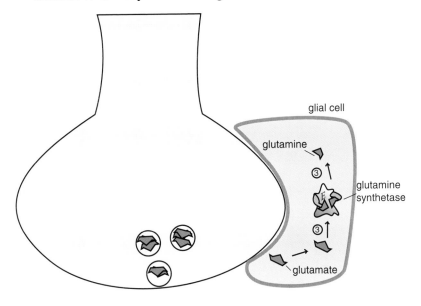

Figure 4-19B. Glutamate is recycled and regenerated, part 2. Once inside the glial cell, glutamate is converted into glutamine by the enzyme glutamine synthetase (3).

Glutamate is Recycled and Regenerated: Part 3

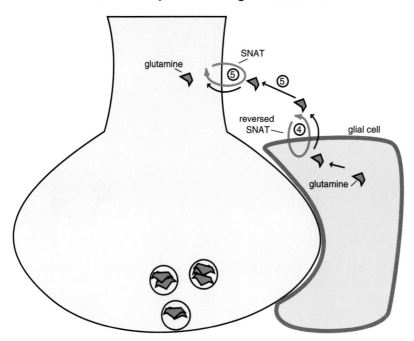

Figure 4-19C. Glutamate is recycled and regenerated, part 3. Glutamine is released from glial cells by a specific neutral amino acid transporter (glial SNAT) through the process of reverse transport (4), and then taken up by SNATs on glutamate neurons (5).

Glutamate is Recycled and Regenerated: Part 4

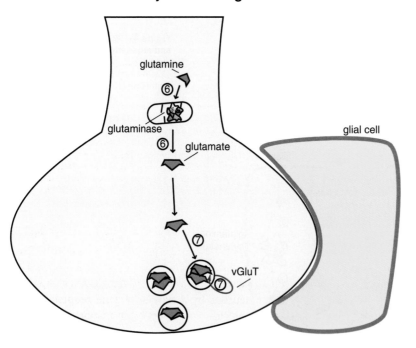

Figure 4-19D. Glutamate is recycled and regenerated, part 4. Glutamine is converted into glutamate within the presynaptic glutamate neuron by the enzyme glutaminase (6) and taken up into synaptic vesicles by the vesicular glutamate transporter (vGluT), where it is stored for future release (7).

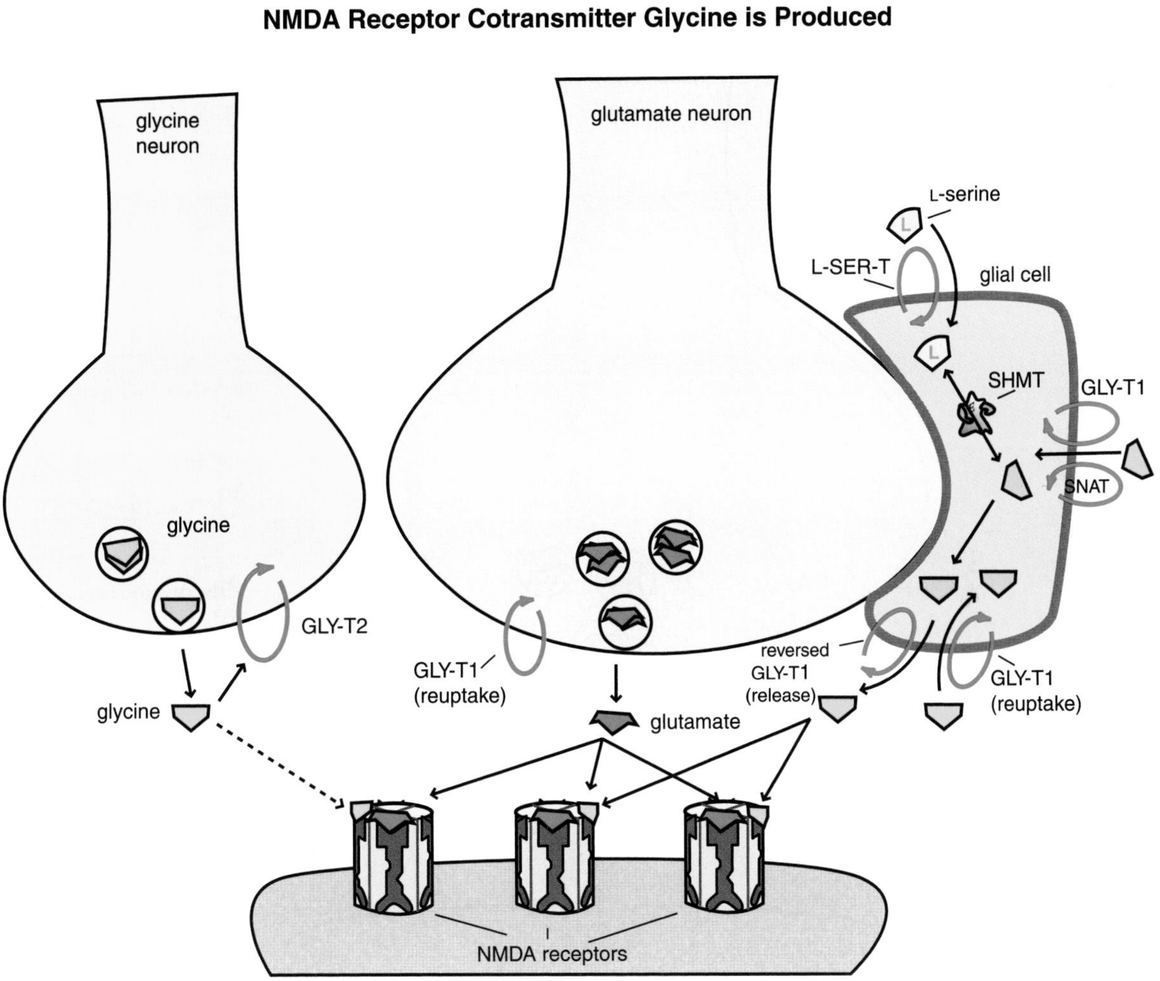

NMDA Receptor Cotransmitter Glycine is Produced

Figure 4-20. *N*-methyl-D-aspartate (NMDA) receptor cotransmitter glycine is produced. Glutamate's actions at NMDA receptors are dependent in part upon the presence of a cotransmitter, either glycine or D-serine. Glycine can be derived directly from dietary amino acids and transported into glial cells either by a glycine transporter (GlyT1) or by a specific neutral amino acid transporter (SNAT). Glycine can also be produced both in glycine neurons and in glial cells. Glycine neurons provide only a small amount of the glycine at glutamate synapses, because most of the glycine released by glycine neurons is used only at glycine synapses and then taken back up into presynaptic glycine neurons via the glycine 2 transporter (GlyT2) before much glycine can diffuse to glutamate synapses. Glycine produced by glial cells plays a larger role at glutamate synapses. Glycine is produced in glial cells when the amino acid L-serine is taken up into glial cells via the L-serine transporter (L-SER-T), and then converted into glycine by the enzyme serine hydroxymethyl-transferase (SHMT). Glycine from glial cells is released into the glutamate synapse through reverse transport by the glycine 1 transporter (GlyT1). Extracellular glycine is then transported back into glial cells via a reuptake pump, namely GlyT1.

That receptor is the NMDA (*N*-methyl-D-aspartate) receptor, described below, and the cotransmitter is either the amino acid glycine (Figure 4-20), or another amino acid closely related to glycine, known as D-serine (Figure 4-21).

Glycine is not known to be synthesized by glutamate neurons, so glutamate neurons must get the glycine they need for their NMDA receptors either from glycine neurons or from glia (Figure 4-20). Glycine neurons release glycine,

but they contribute only a small amount of glycine to glutamate synapses; glycine is unable to diffuse very far from neighboring glycine neurons because the glycine they release is taken back up into those neurons by a type of glycine reuptake pump known as the type 2 glycine transporter or GlyT2 (Figure 4-20).

Thus, neighboring glia are thought to be the source of most of the glycine available for glutamate synapses. Glycine itself can be taken up into glia as

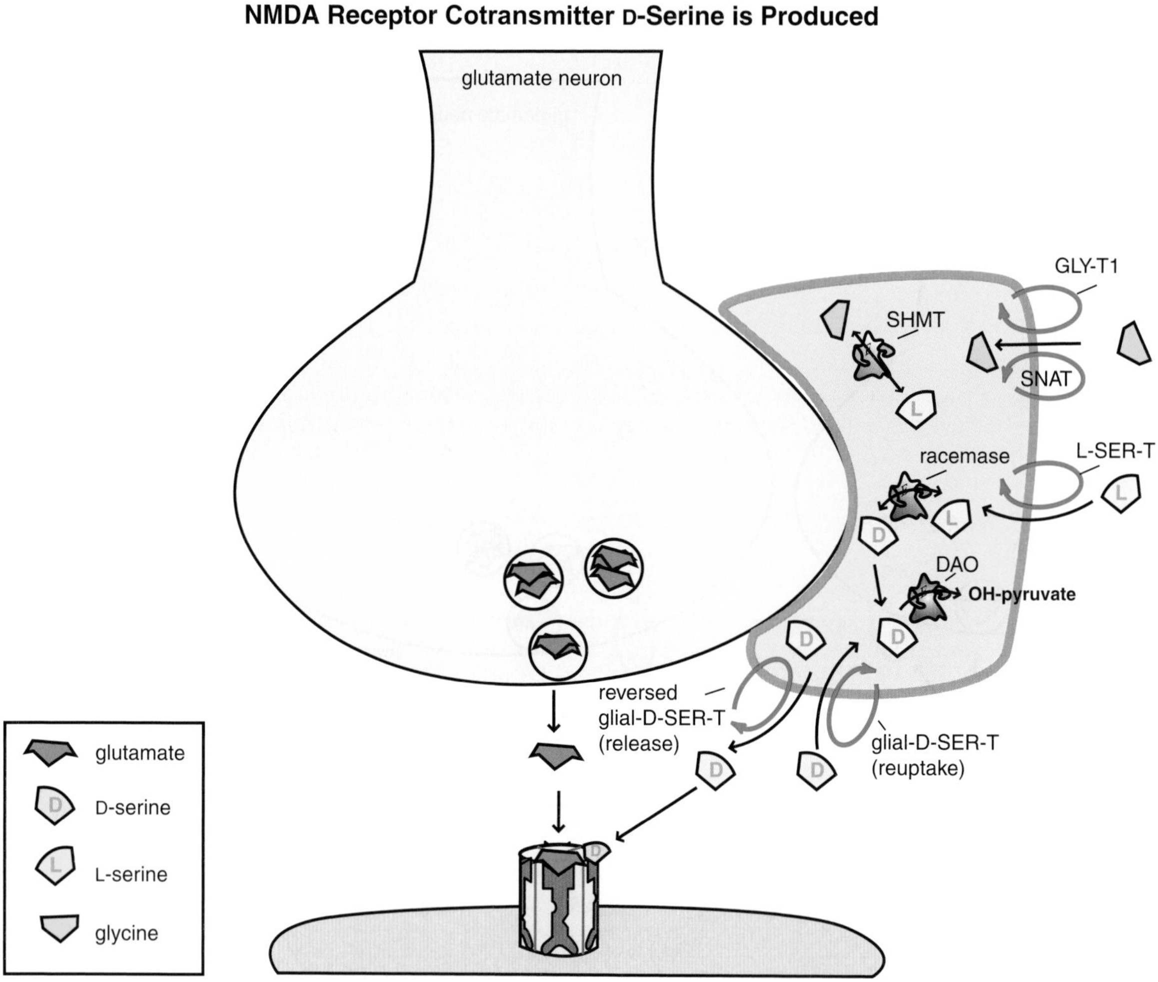

NMDA Receptor Cotransmitter D-Serine is Produced

Figure 4-21. NMDA receptor cotransmitter D-serine is produced. Glutamate requires the presence of either glycine or D-serine at NMDA receptors in order to exert some of its effects there. In glial cells, the enzyme serine racemase converts L-serine into D-serine, which is then released into the glutamate synapse via reverse transport on the glial D-serine transporter (glial D-SER-T). L-Serine's presence in glial cells is a result either of its transport there via the L-serine transporter (L-SER-T) or of its conversion into L-serine from glycine via the enzyme serine hydroxymethyl-transferase (SHMT). Once D-serine is released into the synapse, it is taken back up into the glial cell by a reuptake pump called D-SER-T. Excess D-serine within the glial cell can be destroyed by the enzyme D-amino acid oxidase (DAO), which converts D-serine into hydroxypyruvate (OH-pyruvate).

well as into glutamate neurons from the synapse by a type 1 glycine transporter or GlyT1 (Figure 4-20). Glycine can also be taken up into glia by a glial SNAT (specific neutral amino acid transporter). Glycine is not known to be stored within synaptic vesicles of glia, but as we will learn below, the companion neurotransmitter D-serine is thought possibly to be stored within some type of synaptic vesicle within glia. Glycine in the cytoplasm of glia is nevertheless somehow available for release into synapses, and it escapes from glial cells by riding outside them and into the glutamate synapse on a reversed GlyT1 transporter

(Figure 4-20). Once outside, glycine can get right back into the glia by an inwardly directed GlyT1, which functions as a reuptake pump and is the main mechanism responsible for terminating the action of synaptic glycine (Figure 4-20). GlyT1 transporters are probably also located on the glutamate neuron, but any release or storage from the glutamate neuron is not well characterized (Figure 4-20). Later, in Chapter 5, we will discuss novel treatments for schizophrenia that boost glycine action, and thus glutamate action, at NMDA receptors. Such treatments are in clinical testing and include inhibitors of the key glycine transporter GlyT1, called selective glycine reuptake inhibitors or SGRIs.

Glycine can also be synthesized from the amino acid L-serine, derived from the extracellular space, bloodstream, and diet, transported into glialcells by an L-serine transporter (L-SER-T), and converted from L-serine into glycine by the glial enzyme serine hydroxymethyl-transferase (SHMT) (Figure 4-20). This enzyme works in both directions, either converting L-serine into glycine, or glycine into L-serine.

How is the cotransmitter D-serine produced? D-Serine is unusual in that it is a D-amino acid, whereas the 20 known essential amino acids are all L-amino acids, including D-serine's mirror-image amino acid L-serine. It just so happens that D-serine has high affinity for the glycine site on NMDA receptors, and that glia are equipped with an enzyme called D-serine racemase that can convert regular L-serine into the neurotransmitting amino acid D-serine and vice versa (Figure 4-21). Thus, D-serine can be derived either from glycine or from L-serine, both of which can be transported into glia by their own transporters, and then glycine converted to L-serine by the enzyme SHMT, and finally L-serine converted into D-serine by the enzyme D-serine racemase (Figure 4-21). Interestingly, the D-serine so produced may be stored in some sort of vesicle in glia for subsequent release on a reversed glial D-serine transporter (D-SER-T) for neurotransmitting purposes at glutamate synapses containing NMDA receptors. D-Serine's actions are not only terminated by synaptic reuptake via the inwardly acting glial D-SER-T, but also by an enzyme, D-amino acid oxidase (DAO), that converts D-serine into inactive hydroxypyruvate (Figure 4-21). Below, we will discuss how the brain makes an activator of DAO, known not surprisingly as D-amino acid oxidase activator or DAOA. The gene that makes DAOA may be one of the important regulatory genes that contribute to the genetic basis of schizophrenia, as will be explained below in the section on the neurodevelopmental hypothesis of schizophrenia.

Glutamate receptors

There are several types of glutamate receptors (Figure 4-22 and Table 4-7), including the neuronal presynaptic reuptake pump (EAAT or excitatory amino acid transporter) and the vesicular transporter for glutamate into synaptic vesicles (vGluT), both of which are types of receptors. The properties of various transporters are discussed in Chapter 2. Shown also on the presynaptic neuron as well as the postsynaptic neuron are metabotropic glutamate receptors (Figure 4-22). Metabotropic glutamate receptors are those glutamate receptors which are linked to G proteins. The properties of G-protein-linked receptors are also discussed in Chapter 2.

There are at least eight subtypes of metabotropic glutamate receptors, organized into three separate groups (Table 4-7). Research suggests that group II and group III metabotropic receptors can occur presynaptically, where they function as autoreceptors to block glutamate release (Figure 4-23). Drugs that stimulate these presynaptic autoreceptors as agonists may therefore *reduce* glutamate release and be potentially useful as anticonvulsants and mood stabilizers, and may also protect against glutamate excitotoxicity, as will be explained below. Group I metabotropic glutamate receptors may be located predominantly postsynaptically, where they hypothetically interact with other postsynaptic glutamate receptors to facilitate and strengthen responses mediated by ligand-gated ion-channel receptors for glutamate during excitatory glutamatergic neurotransmission (Figure 4-22).

NMDA (*N*-methyl-D-aspartate), AMPA (α-amino-3-hydroxy-5-methyl-4-isoxazole-propionic acid), and kainate receptors for glutamate, named after the agonists that selectively bind to them, are all members of the ligand-gated ion-channel family of receptors (Figure 4-22 and Table 4-7). These ligand-gated ion channels are also known as ionotropic receptors and ion-channel-linked receptors. The properties of ligand-gated ion channels are discussed in Chapter 3. They tend to be postsynaptic and work together to modulate excitatory postsynaptic neurotransmission triggered by glutamate. Specifically, AMPA and kainate receptors may mediate fast, excitatory neurotransmission, allowing sodium to enter the neuron to depolarize it (Figure 4-24). NMDA receptors in the resting state are normally blocked by magnesium, which plugs a calcium channel (Figure 4-25). NMDA receptors are an interesting type of "coincidence detector" that can open to let calcium into the neuron to trigger postsynaptic actions from glutamate neurotransmission only when three things occur at the same time: glutamate occupies its binding site on the NMDA receptor, glycine or D-serine binds to its site on the NMDA receptor,

Glutamate Receptors

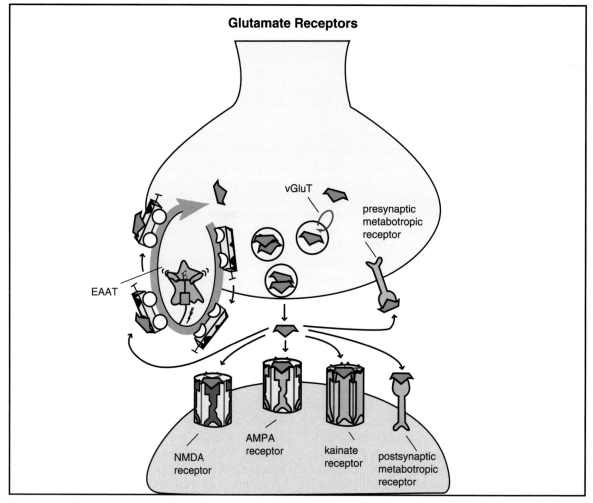

Figure 4-22. Glutamate receptors. Shown here are receptors for glutamate that regulate its neurotransmission. The excitatory amino acid transporter (EAAT) exists presynaptically and is responsible for clearing excess glutamate out of the synapse. The vesicular transporter for glutamate (vGluT) transports glutamate into synaptic vesicles, where it is stored until used in a future neurotransmission. Metabotropic glutamate receptors (linked to G proteins) can occur either pre- or postsynaptically. Three types of postsynaptic glutamate receptors are linked to ion channels, and are known as ligand-gated ion channels: N-methyl-ᴅ-aspartate (NMDA) receptors, α-amino-3-hydroxy-5-methyl-4-isoxazole-propionic acid (AMPA) receptors, and kainate receptors, all named for the agonists that bind to them.

and depolarization occurs, allowing the magnesium plug to be removed (Figures 4-25 and 4-26). Some of the many important signals by NMDA receptors that are activated when NMDA calcium channels are opened include long-term potentiation and synaptic plasticity, as will be explained later in this chapter.

Key glutamate pathways in the brain

Glutamate is a ubiquitous excitatory neurotransmitter that seems to be able to excite nearly any neuron in the brain. That is why it is sometimes called the "master switch." Nevertheless, there are about a half-dozen specific glutamatergic pathways that are of particular relevance to psychopharmacology, and especially to the pathophysiology of schizophrenia (Figure 4-27). They are:

(a) Cortico-brainstem
(b) Cortico-striatal
(c) Hippocampal-striatal
(d) Thalamo-cortical

Table 4-7 Glutamate receptors

Metabotropic			
Group I	mGluR1 mGluR5		
Group II	mGluR2 mGluR3		
Group III	mGluR4 mGluR6 mGluR7 mGluR8		

Ionotropic (ligand-gated ion channels; ion-channel-linked receptors)

Functional class	Gene family	Agonists	Antagonists
AMPA	GluR1 GluR2 GluR3 GluR4	Glutamate AMPA Kainate	
Kainate	GluR5 GluR6 GluR7 KA1 KA2	Glutamate Kainate	
NMDA	NR1 NR2A NR2B NR2C NR2D	Glutamate Aspartate NMDA	MK801 Ketamine PCP (phencyclidine)

(e) Cortico-thalamic

(f) Cortico-cortical (direct)

(g) Cortico-cortical (indirect)

(a) **Cortico-brainstem glutamate pathways.**
A very important descending glutamatergic pathway projects from cortical pyramidal neurons to brainstem neurotransmitter centers, including the raphe for serotonin, the ventral tegmental area (VTA) and substantia nigra for dopamine, and the locus coeruleus for norepinephrine (pathway a in Figure 4-27). This pathway is the cortico-brainstem glutamate pathway, and it is a key regulator of neurotransmitter release. Direct innervation of monoamine neurons in the brainstem by these excitatory cortico-brainstem glutamate neurons *stimulates* neurotransmitter release,

whereas indirect innervation of monoamine neurons by these excitatory cortico-glutamate neurons via GABA interneurons in the brainstem *blocks* neurotransmitter release.

(b) **Cortico-striatal glutamate pathways.** A second descending glutamatergic output from cortical pyramidal neurons projects to the striatal complex (pathway b in Figure 4-27). This pathway is known as the cortico-striatal glutamate pathway when it projects to the dorsal striatum, or the cortico-accumbens glutamate pathway when it projects to a specific area of the ventral striatum known as the nucleus accumbens. In either case, these descending glutamate pathways terminate on GABA neurons destined for a relay station in another part of the striatal complex called the globus pallidus.

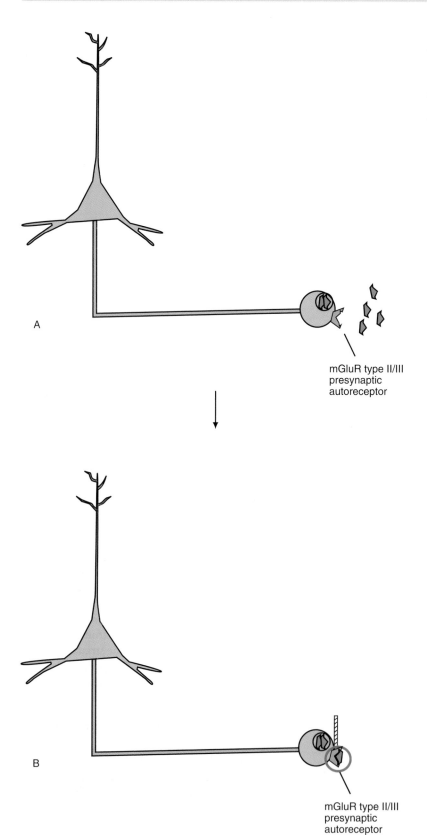

Figure 4-23. Metabotropic glutamate autoreceptors. Groups II and III metabotropic glutamate receptors can exist presynaptically as autoreceptors to regulate the release of glutamate. When glutamate builds up in the synapse (A), it is available to bind to the autoreceptor, which then inhibits glutamate release (B).

A

mGluR type II/III
presynaptic
autoreceptor

B

mGluR type II/III
presynaptic
autoreceptor

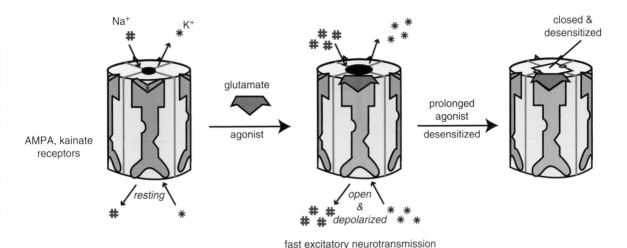

Figure 4-24. Glutamate at AMPA and kainate receptors. Unlike NMDA receptors, AMPA and kainate receptors require only glutamate to bind in order for the channel to open. This leads to fast excitatory neurotransmission and membrane depolarization. Sustained binding of the agonist glutamate will lead to receptor desensitization, causing the channel to close and be transiently unresponsive to agonist.

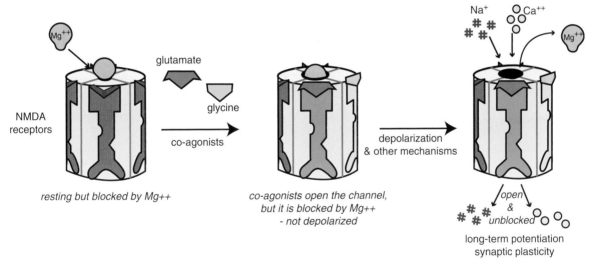

Figure 4-25. Magnesium as a negative allosteric modulator. Magnesium is a negative allosteric modulator (NAM) at NMDA glutamate receptors. Opening of NMDA glutamate receptors requires the presence of both glutamate and glycine, each of which binds to a different site on the receptor. When magnesium is also bound and the membrane is not depolarized, it prevents the effects of glutamate and glycine and thus does not allow the ion channel to open. In order for the channel to open, depolarization must remove magnesium while both glutamate and glycine are bound to their sites on the ligand-gated ion-channel complex.

(c) **Hippocampal-accumbens glutamate pathway.** Another key glutamate pathway projects from the hippocampus to the nucleus accumbens and is known as the hippocampal-accumbens glutamate pathway (c in Figure 4-27). Specific theories link this particular pathway to schizophrenia (see below). Like the cortico-striatal and cortico-accumbens glutamate pathways (b in Figure 4-27), the hippocampal

glutamate projection to the nucleus accumbens also terminates on GABA neurons there that in turn project to a relay station in the globus pallidus.

(d) **Thalamo-cortical glutamate pathway.** This pathway (d in Figure 4-27) brings information from the thalamus back into the cortex, often to process sensory information.

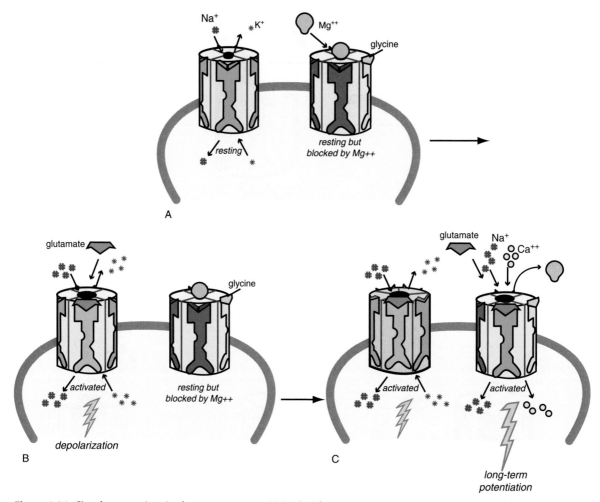

Figure 4-26. Signal propagation via glutamate receptors. (A) On the left is an AMPA receptor with its sodium channel in the resting state, allowing minimal sodium to enter the cell in exchange for potassium. On the right is an NMDA receptor with magnesium blocking the calcium channel and glycine bound to its site. (B) When glutamate arrives, it binds to the AMPA receptor, causing the sodium channel to open, thus increasing the flow of sodium into the dendrite and of potassium out of the dendrite. This causes the membrane to depolarize and triggers a postsynaptic nerve impulse. (C) Depolarization of the membrane removes magnesium from the calcium channel. This, coupled with glutamate binding to the NMDA receptor in the presence of glycine, causes the NMDA receptor to open and allow calcium influx. Calcium influx through NMDA receptors contributes to long-term potentiation, a phenomenon that may be involved in long-term learning, synaptogenesis, and other neuronal functions.

(e) **Cortico-thalamic glutamate pathway.** A fifth glutamate pathway, known as the cortico-thalamic glutamate pathway, projects directly back to the thalamus (pathway e in Figure 4-27), where it may direct the manner in which neurons react to sensory information.

(f) **Direct cortico-cortical glutamate pathways.** Finally, a complex of many cortico-cortical glutamate pathways are present within the cortex (pathways f and g in Figure 4-27).

On the one hand, pyramidal neurons can excite each other within the cerebral cortex via direct synaptic input from their own neurotransmitter glutamate (f in Figure 4-27).

(g) **Indirect cortico-cortical glutamate pathways.** On the other hand, one pyramidal neuron can inhibit another via indirect input, namely via interneurons that release GABA (g in Figure 4-27).

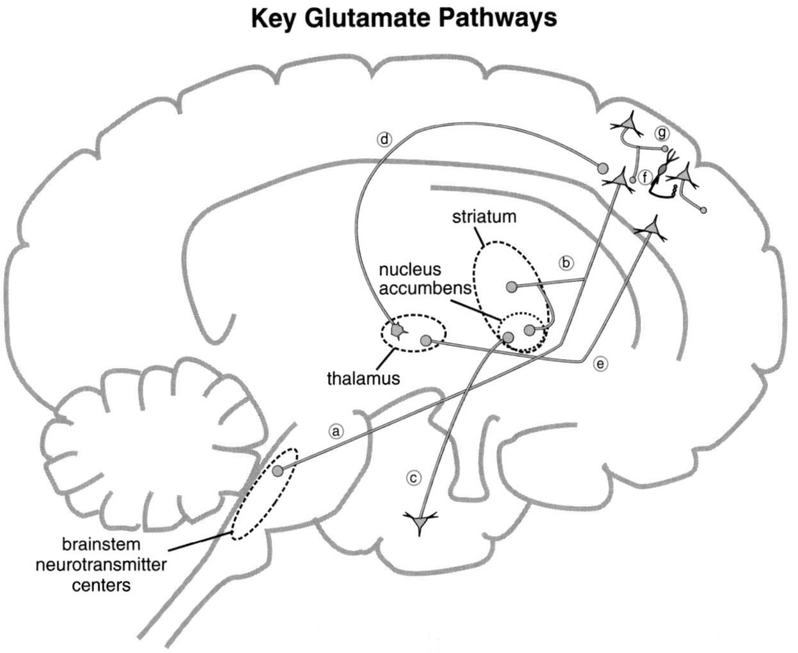

Key Glutamate Pathways

Figure 4-27. Glutamate pathways in the brain. Although glutamate can have actions at virtually all neurons in the brain, there are key glutamate pathways particularly relevant to schizophrenia. (a) The **cortico-brainstem glutamate projection** is a descending pathway that projects from cortical pyramidal neurons in the prefrontal cortex to brainstem neurotransmitter centers (raphe, locus coeruleus, ventral tegmental area, substantia nigra) and regulates neurotransmitter release. (b) Another descending glutamatergic pathway projects from the prefrontal cortex to the striatum (**cortico-striatal glutamate pathway**) and to the nucleus accumbens (cortico-accumbens glutamate pathway), and constitutes the "cortico-striatal" portion of cortico-striato-thalamic loops. (c) There is also a glutamatergic projection from the ventral hippocampus to the nucleus accumbens. (d) **Thalamo-cortical glutamate pathways** are pathways that ascend from the thalamus and innervate pyramidal neurons in the cortex. (e) **Cortico-thalamic glutamate pathways** descend from the prefrontal cortex to the thalamus. (f) Intracortical pyramidal neurons can communicate directly with each other via the neurotransmitter glutamate; these pathways are known as **cortico-cortical glutamatergic pathways**. (g) Intracortical pyramidal neurons can also communicate via GABAergic interneurons.

The NMDA hypofunction hypothesis of schizophrenia: ketamine and phencyclidine

A major current hypothesis for the cause of schizophrenia proposes that glutamate activity at NMDA receptors is hypofunctional due to abnormalities in the formation of glutamatergic NMDA synapses during neurodevelopment. This so-called "NMDA receptor hypofunction hypothesis of schizophrenia" arises in part from observations that when NMDA receptors are made hypofunctional by means of the NMDA receptor antagonists PCP (phencyclidine) or ketamine (Figure 4-28), this produces a psychotic condition in normal humans very similar to symptoms of schizophrenia. Hypothetically, genetic abnormalities also make NMDA receptors and their synapses hypofunctional in order to cause schizophrenia itself. Amphetamine, which releases dopamine, also produces a psychotic condition of delusions and hallucinations in normal humans similar to the positive symptoms of schizophrenia.

What is so attractive about the NMDA receptor hypofunction hypothesis of schizophrenia is that unlike amphetamine, which activates only positive symptoms, PCP and ketamine also mimic the cognitive, negative, and affective symptoms of schizophrenia such as social withdrawal and executive dysfunction. Another attractive aspect of the NMDA hypofunction hypothesis is that it can also explain the dopamine hypothesis of schizophrenia, namely, as a downstream consequence of hypofunctioning NMDA receptors.

The NMDA hypofunction hypothesis of schizophrenia: faulty NMDA synapses on GABA interneurons in prefrontal cortex

Although NMDA receptors and synapses are ubiquitous throughout the brain, and PCP or ketamine block all of them, a current leading theory of schizophrenia suggests that schizophrenia may be caused by neurodevelopmental abnormalities in the formation

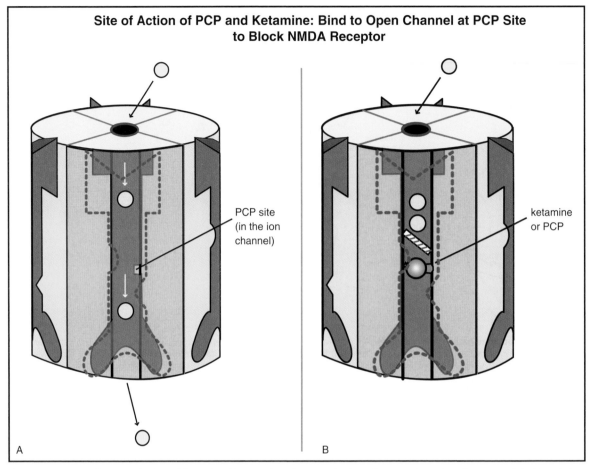

Figure 4-28. Site of action of PCP and ketamine. The anesthetic ketamine binds to the open channel conformation of the *N*-methyl-D-aspartate (NMDA) receptor. Specifically, it binds to a site within the calcium channel of this receptor, which is often termed the PCP site because it is also where phencyclidine (PCP) binds. Blockade of NMDA receptors may prevent the excitatory actions of glutamate.

of glutamate synapses at a specific site: namely, at certain GABA interneurons in the cerebral cortex (see g in Figure 4-27, and also box 1 in both Figure 4-29A and Figure 4-29B). Something appears to be wrong with the genetic programming of those particular GABA interneurons that can be identified in prefrontal cortex as containing a calcium binding protein called parvalbumin (Figure 4-29B). These parvalbumin-containing GABA interneurons appear to be faulty postsynaptic partners to incoming glutamate input from pyramidal neurons in prefrontal cortex, and to form defective NMDA receptor containing synaptic connections with incoming pyramidal neurons (Figure 4-29B, box 1; compare Figure 4-29A, box 1). Thus, they have hypofunctioning NMDA receptors on their dendrites, defective synapses between the glutamate neuronal axons and the GABA interneuronal dendrites, and thus faulty glutamatergic information coming in to the GABA interneuron (Figure 4-29B, box 1). This so-called "dysconnectivity" may be genetically programmed from a variety of faulty genes that all converge on the formation of these particular NMDA synapses.

Parvalbumin-containing GABA interneurons in the prefrontal cortex of patients with schizophrenia have other problems as a consequence of this dysconnectivity, in that they also have deficits in the enzyme that makes their own neurotransmitter GABA (namely, decreased activity of GAD67 (glutamic acid decarboxylase)), causing a compensatory increase in the postsynaptic amount of α_2-subunit-containing $GABA_A$ receptors in the postsynaptic axon initial segment of the pyramidal neurons they innervate (Figure 4-29B, box 2; compare Figure 4-29A, box 2).

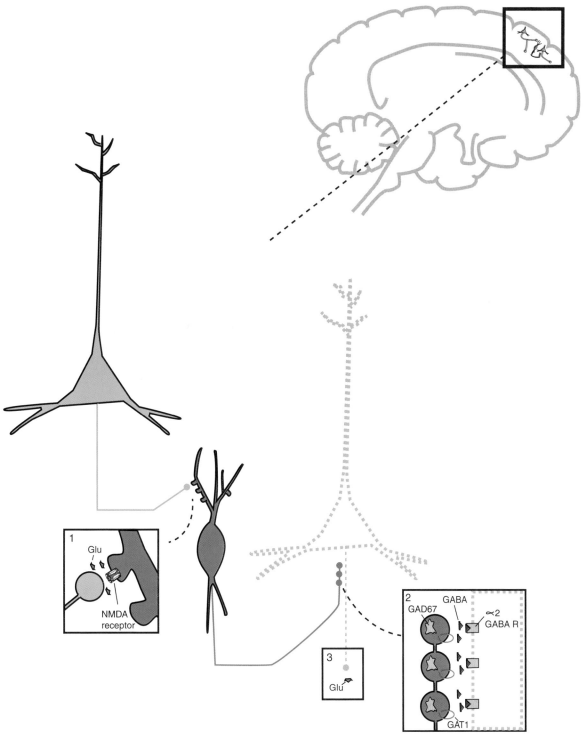

Figure 4-29A. Hypothetical site of glutamate dysfunction in schizophrenia, part 1. Shown here is a close-up of cortical pyramidal neurons communicating via GABAergic interneurons. (1) Glutamate is released from an intracortical pyramidal neuron and binds to an NMDA receptor on a GABAergic interneuron. (2) GABA is then released from the interneuron and binds to GABA receptors of the α₂ subtype that are located on the axon of another glutamate pyramidal neuron. (3) This inhibits the pyramidal neuron, thus reducing the release of downstream glutamate.

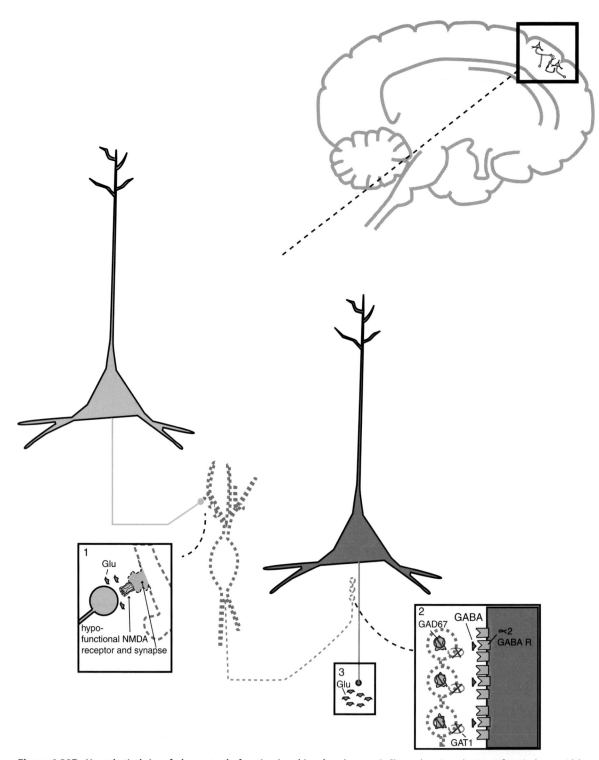

Figure 4-29B. Hypothetical site of glutamate dysfunction in schizophrenia, part 2. Shown here is a close-up of cortical pyramidal neurons communicating via GABAergic interneurons in the presence of hypofunctional NMDA receptors. (1) Glutamate is released from an intracortical pyramidal neuron. However, the NMDA receptor to which it binds is hypofunctional, preventing glutamate from exerting its full effects via the NMDA receptor. (2) This prevents GABA release from the interneuron; thus, stimulation of α_2 GABA receptors on the axon of another glutamate neuron does not occur. (3) When GABA does not bind to the α_2 GABA receptors on its axon, the pyramidal neuron is no longer inhibited. Instead, it is disinhibited and overactive, releasing excessive glutamate downstream.

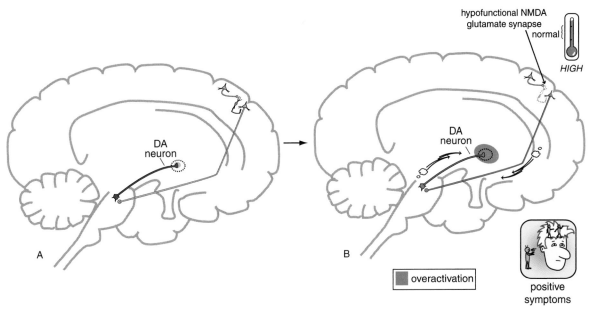

Figure 4-30. NMDA receptor hypofunction and positive symptoms of schizophrenia, part 1. (A) The cortical brainstem glutamate projection communicates with the mesolimbic dopamine pathway in the ventral tegmental area (VTA) to regulate dopamine release in the nucleus accumbens. (B) If NMDA receptors on cortical GABA interneurons are hypoactive, then the cortical brainstem pathway to the VTA will be overactivated, leading to excessive release of glutamate in the VTA. This will lead to excessive stimulation of the mesolimbic dopamine pathway and thus excessive dopamine release in the nucleus accumbens. This is the theoretical biological basis for the mesolimbic dopamine hyperactivity thought to be associated with the positive symptoms of psychosis.

What are the consequences of the hypothetical dysconnectivity of glutamate with these particular GABA interneurons? When parvalbumin-containing GABA interneurons fail to function properly, they do not adequately inhibit key glutamatergic pyramidal neurons in the prefrontal cortex, causing those glutamate neurons to become hyperactive (Figure 4-29B box 3; compare Figure 4-29A box 3). This hypothetically disrupts the functioning of downstream neurons, especially dopamine neurons (Figures 4-30B, 4-31B, and 4-32B, explained below). So, one sick synapse in a neuronal circuit can affect the whole circuit, from GABA interneuron and the glutamate neurons it innervates, to downstream dopamine neurons and beyond.

Linking the NMDA hypofunction hypothesis of schizophrenia with the dopamine hypothesis of schizophrenia: positive symptoms

A complex set of interactions allows glutamate to determine dopamine release. Most relevant to schizophrenia are the glutamate pathways that regulate the mesolimbic and mesocortical dopamine pathways shown in Figures 4-11 through 4-16. Cortico-brainstem glutamate pathways regulate the output of glutamate

from the cortex to the brainstem neurotransmitter center known as the ventral tegmental area (VTA) for both the mesolimbic dopamine projection (pathway a in Figure 4-27 and in Figure 4-30A) and for the mesocortical dopamine projections (pathway a in Figure 4-27 and in Figure 4-32A).

First, we will discuss the glutamate regulation of mesolimbic dopamine neurons (Figure 4-30). It appears that the cortico-brainstem glutamate neurons that innervate only the dopamine neurons projecting from the VTA to the nucleus accumbens – i.e., the mesolimbic dopamine pathway – *directly* innervate those specific dopamine neurons (Figure 4-30A), and thus *stimulate* them. You can imagine what would happen if these upstream glutamate neurons were too active (Figures 4-29B and 4-30B): they would cause hyperactivity of the downstream mesolimbic dopamine neurons (Figure 4-30B). This is exactly what is hypothesized to be happening in schizophrenia. The dopamine hyperactivity of these downstream mesolimbic dopamine neurons is associated with the positive symptoms of schizophrenia but is actually caused hypothetically by dysconnectivity in upstream glutamate neurons, namely, defective and hypofunctional neurodevelopmental glutamate innervation of parvalbumin-containing

111

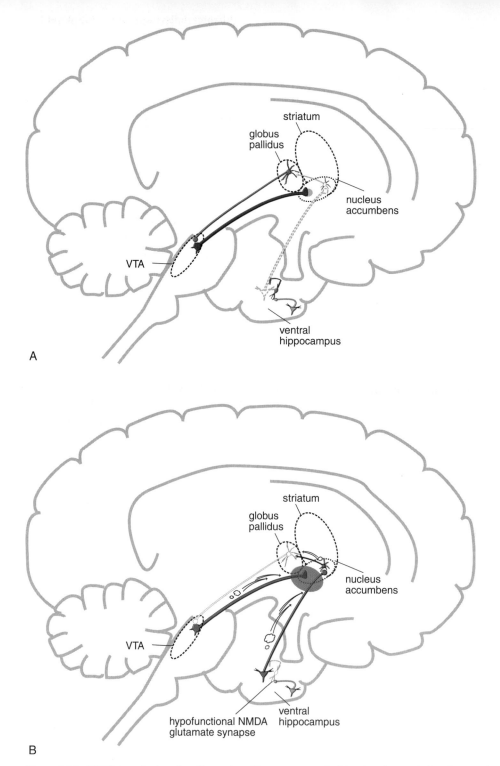

Figure 4-31. NMDA receptor hypofunction and positive symptoms of schizophrenia, part 2. Hypofunctional NMDA receptors at glutamatergic synapses in the ventral hippocampus can also contribute to mesolimbic dopamine hyperactivity. (A) Glutamate released in the ventral hippocampus binds to NMDA receptors on a GABAergic interneuron, stimulating the release of GABA. The GABA binds at receptors on a pyramidal glutamate neuron that projects to the nucleus accumbens; this inhibits glutamate release there. The relative absence of glutamate in the nucleus accumbens allows for normal activation of a GABAergic neuron projecting to the globus pallidus, which in turn allows for normal activation of a GABAergic neuron projecting to the ventral tegmental area (VTA). This leads to normal activation of the mesolimbic dopamine pathway from the VTA to the nucleus accumbens. (B) If NMDA receptors on ventral hippocampal GABA interneurons are hypoactive, then the glutamatergic pathway to the nucleus accumbens will be overactivated, leading to excessive release of glutamate in the nucleus accumbens. This will lead to excessive stimulation of GABAergic neurons projecting to the globus pallidus, which in turn will inhibit release of GABA from the globus pallidus into the VTA. This will lead to disinhibition of the mesolimbic dopamine pathway and thus excessive dopamine release in the nucleus accumbens.

GABA interneurons at NMDA receptor-containing synapses (Figure 4-29B and 4-30B).

It is also possible that the dysconnectivity of upstream glutamate neurons in the *hippocampus* contributes to downstream mesolimbic dopamine hyperactivity via a four-neuron circuit (Figure 4-31A). That circuit consists of (1) the dysconnected and defective hippocampal parvalbumin-containing GABA interneuron, going to (2) the hippocampal glutamate neuron projecting to the nucleus accumbens; then that neuron projecting to two GABA spiny neurons in sequence, (3) the first GABA spiny neuron going from nucleus accumbens to globus pallidus, and finally (4) the second GABA spiny neuron going from globus pallidus to VTA (Figure 4-31A). Loss of adequate glutamate function at parvalbumin-containing GABA interneurons in the hippocampus could lead to hyperactive glutamate output from glutamate neurons that project by this circuit to the mesolimbic dopamine neurons in the VTA, with consequential dopamine hyperactivity and positive symptoms of schizophrenia (Figure 4-31B). Stimulating two GABA neurons in

sequence has the net effect of disinhibition (inhibition of inhibition) at the VTA, the same result as direct stimulation (which was illustrated for the prefrontal cortex in Figure 4-30A). The bottom line is that excessive upstream glutamate output from either the prefrontal cortex or the hippocampus may contribute to downstream dopamine hyperactivity and positive symptoms of schizophrenia.

Linking the NMDA hypofunction hypothesis of schizophrenia with the dopamine hypothesis of schizophrenia: negative symptoms

Next, we will discuss the glutamate regulation of mesocortical dopamine neurons (Figure 4-32). It appears that different cortico-brainstem glutamate neurons regulate those unique dopamine neurons in the VTA that project only to the prefrontal cortex – the mesocortical dopamine pathway (Figure 4-32A) – than regulate those dopamine neurons in the VTA that project to the nucleus accumbens as the mesolimbic dopamine pathway (Figure 4-30A). Thus, different populations of

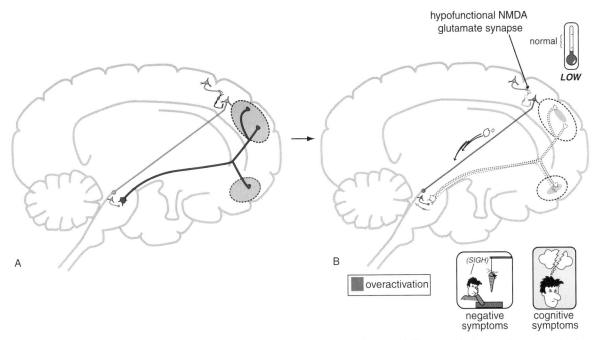

Figure 4-32. NMDA receptor hypofunction and negative symptoms of schizophrenia. (A) The cortical brainstem glutamate projection communicates with the mesocortical dopamine pathway in the ventral tegmental area (VTA) via pyramidal interneurons, thus regulating dopamine release in the prefrontal cortex. (B) If NMDA receptors on cortical GABA interneurons are hypoactive, then the cortical brainstem pathway to the VTA will be overactivated, leading to excessive release of glutamate in the VTA. This will lead to excessive stimulation of the brainstem pyramidal neurons, which in turn leads to inhibition of mesocortical dopamine neurons. This reduces dopamine release in the prefrontal cortex and is the theoretical biological basis for the negative symptoms of psychosis.

glutamate neurons regulate the different populations of dopamine neurons. Cortico-brainstem glutamate neurons destined to regulate mesocortical dopamine neurons in the VTA do not directly innervate them (Figure 4-32A) as do the cortico-brainstem glutamate neurons destined to regulate mesolimbic dopamine neurons in the VTA (Figure 4-30A). Instead, the glutamate neurons regulating mesocortical dopamine neurons do so by indirectly innervating an inhibitory GABA interneuron that itself innervates the mesocortical dopamine neurons (Figure 4-32A). Thus, activation of these particular glutamate neurons leads first to activation of GABA interneurons, which then inhibit mesocortical dopamine neurons (Figure 4-32A). You can imagine what would happen if these glutamate neurons were too active (Figure 4-29B and 4-32B): hypoactivity of the mesocortical dopamine neurons (Figure 4-31B). This is exactly what is hypothesized to be occurring in schizophrenia. The dopamine hypoactivity of these mesocortical dopamine neurons is associated with the negative and cognitive symptoms of schizophrenia. It is hypothetically caused by the same upstream dysconnectivity of glutamate with GABA interneurons that causes the hyperactivity of mesolimbic dopamine neurons, namely, the neurodevelopmental abnormality in glutamate innervation of parvalbumin-containing GABA interneurons at their NMDA synapses (Figures 4-29B and 4-30B). Only in this case, it is affecting a different population of glutamate neurons in the prefrontal cortex and with different downstream consequences: namely, production of negative and cognitive symptoms of schizophrenia rather than positive symptoms.

Different populations of cortico-brainstem glutamate projections thus regulate the release of dopamine from both the mesocortical and the mesolimbic dopamine projections, although it appears that this regulation is the opposite for the glutamate neurons that regulate the mesolimbic dopamine pathway compared with the glutamate neurons that regulate the mesocortical dopamine pathway (compare Figures 4-30A and 4-32A), all due to the presence or absence of a GABA interneuron in the VTA.

Neurodevelopment and genetics in schizophrenia

What causes schizophrenia? Nature (i.e., genetics) or nurture (i.e., the environment or epigenetics)? The modern answer seems to be: both. Modern theories of schizophrenia no longer propose that a single gene causes schizophrenia (pure nature) (Figure 4-33) any more than a bad mother can cause schizophrenia (pure nurture). Instead, it seems more likely that schizophrenia is a "conspiracy" among many genes and many environmental stressors to cause abnormal development of brain connections throughout life. In fact, not only is there no single gene for schizophrenia (or for any other major psychiatric disorder) (Figure 4-33), there is no single gene for any specific psychiatric symptoms, behaviors, personalities, or temperaments (Figure 4-34). Genes do not code for mental illnesses or for psychiatric symptoms. Instead, genes code for proteins (Figure 4-35). Today, mental illnesses are thought to be linked in part to someone inheriting an entire portfolio of many genes that carry risk for a mental illness, especially in combination, and set the stage for a mental illness, but do not cause mental illness per se (Figure 4-36). In schizophrenia, multiple risk genes each hypothetically code for a subtle molecular abnormality (Figure 4-35), any one of which alone may be clinically silent until stress from the environment puts a load on these defective genes, and also causes even normal genes to be expressed when they should be silenced, or silenced when they should be expressed (Figure 4-36), a process called epigenetics (discussed briefly in Chapter 1: Figure 1-30).

Thus, mental illnesses are due not only to genes that are abnormal in their DNA and in the function of the proteins they code, but also to normal genes that make normal functioning proteins but are activated or silenced at the wrong times by the environment (nature and nurture, Figure 4-36). In the case of schizophrenia, the problem seems to be "dysconnectivity" of neurons, particularly in hippocampus and prefrontal cortex, and particularly at glutamate synapses with NMDA receptors that become hypofunctional. Stress, traumatic experiences, learning, sensory experiences, sleep deprivation, toxins, and drugs are all examples of how normal genes, such as those that regulate the formation and removal of synapses, are turned on and off by the environment (Figure 4-36). Cannabis use is a particularly malicious environmental stressor to those vulnerable to schizophrenia. These are all examples of the notion of "experience-dependent" development of synaptic connections, something that is hypothetically abnormal in schizophrenia, both from the experiences that the patient may have and from the genes that

Classic Theory: Genes Cause Mental Illness

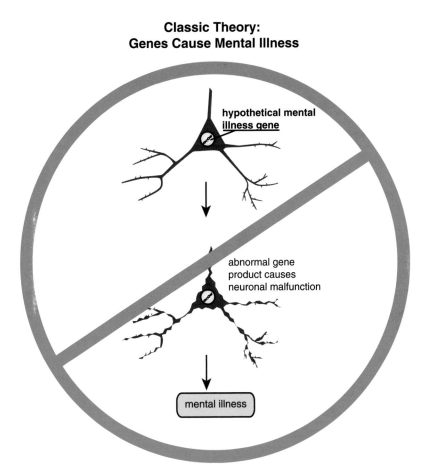

hypothetical mental illness gene

abnormal gene product causes neuronal malfunction

mental illness

Figure 4-33. Classic theory of inherited disease. According to the classic theory of inherited disease, a single abnormal gene can cause a mental illness. That is, an abnormal gene would produce an abnormal gene product, which, in turn, would lead to neuronal malfunction that directly causes a mental illness. However, no such gene has been identified, and there is no longer any expectation that such a discovery might be made. This is indicated by the red cross-out sign over this theory.

respond to these experiences. Thus, in schizophrenia an individual not only hypothetically inherits many abnormal genes, which may converge on the formation of NMDA-receptor-containing glutamate synapses, but theoretically also has notable experiences from a stressful environment that cause the abnormal expression or abnormal silencing of perfectly normal genes, in just the necessary sequence to cause this illness (Figure 4-36).

The best evidence that the environment is involved in schizophrenia is that only half of identical twins of patients with schizophrenia also have schizophrenia. Having identical genes is thus not enough to cause schizophrenia, but presumably epigenetics is also in play such that the affected twin not only expresses some abnormal genes that the unaffected twin might not express, but also expresses some normal genes at the wrong time and silences other normal genes at the wrong time, and together these factors cause schizophrenia in one twin but not the other.

The best evidence for the role of dysconnectivity genes in schizophrenia is the convergence of evidence implicating multiple genes that regulate not only neuronal connectivity in general, but glutamate synapse formation and removal in particular (Table 4-8). This includes *dysbindin, neuregulin, ErbB4*, and *DISC1*, among others (Figures 4-36 and 4-37). Dysbindin, also known as dystrobrevin binding protein 1, is involved in the formation of synaptic structures and regulation of the activity of the vesicular transporter for glutamate, vGluT. Neuregulin is involved in neuronal migration, genesis of glial cells, and subsequent myelination of neurons by glia. Neuregulin also activates an ErbB4 signaling system that is co-localized with NMDA receptors. These ErbB4 receptors also interact with the postsynaptic density of glutamate synapses, and may be involved in mediating the neuroplasticity triggered by NMDA receptors. Both dysbindin and neuregulin impact the formation and function of the postsynaptic density, a set of proteins

Symptom Endophenotype Model:
Genes Cause Psychiatric Symptoms, Behaviors, Personalities, and Temperaments

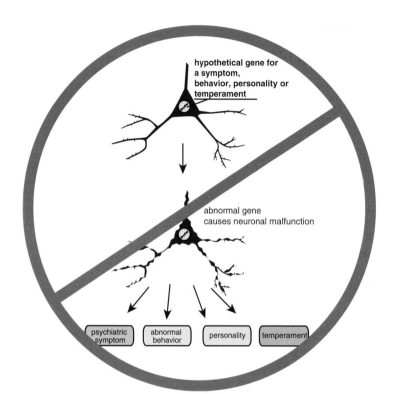

Figure 4-34. Symptom endophenotype model. Another theory, the symptom endophenotype model, posits that, rather than genes causing mental illness, genes instead cause individual symptoms, behaviors, personalities, or temperaments. Thus, an abnormal gene encoding for a symptom, behavior, or trait would cause neuronal malfunction leading to that symptom, behavior, or trait. However, no genes for personality or behavior have been identified, and there is no longer any expectation that such a discovery might be made – as indicated by the red cross-out sign over this theory.

that interacts with the postsynaptic membrane to provide both structural and functional regulatory elements for neurotransmission and for NMDA receptors. DISC1 (disrupted in schizophrenia 1) is aptly named for a disrupted gene linked to schizophrenia that makes a protein involved in neurogenesis, neuronal migration, and dendritic organization, and also affects the transport of synaptic vesicles into presynaptic glutamate nerve terminals and regulates cAMP signaling, which would affect the functions of glutamate neurotransmission mediated by metabotropic glutamate receptors.

Dysbindin, DISC1, and neuregulin all affect normal synapse formation. They all affect NMDA receptor number by altering NMDA receptor trafficking to the postsynaptic membrane, NMDA receptor tethering within that membrane, and NMDA receptor endocytosis that cycles receptors out of the postsynaptic membrane to remove them. Thus, it is easy to see how multiple genetic or epigenetic abnormalities in the expression of these particular genes could lead to dysconnectivity of glutamate neurons in schizophrenia (Figures 4-37 and 4-38).

Other risk genes implicate specific proteins that directly regulate glutamate synapses and, if abnormally expressed, could add to the misery of a disconnected and dysfunctional NMDA glutamate synapse (Figure 4-38). For example, the gene for DAOA (D-amino acid oxidase activator) codes for a protein that activates the enzyme DAO (D-amino acid oxidase). DAO degrades the co-transmitter D-serine that acts at glutamate synapses and at NMDA receptors. DAOA activates this DAO enzyme, so abnormalities in the gene for DAOA would be expected to alter the metabolism of D-serine. This in turn would alter glutamate neurotransmission at NMDA receptors. Another schizophrenia susceptibility gene active directly at glutamate synapses is RSG4 (regulator of G-protein signaling), and this gene product also impacts metabotropic glutamate receptor signaling through the G-protein-coupled signal transduction system.

Normally, when glutamate synapses are active, their NMDA receptors trigger an electrical phenomenon known as long-term potentiation (LTP).

Hypothetical Gene for Subtle Molecular Abnormalities

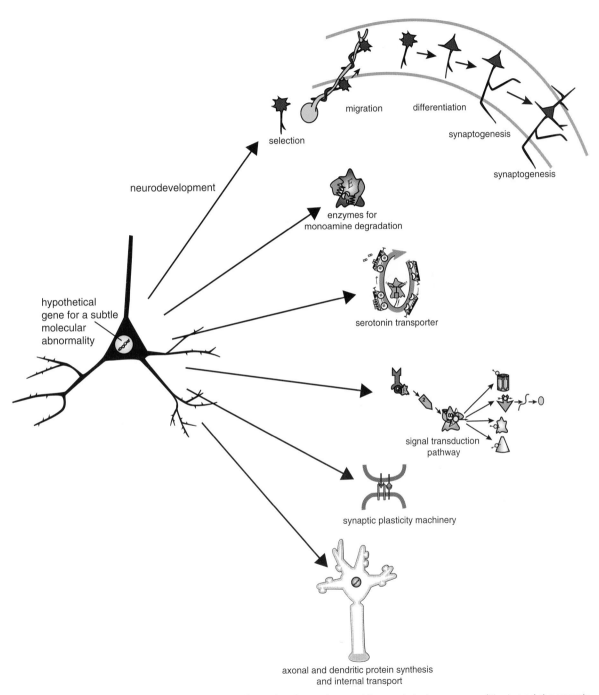

Figure 4-35. Subtle molecular abnormalities. Genes do not directly encode mental illnesses, behaviors, or personalities. Instead, they encode proteins. In some cases, genes may produce genetically altered proteins that code for subtle molecular abnormalities, which in turn may be linked to the development of psychiatric symptoms. Thus, a gene may code for an abnormality in the neurodevelopmental process or in the synthesis or activity of enzymes, transporters, receptors, components of signal transduction, synaptic plasticity machinery, and other neuronal components. Each subtle molecular abnormality may convey risk for the development of mental illness, rather than directly causing a mental illness.

Nature vs. Nurture: Genetics plus Epigenetics as the Stress - Diathesis Model of Schizophrenia:
too many genetic biases combined with too many stressors results in schizophrenia

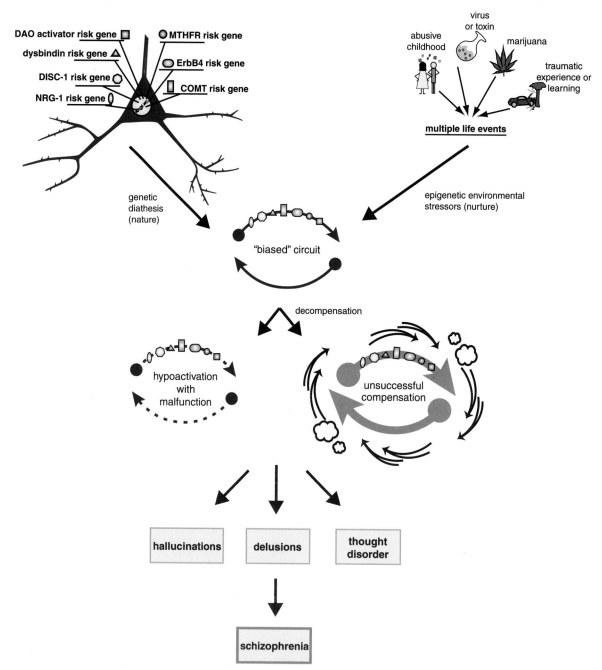

Figure 4-36. Stress–diathesis model of schizophrenia. Schizophrenia may occur as the result of both genetic (nature) and epigenetic (nurture) factors. That is, an individual with multiple genetic risk factors, combined with multiple stressors causing epigenetic changes, may not have sufficient backup mechanisms to compensate for inefficient information processing within a genetically "biased" circuit. The circuit may be unsuccessfully compensated by overactivation, or it may break down and not activate at all. In either case, the abnormal biological endophenotype would be associated with an abnormal behavioral phenotype, and thus with psychiatric symptoms such as hallucinations, delusions, and thought disorder. Such abnormal circuit activation would be potentially detectable with functional brain scanning, and psychiatric symptoms would be manifest on clinical interview.

Table 4-8 Susceptibility genes for schizophrenia

Genes for
Dysbindin (dystrobrevin binding protein 1 or DTNBP1)
Neuregulin (NRG1)
DISC1 (disrupted in schizophrenia 1)
DAOA (D-amino acid oxidase activator; G72/G30)
DAAO (D-amino acid oxidase)
RGS4 (regulator of G protein signaling 4)
COMT (catechol-O-methyl-transferase)
CHRNA7 (α_7-nicotinic cholinergic receptor)
GAD1 (glutamic acid decarboxylase 1)
GRM3 (mGluR$_3$)
PPP3CC
PRODH2
AKT1
ErbB4
FEZ1
MUTED
MRDS1 (OFCC1)
BDNF (brain-derived neurotrophic factor)
Nur77
MAO-A (monoamine oxidase A)
Spinophylin
Calcyon
Tyrosine hydroxylase
Dopamine D$_2$ receptor (D$_2$R)
Dopamine D$_3$ receptor (D$_3$R)

With the help of dysbindin, DISC1, and neuregulin, LTP leads to structural and functional changes of the synapse that make neurotransmission more efficient, sometimes called "strengthening" of synapses (Figure 4-39). This includes increasing the number of AMPA receptors. AMPA receptors are important for mediating excitatory neurotransmission and depolarization at glutamate synapses. Thus, more AMPA receptors can mean a "strengthened" synapse. Synaptic connections that are frequently used develop recurrent LTP and consequential robust neuroplastic influences, thus strengthening them according to the old saying "nerves that fire together wire together." However, if something is wrong with the genes that regulate synaptic strengthening, it is possible that this causes less effective use of these synapses, makes the NMDA receptors hypoactive, leading to ineffective LTP and fewer AMPA receptors trafficking into the postsynaptic neuron (Figure 4-39). Such a synapse would be "weak," theoretically causing inefficient information processing in its circuit and possibly also causing symptoms of schizophrenia. The strengthening or weakening of a glutamate synapse is an example of "activity-dependent" or "use-dependent" or "experience-dependent" regulation of NMDA receptors and functionality at glutamate synapses. This not only occurs when these synapses first form, but continues throughout life as a sort of ongoing remodeling in response to what experiences the individual has, and thus how much that synapse is used or neglected. Abnormalities in these continuing dynamics at NMDA receptors and glutamate synapses may explain why the course of schizophrenia is progressive and changes over time for most patients, namely, from an asymptomatic period, to a prodrome, to a first break psychosis with robust treatment responsiveness, to multiple psychotic episodes with declining treatment responsiveness, to a state of pervasive negative and cognitive symptoms without recovery.

Another important aspect of synaptic strength is that it likely determines whether a given synapse is eliminated or maintained. Specifically, "strong" synapses with efficient NMDA neurotransmission and many AMPA receptors survive whereas "weak" synapses with few AMPA receptors may be targets for elimination (Figure 4-39). This normally shapes the brain's circuits so that the most critical synapses are not only strengthened but also survive the ongoing selection process, keeping the most efficient and most frequently utilized synapses, while eliminating inefficient and rarely utilized synapses. However, if critical synapses are not adequately strengthened in schizophrenia, it could lead to their wrongful elimination, causing dysconnectivity that disrupts information flow from circuits now deprived of synaptic connections where communication needs to be efficient (Figure 4-39). Competitive elimination of "weak" but critical synapses during adolescence could even explain why schizophrenia has onset at this time. Normally, almost half of the brain's synapses are eliminated in adolescence (Figure 4-40). In adulthood, you may lose (and replace elsewhere) about 7% of the synapses in your cortex every week! If abnormalities in genes for dysbindin, neuregulin, and/or DISC1 lead to

Overview of Neurodevelopment

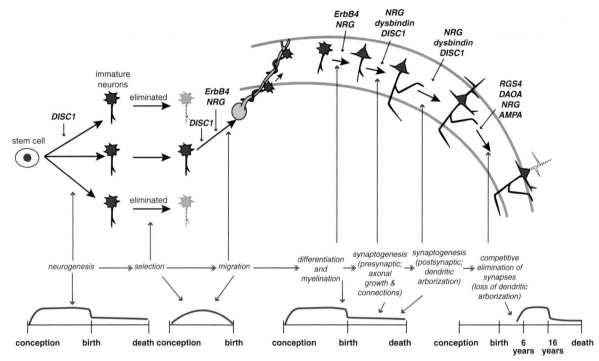

Figure 4-37. Overview of neurodevelopment. The process of brain development is shown here. After conception, stem cells differentiate into immature neurons. Those that are selected migrate and then differentiate into different types of neurons, after which synaptogenesis occurs. Most neurogenesis, neuronal selection, and neuronal migration occur before birth, although new neurons can form in some brain areas even in adults. After birth, differentiation and myelination of neurons as well as synaptogenesis continue throughout a lifetime. Brain restructuring also occurs throughout life, but is most active during childhood and adolescence in a process known as competitive elimination. Key genes involved in the process of neurodevelopment include DISC1 (disrupted in schizophrenia 1), ErbB4, neuregulin (NRG), dysbindin, regulator of G protein signaling 4 (RGS4), D-amino acid oxidase activator (DAOA), and genes for AMPA.

the lack of critical synapses being strengthened, these critical synapses may be mistakenly eliminated during adolescence with disastrous consequences, namely the onset of symptoms of schizophrenia. Also, it may be that the dysconnectivity of abnormal glutamate synapses present from birth is masked by the presence of many additional weak connections prior to adolescence, acting with exuberance to compensate for defective glutamate connectivity, and with that compensation destroyed by the normal competitive elimination of synapses in adolescence, schizophrenia emerges.

Neuroimaging circuits in schizophrenia

Imaging brain circuits in patients with schizophrenia with functional magnetic resonance imaging (fMRI) uncovers abnormal information processing in brain areas linked to cognition and emotion. Modern

psychiatric research techniques can put a "load" on brain circuits, and thereby perform a type of psychiatric "stress test" while visualizing the activity of the brain circuits. fMRI brain scanners can most readily detect the activity of neurons near the surface of the brain, which are mostly pyramidal neurons in the cortex, although some deeper gray-matter areas such as the striatum and amygdala can also be imaged. The activity of neurons so visualized in the cortex is the first leg of various brain circuits, especially glutamate neurons, as shown in Figure 4-27, acting within feedback loops from the cortex to the striatal complex, with that information relayed to the thalamus via a GABA neuron, then back to the cortex again via another glutamate neuron as cortico-striato-thalamo-cortical or CSTC feedback loops. Brain circuits like this are information-processing "engines" that are activated by various tasks or loads placed upon them, and seeing them light up may be literally watching the brain "think."

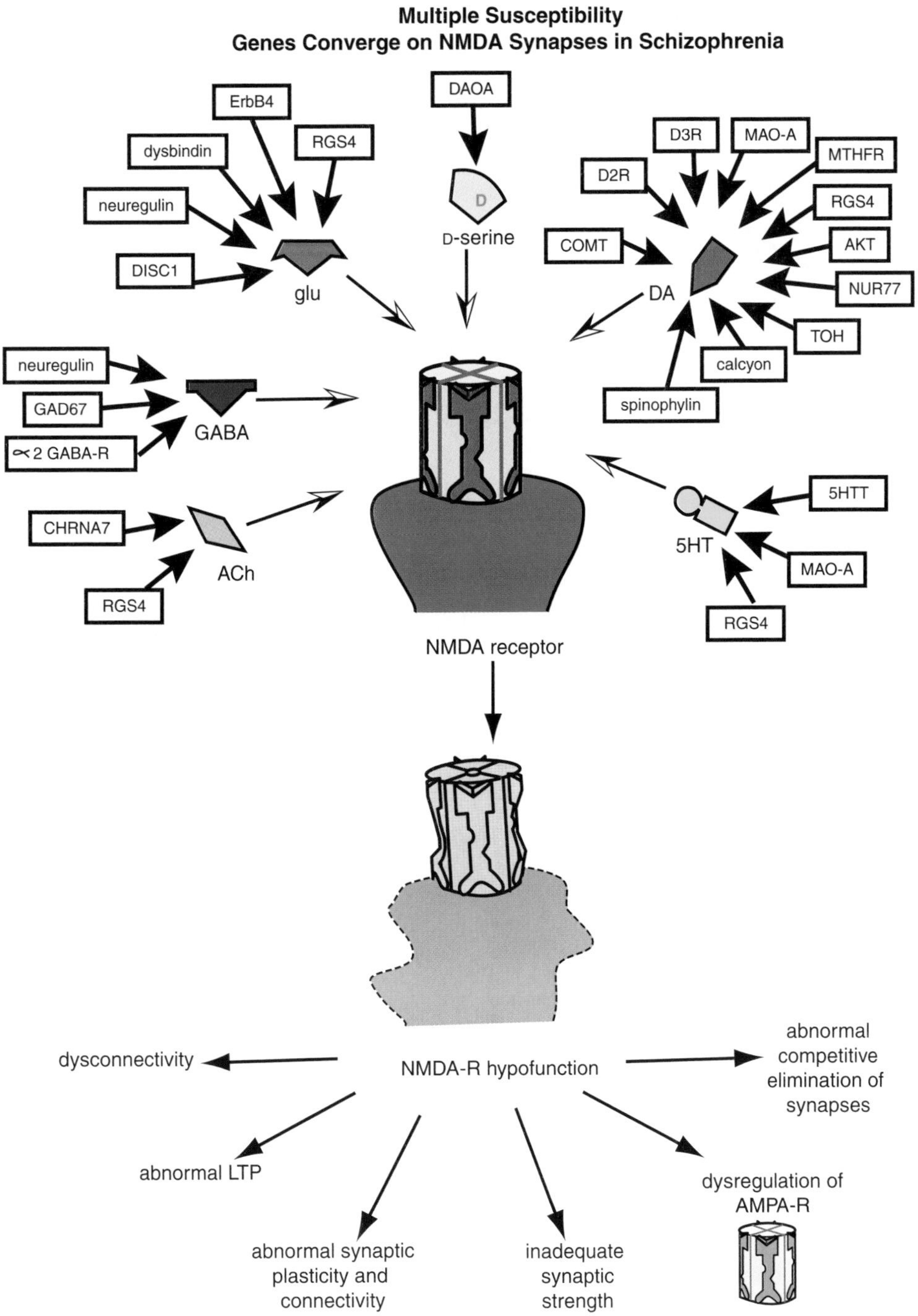

Figure 4-38. Multiple susceptibility genes converge on NMDA synapses in schizophrenia. There is a powerful convergence of susceptibility genes for schizophrenia upon the connectivity, synaptogenesis, and neurotransmission at glutamate synapses, and specifically at NMDA receptors. Susceptibility genes shown here include those that affect various neurotransmitters involved in modulating NMDA receptors, namely glutamate, γ-aminobutyric acid (GABA), acetylcholine (ACh), dopamine (DA), and serotonin (5HT). That is, abnormalities in genes for various neurotransmitters that regulate NMDA receptors could have additional downstream actions on glutamate functioning at NMDA receptors. Thus, genes that regulate these other neurotransmitters may also constitute susceptibility genes for schizophrenia. The idea is that any of these susceptibility genes could conspire to cause NMDA receptor hypofunction, which would lead to abnormal long-term potentiation (LTP), abnormal synaptic plasticity and connectivity, inadequate synaptic strength, and/or dysregulation of α-amino-3-hydroxy-5-methyl-4-isoxazole-propionic acid (AMPA) receptors. Any combination of sufficient genetic risk factors with sufficient stress or environmental risk will result in the susceptibility for schizophrenia to become manifest as the disease of schizophrenia with the presence of full syndrome symptoms.

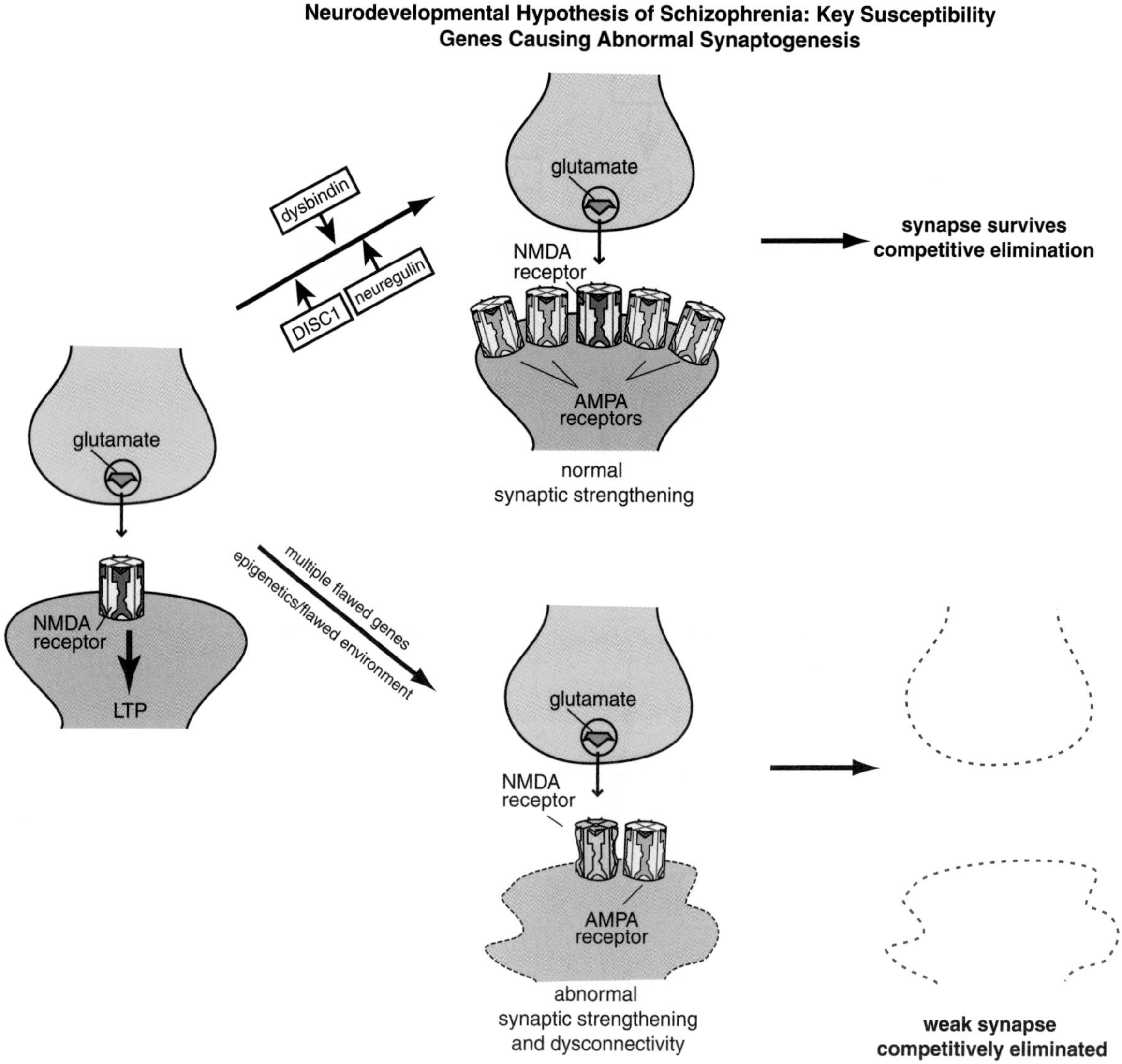

Neurodevelopmental Hypothesis of Schizophrenia: Key Susceptibility Genes Causing Abnormal Synaptogenesis

Figure 4-39. Neurodevelopmental hypothesis of schizophrenia. Dysbindin, DISC1 (disrupted in schizophrenia 1), and neuregulin are all involved in "strengthening" of glutamate synapses. Under normal circumstances, N-methyl-ᴅ-aspartate (NMDA) receptors in active glutamate synapses trigger long-term potentiation (LTP), which leads to structural and functional changes of the synapse to make it more efficient, or "strengthened." In particular, this process leads to an increased number of α-amino-3-hydroxy-5-methyl-4-isoxazole-propionic acid (AMPA) receptors, which are important for mediating glutamatergic neurotransmission. Normal synaptic strengthening means that the synapse will survive during competitive elimination. If the genes that regulate strengthening of glutamate synapses are abnormal, then this could cause hypofunctioning of NMDA receptors, with a resultant decrease in LTP and fewer AMPA receptors. This abnormal synaptic strengthening and dysconnectivity would lead to weak synapses that would not survive competitive elimination. This would theoretically lead to increased risk of developing schizophrenia, and these abnormal synapses could mediate the symptoms of schizophrenia.

Function in the brain is topographical, meaning different brain circuits process different kinds of information. For example, the dorsolateral prefrontal cortex (DLPFC) is thought to be most closely linked to cognitive functioning such as problem solving, whereas the ventromedial prefrontal cortex (VMPFC) – along with the amygdala – is thought to be most closely linked to emotional functioning, such as mood. Neurons in various brain areas "stressed" with an information-processing "load" literally light up a specific brain area that can be visualized with current neuroimaging techniques. Thus, doing a calculation can light up the DLPFC and seeing a sad face can activate the VMPFC and amygdala.

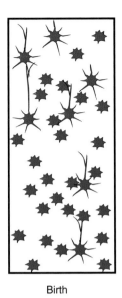
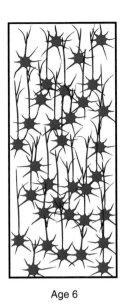
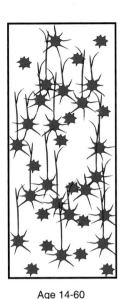

Birth   Age 6   Age 14-60

Figure 4-40. Synapse formation by age. Synapses are formed at a furious rate between birth and age 6. Competitive elimination and restructuring of synapses peaks during pubescence and adolescence, leaving about half to two-thirds of the synapses present in childhood to survive into adulthood.

Studies in patients with schizophrenia suggest that they cannot adequately recruit the hippocampus during memory recall, even though output from the hippocampus seems to be high in the first place. Also, patients with schizophrenia do not seem to be able to appropriately activate the DLPFC during a working memory task (compare Figures 4-41A and 4-41B), with decreased recruitment correlated with worsening cognitive symptoms (Figure 4-41C). Actually, the results are somewhat inconsistent across studies, and it appears that prefrontal cortical or hippocampal dysfunction in schizophrenia is likely to be more complicated than just "up" (hyperactivation) or "down" (hypoactivation), but might be better characterized as "out of tune." According to this concept, either too much or too little activation of neuronal activity in the prefrontal cortex is suboptimal and can potentially be symptomatic, just as a guitar string is out of tune whether it has too much or too little tension on it.

How can circuits in schizophrenia be both hyperactive and hypoactive? Patients with schizophrenia appear to utilize greater prefrontal resources when performing cognitive tasks and yet achieve lower accuracy because they have cognitive impairment despite their best efforts. To perform near normal, patients with schizophrenia engage the DLPFC, but do so inefficiently, recruiting greater neural resources and hyperactivating the DLPFC. When performing poorly, schizophrenia patients do not appropriately

engage and sustain the DLPFC, and thus show hypoactivation. Thus, DLPFC circuits in schizophrenia patients can either be underactive and hypofrontal or overactive and inefficient.

It is interesting to note that unaffected siblings of patients with schizophrenia may have the very same inefficient information processing in DLPFC that schizophrenia patients have. Although unaffected siblings of schizophrenia patients might have some mild degree of cognitive impairment, they do not share the full syndrome of schizophrenia; however, neuroimaging reveals that they may share the same inefficient DLPFC functioning while performing cognitive tasks that characterizes their sibling with schizophrenia. The unaffected siblings of a schizophrenia patient may thus share some of the susceptibility genes for schizophrenia with their affected sibling, but not enough of these risk genes to have the full syndrome of schizophrenia itself. Functional neuroimaging also has the potential of unmasking inefficient information processing in clinically silent presymptomatic patients destined to progress to the full schizophrenia syndrome, but much further research is required to see if this will become clinically useful.

Schizophrenia has also long been recognized as having impairments in the ability to identify and accurately interpret emotions from overt sources, including facial expressions. This may be due to inefficient information processing within the VMPFC and amygdala and can be measured by imaging

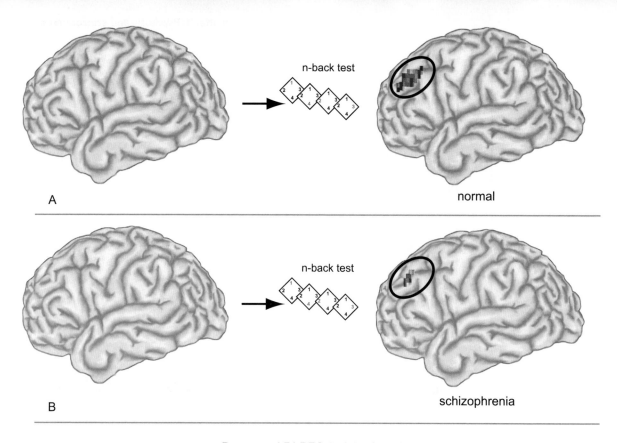

A

normal

B

schizophrenia

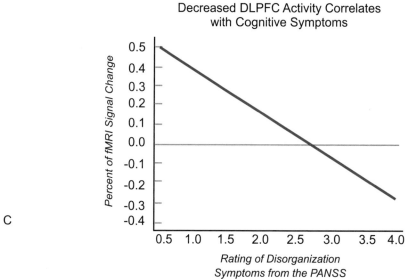

Decreased DLPFC Activity Correlates
with Cognitive Symptoms

C

*Rating of Disorganization
Symptoms from the PANSS*

Figure 4-41. *n*-back test in schizophrenia. (A) Functional neuroimaging studies have suggested that information processing in schizophrenia is abnormal in certain brain regions. Information processing during cognitive tasks has been evaluated using the *n*-back test. In the 0-back variant of the test, participants view a number on a screen and then indicate what the number was. In the 1-back test, participants are shown a stimulus but do not respond; after viewing the second stimulus, the participant then pushes a button corresponding to the first stimulus. The *n* can be any number, with higher numbers associated with greater difficulty. Performing the *n*-back test results in activation of the dorsolateral prefrontal cortex (DLPFC). The degree of activation indicates how efficient the information processing is in DLPFC, with both overactivation and hypoactivation associated with inefficient information processing. (B) Patients with schizophrenia exhibit inefficient information processing during cognitive challenges such as the *n*-back test. To perform near normal, these individuals must recruit greater neuronal resources, initially resulting in hyperactivation of the dorsolateral prefrontal cortex (DLPFC). Under increased cognitive load, however, schizophrenia patients do not appropriately engage and sustain the DLPFC, with resultant hypoactivation. (C) The degree of DLPFC activity, as measured by functional neuroimaging, correlates with the number of cognitive symptoms that a patient exhibits.

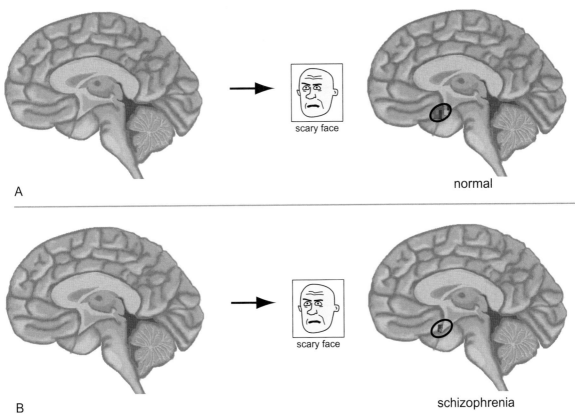

Figure 4-42. Fearful stimuli and schizophrenia. (A) Normally, exposure to an emotional stimulus, such as a scary face, causes hyperactivation in the amygdala. (B) Patients with schizophrenia often have impairments in the ability to identify and interpret emotional stimuli. The underlying neurobiological explanation for this may be inefficient information processing within the ventral system. In this example, the amygdala is not appropriately engaged during exposure to an emotional stimulus.

the response of the amygdala to emotional input, especially from facial expressions. The amygdala is normally activated by looking at scary, threatening faces, or by assessing how happy or sad a face may be and while attempting to match emotions to faces (Figure 4-42). Whereas healthy controls may activate the amygdala in response to scary or fearful or emotionally charged faces (Figure 4-42A), patients with schizophrenia may not (Figure 4-42B). This may represent distortion of reality as well as impairment in recognizing negative emotions and in decoding negative emotions in schizophrenia. Failure to mount the "normal" emotional response to a scary face can also represent an inability to interpret social cues and lead to distortions in judgment and reasoning in schizophrenia. Thus, these negative and affective symptoms of schizophrenia may be due in part to lack of emotional processing under circumstances when this should be occurring.

On the other hand, a neutral face or neutral stimulus may provoke little activation of the amygdala in a healthy person (Figure 4-43A), yet an over-reaction in a patient with schizophrenia (Figure 4-43B), who may mistakenly judge people negatively or conclude wrongly that another holds strong unfavorable impressions of them or may even be threatening them. Activating emotional processing in the amygdala when it is inappropriate may accompany the symptom of paranoia, and lead to impaired interpersonal functioning including problems in social communication. Thus, patients with schizophrenia may exhibit deficits in recognizing emotions that may be manifested either as positive or negative symptoms of this disorder. The underlying biological endophenotype of amygdala activation (or lack of activation) can be assessed with neuroimaging whether the patient is experiencing these symptoms or not. Looking at the efficiency of emotional information processing may help clinicians

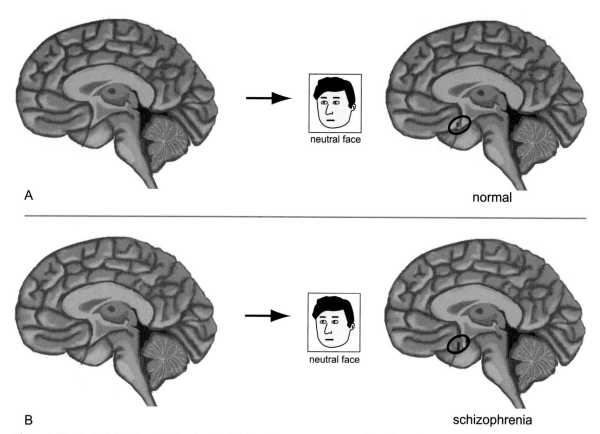

Figure 4-43. Neutral stimuli and schizophrenia. (A) Normally, exposure to a neutral stimulus, such as a neutral face, causes little activation of the amygdala. (B) Schizophrenia patients may mistakenly judge others as threatening, with associated inappropriate hyperactivation of the amygdala.

identify and understand emotional symptoms that are difficult for patients with schizophrenia to express.

Imaging genetics and epistasis

Not only can the impact of a mental illness such as schizophrenia be imaged today, so can the impact of certain genes. That is, single genes can alter the efficiency of information processing in everyone, and as such may endow risk for mental illness, but not cause mental illness by themselves, as discussed above (Figure 4-36). Thus, individuals with the gene for catechol-O-methyl-transferase (COMT) that has higher enzyme activity (called Val, for the amino acid valine substituted at a critical site) have lower dopamine levels in DLPFC, and thus less efficient information processing there compared to individuals with the gene for COMT with lower enzyme activity and higher dopamine levels (called Met) (Figure 4-44). This difference in neuronal "effort" is usually not

apparent as cognitive difficulties in the normal population, but may serve as one of many risk factors for schizophrenia (Table 4-8 and Figure 4-38).

Don't have T with Val

The effects of two or more risk genes working together to increase the risk of schizophrenia can now be demonstrated with neuroimaging that shows how certain risk genes "conspire" to decrease the efficiency of information processing in the DLPFC during a cognitive load in schizophrenia (Figure 4-44). That is, the Val variant of COMT by itself may or may not consistently alter DLPFC activity during a working memory test in schizophrenia compared to individuals with the Met variant of COMT, but when combined with another genetic variant of another enzyme that independently reduces the availability of dopamine in prefrontal cortex, there is a more robust increase in DLPFC activity during a working memory load (Figure 4-44).

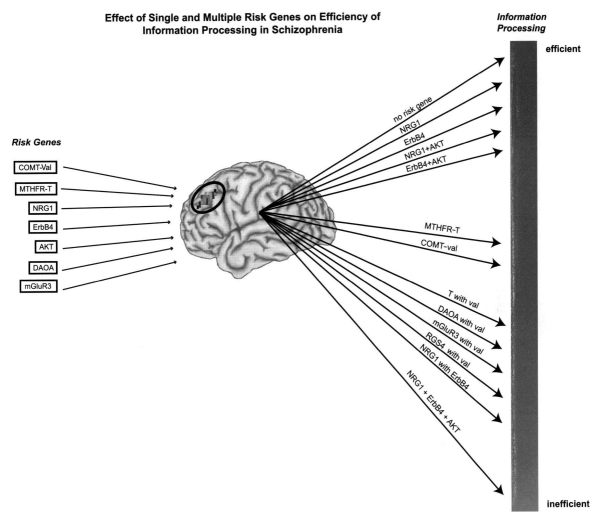

Effect of Single and Multiple Risk Genes on Efficiency of Information Processing in Schizophrenia

Figure 4-44. Risk genes and efficiency of information processing in schizophrenia. Several genes have been identified that may confer risk of inefficient information processing in schizophrenia. The single genes with the greatest risk may be the catechol-*O*-methyl-transferase Val allele (COMT-Val) and the methylene tetrahydrofolate reductase T allele (MTHFR-T). Risk may be even greater for individuals with multiple risk genes, and in particular for patients with both the COMT-Val allele and another risk gene. Perhaps the greatest risk has been seen for individuals who carry the neuregulin 1 (NRG1), ErbB4, and AKT risk genes.

That variant is the T form of the enzyme MTHFR (methylene tetrahydrofolate reductase), involved in the formation of dopamine and in regulating the activity of COMT at the level of gene expression. There can be reduced efficiency of information processing during a working memory load with the T form of MTHFR alone, but combined with the Val form of COMT, the change in information processing is more robust, thus demonstrating the epistatic interaction of MTHFR-T with COMT-Val (Figure 4-44). So, you may want to have tea with Valerie, but you don't necessarily want to have T with Val, or your cognitive

difficulties may be epistatically worsened if you have schizophrenia.

Be careful of having your alphabet soup

Another example of epistasis is how the efficiency of information processing in DLPFC gets worse if you combine two or three of several of the schizophrenia risk genes that have horrible-sounding names from various letters of the alphabet: NRG1 (neuregulin), ErbB4, and AKT. We have already mentioned above that NRG1 is involved in neuronal migration and synapse formation, and can impact the formation and function of the postsynaptic density, a set of proteins that interacts with the postsynaptic membrane to provide both structural and functional regulatory elements for neurotransmission and for NMDA receptors. NRG1 also affects NMDA receptor number by altering NMDA receptor trafficking to the postsynaptic membrane, NMDA receptor tethering within that membrane, and NMDA receptor endocytosis that cycles receptors out of the postsynaptic membrane to remove them. NRG1 directly interacts with ErbB4, and activates the ErbB4 signaling system that is co-localized with NMDA receptors and interacts with the postsynaptic density of glutamate synapses and is involved in mediating the neuroplasticity triggered by NMDA receptors. Thus, it is easy to see how a genetic abnormality in the NRG1 protein could readily interact in an undesirable way with a genetic abnormality in its receptor ErbB4, to cause problems with information processing and to increase the risk for schizophrenia. In fact, when patients with schizophrenia have the risk genes both for NRG1 and for ErbB4, but not when they have just one of them, their information processing in DLPFC is abnormal (Figure 4-44).

How about AKT? AKT is a kinase enzyme, part of the intracellular signal transduction cascades discussed in Chapter 1 (Figures 1-9, 1-16, 1-18, 1-28). This particular kinase specifically interacts with β-arrestin 2 and GSK-3 during signal transduction and has been shown to regulate neuronal cell size and cell survival, and to increase synaptic plasticity. Malfunctioning of AKT can lead to overactivation of GSK-3 and lack of internalization of dopamine D_2 receptors, contributing to dopamine hyperactivity and the risk of schizophrenia. By itself or in combination with the risk gene for either NRG1 or ErbB4, the risk gene for AKT does not appear to compromise the efficiency of information processing in the DLPFC of patients with schizophrenia (Figure 4-44). However, when combined with both the risk genes for NRG1 and ErbB4, the risk gene for AKT further increases the activation and inefficiency of information processing in DLPFC of patients with schizophrenia who have both the risk genes for NRG1 plus ErbB4, a further example of epistasis, but here among three risk genes (Figure 4-44). Thus, it is apparent that the more risk genes, the more the bias towards circuit breakdown in schizophrenia, and the more likely the illness will manifest, as shown in the hypothetical interactions of Figures 4-36 and 4-38.

Summary

This chapter has provided a clinical description of psychosis, with special emphasis on the psychotic illness schizophrenia. We have explained the dopamine hypothesis of schizophrenia, and the related NMDA receptor hypofunction hypothesis of schizophrenia, which are the major hypotheses for explaining the mechanism for the symptoms of schizophrenia. The major dopamine pathways and the major glutamate pathways in the brain have all been described. Overactivity of the mesolimbic dopamine system may mediate the positive symptoms of psychosis and may be linked to hypofunctioning NMDA glutamate receptors in parvalbumin-containing GABA interneurons in the prefrontal cortex and hippocampus. Underactivity of the mesocortical dopamine system may mediate the negative, cognitive, and affective symptoms of schizophrenia and could also be linked to hypofunctioning NMDA receptors at different GABA interneurons.

The synthesis, metabolism, reuptake, and receptors for both dopamine and glutamate are described in this chapter. Dopamine D_2 receptors are targets of all known antipsychotic drugs. NMDA glutamate receptors require interaction not only with the neurotransmitter glutamate, but also with the cotransmitters glycine or D-serine. Dysconnectivity of NMDA-receptor-containing synapses caused by genetic and environmental/epigenetic influences is a major hypothesis for the cause of schizophrenia, including its upstream glutamate hyperactivity and NMDA receptor hypofunction, as well as its downstream increases in mesolimbic dopamine but decreases in mesocortical dopamine. A whole host of susceptibility genes that regulate neuronal connectivity and synapse formation also increase the risk for schizophrenia and converge upon the NMDA-receptor-containing glutamate synapse as a hypothetical central biological flaw in schizophrenia. Malfunctioning neural circuits can be imaged in schizophrenic patients, including those in the dorsolateral prefrontal cortex that are linked to cognitive symptoms, and those in the amygdala that are linked to symptoms of emotional dysregulation. The effects of risk genes on the efficient functioning of brain circuits can also be imaged, including the epistatic interaction of two or more risk genes.

This chapter will explore antipsychotic drugs, with an emphasis on treatments for schizophrenia. These treatments include not only conventional antipsychotic drugs, but also the newer atypical antipsychotic drugs that have largely replaced the older conventional agents. Atypical antipsychotics are really misnamed, since they are also used as treatments for both the manic and depressed phases of bipolar disorder, as augmenting agents for treatment-resistant depression, and "off-label" for various other disorders, such as treatment-resistant anxiety disorders. The reader is referred to standard reference manuals and textbooks for practical prescribing information, such as drug doses, because this chapter on antipsychotic drugs will

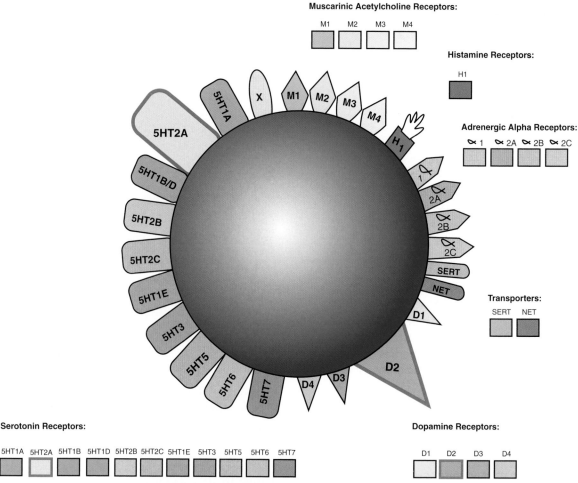

Figure 5-1. Qualitative and semi-quantitative representation of receptor binding properties. Throughout this chapter, the receptor binding properties of the atypical antipsychotics are represented both graphically and semi-quantitatively. Each drug is represented as a blue sphere, with its most potent binding properties depicted along the outer edge of the sphere. Additionally, each drug has a series of colored boxes associated with it. Each colored box represents a different binding property, and binding strength is indicated by the size of the box and the number of plus signs. Within the colored box series for any particular antipsychotic, larger boxes with more plus signs (positioned to the left) indicate stronger binding affinity, while smaller boxes with fewer plus signs (positioned to the right) represent weaker binding affinity. The series of boxes associated with each drug are arranged such that the size and positioning of a box reflect the binding potency for a particular receptor. The vertical dotted line cuts through the dopamine 2 (D_2) receptor binding box, with binding properties that are more potent than D_2 on the left and those that are less potent than D_2 on the right. All binding properties are based on the mean values of published K_i (binding affinity) data (http://pdsp.med.unc.edu). The semi-quantitative depiction used throughout this chapter provides a quick visual reference of how strongly a particular drug binds to a particular receptor. It also allows for easy comparison of a drug's binding properties with those of other atypical antipsychotics.

emphasize basic pharmacologic concepts of mechanism of action and not practical issues such as how to prescribe these drugs (for that information see for example *Stahl's Essential Psychopharmacology: the Prescriber's Guide*, which is a companion to this textbook).

Antipsychotic drugs exhibit possibly the most complex pharmacologic mechanisms of any drug class within the field of clinical psychopharmacology. The pharmacologic concepts developed here

should help the reader understand the rationale for how to use each of the different antipsychotic agents, based upon their interactions with different neurotransmitter systems (Figure 5-1). Such interactions can often explain both the therapeutic actions and the side effects of various antipsychotic medications and thus can be very helpful background information for prescribers of these therapeutic agents.

Conventional antipsychotics
What makes an antipsychotic "conventional"?

In this section we will discuss the pharmacologic properties of the first drugs that were proven to effectively treat schizophrenia. A list of many conventional antipsychotic drugs is given in Table 5-1. These drugs are usually called *conventional* antipsychotics, but they are sometimes also called *classical* antipsychotics, or *typical* antipsychotics, or *first-generation* antipsychotics. The earliest effective treatments for schizophrenia and other psychotic illnesses arose from serendipitous clinical observations more than 60 years ago, rather than from scientific knowledge of the neurobiological basis of psychosis, or of the mechanism of action of effective antipsychotic agents. Thus, the first antipsychotic drugs were discovered by accident in the 1950s when a drug with antihistamine properties (chlorpromazine) was serendipitously observed to have antipsychotic effects when this putative antihistamine was tested in schizophrenia patients. Chlorpromazine indeed has antihistaminic activity, but its therapeutic actions in schizophrenia are not mediated by this property. Once chlorpromazine was observed to be an effective antipsychotic agent, it was tested experimentally to uncover its mechanism of antipsychotic action.

Early in the testing process, chlorpromazine and other antipsychotic agents were all found to cause "neurolepsis," known as an extreme form of slowness or absence of motor movements as well as behavioral indifference in experimental animals. The original antipsychotics were first discovered largely by their ability to produce this effect in experimental animals, and are thus sometimes called "neuroleptics." A human counterpart of neurolepsis is also caused by these original (i.e., conventional) antipsychotic drugs and is characterized by psychomotor slowing, emotional quieting, and affective indifference.

Table 5-1 Some conventional antipsychotics still in use

Generic name	Trade name	Comment
Chlorpromazine	Thorazine	Low potency
Cyamemazine	Tercian	Atypical at low doses; popular in France; not available in the US
Flupenthixol	Depixol	Depot; not available in the US
Fluphenazine	Prolixin	High potency; depot
Haloperidol	Haldol	High potency; depot
Loxapine	Loxitane	Atypical at low doses
Mesoridazine	Serentil	Low potency; QT$_c$ issues; second line
Perphenazine	Trilafon	High potency
Pimozide	Orap	High potency; Tourette's syndrome; QT$_c$ issues; second line
Pipothiazine	Piportil	Depot; not available in the US
Sulpiride	Dolmatil	May have some atypical properties; not available in the US
Thioridazine	Mellaril	Low potency; QT$_c$ issues; second line
Thiothixene	Navane	High potency
Trifluoperazine	Stelazine	High potency
Zuclopenthixol	Clopixol	Depot; not available in the US

What Makes an Antipsychotic Conventional?

D2 Antagonist Actions

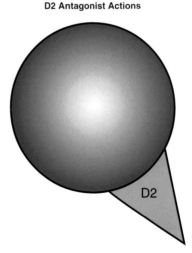

Figure 5-2. D$_2$ antagonist. Conventional antipsychotics, also called first-generation antipsychotics or typical antipsychotics, share the primary pharmacological property of D$_2$ antagonism, which is responsible not only for their antipsychotic efficacy but also for many of their side effects. Shown here is an icon representing this single pharmacological action.

D$_2$ receptor antagonism makes an antipsychotic conventional

By the 1970s it was widely recognized that the key pharmacologic property of all "neuroleptics" with antipsychotic properties was their ability to block dopamine D$_2$ receptors (Figure 5-2). This action has proven to be responsible not only for the antipsychotic efficacy of conventional antipsychotic drugs, but also for most of their undesirable side effects, including "neurolepsis."

The therapeutic actions of conventional antipsychotic drugs are hypothetically due to blockade of D$_2$ receptors specifically in the mesolimbic dopamine pathway (Figure 5-3). This has the effect of reducing the hyperactivity in this pathway that is postulated to cause the positive symptoms of psychosis, as discussed in Chapter 4 (Figures 4-12 and 4-13). All conventional antipsychotics reduce positive psychotic symptoms about equally well in schizophrenia patients studied in large multicenter trials if they are dosed to block a substantial number of D$_2$ receptors there (Figure 5-4). Unfortunately, in order to block adequate numbers of D$_2$ receptors in the mesolimbic dopamine pathway to

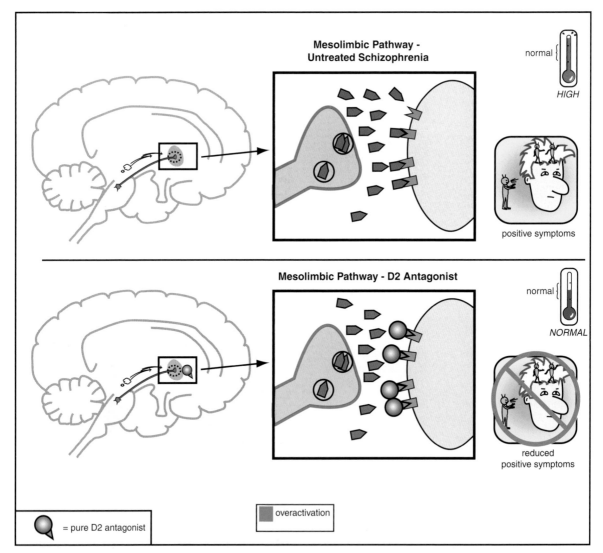

Figure 5-3. Mesolimbic dopamine pathway and D$_2$ antagonists. In untreated schizophrenia, the mesolimbic dopamine pathway is hypothesized to be hyperactive, indicated here by the pathway appearing red as well as by the excess dopamine in the synapse. This leads to positive symptoms such as delusions and hallucinations. Administration of a D$_2$ antagonist, such as a conventional antipsychotic, blocks dopamine from binding to the D$_2$ receptor, which reduces hyperactivity in this pathway and thereby reduces positive symptoms as well.

Hypothetical Thresholds for Conventional Antipsychotic Drug Effects

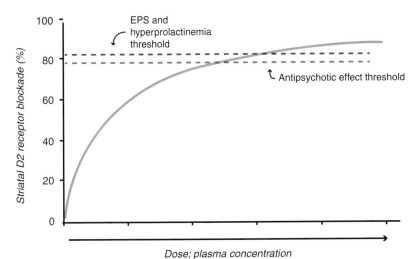

Figure 5-4. **Hypothetical thresholds for conventional antipsychotic drug effects.** All known antipsychotics bind to the dopamine 2 receptor, with the degree of binding determining whether one experiences therapeutic and/or side effects. For most conventional antipsychotics, the degree of D2 receptor binding in the mesolimbic pathway needed for antipsychotic effects is close to 80%, while D2 receptor occupancy greater than 80% in the dorsal striatum is associated with extrapyramidal side effects (EPS) and in the pituitary is associated with hyperprolactinemia. For conventional antipsychotics (i.e,. pure D2 antagonists) it is assumed that the same number of D2 receptors is blocked in all brain areas. Thus, there is a narrow window between the threshold for antipsychotic efficacy and that for side effects in terms of D2 binding.

quell positive symptoms, one must simultaneously block the same number of D_2 receptors throughout the brain, and this causes undesirable side effects as a "high cost of doing business" with conventional antipsychotics (Figures 5-5 through 5-8). Although modern neuroimaging techniques are able to measure directly the blockade of D_2 receptors in the dorsal (motor) striatum of the nigrostriatal pathway, as shown in Figure 5-4, for conventional antipsychotics it is assumed that the same number of D_2 receptors is blocked in all brain areas, including the ventral limbic area of striatum known as the nucleus accumbens of the mesolimbic dopamine pathway, the prefrontal cortex of the mesocortical dopamine pathway, and the pituitary gland of the tuberoinfundibular dopamine pathway.

Neurolepsis

D_2 receptors in the mesolimbic dopamine system are postulated to mediate not only the positive symptoms of psychosis, but also the normal reward system of the brain, and the nucleus accumbens is widely considered to be the "pleasure center" of the brain. It may be the final common pathway of all reward and reinforcement, including not only normal reward (such as the pleasure of eating good food, orgasm, listening to music) but also the artificial reward of substance abuse. If D_2 receptors are stimulated in some parts of the mesolimbic pathway, this can lead to the experience of pleasure. Thus, if D_2 receptors in the mesolimbic system are blocked, this may not only reduce positive symptoms

of schizophrenia, but also block reward mechanisms, leaving patients apathetic, anhedonic, lacking motivation, interest, and joy from social interactions, a state very similar to that of negative symptoms of schizophrenia. The near shutdown of the mesolimbic dopamine pathway necessary to improve the positive symptoms of psychosis (Figure 5-4) may contribute to worsening of anhedonia, apathy, and negative symptoms, and this may be a partial explanation for the high incidence of smoking and drug abuse in schizophrenia.

Antipsychotics also block D_2 receptors in the mesocortical DA pathway (Figure 5-5), where DA may already be deficient in schizophrenia (see Figures 4-14 through 4-16). This can cause or worsen negative and cognitive symptoms even though there is only a low density of D_2 receptors in the cortex. An adverse behavioral state can be produced by conventional antipsychotics, and is sometimes called the "neuroleptic-induced deficit syndrome" because it looks so much like the negative symptoms produced by schizophrenia itself, and is reminiscent of "neurolepsis" in animals.

Extrapyramidal symptoms and tardive dyskinesia

When a substantial number of D_2 receptors are blocked in the nigrostriatal DA pathway, this will produce various disorders of movement that can appear very much like those in Parkinson's disease; this is why these movements are sometimes called drug-induced

133

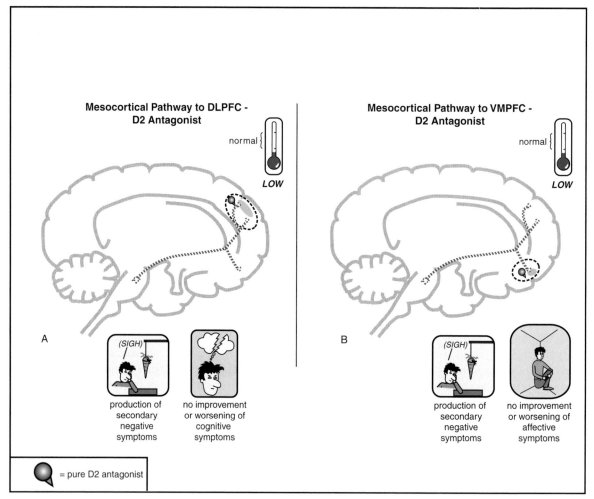

Figure 5-5. Mesocortical dopamine pathway and D$_2$ antagonists. In untreated schizophrenia, the mesocortical dopamine pathways to dorsolateral prefrontal cortex (DLPFC) and to ventromedial prefrontal cortex (VMPFC) are hypothesized to be hypoactive, indicated here by the dotted outlines of the pathway. This hypoactivity is related to cognitive symptoms (in the DLPFC), negative symptoms (in the DLPFC and VMPFC), and affective symptoms of schizophrenia (in the VMPFC). Administration of a D$_2$ antagonist could further reduce activity in this pathway and thus not only not improve such symptoms but actually potentially worsen them.

parkinsonism. Since the nigrostriatal pathway is part of the extrapyramidal nervous system, these motor side effects associated with blocking D$_2$ receptors in this part of the brain are sometimes also called extrapyramidal symptoms, or EPS (Figures 5-4 and 5-6).

Worse yet, if these D$_2$ receptors in the nigrostriatal DA pathway are blocked chronically (Figure 5-7), they can produce a hyperkinetic movement disorder known as tardive dyskinesia. This movement disorder causes facial and tongue movements, such as constant chewing, tongue protrusions, facial grimacing, and also limb movements that can be quick, jerky, or choreiform (dancing). Tardive dyskinesia is thus caused by long-

term administration of conventional antipsychotics and is thought to be mediated by changes, sometimes irreversible, in the D$_2$ receptors of the nigrostriatal DA pathway. Specifically, these receptors are hypothesized to become supersensitive or to "upregulate" (i.e., increase in number), perhaps in a futile attempt to overcome drug-induced blockade of D$_2$ receptors in the striatum (Figure 5-7).

About 5% of patients maintained on conventional antipsychotics will develop tardive dyskinesia every year (i.e., about 25% of patients by 5 years), not a very encouraging prospect for a lifelong illness starting in the early twenties. The risk of developing tardive

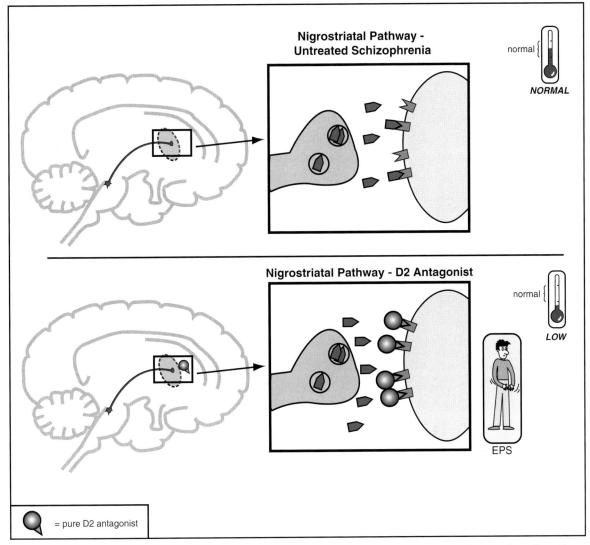

Figure 5-6. Nigrostriatal dopamine pathway and D₂ antagonists. The nigrostriatal dopamine pathway is theoretically unaffected in untreated schizophrenia. However, blockade of D₂ receptors, as with a conventional antipsychotic, prevents dopamine from binding there and can cause motor side effects that are often collectively termed extrapyramidal symptoms (EPS).

dyskinesia in elderly subjects may be as high as 25% within the first year of exposure to conventional antipsychotics. However, if D₂ receptor blockade is removed early enough, tardive dyskinesia may reverse. This reversal is theoretically due to a "resetting" of these D₂ receptors by an appropriate decrease in the number or sensitivity of them in the nigrostriatal pathway once the antipsychotic drug that had been blocking these receptors is removed. However, after long-term treatment, the D₂ receptors apparently cannot or do not reset back to normal, even when conventional antipsychotic drugs are discontinued. This leads to tardive dyskinesia

that is irreversible, continuing whether conventional antipsychotic drugs are administered or not.

Is there any way to predict those who will be harmed with the development of tardive dyskinesia after chronic treatment with conventional antipsychotics? Patients who develop EPS early in treatment may be twice as likely to develop tardive dyskinesia if treatment with a conventional antipsychotic is continued chronically. Also, specific genotypes of dopamine receptors may confer important genetic risk factors for developing tardive dyskinesia with chronic treatment using a conventional antipsychotic. Risk of new cases of tardive

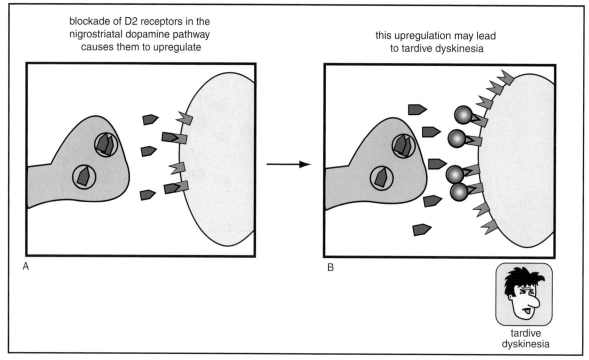

Figure 5-7. Tardive dyskinesia. Long-term blockade of D_2 receptors in the nigrostriatal dopamine pathway can cause upregulation of those receptors, which may lead to a hyperkinetic motor condition known as tardive dyskinesia, characterized by facial and tongue movements (e.g., tongue protrusions, facial grimaces, chewing) as well as quick, jerky limb movements. This upregulation may be the consequence of the neuron's futile attempt to overcome drug-induced blockade of its dopamine receptors.

dyskinesia, however, can diminish considerably after 15 years of treatment, presumably because patients who have not developed tardive dyskinesia despite 15 years of treatment with a conventional antipsychotic have lower genetic risk factors for it.

A rare but potentially fatal complication called the "neuroleptic malignant syndrome," associated with extreme muscular rigidity, high fevers, coma, and even death, and possibly related in part to D_2 receptor blockade in the nigrostriatal pathway, can also occur with conventional antipsychotic agents.

Prolactin elevation

Dopamine D_2 receptors in the tuberoinfundibular DA pathway are also blocked by conventional antipsychotics, and this causes plasma prolactin concentrations to rise, a condition called hyperprolactinemia (Figure 5-8). This is associated with conditions called galactorrhea (i.e., breast secretions) and amenorrhea (i.e., irregular or lack of menstrual periods). Hyperprolactinemia may thus interfere with fertility, especially in women. Hyperprolactinemia might lead to more

rapid demineralization of bones, especially in postmenopausal women who are not taking estrogen replacement therapy. Other possible problems associated with elevated prolactin levels may include sexual dysfunction and weight gain, although the role of prolactin in causing such problems is not clear.

The dilemma of blocking D_2 dopamine receptors in all dopamine pathways

It should now be obvious that the use of conventional antipsychotic drugs presents a powerful dilemma. That is, there is no doubt that conventional antipsychotic medications exert dramatic therapeutic actions upon positive symptoms of schizophrenia by blocking hyperactive dopamine neurons in the mesolimbic dopamine pathway. However, there are *several* dopamine pathways in the brain, and it appears that blocking dopamine receptors in *only one* of them is useful (Figure 5-3), whereas blocking dopamine receptors in the remaining pathways may be harmful (Figures 5-4 through 5-8). The pharmacologic

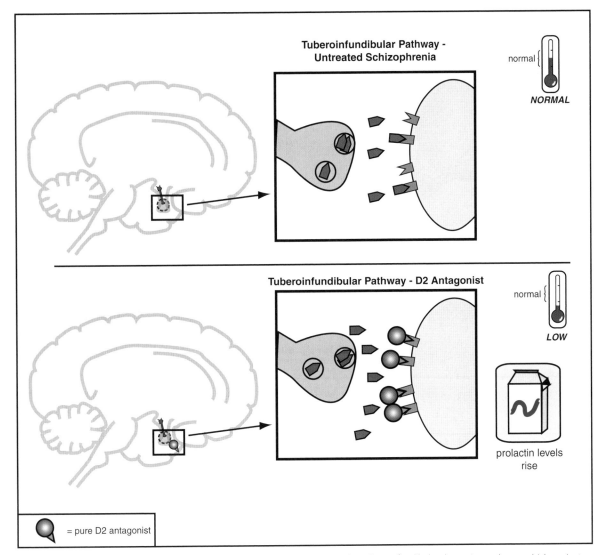

Figure 5-8. Tuberoinfundibular dopamine pathway and D₂ antagonists. The tuberoinfundibular dopamine pathway, which projects from the hypothalamus to the pituitary gland, is theoretically "normal" in untreated schizophrenia. D₂ antagonists reduce activity in this pathway by preventing dopamine from binding to D₂ receptors. This causes prolactin levels to rise, which is associated with side effects such as galactorrhea (breast secretions) and amenorrhea (irregular menstrual periods).

quandary here is what to do if one wishes simultaneously to *decrease* dopamine in the mesolimbic dopamine pathway in order to treat positive psychotic symptoms theoretically mediated by hyperactive mesolimbic dopamine neurons and yet *increase* dopamine in the mesocortical dopamine pathway to treat negative and cognitive symptoms, while leaving dopaminergic tone unchanged in both the nigrostriatal and tuberoinfundibular dopamine pathways to avoid side effects. This dilemma may have been addressed in part by the atypical antipsychotic drugs described in the following

sections, and is one of the reasons why the atypical antipsychotics have largely replaced conventional antipsychotic agents in the treatment of schizophrenia and other psychotic disorders throughout the world.

Muscarinic cholinergic blocking properties of conventional antipsychotics

In addition to blocking D₂ receptors in all dopamine pathways (Figures 5-3 through 5-8), conventional antipsychotics have other important pharmacologic

Various Binding Properties of Conventional Antipsychotics

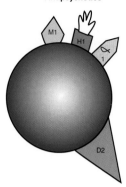

Figure 5-9. Conventional antipsychotic. Shown here is an icon representing a conventional antipsychotic drug. Conventional antipsychotics have pharmacological properties in addition to dopamine D_2 antagonism. The receptor profiles differ for each agent, contributing to divergent side-effect profiles. However, some important characteristics that multiple agents share are the ability to block muscarinic cholinergic receptors, histamine H_1 receptors, and/or α_1-adrenergic receptors.

properties (Figure 5-9). One particularly important pharmacologic action of some conventional antipsychotics is their ability to block muscarinic M_1-cholinergic receptors (Figures 5-9 through 5-11). This can cause undesirable side effects such as dry mouth, blurred vision, constipation, and cognitive blunting (Figure 5-10). Differing degrees of muscarinic cholinergic blockade may also explain why some conventional antipsychotics have a lesser propensity to produce extrapyramidal side effects (EPS) than others. That is, those conventional antipsychotics that cause more EPS are the agents that have only *weak* anticholinergic properties, whereas those conventional antipsychotics that cause fewer EPS are the agents that have *stronger* anticholinergic properties.

How does muscarinic cholinergic receptor blockade reduce the EPS caused by dopamine D_2 receptor blockade in the nigrostriatal pathway? The reason seems to be based on the fact that dopamine and acetylcholine have a reciprocal relationship with each other in the nigrostriatal pathway (Figure 5-11).

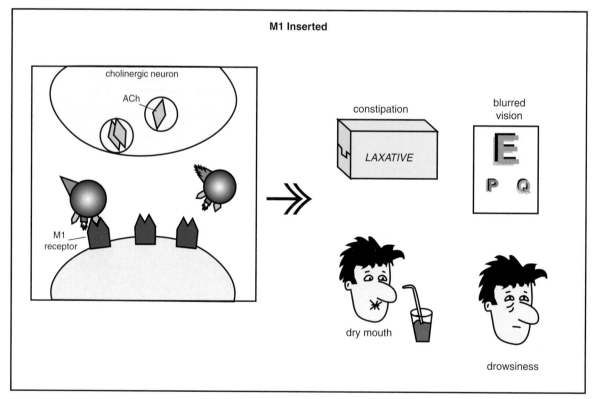

Figure 5-10. Side effects of muscarinic cholinergic receptor blockade. In this diagram, the icon of a conventional antipsychotic drug is shown with its M_1 anticholinergic/antimuscarinic portion inserted into acetylcholine receptors, causing the side effects of constipation, blurred vision, dry mouth, and drowsiness.

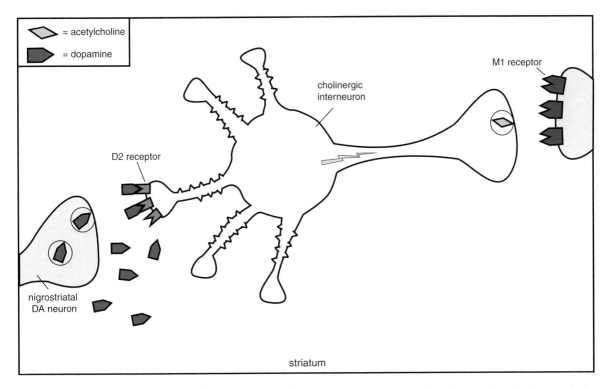

Figure 5-11A. Reciprocal relationship of dopamine and acetylcholine. Dopamine and acetylcholine have a reciprocal relationship in the nigrostriatal dopamine pathway. Dopamine neurons here make postsynaptic connections with the dendrite of a cholinergic neuron. Normally, dopamine suppresses acetylcholine activity (no acetylcholine being released from the cholinergic axon on the right).

Dopamine neurons in the nigrostriatal dopamine pathway make postsynaptic connections with cholinergic neurons (Figure 5-11A). Dopamine normally *inhibits* acetylcholine release from postsynaptic nigrostriatal cholinergic neurons, thus suppressing acetylcholine activity there (Figure 5-11A). If dopamine can no longer suppress acetylcholine release because dopamine receptors are being blocked by a conventional antipsychotic drug, then acetylcholine becomes overly active (Figure 5-11B).

One compensation for this overactivity of acetylcholine is to block it with an anticholinergic agent (Figure 5-11C). Thus, drugs with anticholinergic actions will diminish the excess acetylcholine activity caused by removal of dopamine inhibition when dopamine receptors are blocked (Figures 5-10 and 5-11C). If anticholinergic properties are present in the same drug with D_2 blocking properties, they will tend to mitigate the effects of D_2 blockade in the nigrostriatal dopamine pathway. Thus, conventional antipsychotics with potent anticholinergic properties have lower EPS than conventional antipsychotics with weak anticholinergic properties. Furthermore, the effects of D_2 blockade in the nigrostriatal system can be mitigated by co-administering an agent with anticholinergic properties. This has led to the common strategy of giving anticholinergic agents along with conventional antipsychotics in order to reduce EPS. Unfortunately, this concomitant use of anticholinergic agents does not lessen the ability of the conventional antipsychotics to cause tardive dyskinesia. It also causes the well-known side effects associated with anticholinergic agents, such as dry mouth, blurred vision, constipation, urinary retention, and cognitive dysfunction (Figure 5-10).

Other pharmacologic properties of conventional antipsychotic drugs

Still other pharmacologic actions are associated with the conventional antipsychotic drugs. These include generally undesired blockade of histamine H_1 receptors (Figure 5-9) causing weight gain and drowsiness, as well as blockade of α_1-adrenergic receptors causing

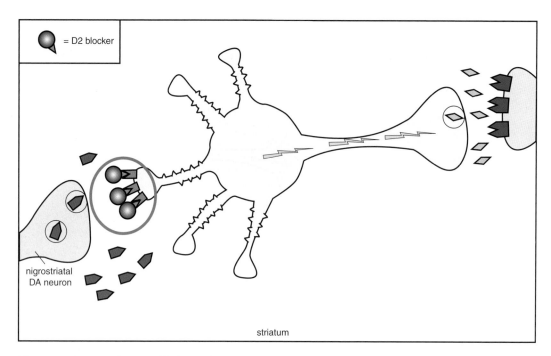

Figure 5-11B. Dopamine, acetylcholine, and D$_2$ antagonism. This figure shows what happens to acetylcholine activity when dopamine receptors are blocked. As dopamine normally suppresses acetylcholine activity, removal of dopamine inhibition causes an increase in acetylcholine activity. Thus if dopamine receptors are blocked at the D$_2$ receptors on the cholinergic dendrite on the left, then acetylcholine becomes overly active, with enhanced release of acetylcholine from the cholinergic axon on the right. This is associated with the production of extrapyramidal symptoms (EPS). The pharmacological mechanism of EPS therefore seems to be a relative dopamine deficiency and a relative acetylcholine excess.

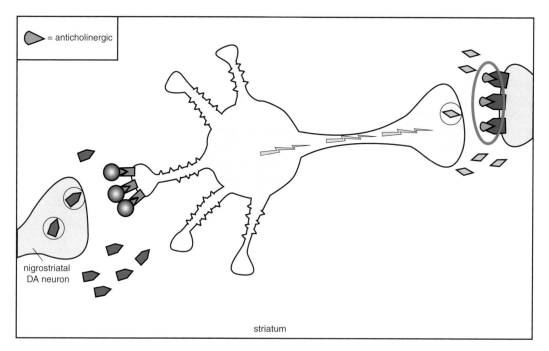

Figure 5-11C. D$_2$ antagonism and anticholinergic agents. One compensation for the overactivity that occurs when dopamine receptors are blocked is to block the acetylcholine receptors with an anticholinergic agent (M$_1$ receptors being blocked by an anticholinergic on the far right). Thus, anticholinergics overcome excess acetylcholine activity caused by removal of dopamine inhibition when dopamine receptors are blocked by conventional antipsychotics. This also means that extrapyramidal symptoms (EPS) are reduced.

cardiovascular side effects such as orthostatic hypotension and drowsiness. Conventional antipsychotic agents differ in terms of their ability to block these various receptors represented in Figure 5-9. For example, the popular conventional antipsychotic haloperidol has relatively little anticholinergic or antihistaminic binding activity, whereas the classic conventional antipsychotic chlorpromazine has potent anticholinergic and antihistaminic binding. Because of this, conventional antipsychotics differ somewhat in their side-effect profiles, even if they do not differ overall in their therapeutic profiles. That is, some conventional antipsychotics are more sedating than others, some have more ability to cause cardiovascular side effects than others, some have more ability to cause EPS than others.

A somewhat old-fashioned way to subclassify conventional antipsychotics is "low potency" versus "high potency" (Table 5-1). In general, as the name implies, low-potency agents require higher doses than high-potency agents, but, in addition, low-potency agents tend to have more of the additional properties discussed here than do the so-called high-potency agents: namely, low-potency agents have greater anticholinergic, antihistaminic, and α_1 antagonist properties than high-potency agents, and thus are probably more sedating in general. A number of conventional antipsychotics are available in long-acting depot formulations (Table 5-1).

Atypical antipsychotics
What makes an antipsychotic "atypical"?

From a clinical perspective, an "atypical antipsychotic" is defined in part by the "atypical" clinical properties that distinguish such drugs from conventional antipsychotics. That is, atypical antipsychotics have the clinical profile of *equal positive symptom antipsychotic actions*, but *low extrapyramidal symptoms* and *less hyperprolactinemia* compared to conventional antipsychotics. Thus, they are "atypical" from what is expected from a classical, conventional, first-generation antipsychotic. Since almost all of the agents with this atypical profile came after the introduction of clozapine, sometimes the atypical antipsychotics are also called *second-generation antipsychotics*.

From a pharmacological perspective, the current atypical antipsychotics as a class are defined as *serotonin–dopamine antagonists*, with simultaneous serotonin $5HT_{2A}$ receptor antagonism that accompanies D_2 antagonism (Figure 5-12). Pharmacologic actions in addition to $5HT_{2A}$ antagonism that can hypothetically also mediate the atypical antipsychotic clinical profile of low EPS and less hyperprolactinemia with comparable antipsychotic actions include partial agonist actions at $5HT_{1A}$ receptors and partial agonist actions at D_2 receptors. Each of these mechanisms will be discussed here. In order to understand the

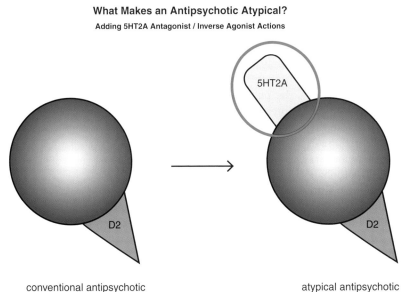

What Makes an Antipsychotic Atypical?

Adding 5HT2A Antagonist / Inverse Agonist Actions

conventional antipsychotic   atypical antipsychotic

Figure 5-12. Serotonin–dopamine antagonist. The "atypicality" of atypical antipsychotics has often been attributed to the coupling of D_2 antagonism with serotonin $5HT_{2A}$ antagonism. On the right is an icon representing this dual pharmacological action.

Serotonin is Produced

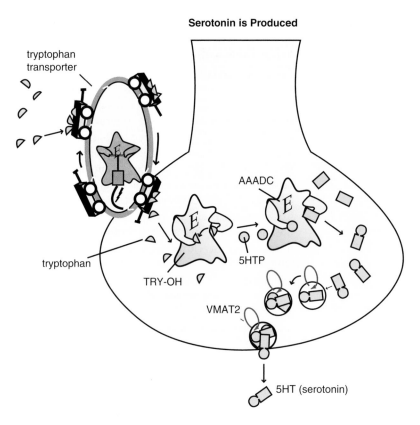

AAADC

5HTP

TRY-OH

VMAT2

tryptophan
transporter

tryptophan

5HT (serotonin)

Figure 5-13. Serotonin is produced. Serotonin (5-hydroxytryptamine [5HT]) is produced from enzymes after the amino acid precursor tryptophan is transported into the serotonin neuron. The tryptophan transport pump is distinct from the serotonin transporter. Once transported into the serotonin neuron, tryptophan is converted by the enzyme tryptophan hydroxylase (TRY-OH) into 5-hydroxytryptophan (5HTP), which is then converted into 5HT by the enzyme aromatic amino acid decarboxylase (AAADC). Serotonin is then taken up into synaptic vesicles via the vesicular monoamine transporter (VMAT2), where it stays until released by a neuronal impulse.

mechanism of action of atypical antipsychotics and how this differs from conventional antipsychotics, it is necessary to have a somewhat detailed understanding of the neurotransmitter serotonin and its receptors; thus serotonin pharmacology will be discussed in detail throughout this chapter.

Serotonin synthesis and termination of action

Serotonin is also known as 5-hydroxytryptamine and abbreviated as 5HT. Synthesis of 5HT begins with the amino acid tryptophan, which is transported into the brain from the plasma to serve as the 5HT precursor (Figure 5-13). Two synthetic enzymes then convert tryptophan into serotonin: firstly tryptophan hydroxylase (TRY-OH) converts tryptophan into 5-hydroxytryptophan, and then aromatic amino acid decarboxylase (AAADC) converts 5HTP into 5HT (Figure 5-13). After synthesis, 5HT is taken up into synaptic vesicles by a vesicular monoamine transporter (VMAT2) and stored there until it is used during neurotransmission.

5HT action is terminated when it is enzymatically destroyed by monoamine oxidase (MAO), and converted into an inactive metabolite (Figure 5-14). Serotonergic neurons themselves contain MAO-B, which has low affinity for 5HT, so much of 5HT is thought to be enzymatically degraded by MAO-A outside of the neuron once 5HT is released. The 5HT neuron also has a presynaptic transport pump for serotonin called the serotonin transporter (SERT) that is unique for 5HT and that terminates serotonin's actions by pumping it out of the synapse and back into the presynaptic nerve terminal where it can be re-stored in synaptic vesicles for subsequent use in another neurotransmission (Figure 5-14).

$5HT_{2A}$ receptors

The key to understanding why antipsychotics are atypical is to understand the pharmacology of $5HT_{2A}$ receptors, and the significance of what happens when they are blocked by atypical antipsychotics. All $5HT_{2A}$ receptors are postsynaptic, and $5HT_{2A}$ receptors are located in many brain regions. When they are located on cortical

Serotonin Action is Terminated

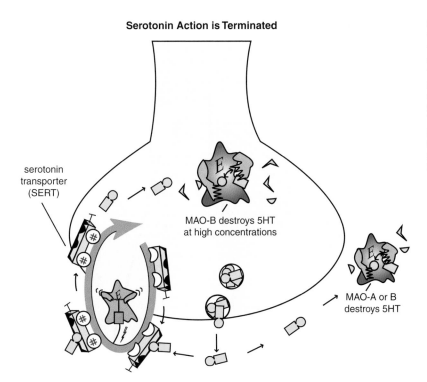

serotonin transporter (SERT)

MAO-B destroys 5HT at high concentrations

MAO-A or B destroys 5HT

Figure 5-14. Serotonin's action is terminated. Serotonin (5HT) action is terminated by the enzymes monoamine oxidase A (MAO-A) and MAO-B outside the neuron, and by MAO-B within the neuron when it is present in high concentrations. These enzymes convert serotonin into an inactive metabolite. There is also a presynaptic transport pump selective for serotonin, called the serotonin transporter or SERT, that clears serotonin out of the synapse and back into the presynaptic neuron.

pyramidal neurons, they are excitatory (Figure 5-15A, box 1) and can thus enhance downstream glutamate release (Figure 5-15A, box 2). As discussed in Chapter 4, glutamate regulates downstream dopamine release, so stimulating (Figure 5-15A) or blocking (Figure 5-15B) $5HT_{2A}$ receptors can therefore also regulate downstream dopamine release. Cortical $5HT_{1A}$ receptors also regulate downstream dopamine release (Figure 5-15C, discussed below).

$5HT_{2A}$ receptors are brakes on dopamine release in the striatum

$5HT_{2A}$ stimulation of cortical pyramidal neurons by serotonin (Figure 5-15A, box 1) hypothetically *blocks downstream dopamine release* in the striatum. It does this via stimulation of glutamate release in the brainstem that triggers release of inhibitory GABA there (Figure 5-15A, box 2). Release of dopamine from neurons in the striatum is thus inhibited (Figure 5-15A).

$5HT_{2A}$ antagonism cuts the brake cable

$5HT_{2A}$ antagonism of cortical pyramidal neurons by an atypical antipsychotic interferes with serotonin applying its braking action to dopamine release via

$5HT_{2A}$ receptors (Figure 5-15B, box 1). Thus, $5HT_{2A}$ antagonism in the cortex hypothetically *stimulates downstream dopamine release* in the striatum (Figure 5-15B). It does this by reducing glutamate release in the brainstem, which in turn fails to trigger the release of inhibitory GABA at dopamine neurons there (Figure 5-15B, box 2). Release of dopamine from neurons downstream in the striatum is thus disinhibited, which should theoretically mitigate EPS.

$5HT_{2A}$ receptors in other brain areas are also a brake on dopamine release in the striatum

$5HT_{2A}$ receptors theoretically regulate dopamine release from nigrostriatal dopamine neurons by additional mechanisms in additional brain areas. That is, serotonin neurons whose cell bodies are in the midbrain raphe may innervate nigrostriatal dopamine neurons both at the level of the dopamine neuronal cell bodies in the substantia nigra (Figure 5-16A, box 2) and at the dopamine neuronal axon terminals in the striatum (Figure 5-16A, box 1). This innervation may be either via a direct connection between the serotonin neuron and the dopamine neuron, or via an indirect connection with a GABA interneuron. *$5HT_{2A}$ receptor stimulation*

Cortical 5HT2A Receptors Decrease Dopamine Release

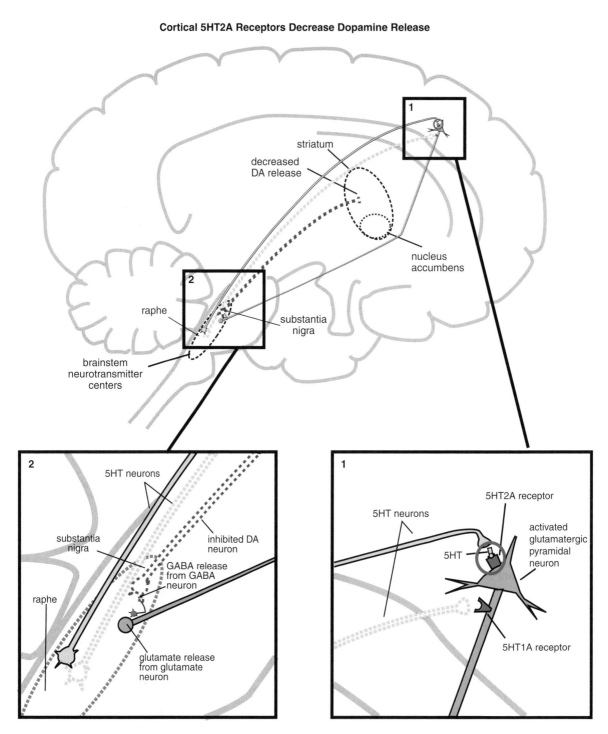

Figure 5-15A. Cortical 5HT₂ₐ receptors decrease dopamine release. Shown here is the mechanism by which serotonin release in the cortex can lead to decreased dopamine release in the striatum. (1) Serotonin is released in the cortex and binds to 5HT₂ₐ receptors on glutamatergic pyramidal neurons, causing activation of those neurons. (2) Activation of glutamatergic pyramidal neurons leads to glutamate release in the brainstem, which in turn stimulates GABA release. GABA binds to dopaminergic neurons projecting from the substantia nigra to the striatum, inhibiting dopamine release (indicated by the dotted outline of the dopaminergic neuron).

Blocking Cortical 5HT2A Receptors Increases Dopamine Release

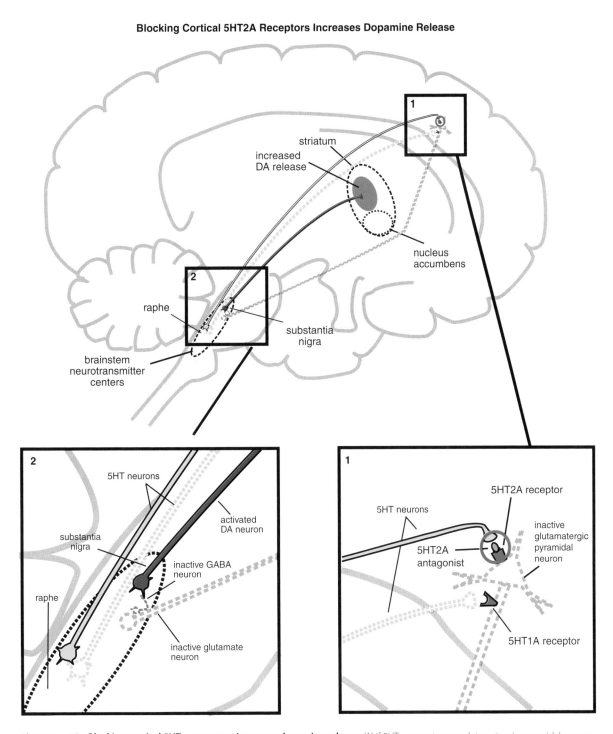

Figure 5-15B. Blocking cortical 5HT$_{2A}$ receptors increases dopamine release. (1) If 5HT$_{2A}$ receptors on glutamatergic pyramidal neurons are blocked, then these neurons cannot be activated by serotonin release in the cortex (indicated by the dotted outline of the glutamatergic neuron). (2) If glutamate is not released from glutamatergic pyramidal neurons into the brainstem, then GABA release is not stimulated and in turn cannot inhibit dopamine release from the substantia nigra into the striatum.

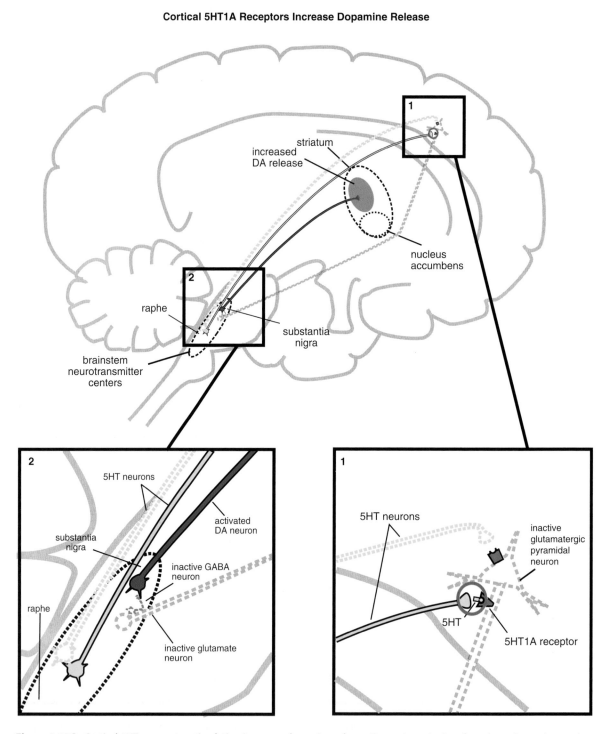

Figure 5-15C. Cortical 5HT$_{1A}$ receptor stimulation increases dopamine release. Serotonin projections from the raphe nucleus to the cortex also make axoaxonic connections with glutamatergic pyramidal neurons. (1) Serotonin released at these synapses can bind to 5HT$_{1A}$ receptors, which causes inhibition of the glutamatergic neuron (indicated by the dotted outline of the glutamatergic neuron). (2) If glutamate is not released from glutamatergic pyramidal neurons into the brainstem, then GABA release is not stimulated and in turn cannot inhibit dopamine release from the substantia nigra into the striatum. Thus, cortical 5HT$_{1A}$ receptor *stimulation* is functionally analogous to cortical 5HT$_{2A}$ receptor *blockade*, in that both lead to increased dopamine release in the striatum.

Nigral and Striatal 5HT2A Receptors Decrease Dopamine Release

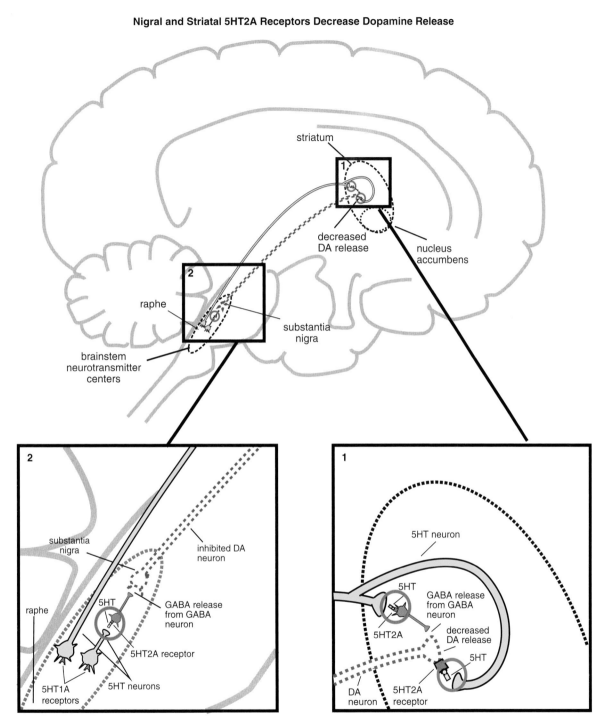

Figure 5-16A. Nigral and striatal 5HT$_{2A}$ receptor stimulation decreases dopamine release. (1) In the striatum, serotonergic projections synapse directly with dopaminergic neurons and indirectly via GABAergic neurons. At GABAergic neurons, serotonin binding to 5HT$_{2A}$ receptors disinhibits GABA release, which in turn decreases release of dopamine (indicated by the dotted outline of the dopaminergic neuron). Similarly, when serotonin binds to 5HT$_{2A}$ receptors directly on dopamine neurons, this causes a decrease in dopamine release. (2) Serotonin can also decrease dopamine release in the striatum via 5HT$_{2A}$ binding in the brainstem. That is, serotonin released in the raphe nucleus binds to 5HT$_{2A}$ receptors on GABAergic interneurons. This causes GABA to be released onto dopaminergic neurons in the substantia nigra, thus inhibiting dopamine release into the striatum (indicated by the dotted outline of the dopaminergic neuron).

Blocking Nigral and Striatal 5HT2A Receptors Increases Dopamine Release

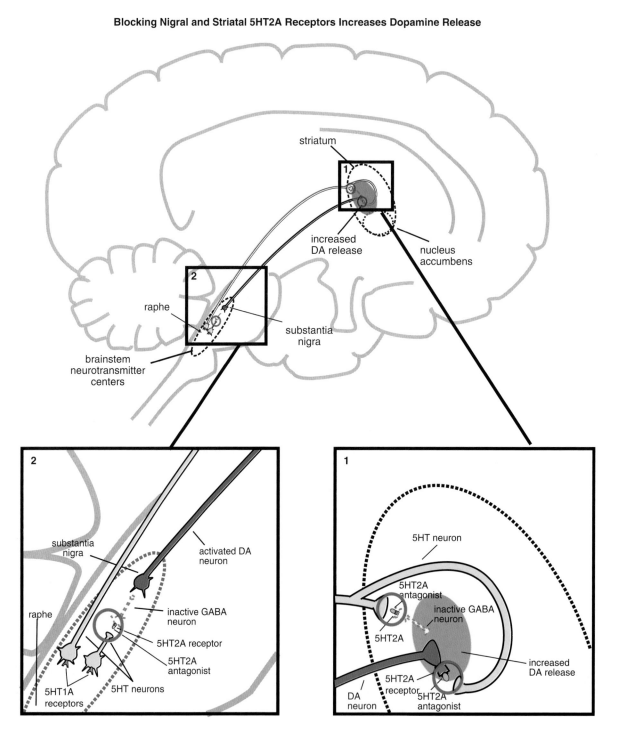

Figure 5-16B. Blocking nigral and striatal 5HT$_{2A}$ receptors increases dopamine release. (1) If 5HT$_{2A}$ receptors on GABAergic interneurons in the striatum are blocked, then serotonin is unable to stimulate these receptors to cause release of GABA (indicated by the dotted outline of the GABAergic neuron). Thus, GABA is unable to inhibit dopamine release. Likewise, blockade of 5HT$_{2A}$ receptors directly on striatal dopaminergic neurons prevents inhibition of dopamine release, thereby increasing striatal dopamine. (2) In the brainstem, blockade of 5HT$_{2A}$ receptors on GABAergic interneurons prevents GABA release onto dopaminergic neurons in the substantia nigra (indicated by the dotted outline of the GABAergic neuron). Thus, dopamine can be released into the striatum.

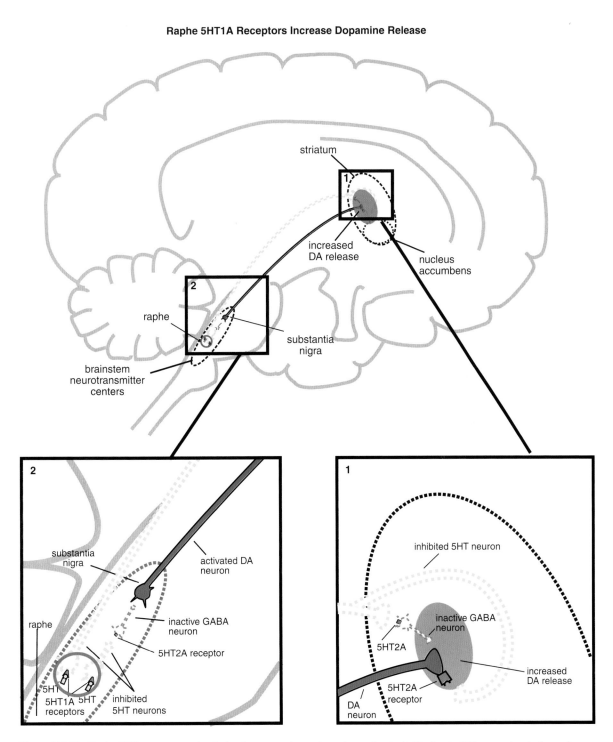

Figure 5-16C. Raphe 5HT$_{1A}$ receptor stimulation increases dopamine release. Serotonin binding to 5HT$_{1A}$ receptors in the raphe nucleus inhibits serotonin release (indicated by the dotted outline of the serotonin neurons). (1) In the striatum, reduced serotonin release means that 5HT$_{2A}$ receptors on GABAergic and dopaminergic neurons are not stimulated, which in turn means that dopamine release is not inhibited. (2) Similarly, in the brainstem, reduced serotonin release means that 5HT$_{2A}$ receptors on GABAergic interneurons are not stimulated and therefore GABA is not released (indicated by the dotted outline of the GABAergic neuron). Thus, dopamine can be released into the striatum.

Nigrostriatal Pathway

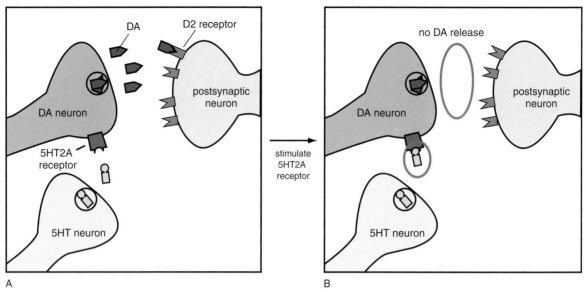

A   B

Figure 5-17. **Enlarged view of serotonin (5HT) and dopamine (DA) interactions in the nigrostriatal DA pathway at axon terminals in the striatum.** Normally, 5HT inhibits DA release. (A) DA is being released because no 5HT is stopping it. Specifically, no 5HT is present at its $5HT_{2A}$ receptor on the nigrostriatal DA neuron. (B) Now DA release is being inhibited by 5HT in the nigrostriatal dopamine pathway. When 5HT occupies its $5HT_{2A}$ receptor on the DA neuron (lower red circle), this inhibits DA release, so there is no DA in the synapse (upper red circle).

by serotonin at either end of substantia nigra neurons hypothetically *blocks dopamine release* in the striatum (Figure 5-16A). On the other hand, $5HT_{2A}$ *receptor antagonism* by an atypical antipsychotic at these same sites hypothetically *stimulates downstream dopamine release* in the striatum (Figure 5-16B). Such release of dopamine in the striatum should mitigate EPS, which is theoretically why antipsychotics with $5HT_{2A}$ antagonist properties are atypical. $5HT_{1A}$ receptors also regulate dopamine release in the striatum (Figure 5-16C, discussed below).

$5HT_{2A}$ receptor antagonism theoretically makes an antipsychotic atypical: low EPS

So, exactly how does this dopamine release by $5HT_{2A}$ antagonism reduce EPS? The answer to this is shown in Figures 5-17 and 5-18. Normally, serotonin reduces dopamine release from the striatum by actions of serotonin at the various $5HT_{2A}$ receptors discussed above (Figures 5-15A, 5-16A, 5-17). By contrast, the two actions of an atypical antipsychotic, namely blocking both D_2 receptors and $5HT_{2A}$ receptors, are shown in Figure 5-18, one at a time. On the left, D_2 receptors are blocked by the D_2 antagonist actions of the atypical antipsychotic, just like a conventional antipsychotic

(Figure 5-18A). If this were the only action of the drug, there would be EPS if occupancy of D_2 receptors reached 80% or more (Figure 5-18A). This is exactly what happens with a conventional antipsychotic. However, atypical antipsychotics have a second property, namely to block $5HT_{2A}$ receptors, which as discussed above have multiple mechanisms by which they increase dopamine release in the striatum (Figures 5-15B, 5-16B, 5-18B). The result of this increased dopamine release is that dopamine competes with D_2 receptor antagonists in the striatum, and reduces the D_2 receptor binding there below 80% to more like 60%, enough to eliminate extrapyramidal symptoms (Figure 5-18B). This is the hypothesis most frequently linked to the explanation for the mechanism of the most important distinguishing clinical properties of atypical antipsychotics, namely *low extrapyramidal symptoms* (EPS) with comparable antipsychotic actions.

$5HT_{2A}$ receptor antagonism theoretically makes an antipsychotic atypical: low hyperprolactinemia

How do $5HT_{2A}$ antagonist actions reduce hyperprolactinemia? Serotonin and dopamine have reciprocal roles in the regulation of prolactin secretion from the pituitary lactotroph cells. That is, dopamine inhibits prolactin

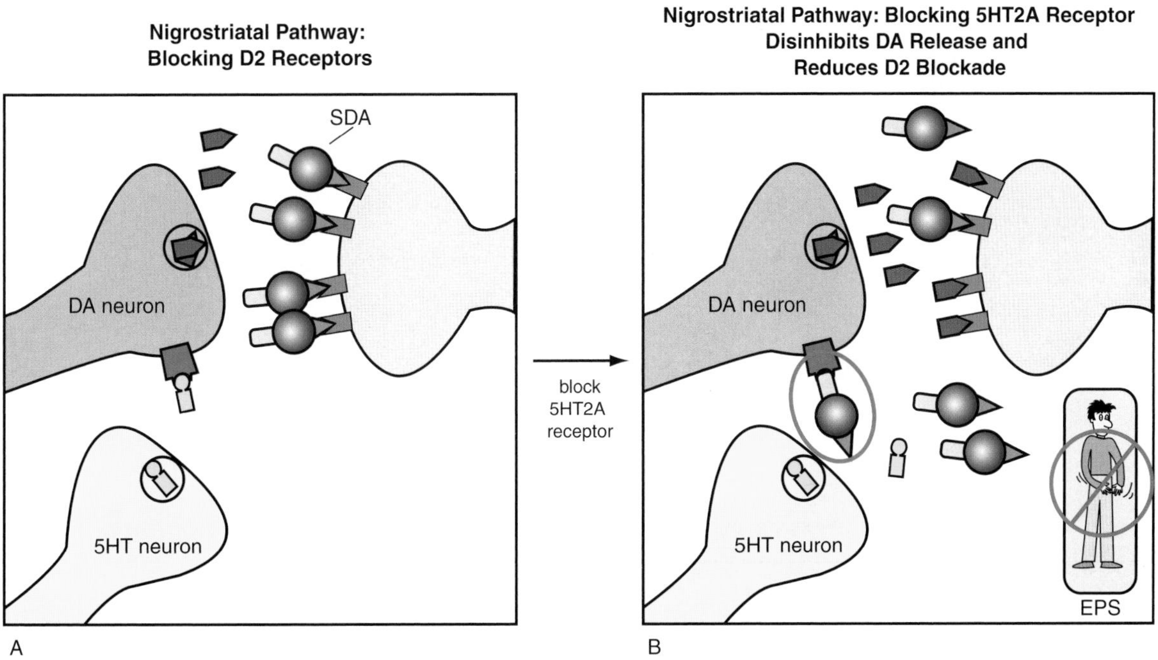

Nigrostriatal Pathway:
Blocking D2 Receptors

Nigrostriatal Pathway: Blocking 5HT2A Receptor
Disinhibits DA Release and
Reduces D2 Blockade

Figure 5-18. Serotonin 2A antagonists in the nigrostriatal pathway. (A) Postsynaptic dopamine 2 (D_2) receptors are being blocked by a serotonin–dopamine antagonist (SDA) in the nigrostriatal dopamine pathway. This shows what would happen if D_2 blockade were the only active action of an atypical antipsychotic – the drug would only bind to postsynaptic D_2 receptors and block them. In contrast, (B) shows the dual action of the SDAs, in which both D_2 and $5HT_{2A}$ receptors are blocked. The interesting thing is that the second action of $5HT_{2A}$ antagonism actually reverses the first action of D_2 antagonism. This happens because dopamine is released when serotonin can no longer inhibit its release. Another term for this is disinhibition. Thus, blocking a $5HT_{2A}$ receptor disinhibits the dopamine neuron, causing dopamine to pour out of it. The consequence of this is that dopamine can then compete with the SDA for the D_2 receptor and reverse the inhibition there. As D_2 blockade is thereby reversed, SDAs cause little or no extrapyramidal symptoms (EPS) or tardive dyskinesia.

release via stimulating D_2 receptors (Figure 5-19), whereas serotonin promotes prolactin release via stimulating $5HT_{2A}$ receptors (Figure 5-20). Thus, when D_2 receptors alone are blocked by a conventional antipsychotic, dopamine can no longer inhibit prolactin release, so prolactin levels rise (Figure 5-21). However, in the case of an atypical antipsychotic, there is simultaneous inhibition of $5HT_{2A}$ receptors, so serotonin can no longer stimulate prolactin release (Figure 5-22). This mitigates the hyperprolactinemia of D_2 receptor blockade. Although this is interesting theoretical pharmacology, in practice, not all serotonin–dopamine antagonists reduce prolactin secretion to the same extent, and others do not reduce prolactin elevations at all.

$5HT_{2A}$ receptor antagonism theoretically makes an antipsychotic atypical: comparable antipsychotic actions

Why doesn't $5HT_{2A}$ antagonism reverse antipsychotic actions? Although a conventional antipsychotic can only decrease dopamine, and will do this at D_2 receptors throughout the brain, atypical antipsychotics with their additional $5HT_{2A}$ antagonist properties have much more complicated net actions on dopamine activity, since they not only decrease dopamine activity by blocking D_2 receptors but they can also increase dopamine release and thus increase dopamine activity by indirectly stimulating dopamine receptors. However, these actions seem to be very different in different parts of the brain. In the nigrostriatal dopamine pathway and in the tuberoinfundibular dopamine pathway, there is sufficient dopamine release by atypical antipsychotics to reverse, in part, the unwanted actions of EPS and hyperprolactinemia. This does not appear to occur in the mesolimbic dopamine pathway, as antipsychotic actions of atypical antipsychotics are just as robust as those of conventional antipsychotics, presumably due to regional differences in the way in which $5HT_{2A}$ receptors can or cannot exert control over dopamine release. The trick has been to exploit these differing regional pharmacological mechanisms to get the best clinical

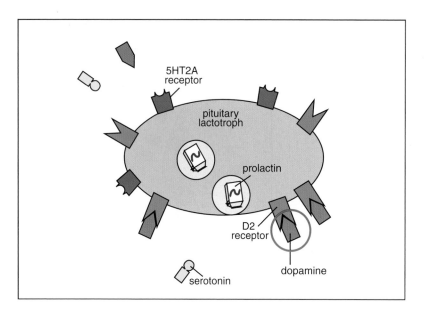

Figure 5-19. Dopamine inhibits prolactin. Dopamine inhibits prolactin release from pituitary lactotroph cells in the pituitary gland when it binds to D_2 receptors (red circle).

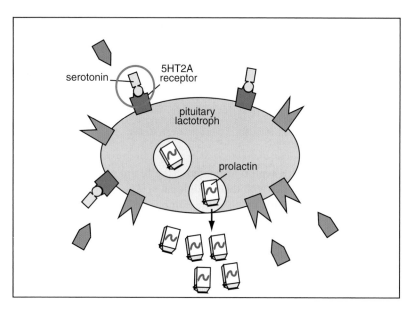

Figure 5-20. Serotonin stimulates prolactin. Serotonin (5HT) stimulates prolactin release from pituitary lactotroph cells in the pituitary gland when it binds to $5HT_{2A}$ receptors (red circle). Thus, serotonin and dopamine have a reciprocal regulatory action on prolactin release.

results by simultaneous blockade of D_2 receptors and $5HT_{2A}$ receptors that can fortuitously have net blockade of differing amounts of D_2 receptors in different areas of the same brain at the same time with the same drug! Although there are obviously many other factors at play here, and this is an overly simplistic explanation, it is a useful starting point for beginning to appreciate the pharmacological actions of serotonin–dopamine antagonists as a unique class of atypical antipsychotic drugs.

The making of a therapeutic window

One way to display this phenomenon of the atypical antipsychotics' differing clinical actions is to contrast what happens to dopamine D_2 binding in the striatum when a pure D_2 antagonist is given (Figure 5-4) versus when an atypical antipsychotic that combines equal or greater potency for blocking $5HT_{2A}$ receptors with D_2 antagonism is given (Figure 5-23). In the case of a pure D_2 antagonist like a conventional antipsychotic, the amount of D_2 receptor antagonism shown in

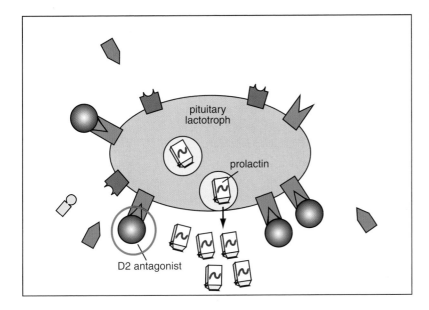

Figure 5-21. Conventional antipsychotics and prolactin. Conventional antipsychotic drugs are D$_2$ antagonists and thus oppose dopamine's inhibitory role on prolactin secretion from pituitary lactotrophs. Thus, these drugs increase prolactin levels (red circle).

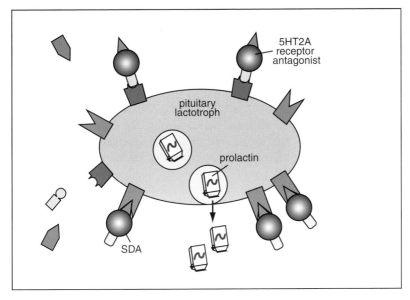

Figure 5-22. Atypical antipsychotics and prolactin. This figure shows how 5HT$_{2A}$ antagonism reverses the ability of D$_2$ antagonism to increase prolactin secretion. As dopamine and serotonin have reciprocal regulatory roles in the control of prolactin secretion, one cancels the other. Thus, stimulating 5HT$_{2A}$ receptors reverses the effects of stimulating D$_2$ receptors. The same thing works in reverse, namely, blockade of 5HT$_{2A}$ receptors (shown here) reverses the effects of blocking D$_2$ receptors (shown in Figure 5-21).

Figure 5-4 for the striatum is assumed to be the *same amount* in the limbic area and in the pituitary. This is why you get EPS and hyperprolactinemia at the *same dose* as you get antipsychotic actions, namely when all of these D$_2$ receptors in all of these brain areas are blocked substantially (many estimate this to be approximately 80%). There is little if any wiggle room between therapeutic actions and side effects (Figure 5-4).

However, in the case of an atypical antipsychotic, where essentially all of these drugs have an affinity for blocking 5HT$_{2A}$ that is equal to or greater than their affinity for blocking D$_2$ receptors, the amount of D$_2$ antagonism in the striatum is *lowered* at the same dose where the drugs have antipsychotic actions. This creates a *window between the dose that exerts antipsychotic actions and the dose that causes EPS or elevated prolactin levels* (Figure 5-23). While D$_2$ receptors are assumed to be blocked by 80% in the limbic areas to cause antipsychotic actions, the D$_2$ receptors in both the striatum and the pituitary are assumed to be blocked by only approximately 60%, below the threshold for side effects. Of course, if an

Hypothetical Thresholds for Atypical Antipsychotic Drug Effects

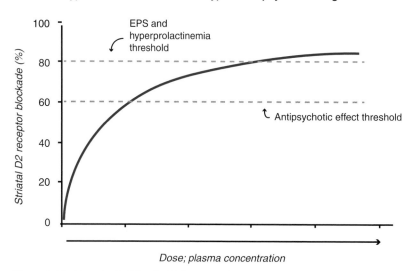

Figure 5-23. Hypothetical thresholds for atypical antipsychotic drug effects. All known antipsychotics bind to the dopamine 2 receptor, with the degree of binding determining whether one experiences therapeutic and/or side effects. For most atypical antipsychotics, D2 receptor occupancy greater than 80% in the mesolimbic pathway is needed for therapeutic effects, while D2 occupancy greater than 80% in the dorsal striatum is associated with extrapyramidal side effects (EPS) and D2 occupancy greater than 80% in the pituitary is associated with hyperprolactinemia. For conventional antipsychotics (i.e,. pure D2 antagonists) it is assumed that the same number of D2 receptors is blocked in all brain areas (see Figure 5-4). However, the 5HT2A and 5HT1A properties of atypical antipsychotics can presumably lower the amount of D2 antagonism in the dorsal striatum and in the pituitary but not in the limbic area; thus, there may be greater occupancy of D2 receptors in the limbic area of nucleus accumbens (not shown), perhaps up to 80% occupancy, while nigrostriatal and pituitary D2 receptors are only occupied at 60% due to the 5HT2A and 5HT1A properties of atypical antipsychotics.

atypical antipsychotic has its dose raised high enough, there will eventually be 80% blockade of even the striatum and pituitary, and the drug will lose its atypical properties. Thus, the drug is only "atypical" in the dosing window shown in Figure 5-23. This window is created by the fact that atypical antipsychotics almost always have higher affinity for $5HT_{2A}$ receptors than they do for D_2 receptors.

You can visualize the relative receptor actions of atypical antipsychotics on $5HT_{2A}$ receptors versus D_2 receptors by viewing simultaneously the relative potencies of the individual atypical antipsychotic drugs for binding $5HT_{2A}$ receptors versus D_2 receptors (Figure 5-24). The atypical antipsychotics can be categorized many ways, but for our discussion throughout this chapter, we will organize them as either the "pines" (peens) (Figure 5-24A), the "dones" (Figure 5-24B), or "two pips and a rip" (Figure 5-24C). Specifically, the pharmacologic binding properties of each drug are represented as a row of semi-quantitative and rank-order relative binding potencies at numerous neurotransmitter receptors. These figures are conceptual and not precisely quantitative, can differ from one laboratory to another, from species to species, and from method to

method, and the consensus values for binding properties evolve over time. More potent binding (higher affinity) is shown to the left of the value for the D_2 receptor, less potent binding (lower affinity) is shown to the right. Since these agents are all dosed to occupy about 60% or more of striatal D_2 receptors (Figure 5-23), all receptors to the left of D_2 in Figure 5-24 are occupied at the level of 60% or more at antipsychotic dosing levels. For these receptors to the left, there are also potentially clinically relevant receptor actions even at doses below those for treating psychosis. The receptors to the right of D_2 in Figure 5-24 are occupied at a level of less than 60% at antipsychotic dosing levels. Only those receptors that are bound by drug within an order of magnitude of potency of D_2 affinity are shown to the right of D_2. These receptor actions have potentially relevant clinical actions despite lower levels of occupancy than D_2 receptors, with dwindling occupancy levels as the receptor is listed further and further to the right, and also when given at lower doses than normal antipsychotic dosing levels.

The point is that although no two atypical antipsychotics have exactly the same pharmacologic binding profiles, it is easy to see that for the pines

5HT2A binding by pines

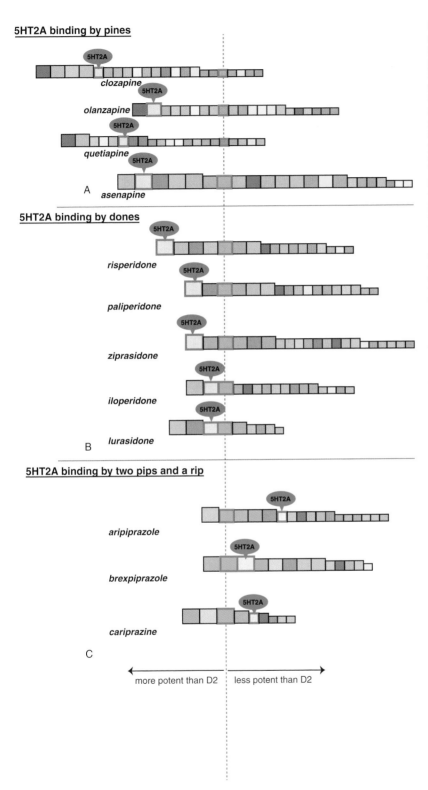

5HT2A binding by dones

5HT2A binding by two pips and a rip

Figure 5-24. 5HT₂ₐ binding by atypical antipsychotics. Shown here is a visual depiction of the binding profiles of atypical antipsychotics (see Figure 5-1). Each colored box represents a different binding property, with the size and positioning of the box reflecting the binding potency of the property (i.e., size indicates potency relative to a standard K_i scale, while position reflects potency relative to the other binding properties of that drug). The vertical dotted line cuts through the dopamine 2 (D_2) receptor binding box, with binding properties that are more potent than D_2 on the left and those that are less potent than D_2 on the right. Interestingly, D_2 binding is not the most potent property for any of the atypical antipsychotics. (A) The "pines" (clozapine, olanzapine, quetiapine, asenapine) all bind much more potently to the 5HT₂ₐ receptor than they do to the D_2 receptor. (B) The "dones" (risperidone, paliperidone, ziprasidone, iloperidone, lurasidone) also bind more potently to the 5HT₂ₐ receptor than to the D_2 receptor, or show similar potency at both receptors. (C) Aripiprazole and cariprazine both bind more potently to the D_2 receptor than to the 5HT₂ₐ receptor, while brexpiprazole has similar potency at both receptors.

(Figure 5-24A) and for the dones (Figure 5-24B), $5HT_{2A}$ receptor binding is always to the left of D_2 binding. This binding property of greater $5HT_{2A}$ than D_2 binding potency is what is widely thought to make these drugs "atypical" antipsychotics and to create the "window" of atypical antipsychotic action that is theoretically linked to low EPS as well as to low propensity to elevate prolactin. Note that for two pips and a rip, the $5HT_{2A}$ binding potency is to the right of D_2 binding, and thus less potent than D_2 binding (Figure 5-24C). The fact that the two pips and a rip are still atypical antipsychotics in their clinical properties is attributed to other actions, as will be explained in the sections below on $5HT_{1A}$ receptors and partial agonism of D_2 receptors. Rather than having more potent $5HT_{2A}$ than D_2 binding, as is the case for the pines and the dones, binding at $5HT_{1A}$ receptors and partial agonism of D_2 receptors may account for the atypical properties of the two pips and a rip.

$5HT_{1A}$ partial agonism can also make an antipsychotic atypical

In order to understand how $5HT_{1A}$ partial agonism can also reduce EPS, it is important to grasp how $5HT_{1A}$ receptors function in various parts of the brain, and how they can regulate dopamine release in the striatum.

Postsynaptic $5HT_{1A}$ receptors in prefrontal cortex are accelerators for dopamine release in striatum

If $5HT_{2A}$ stimulation is the "brake" *stopping* downstream dopamine release (Figure 5-15A), and $5HT_{2A}$ antagonism "cuts the brake cable," *enhancing* dopamine release (Figure 5-15B), what is the accelerator for downstream dopamine release in the striatum? The answer is postsynaptic $5HT_{1A}$ receptors on pyramidal neurons in the cortex (Figure 5-15C, box 1). $5HT_{1A}$ receptor stimulation in the cortex hypothetically *stimulates downstream dopamine release* in the striatum, by reducing glutamate release in the brainstem, which in turn fails to trigger the release of inhibitory GABA at dopamine neurons there (Figure 5-15C, box 2). Dopamine neurons are thus disinhibited, just as they are by a $5HT_{2A}$ antagonist. This would theoretically cause dopamine release in striatum, and mitigate EPS.

Presynaptic $5HT_{1A}$ receptors in raphe are also accelerators for dopamine release in the striatum

$5HT_{1A}$ receptors can not only be postsynaptic throughout the brain (Figures 5-15C, 5-16B, 5-16C), but also they can be presynaptic on the dendrites and

cell bodies of serotonin neurons in the midbrain raphe (Figure 5-25A). In fact, the only type of presynaptic 5HT receptor at the somatodendritic end of a serotonin neuron is a $5HT_{1A}$ receptor (Figure 5-25A). When 5HT is detected at presynaptic somatodendritic $5HT_{1A}$ receptors on neuronal dendrites and on the neuronal cell body, this activates an autoreceptor function that causes a slowing of neuronal impulse flow through the serotonin neuron and a reduction of serotonin release from its axon terminal (Figure 5-25B). Downregulation and desensitization of these presynaptic $5HT_{1A}$ somatodendritic autoreceptors are thought to be critical to the antidepressant actions of drugs that block serotonin reuptake, and this is discussed in Chapter 7 on antidepressants.

When serotonin occupies a presynaptic $5HT_{1A}$ somatodendritic autoreceptor in the midbrain raphe, where they are located (Figure 5-15C, box 2; Figure 5-16C, box 2), this turns off serotonin neurons. The serotonin pathways from raphe (Figure 5-16C, box 2) to substantia nigra (Figure 5-16C, box 2) and to striatum (Figure 5-16C, box 1) are thus "off" in the presence of serotonin at presynaptic $5HT_{1A}$ receptors; as a consequence, serotonin is not released onto postsynaptic $5HT_{2A}$ receptors on nigrostriatal neurons, activation of which would ordinarily inhibit dopamine release in the striatum (Figure 5-16A). Lack of serotonin release due to stimulation of presynaptic $5HT_{1A}$ receptors thereby allows the nigrostriatal dopamine neurons to be active and thus to release dopamine in the striatum (Figure 5-16C). Pre- and postsynaptic $5HT_{1A}$ receptors work together to enhance dopamine release in the striatum, and when both are stimulated by certain atypical antipsychotics, this theoretically mitigates EPS.

Some, but not all, atypical antipsychotics have potent $5HT_{1A}$ partial agonist properties (Figure 5-26). In particular, the two pips and a rip, namely aripiprazole and the experimental antipsychotics brexpiprazole and cariprazine, all have $5HT_{1A}$ partial agonist actions not only more potent than their $5HT_{2A}$ antagonist actions, but comparable to their D_2 antagonist actions (Figure 5-26C). The $5HT_{2A}$ antagonist actions may also contribute to the atypical properties of these three agents (Figure 5-26C), but the reduction of EPS for these agents is likely given a major boost by the additional presence of potent $5HT_{1A}$ partial agonist actions. In addition, note that potentially clinically relevant $5HT_{1A}$ partial agonist actions are present for a few of the pines (especially clozapine and quetiapine)

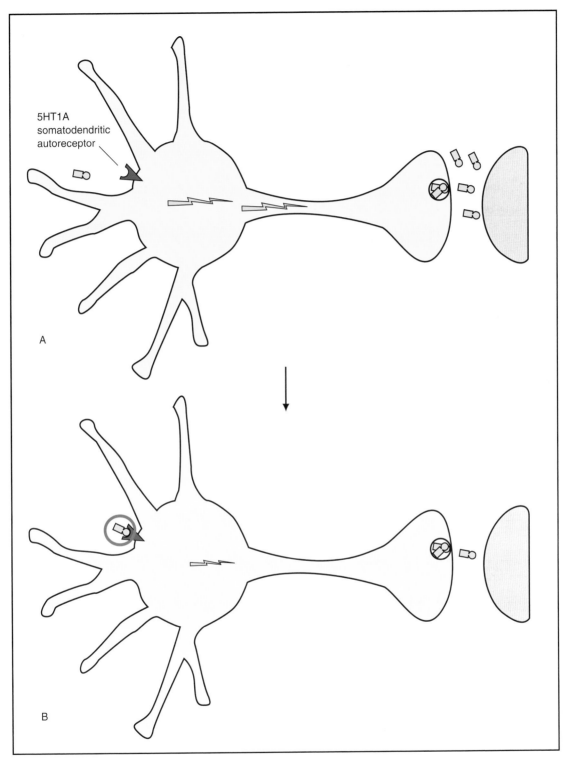

Figure 5-25. 5HT_{1A} autoreceptors. Presynaptic $5HT_{1A}$ receptors are autoreceptors located on the cell body and dendrites, and are therefore called somatodendritic autoreceptors (A). When serotonin (5HT) binds to these $5HT_{1A}$ receptors, it causes a shutdown of 5HT neuronal impulse flow, depicted here as decreased electrical activity and a reduction in the release of 5HT from the synapse on the right (B).

5HT1A binding by pines

5HT1A binding by dones

5HT1A binding by two pips and a rip

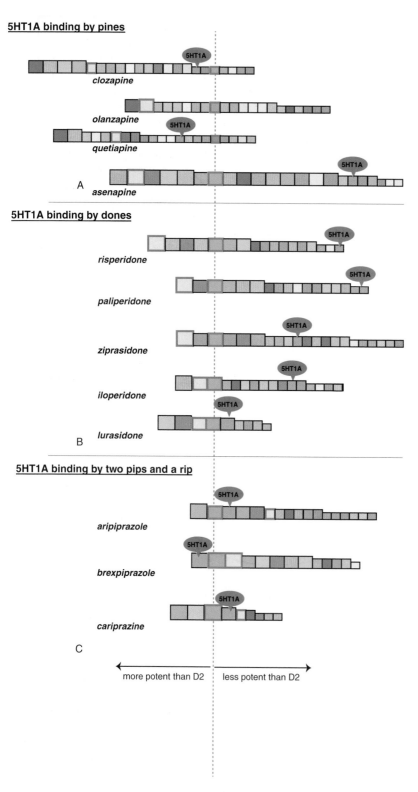

Figure 5-26. 5HT$_{1A}$ binding by atypical antipsychotics. Shown here is a visual depiction of the binding profiles of atypical antipsychotics (see Figure 5-1). (A) Clozapine and quetiapine both bind more potently to the 5HT$_{1A}$ receptor than they do to the D$_2$ receptor, while asenapine binds less potently to the 5HT$_{1A}$ receptor and olanzapine does not bind to it at all. (B) All of the "dones" (risperidone, paliperidone, ziprasidone, iloperidone, lurasidone) bind to the 5HT$_{1A}$ receptor with less potency than they do to the D$_2$ receptor. (C) Aripiprazole, brexpiprazole, and cariprazine each have similar relative potency for the D$_2$ and 5HT$_{1A}$ receptors. 5HT$_{1A}$ binding is actually the most potent property of brexpiprazole.

(Figure 5-26A) and some of the dones (especially lurasidone, iloperidone, and ziprasidone) (Figure 5-26B), with those binding properties further to the left being relatively more potent and thus potentially more clinically relevant as well at antipsychotic dosing levels.

The most dopamine release in striatum and fewest EPS may come when you take your foot off the brake and also step on the accelerator

If blocking $5HT_{2A}$ receptors is like taking your foot off the brake, and if stimulating $5HT_{1A}$ receptors is like stepping on the accelerator, this could account for why both of these actions that release dopamine from the striatum might be additive. It may also potentially explain why atypical antipsychotics with either potent $5HT_{2A}$ antagonism (Figure 5-24) or potent $5HT_{1A}$ agonist/partial agonist properties (Figure 5-26), or with both actions, have a reduced incidence of EPS. Thus, either pharmacologic action alone or both pharmacologic actions together seem to contribute to the atypical antipsychotic profiles of specific atypical antipsychotic drugs.

Not only do several atypical antipsychotics have $5HT_{1A}$ partial agonist actions (Figure 5-26), but so do various agents with known or suspected antidepressant actions, from vilazodone to buspirone (augmentation of selective serotonin reuptake inhibitors [SSRIs]/serotonin–norepinephrine reuptake inhibitors [SNRIs]), to experimental agents with selective or mixed $5HT_{1A}$ partial agonism (e.g., vortioxetine). This has led to speculation that those atypical antipsychotics with $5HT_{1A}$ partial agonist actions that are proven antidepressants (such as quetiapine and aripiprazole) may be working in part through this mechanism, and that other atypical antipsychotics with $5HT_{1A}$ partial agonist actions are also potential antidepressants (such as brexpiprazole, cariprazine, lurasidone, iloperidone, and others). The mechanism of how $5HT_{1A}$ partial agonism exerts its possible antidepressant efficacy is unknown, but could be linked to release of dopamine and norepinephrine in prefrontal cortex or to the potentiation of serotonin levels in the presence of a serotonin reuptake inhibitor, which would be theoretically linked to antidepressant actions.

$5HT_{1B/D}$ receptors

Presynaptic 5HT receptors are autoreceptors, and detect the presence of 5HT, causing a shutdown of further 5HT release and 5HT neuronal impulse flow. Discussed above are the $5HT_{1A}$ presynaptic receptors at the somatodendritic end of the serotonin neuron (Figure 5-25). There is also another type of presynaptic serotonin receptor, and it is located at the other end of the neuron, on the axon terminals (Figure 5-27). When 5HT is detected in the synapse by presynaptic 5HT receptors on axon terminals, it occurs via a $5HT_{1B/D}$ receptor which is also called a *terminal autoreceptor* (Figure 5-27). In the case of the $5HT_{1B/D}$ terminal autoreceptor, 5HT occupancy of this receptor causes a blockade of 5HT release (Figure 5-27B). On the other hand, drugs that block the $5HT_{1B/D}$ autoreceptor can promote 5HT release, and this could hypothetically result in antidepressant actions, as for the experimental antidepressant vortioxetine discussed in Chapter 7. Among the atypical antipsychotics, only iloperidone, ziprasidone (Figure 5-28B), and asenapine (Figure 5-28A), unproven yet as antidepressants, have $5HT_{1B/D}$ binding more potent than or comparably potent to D_2 binding, although many other agents have low potency at this receptor (Figure 5-28), including the proven antidepressants olanzapine, quetiapine, and aripiprazole. However, the link of $5HT_{1B/D}$ to the antidepressant actions of these agents, although plausible, remains unproven.

$5HT_{2C}$ receptors

$5HT_{2C}$ receptors are postsynaptic, and regulate both dopamine and norepinephrine release. *Stimulation* of $5HT_{2C}$ receptors is one experimental approach to a novel antipsychotic, since this suppresses dopamine release, curiously more from the mesolimbic than from the nigrostriatal pathways, yielding an excellent preclinical profile: namely, an antipsychotic without EPS. One such agent, the $5HT_{2C}$ selective agonist vabacaserin, has entered clinical trials for the treatment of schizophrenia. *Stimulating* $5HT_{2C}$ receptors is also an experimental approach to the treatment of obesity, since this leads to weight loss in both preclinical and clinical studies. Another $5HT_{2C}$ selective agonist, lorcaserin, is now approved for the treatment of obesity. Psychopharmacological treatments for obesity, including lorcaserin, are discussed in Chapter 14.

Blocking $5HT_{2C}$ receptors stimulates dopamine and norepinephrine release in prefrontal cortex, and has pro-cognitive but particularly antidepressant actions in experimental animals. Several known and experimental antidepressants are $5HT_{2C}$ antagonists, ranging from certain tricyclic antidepressants to mirtazapine, to agomelatine, and these are discussed in Chapter 7 on

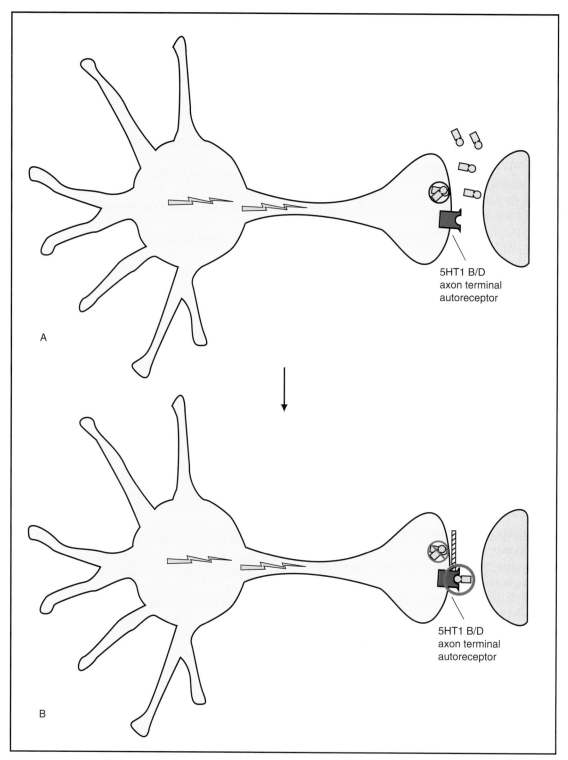

Figure 5-27. 5HT$_{1B/D}$ autoreceptors. Presynaptic 5HT$_{1B/D}$ receptors are autoreceptors located on the presynaptic axon terminal. They act by detecting the presence of serotonin (5HT) in the synapse and causing a shutdown of further 5HT release. When 5HT builds up in the synapse (A), it is available to bind to the autoreceptor, which then inhibits serotonin release (B).

5HT1 B/D
axon terminal
autoreceptor

5HT1 B/D
axon terminal
autoreceptor

A

B

5HT1B/D binding by pines

5HT1B/D binding by dones

5HT1B/D binding by two pips and a rip

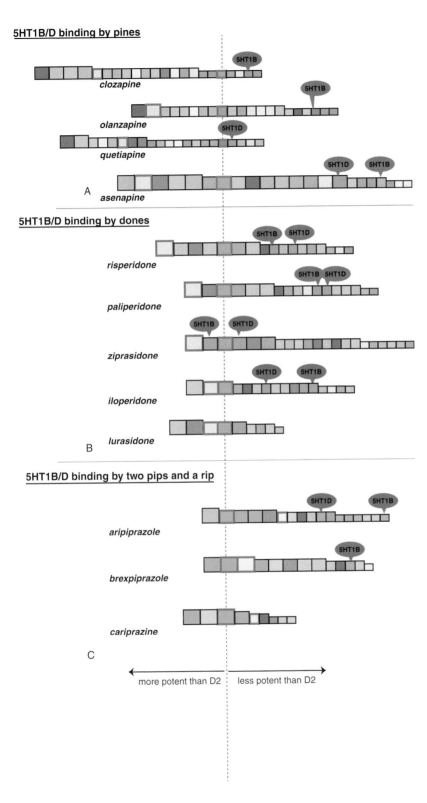

Figure 5-28. 5HT$_{1B/D}$ **binding by atypical antipsychotics.** Shown here is a visual depiction of the binding profiles of atypical antipsychotics (see Figure 5-1). (A) Clozapine, olanzapine, and asenapine all bind relatively weakly to the 5HT$_{1B}$ receptor, while quetiapine and asenapine bind to the 5HT$_{1D}$ receptor. (B) Risperidone, paliperidone, ziprasidone, and iloperidone all have some affinity for the 5HT$_{1B}$ and 5HT$_{1D}$ receptors. In particular, ziprasidone binds more potently to the 5HT$_{1B}$ receptor than to the D$_2$ receptor. Lurasidone does not bind to 5HT$_{1B/D}$. (C) Aripiprazole and brexpiprazole each bind weakly to the 5HT$_{1B}$ receptor; aripiprazole also binds to the 5HT$_{1D}$ receptor; cariprazine does not bind to 5HT$_{1B/D}$.

antidepressants. Some atypical antipsychotics have potent $5HT_{2C}$ antagonist properties, especially the pines, including those with known antidepressant action, namely quetiapine and olanzapine (Figure 5-29A). Olanzapine is often combined with fluoxetine to boost olanzapine's antidepressant actions in treatment-resistant and bipolar depression. Fluoxetine is not only a well-known SSRI, but also has potent $5HT_{2C}$ antagonist properties that may not only contribute to its antidepressant effects as monotherapy, but also add to the $5HT_{2C}$ antagonist actions of olanzapine when an olanzapine–fluoxetine combination is given. For quetiapine, there is some evidence for pharmacologic synergism between its norepinephrine reuptake blocking properties and its $5HT_{2C}$ antagonist properties (see NET for quetiapine in Figure 5-47, to the left and more potent than $5HT_{2C}$ antagonism). These two mechanisms can each boost dopamine and norepinephrine release in prefrontal cortex, something theoretically linked to antidepressant actions. This is discussed as well in Chapter 7 on antidepressants. Potent $5HT_{2C}$ antagonist actions suggests theoretical antidepressant effects for asenapine (Figure 5-29A), but there are only relatively weak $5HT_{2C}$ binding potencies for most of the other atypical antipsychotics (Figure 5-29B and C).

$5HT_3$ receptors

$5HT_3$ receptors are postsynaptic and regulate inhibitory GABA interneurons in various brain areas that in turn regulate the release of a number of neurotransmitters, from serotonin itself to acetylcholine, norepinephrine, dopamine, and histamine. $5HT_3$ receptors are also involved in centrally mediated vomiting and possibly also in nausea. Peripheral $5HT_3$ receptors in the gut regulate bowel motility.

Blocking $5HT_3$ receptors in the chemoreceptor trigger zone of the brainstem is an established therapeutic approach to mitigating the nausea and vomiting caused by cancer chemotherapy. Blocking $5HT_3$ receptors on GABA interneurons increases the release of serotonin, dopamine, norepinephrine, acetylcholine, and histamine in the cortex and is thus a novel approach to an antidepressant and to a pro-cognitive agent. The proven antidepressant mirtazapine and the experimental antidepressant vortioxetine are potent $5HT_3$ antagonists, and this may contribute to the antidepressant actions of such agents, especially in combination with inhibition of serotonin, norepinephrine, and/or dopamine

reuptake. Antidepressant actions linked to $5HT_3$ receptors and other serotonin receptors are discussed in Chapter 7 on antidepressants. Among the atypical antipsychotics, only clozapine has $5HT_3$ binding potency comparable to its D_2 binding potency, and the others have very weak or essentially no affinity for this receptor, so $5HT_3$ antagonism does not likely contribute to the clinical actions of atypical antipsychotics.

$5HT_6$ receptors

$5HT_6$ receptors are postsynaptic and may be key regulators of the release of acetylcholine and cognitive processes. Blocking this receptor improves learning and memory in experimental animals. $5HT_6$ antagonists have been proposed as novel pro-cognitive agents for the cognitive symptoms of schizophrenia when added on to an atypical antipsychotic. Some atypical antipsychotics are potent $5HT_6$ antagonists (clozapine, olanzapine, asenapine) relative to D_2 binding (Figure 5-30A) and other atypical antipsychotics have moderate or weak binding to $5HT_6$ receptors relative to D_2 binding (quetiapine, ziprasidone, iloperidone, aripiprazole, brexpiprazole) (Figure 5-30A, B, C), but it remains unclear how this action contributes to any of their clinical profiles.

$5HT_7$ receptors

$5HT_7$ receptors are postsynaptic and are important regulators of serotonin release. When blocked, serotonin release is disinhibited, especially when $5HT_7$ antagonism is combined with serotonin reuptake inhibition. This is discussed in further detail later in this chapter and also in Chapter 7 on antidepressants. Novel $5HT_7$-selective antagonists are thought to be regulators of circadian rhythms, sleep, and mood in experimental animals. Several proven antidepressants have at least moderate affinity for $5HT_7$ receptors as antagonists, including amoxapine, desipramine, imipramine, mianserin, fluoxetine, and the experimental antidepressant vortioxetine. Several of the pines and dones are potent $5HT_7$ antagonists relative to D_2 binding (to the left of D_2 for clozapine, quetiapine, and asenapine in Figure 5-30A, and to the left of D_2 for risperidone, paliperidone, and lurasidone in Figure 5-30B). Other pines, dones, and the two pips and a rip have moderate affinities as well (to the right in Figure 5-30A, B, C) which are potentially clinically relevant.

5HT2C binding by pines

5HT2C binding by dones

5HT2C binding by two pips and a rip

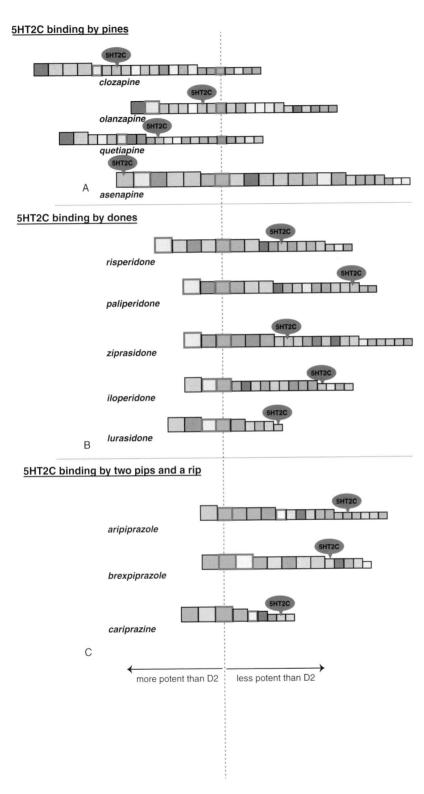

more potent than D2 | less potent than D2

Figure 5-29. 5HT_{2C} binding by atypical antipsychotics. Shown here is a visual depiction of the binding profiles of atypical antipsychotics (see Figure 5-1). (A) All of the "pines" (clozapine, olanzapine, quetiapine, asenapine) bind more potently to the 5HT_{2C} receptor than they do to the D_2 receptor. (B) All of the "dones" (risperidone, paliperidone, ziprasidone, iloperidone, lurasidone) have some affinity for the 5HT_{2C} receptor, though none with more potency than at the D_2 receptor. (C) Aripiprazole, brexpiprazole, and cariprazine all have relatively weak affinity for the 5HT_{2C} receptor.

5HT6 and 5HT7 binding by pines

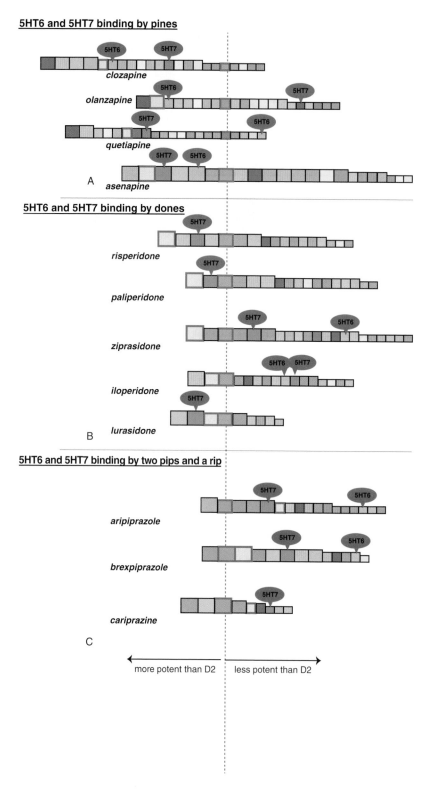

A

5HT6 and 5HT7 binding by dones

B

5HT6 and 5HT7 binding by two pips and a rip

C

more potent than D2 | less potent than D2

Figure 5-30. 5HT$_6$ and 5HT$_7$ binding by atypical antipsychotics. Shown here is a visual depiction of the binding profiles of atypical antipsychotics (see Figure 5-1). (A) Clozapine, olanzapine, and asenapine each bind more potently to the 5HT$_6$ receptor, whereas binding of quetiapine to 5HT$_6$ receptors is relatively weak. Clozapine, quetiapine, and asenapine each have greater affinity for the 5HT$_7$ receptor compared to the D$_2$ receptor. Olanzapine also binds to the 5HT$_7$ receptor, but with relatively weak potency. (B) Of the dones, only ziprasidone and iloperidone bind to 5HT$_6$, and in both cases this 5HT$_6$ affinity is weaker than for the D$_2$ receptor. Risperidone, paliperidone, and lurasidone have greater affinity for the 5HT$_7$ receptor than for the D$_2$ receptor. Ziprasidone also has relatively potent binding at the 5HT$_7$ receptor, though with less affinity than for D$_2$ receptors. (C) Aripiprazole and brexpiprazole have relatively weak affinity for 5HT$_6$ receptors. Aripiprazole, brexpiprazole, and cariprazine all bind to the 5HT$_7$ receptor, though none with more potency than for the D$_2$ receptor.

It is plausible but unproven that $5HT_7$ antagonism contributes to the known antidepressant actions of quetiapine, especially in combination with SSRIs/ SNRIs, and in combination with its other potential antidepressant mechanisms discussed above for quetiapine such as NET inhibition, $5HT_{2C}$ antagonism, and $5HT_{1A}$ partial agonism. It is also plausible but unproven that $5HT_7$ antagonism could contribute to the known antidepressant actions of aripiprazole, especially in combination with SSRIs/SNRIs and in combination with its $5HT_{1A}$ partial agonism. This leads to speculation that lurasidone, asenapine, brexpiprazole, and others could have antidepressant potential in unipolar major depressive disorder, especially in combination with SSRIs/SNRIs, but more clinical trials are necessary at this time to prove this. Recent data already indicate antidepressant actions of lurasidone in bipolar depression.

D_2 partial agonism (DPA) makes an antipsychotic atypical

Some antipsychotics act to stabilize dopamine neurotransmission in a state between silent antagonism and full stimulation/agonist action by acting as partial agonists at D_2 receptors (Figure 5-31). Partial agonist actions at G-protein-linked receptors, which is how D_2 receptors are categorized, are explained in Chapter 2 and illustrated in Figures 2-3 through 2-10. Dopamine partial agonists (DPAs) theoretically bind to the D_2 receptor in a manner that is neither too antagonizing like a conventional antipsychotic ("too cold," with antipsychotic actions but extrapyramidal symptoms: Figure 5-32A), nor too stimulating like a stimulant or dopamine itself ("too hot," with positive symptoms of psychosis: Figure 5-32B). Instead, a partial agonist binds in an intermediary manner ("just right," with antipsychotic actions but no extrapyramidal symptoms: Figure 5-32C). For this reason, partial agonists are sometimes called "Goldilocks" drugs if they get the balance "just right" between full agonism and complete antagonism. However, as we shall see, this explanation is an oversimplification and the balance is different for each drug in the D_2 partial agonist class.

Partial agonists have the intrinsic ability to bind receptors in a manner that causes signal transduction from the receptor to be intermediate between full output and no output (Figure 5-33). The naturally occurring neurotransmitter generally functions as a

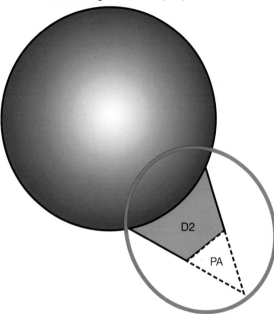

What Makes an Antipsychotic Atypical?

D2 Partial Agonist Actions (DPA)

Figure 5-31. D_2 partial agonism. A third property that may render an antipsychotic atypical is that of dopamine 2 partial agonism (DPA). These agents may stabilize dopamine neurotransmission in a state between silent antagonism and full stimulation.

full agonist, and causes maximum signal transduction from the receptor it occupies (Figure 5-33, top) whereas antagonists essentially shut down all output from the receptor they occupy and make them "silent" in terms of communicating with downstream signal transduction cascades (Figure 5-33, middle). Partial agonists cause receptor output that is more than the silent antagonist, but less than the full agonist (Figure 5-33, bottom). Thus, many degrees of partial agonism are possible between these two extremes. Full agonists, antagonists, and partial agonists may cause different changes in receptor conformation that lead to a corresponding range of signal transduction output from the receptor (Figure 5-34).

An amazing characteristic of D_2 receptors is that it only takes a very small amount of signal transduction through D_2 receptors in the striatum for a dopamine D_2 receptor partial agonist to avoid extrapyramidal side effects. Thus a very slight degree of partial agonist property, sometimes called "intrinsic activity," can have a very different set of clinical consequences compared to a fully silent and completely blocked D_2 receptor, which is what almost all known

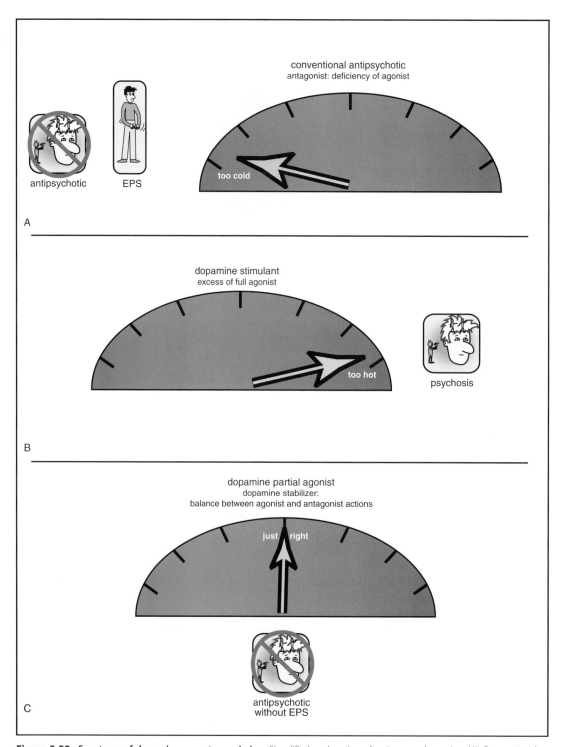

Figure 5-32. Spectrum of dopamine neurotransmission. Simplified explanation of actions on dopamine. (A) Conventional antipsychotics bind to the D_2 receptor in a manner that is "too cold"; that is, they have powerful antagonist actions while preventing agonist actions and thus can reduce positive symptoms of psychosis but also cause extrapyramidal symptoms (EPS). (B) D_2 receptor agonists, such as dopamine itself, are "too hot" and can therefore lead to positive symptoms. (C) D_2 partial agonists bind in an intermediary manner to the D_2 receptor and are therefore "just right," with antipsychotic actions but no EPS.

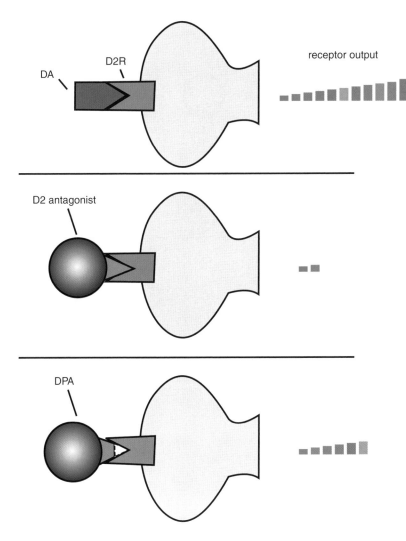

receptor output

Figure 5-33. Dopamine receptor output. Dopamine itself is a full agonist and causes full receptor output (top). Conventional antipsychotics are full antagonists and allow little if any receptor output (middle). The same is true for atypical antipsychotics that are serotonin–dopamine antagonists. However, D_2 partial agonists (DPAs) can partially activate dopamine receptor output and cause a stabilizing balance between stimulation and blockade of dopamine receptors (bottom).

conventional and atypical antipsychotics do. Those agents all lie to the far left on the D_2 partial agonist spectrum in Figure 5-35. Partial agonists capable of treating schizophrenia lie far to the left on the D_2 partial agonist spectrum, but not all the way to full antagonist. By contrast, dopamine itself, the naturally occurring full agonist, is all the way to the right on the D_2 partial agonist spectrum in Figure 5-35. Agents capable of treating Parkinson's disease (such as ropinirole and pramipexole) lie far to the right on the D_2 partial agonist spectrum.

What is so interesting is how very small movements off the far left and up the partial agonist spectrum in Figure 5-35 can have profound effects upon the clinical properties of an antipsychotic: just slightly too close to a pure antagonist (too far to the left), and it is just a conventional antipsychotic with EPS and

akathisia unless it has other $5HT_{2A}/5HT_{1A}$ properties that compensate for being too far to the left (comparable to "too cold" in Figure 5-32A). On the other hand, just slightly too far to the right, and it is an atypical antipsychotic without EPS or akathisia, but one that is too activating, capable of worsening positive symptoms of schizophrenia and also causing intolerable nausea and vomiting (comparable to "too hot" in Figure 5-32B). The elusive Goldilocks solution of a drug that is a tolerable high-dose antipsychotic without EPS and a tolerable low-dose antidepressant is being sought empirically by iterative introduction of a series of partial agonists each differing in their intrinsic activity that demonstrate the consequences of being either too close to the antagonist end of the spectrum, or too far off that end of the spectrum. This is just a theory of how building tiny bits of partial agonism into

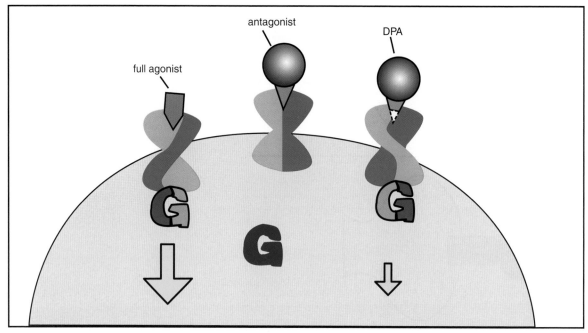

Figure 5-34. Agonist spectrum and receptor conformation. This figure depicts changes in receptor conformation in response to full agonists versus antagonists versus partial agonists. With full agonists, the receptor conformation is such that there is robust signal transduction through the G-protein-linked second-messenger system of D_2 receptors (on the left). Antagonists, on the other hand, bind to the D_2 receptor in a manner that produces a receptor conformation that is not capable of any signal transduction (middle). Partial agonists, such as a dopamine partial agonist (DPA), cause a receptor conformation such that there is an intermediate amount of signal transduction (on the right). However, the partial agonist does not induce as much signal transduction as a full agonist.

a D_2 antagonist can dramatically change its clinical properties, but there is some reasonable evidence for this possibility, given that there are several agents with significant clinical testing or experience that are available and that have tested this pharmacological concept in patients with schizophrenia.

For example, it is possible that the older agents sulpiride and amisulpride (not available in the US) are just barely off the antagonist part of the spectrum, without sufficient $5HT_{2A}$ or $5HT_{1A}$ actions to forgive this, and thus have low but not zero EPS with robust antipsychotic activities at high doses, plus anecdotal but not well-tested antidepressant and negative symptom clinical actions at low doses (Figure 5-35). Fairly extensive testing has been carried out of five other partial agonists shown in Figure 5-35, with progressively increasing amounts of partial agonist action as they go from left to right. The first dart thrown at the partial agonist spectrum was OPC4392 (structurally and pharmacologically related to both aripiprazole and brexpiprazole, which were tested later). OPC4392 landed too close to the agonist part of the curve, although it had relatively little intrinsic activity. This surprised investigators, who discovered that although OPC4392 improved negative symptoms of schizophrenia, it also activated rather than consistently improved positive symptoms of schizophrenia, and in balance did not have the profile of an acceptable antipsychotic so was never marketed.

However, investigators threw another dart closer to the antagonist part of the spectrum and it landed as aripiprazole. This agent is indeed an atypical antipsychotic in which the balance was improved so that it ameliorated positive symptoms without activating negative symptoms at higher antipsychotic doses, while proving to be an antidepressant at lower doses. Aripiprazole still has some akathisia, and some thought this was because it might be a bit too close to the antagonist end of the spectrum. Thus another dart, called bifeprunox, was aimed further up the spectrum, landing as more of an agonist than aripiprazole but less of an agonist than OPC4392, hoping for an improvement compared with aripiprazole, with less akathisia. What happened is that bifeprunox is too much of an agonist: it causes nausea and vomiting from dopamine agonist

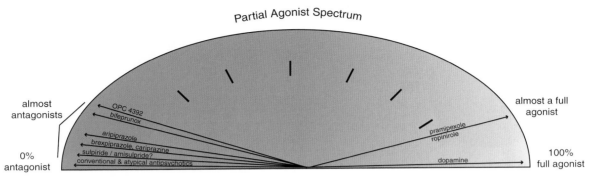

Figure 5-35. Spectrum of dopamine partial agonists. Dopamine partial agonists may themselves fall along a spectrum, with some having actions closer to a silent antagonist and others having actions closer to a full agonist. Agents with too much agonism may be psychotomimetic and thus not effective antipsychotics. Instead, partial agonists that are closer to the antagonist end of the spectrum (such as aripiprazole, cariprazine, or brexpiprazole, but not bifeprunox) seem to have favorable profiles. Amisulpride and sulpiride may be very partial agonists, with their partial agonist clinical properties more evident at lower doses.

actions (and $5HT_{1A}$ partial agonist actions), and bifeprunox's antipsychotic actions, although better than placebo, were not as robust as a full antagonist atypical antipsychotic, so the US Food and Drug Administration (FDA) did not approve it.

Two more agents with antagonist actions greater than aripiprazole are in late-stage clinical testing, namely a second "pip," brexpiprazole, and the "rip" cariprazine (Figure 5-35). So far, both appear to have efficacy in schizophrenia, and clinical trials and dose finding in mania and depression are ongoing, but both agents, although having subtle pharmacologic differences, are looking as though they will have significant clinical differences not only from aripiprazole but also from each other. The take-away point here is that D_2 partial agonism can make an antipsychotic atypical, and that subtle changes in the degree of intrinsic efficacy along the partial agonist scale at the full antagonist end of the spectrum can have profound clinical consequences.

Links between antipsychotic binding properties and clinical actions

Although D_2 antagonist/partial agonist properties can explain the antipsychotic efficacy for positive symptoms as well as many side effects of antipsychotics, and the $5HT_{2A}$ antagonist, $5HT_{1A}$ partial agonist and muscarinic antagonist properties can explain the reduced propensity for EPS or elevating prolactin of various antipsychotics, there are many additional pharmacologic properties of these drugs. In fact, the atypical antipsychotics as a class have perhaps the most complicated pattern of binding to neurotransmitter

receptors of any drug class in psychopharmacology, and no two agents have an identical portfolio of these additional properties (Figure 5-24). Binding properties of each individual atypical antipsychotic are discussed later in this chapter. In this section, we will review a number of other receptor interactions for the class of atypical antipsychotic drugs in general, and show where the potential links may exist between pharmacology and clinical actions. Although many of the actions of these drugs on the various receptors are fairly well established, the link between receptor binding and clinical actions remains hypothetical, with some links better established than others.

Antidepressant actions in bipolar and unipolar depression

Atypical antipsychotics are really misnamed, because they also have antidepressant actions alone and in combination with other antidepressants. It does not seem likely that D_2 antagonism or $5HT_{2A}$ antagonism are the mechanisms for this, because agents with only those properties are not effective antidepressants, and antipsychotics with these properties often work at doses lower than those necessary for antipsychotic actions, perhaps due to other pharmacologic actions. The actions hypothetically linked to antidepressant effects are those that exist for proven antidepressants, although not every atypical antipsychotic with a potential antidepressant mechanism is proven to be an antidepressant in clinical trials. The hypothetical antidepressant actions of one or more of the atypical antipsychotics are shown in Figure 5-36, and

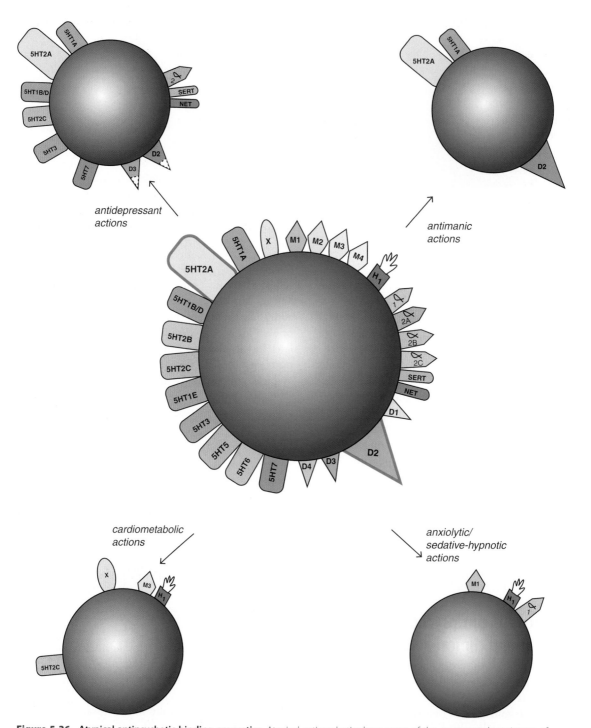

Figure 5-36. Atypical antipsychotic binding properties. Atypical antipsychotics have some of the most complex mixtures of pharmacological properties in psychopharmacology. Beyond antagonism of $5HT_{2A}$ and D_2 receptors, agents in this class interact with multiple other receptor subtypes for both dopamine and serotonin, and have effects on other neurotransmitter systems as well. Some of these multiple pharmacological properties can contribute to the therapeutic effects of atypical antipsychotics (e.g., antidepressant, antimanic, and anxiolytic effects), whereas others can contribute to their side effects (e.g,. sedative-hypnotic and cardiometabolic effects). No two atypical antipsychotics have identical binding properties, which probably helps to explain why they all have distinctive clinical properties.

each of these pharmacologic actions is discussed in more detail in Chapter 7. Numerous receptor binding properties linked to various serotonin receptors have already been mentioned, including $5HT_{1A}$ partial agonist actions and antagonism of $5HT_{1B/D}$, $5HT_{2C}$, $5HT_3$, and $5HT_7$ receptors. Additional mechanisms linked to antidepressant actions that are shared by various atypical antipsychotics include:

- **Serotonin and/or norepinephrine reuptake inhibition** – Only quetiapine has potency greater than its D_2 binding, but ziprasidone and zotepine have weak binding at these sites.
- **Alpha-2 (α_2) antagonism** – The proven antidepressant mirtazapine is best known for α_2 antagonism, but several atypical antipsychotics also have this action with variable degrees of potency, including essentially all the pines (higher potency especially for quetiapine and clozapine: Figure 5-37A) and dones (higher potency especially for risperidone: Figure 5-37B) as well as aripiprazole (Figure 5-37C).

Antimanic actions

All antipsychotics are effective for psychotic mania, but atypical antipsychotics appear to have greater efficacy, or at least greater documentation of efficacy, for nonpsychotic mania, leading to the major hypothesis that it is the D_2 antagonism/partial agonism combined with $5HT_{2A}$ antagonism that is the mechanism of this (Figure 5-36). However, proven for aripiprazole and with preliminary evidence of efficacy for cariprazine, agents with D_2 partial agonism and with $5HT_{1A}$ partial agonism more potent than $5HT_{2A}$ antagonism are also effective for mania, so $5HT_{1A}$ agonist/partial agonist actions may contribute to antimanic efficacy as well (Figure 5-36).

Anxiolytic actions

A somewhat controversial use of atypical antipsychotics is for the treatment of various anxiety disorders. Some studies suggest efficacy of various atypical antipsychotics for generalized anxiety disorder, and to augment other agents for other anxiety disorders, but perhaps more controversial is their use for posttraumatic stress disorder (PTSD). Furthermore, side effects and cost considerations and the lack of regulatory approval have tended to restrict this application of the atypical antipsychotics. It is possible that the antihistamine and anticholinergic sedative properties of some of these agents are calming in some patients and responsible for anxiolytic action in them (Figure 5-36). Agents with these properties are listed in the following section on sedation. Anecdotal use as well as clinical evidence for utility in various anxiety disorders is probably greatest for quetiapine.

Sedative-hypnotic and sedating actions

There has been a longstanding debate as to whether sedation is a good or a bad property for an antipsychotic. The answer seems to be that sedation is both good and bad. In some cases, particularly for short-term treatment, sedation is a desired therapeutic effect, especially early in treatment, during hospitalization, and when patients are aggressive, agitated, or needing sleep induction. In other cases, particularly for long-term treatment, sedation is generally a side effect to be avoided because diminished arousal, sedation, and somnolence can lead to cognitive impairment. When cognition is impaired, functional outcomes are compromised.

Blocking one or more of three particular receptors is held theoretically responsible for causing sedation: M_1-muscarinic cholinergic receptors, H_1-histaminic receptors, and α_1-adrenergic receptors (Figures 5-36 and 5-38). Blocking central α_1-adrenergic receptors is associated with sedation, and blocking peripheral α_1-adrenergic receptors is associated with orthostatic hypotension. Central dopamine, acetylcholine, histamine, and norepinephrine are all involved in arousal pathways (Figure 5-38), so it is not surprising that blocking one or more of these systems can lead to sedation as well as to cognitive problems. Arousal pathways are discussed in detail in the chapters on sleep (Chapter 11) and cognition (Chapter 13). Pharmacologic evidence suggests that the best long-term outcomes in schizophrenia result when adequate $D_2/5HT_{2A}/5HT_{1A}$ receptor occupancy improves positive symptoms of psychosis, rather than from nonspecific sedation resulting from muscarinic, histaminic, and adrenergic receptor blockade. All atypical antipsychotics are not equally sedating because they do not all have potent antagonist properties at H_1 histamine, muscarinic cholinergic, and α_1-adrenergic receptors. Obviously drugs that combine potent actions at all three receptors will be the most sedating:

- **Potent antihistamine actions** – Clozapine, quetiapine, olanzapine, and iloperidone are all

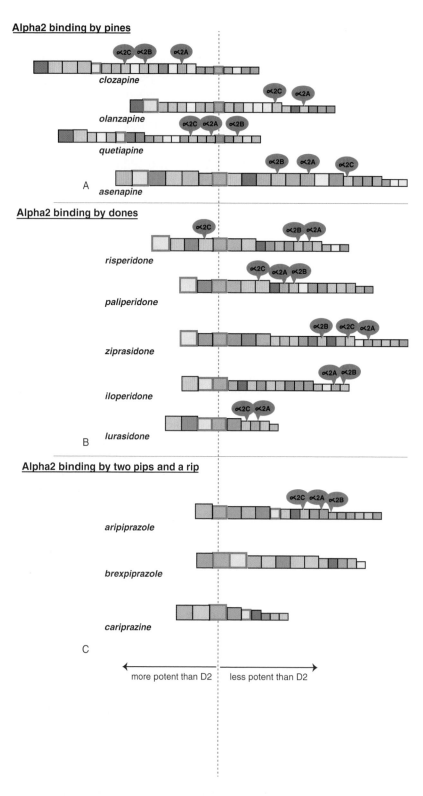

Alpha2 binding by pines

clozapine

olanzapine

quetiapine

A *asenapine*

Alpha2 binding by dones

risperidone

paliperidone

ziprasidone

iloperidone

B *lurasidone*

Alpha2 binding by two pips and a rip

aripiprazole

brexpiprazole

cariprazine

C

more potent than D2 | less potent than D2

Figure 5-37. Alpha-2 binding by atypical antipsychotics. Shown here is a visual depiction of the binding profiles of atypical antipsychotics (see Figure 5-1). (A) All of the "pines" (clozapine, olanzapine, quetiapine, asenapine) bind to α₂ receptors to varying degrees. Clozapine and quetiapine in particular bind to some α₂ receptor subtypes with greater potency than they do to the D₂ receptor. (B) All of the "dones" (risperidone, paliperidone, ziprasidone, iloperidone, lurasidone) bind to α₂ receptors to varying degrees. Risperidone binds to the α₂c receptor with greater potency than it does to the D₂ receptor. (C) Aripiprazole binds to α₂ receptors with less potency than it does to the D₂ receptor. Brexpiprazole and cariprazine do not bind to α₂ receptors.

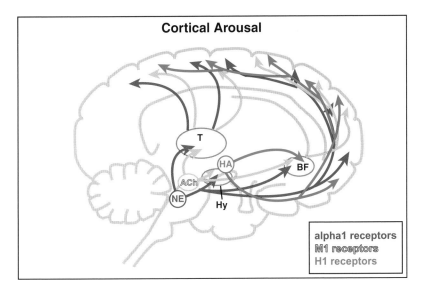

Cortical Arousal

alpha1 receptors
M1 receptors
H1 receptors

Figure 5-38. Neurotransmitters of cortical arousal. The neurotransmitters acetylcholine (ACh), histamine (HA), and norepinephrine (NE) are all involved in arousal pathways connecting neurotransmitter centers with the thalamus (T), hypothalamus (Hy), basal forebrain (BF), and cortex. Thus, pharmacological actions at their receptors could influence arousal. In particular, antagonism of M_1-muscarinic, H_1-histamine, and α_1-adrenergic receptors are all associated with sedating effects.

more potent H_1 antagonists than D_2 antagonists (all to the left in Figure 5-39A and B). All other antipsychotics have moderate potency, except lurasidone, which has essentially no binding to H_1 (Figure 5-39).

- **Potent anticholinergic actions** – Only the pines clozapine, quetiapine, and olanzapine have high potency for muscarinic receptors, whereas there is essentially no muscarinic cholinergic receptor binding for the other atypical antipsychotics, including asenapine (Figure 5-39A).

- **Potent α_1-adrenergic antagonism** – All atypical antipsychotics have at least moderate binding potency to α_1-adrenergic receptors, but the most potent relative to their D_2 binding are clozapine, quetiapine, risperidone, and iloperidone (Figure 5-40).

Given this portfolio of findings, it is not surprising that in general the pines are more sedating than the dones, and furthermore, the presence of antihistamine and antimuscarinic binding has implications for how fast one can taper and switch these agents. Alpha-1 antagonist properties may have theoretical implications for lowering EPS by a novel mechanism. These points are discussed in further detail later in this chapter.

Cardiometabolic actions

Although all atypical antipsychotics share a class warning for causing weight gain and risks for obesity, dyslipidemia, diabetes, accelerated cardiovascular disease, and even premature death, there is actually a spectrum of risk among the various agents.

- **High metabolic risk** – clozapine, olanzapine
- **Moderate metabolic risk** – risperidone, paliperidone, quetiapine, iloperidone (weight only)
- **Low metabolic risk** – ziprasidone, aripiprazole, lurasidone, iloperidone (low for dyslipidemia), asenapine, brexpiprazole?, cariprazine?

The pharmacologic mechanisms for what propels a patient taking an atypical antipsychotic along the "metabolic highway" (Figure 5-41) of these risks are only beginning to be understood. The "metabolic highway" begins with increased appetite and weight gain, and progresses to obesity, insulin resistance, and dyslipidemia with increases in fasting triglyceride levels (Figure 5-41). Ultimately, hyperinsulinemia advances to pancreatic β-cell failure, prediabetes and then diabetes. Once diabetes is established, risk for cardiovascular events is further increased, as is the risk of premature death (Figure 5-41). Receptors associated with increased weight are the H_1 histamine receptor and the $5HT_{2C}$ serotonin receptor, and when these receptors are blocked, particularly at the same time, patients can experience weight gain. Since weight gain can lead to obesity, and obesity to diabetes, and diabetes to cardiac disease along the metabolic highway (Figure 5-41), it seemed feasible at first that weight gain might explain all the other cardiometabolic complications associated with treatment with those atypical antipsychotics that cause weight gain. This may be true, but only in part,

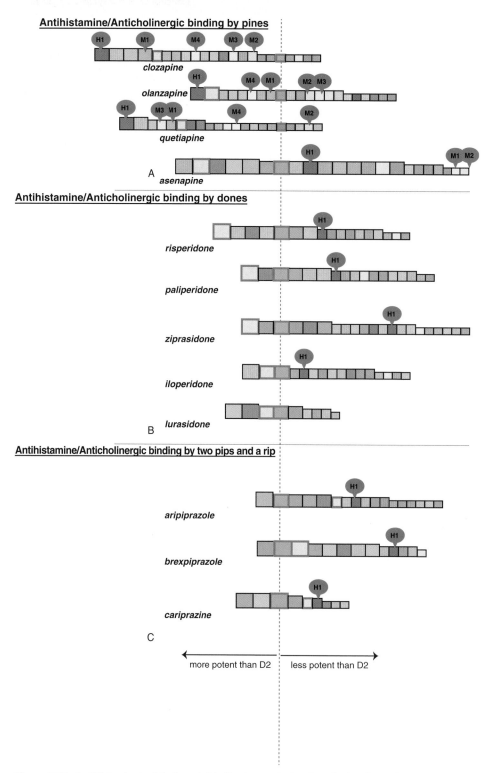

Figure 5-39. Antihistamine/anticholinergic binding by atypical antipsychotics. Shown here is a visual depiction of the binding profiles of atypical antipsychotics (see Figure 5-1). (A) Clozapine, olanzapine, and quetiapine all have strong potency for histamine 1 and muscarinic receptors. Asenapine has some affinity for histamine 1 receptors and weak affinity for muscarinic receptors. (B) Risperidone, paliperidone, ziprasidone, and iloperidone all have some potency for histamine 1 receptors, though with less potency than for D_2 receptors. Lurasidone does not bind to histamine 1 or muscarinic receptors. (C) Aripiprazole, brexpiprazole, and cariprazine all bind at the histamine 1 receptor with less potency than they do to the D_2 receptor, and do not bind to muscarinic receptors.

Alpha1 binding by pines

Alpha1 binding by dones

Alpha1 binding by two pips and a rip

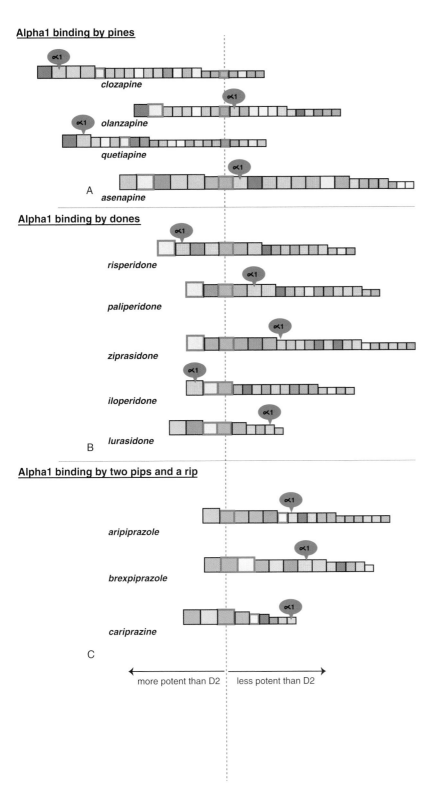

Figure 5-40. Alpha-1 binding by atypical antipsychotics. Shown here is a visual depiction of the binding profiles of atypical antipsychotics (see Figure 5-1). (A) Clozapine and quetiapine each have greater potency for the α_1 receptor than for the D_2 receptor, while olanzapine and asenapine each bind with similar potency to the α_1 and the D_2 receptors. (B) All of the "dones" (risperidone, paliperidone, ziprasidone, iloperidone, lurasidone) bind to the α_1 receptor. In particular, risperidone and iloperidone bind with greater potency than they do to the D_2 receptor. (C) Aripiprazole, brexpiprazole, and cariprazine each have some binding potency at the α_1 receptor.

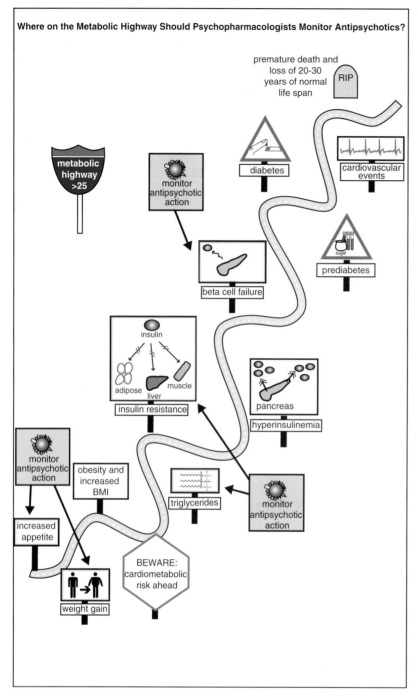

Where on the Metabolic Highway Should Psychopharmacologists Monitor Antipsychotics?

Figure 5-41. Monitoring on the metabolic highway. Where on the metabolic highway should psychopharmacologists monitor antipsychotics? Key stages along the metabolic highway where antipsychotics can produce cardiometabolic risks are the places where the actions of these drugs should be monitored. Thus, there are at least three "on" ramps where the cardiometabolic risk of some atypical antipsychotics can enter the metabolic highway, and they are all shown here. First, increased appetite and weight gain can lead to elevated body mass index (BMI) and ultimately obesity. Thus, weight and BMI should be monitored here. Second, atypical antipsychotics can cause insulin resistance by an unknown mechanism; this can be detected by measuring fasting plasma triglyceride levels. Finally, atypical antipsychotics can cause sudden onset of diabetic ketoacidosis (DKA) or hyperglycemic hyperosmolar syndrome (HHS) by unknown mechanisms, possibly including blockade of M_3-cholinergic receptors. This can be detected by informing patients of the symptoms of DKA/HHS and by measuring fasting glucose levels.

and perhaps mostly for those agents that have both potent antihistamine properties (Figure 5-39) and potent $5HT_{2C}$ antagonist properties (Figure 5-29), notably clozapine, olanzapine, quetiapine, as well as the antidepressant mirtazapine (discussed in Chapter 7).

However, it now appears that the cardiometabolic risk of certain atypical antipsychotics cannot simply be explained by increased appetite and weight gain, even though they certainly do represent the first steps down the slippery slope towards cardiometabolic complications. That is, some atypical antipsychotics can elevate fasting triglyceride levels and cause increased insulin resistance in a manner that cannot be explained by weight gain alone. When dyslipidemia and insulin resistance occur, this moves a patient along the metabolic highway towards diabetes and cardiovascular disease (Figure 5-41). Although this happens in many patients with weight gain alone, it also occurs in some patients who take atypical antipsychotics and prior to their gaining significant weight, as if there is an acute receptor-mediated action of these drugs on insulin regulation.

This hypothesized mechanism is indicated as receptor "X" on the drug icon in Figure 5-36 and on the icons for those agents hypothesized to have this action on insulin resistance and fasting triglycerides shown later in this chapter. To date, the mechanism of this increased insulin resistance and elevation of fasting triglycerides has been vigorously pursued but has not yet been identified. The rapid elevation of fasting triglycerides upon initiation of some antipsychotics, and the rapid fall of fasting triglycerides upon discontinuation of such drugs, is highly suggestive that an unknown pharmacologic mechanism causes these changes, although this remains speculative. The hypothetical actions of atypical antipsychotics with this postulated receptor action are shown in Figure 5-42, where adipose tissue, liver, and skeletal

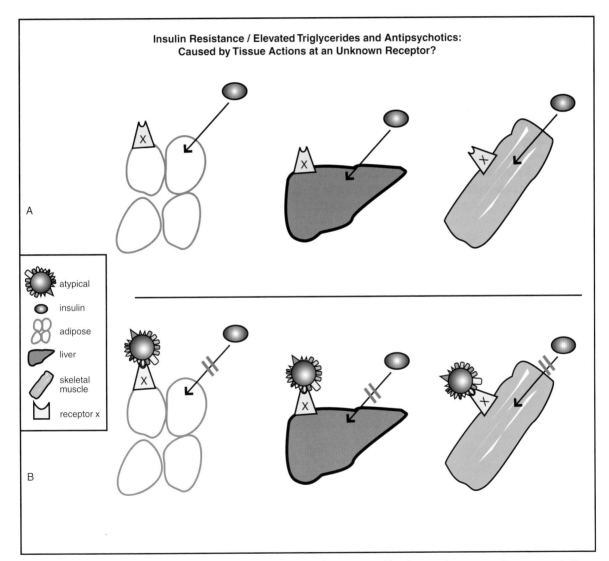

Figure 5-42. Insulin resistance, elevated triglycerides, and antipsychotics: caused by tissue actions at an unknown receptor? Some atypical antipsychotics may lead to insulin resistance and elevated triglycerides independently of weight gain, although the mechanism is not yet established. This figure depicts a hypothesized mechanism in which antipsychotic binds to receptor X at adipose tissue, liver, and skeletal muscle to cause insulin resistance.

muscle all develop insulin resistance in response to administration of certain antipsychotic drugs (e.g., high-risk drugs but not "metabolically friendly" low-risk drugs) at least in certain patients. Whatever the mechanism of this effect, it is clear that fasting plasma triglycerides and insulin resistance can be elevated significantly in some patients taking certain antipsychotics, and that this enhances cardiometabolic risk, moves such patients along the metabolic highway (Figure 5-41), and functions as another step down the slippery slope towards the diabolical destination of cardiovascular events and premature death. This does not happen in all patients taking any antipsychotic, but the development of this problem can be detected by monitoring (Figure 5-43), and it can be managed easily when it does occur (Figure 5-44).

Another rare but life-threatening cardiometabolic problem is known to be associated with atypical antipsychotics: namely, an association with the sudden occurrence of diabetic ketoacidosis (DKA) or the related condition hyperglycemic hyperosmolar syndrome (HHS). The mechanism of this complication is under intense investigation, and is probably complex and multifactorial. In some cases, it may be that patients with undiagnosed insulin resistance, prediabetes or diabetes, who are in a state of compensated hyperinsulinemia on the metabolic highway (Figure 5-41), when given an atypical antipsychotic agent, become decompensated because of some pharmacologic mechanism associated with these drugs. Because of the risk of DKA/HHS, it is important to know the patient's location along the metabolic highway prior to prescribing an antipsychotic, particularly if the patient has hyperinsulinemia, prediabetes, or diabetes. It is also important to monitor (Figures 5-41 and 5-43) and manage (Figure 5-44) these risk factors.

Specifically, there are at least three stops along the metabolic highway where a psychopharmacologist should monitor a patient taking an atypical antipsychotic and manage the cardiometabolic risks of atypical antipsychotics (Figure 5-41). This starts with monitoring weight and body mass index to detect weight gain, and fasting glucose to detect the development of diabetes (Figures 5-41 and 5-43). It also means getting a baseline of fasting triglyceride levels and determining whether there is a family history of diabetes. The second action to monitor is whether atypical antipsychotics are causing dyslipidemia and increased insulin resistance, by measuring fasting triglyceride levels before and after starting an atypical antipsychotic (Figure 5-41). If body mass index or

Psychopharmacologist's Metabolic Monitoring Toolkit

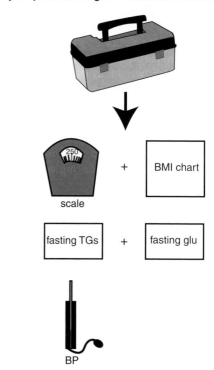

Figure 5-43. Metabolic monitoring toolkit. The psychopharmacologist's metabolic monitoring toolkit includes items for tracking four major parameters: weight/body mass index (BMI), fasting triglycerides (TGs), fasting glucose (glu), and blood pressure (BP). These items are simply a flowchart that can appear at the beginning of a patient's chart with entries for each visit, a scale, a BMI chart to convert weight into BMI, a blood pressure cuff, and laboratory results for fasting triglycerides and fasting glucose.

fasting triglycerides increase significantly, a switch to a different antipsychotic that does not cause these problems should be considered. In patients who are obese, with dyslipidemia, and either in a prediabetic or diabetic state, it is especially important to monitor blood pressure, fasting glucose, and waist circumference before and after initiating an atypical antipsychotic. Best practices are to monitor these parameters in anyone taking any atypical antipsychotic. In high-

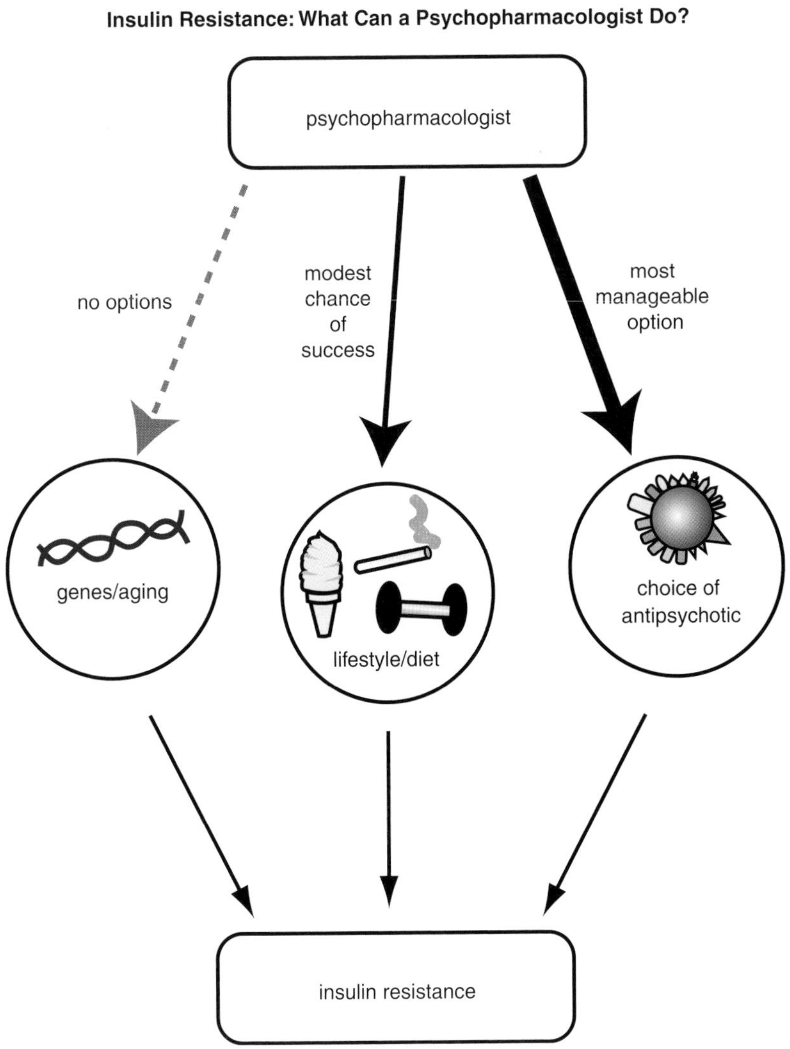

Insulin Resistance: What Can a Psychopharmacologist Do?

Figure 5-44. Insulin resistance: what can a psychopharmacologist do? Several factors influence whether or not an individual develops insulin resistance, some of which are manageable by a psychopharmacologist and some of which are not. Unmanageable factors include genetic makeup and age, while items that are modestly manageable include lifestyle (e.g., diet, exercise, smoking). Psychopharmacologists exert their greatest influence on managing insulin resistance through selection of antipsychotics that either do or do not cause insulin resistance.

risk patients, it is especially important to be vigilant for DKA/HHS, and possibly to reduce that risk by maintaining the patient on an antipsychotic with lower cardiometabolic risk. In high-risk patients, especially those with pending or actual pancreatic β-cell failure as manifested by hyperinsulinemia, pre-diabetes, or diabetes, fasting glucose and other chemical and clinical parameters can be monitored to detect early signs of rare but potentially fatal DKA/HHS.

The psychopharmacologist's metabolic toolkit is quite simple (Figure 5-43). It involves a flowchart that tracks perhaps as few as four parameters over time, especially before and after switches from one antipsychotic to another, or as new risk factors

evolve. These four parameters are weight (as body mass index), fasting triglycerides, fasting glucose, and blood pressure.

The management of patients at risk for cardiometabolic disease can be quite simple as well, although patients who already have developed dyslipidemia, hypertension, diabetes, and heart disease will likely require management of these problems by a medical specialist. However, the psychopharmacologist is left with a very simple set of options for managing patients with cardiometabolic risk who are prescribed an atypical antipsychotic (Figure 5-44). The major factors that determine whether a patient progresses along the metabolic highway to premature death include those that are unmanageable (e.g., the patient's genetic makeup and age), those that are modestly manageable (e.g., change in lifestyle such as diet, exercise, and stopping smoking), and those that are most manageable, namely the selection of antipsychotic and perhaps switching from one that is causing increased risk in a particular patient, to one that monitoring demonstrates reduces that risk.

Pharmacologic properties of individual antipsychotics: the pines, the dones, two pips and a rip, plus more

Here we will review some of the differences among 17 selected antipsychotic agents, based both on the art and the science of psychopharmacology. Further details on how to prescribe these individual drugs are available in the companion *Stahl's Essential Psychopharmacology: the Prescriber's Guide* and other standard references. The pharmacologic properties represented in the icons shown in the next section are conceptual and not precisely quantitative and are shown in two ways: a rank order of binding potencies in a strip below an icon containing the most important binding properties. For each individual drug, these are the same strips shown earlier in this chapter in several figures containing all the drugs in the various categories (e.g., Figure 5-24). As before, more potent binding is shown to the left of the value for the D_2 receptor, less potent binding is shown to the right. As mentioned earlier, these agents are all dosed to treat psychosis in order to occupy about 60% or more of D_2 receptors (Figure 5-23). Thus, all receptors to the left of D_2 are occupied at the level of 60% or more at antipsychotic dosing levels. For those receptors to the left of D_2, there are also potentially clinically relevant receptor actions even at doses below those for treating psychosis. The receptors to the right of D_2 are occupied at a level of less than 60% at antipsychotic dosing levels. Those that are within an order of magnitude of potency of D_2 are shown to the right of D_2, and have potentially relevant clinical action despite lower levels of occupancy than D_2 receptors, with declining occupancy levels as the receptor is listed further to the right, and also at lower than antipsychotic dosing levels. The point is really that no two atypical antipsychotics have exactly the same pharmacologic binding profiles, even though many of their properties overlap. The distinctive pharmacologic properties of each

atypical antipsychotic are worth noting in order to match the best antipsychotic agent to each individual patient.

The pines (peens)

Clozapine

Clozapine, a serotonin $5HT_{2A}$–dopamine D_2 antagonist or serotonin–dopamine antagonist (SDA) (Figure 5-45) is considered to be the "prototypical" atypical antipsychotic, and has one of the most complex pharmacologic profiles of any of the atypical antipsychotics. Although antipsychotics are generally dosed so that about 60% of D_2 receptors are occupied (Figure 5-23), this may be lower for clozapine for unknown reasons. Clozapine was the first antipsychotic to be recognized as "atypical" and thus to cause few if any extrapyramidal side effects, not to cause tardive dyskinesia, and not to elevate prolactin. Despite its complex pharmacology, these atypical properties were linked particularly to the presence of serotonin $5HT_{2A}$ antagonism added to the dopamine D_2 antagonism of conventional antipsychotics, and this has become the prototypical binding characteristic of the entire class of atypical antipsychotics, namely $5HT_{2A}$ antagonism combined with D_2 antagonism. Interesting, however, is how complex the binding pattern is for all the various receptors for clozapine (Figure 5-45) and how clozapine actually has higher potency for so many of them than it even does for D_2 receptors!

Clozapine, however, is the one atypical antipsychotic recognized as particularly effective when other antipsychotic agents have failed, and is thus the "gold standard" for efficacy in schizophrenia. It may have a particular niche in treating aggression and violence in psychotic patients. It is unknown what pharmacologic property accounts for this gold-standard enhanced efficacy of clozapine, but it is unlikely to be simply $5HT_{2A}$ antagonism, since clozapine can show greater efficacy than other atypical antipsychotics that share this pharmacologic property. Although patients treated with clozapine may occasionally experience an "awakening" (in the Oliver Sachs sense), characterized by return to a near-normal level of cognitive, interpersonal, and vocational functioning, and not just significant improvement in positive symptoms of psychosis, this is unfortunately rare. The fact that awakenings can be observed at all, however, gives hope for the possibility that a state of wellness might some day be achieved in schizophrenia by the right

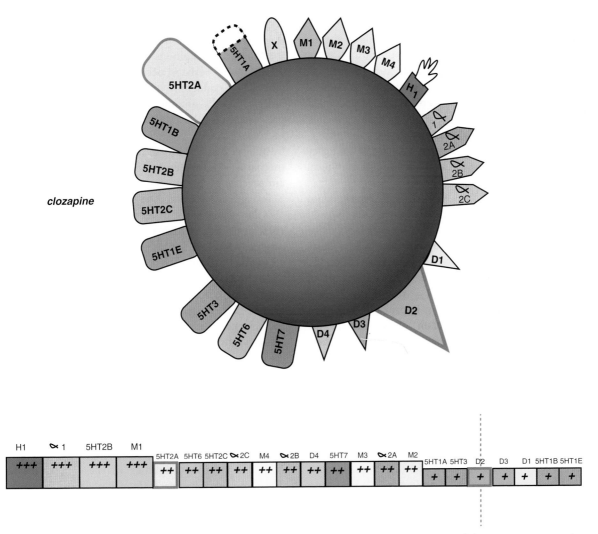

Figure 5-45. Clozapine's pharmacological and binding profile. The most prominent binding properties of clozapine are represented here; this is perhaps one of the most complex binding portfolios in all of psychopharmacology. Clozapine's binding properties vary greatly with technique and species and from one laboratory to another. This icon portrays a qualitative consensus of current thinking about the binding properties of clozapine, which are constantly being revised and updated. In addition to serotonin $5HT_{2A}$–dopamine D_2 antagonism (SDA properties), numerous other binding properties have been identified for clozapine, most of which are more potent than its binding at the D_2 receptor. It is unknown which of these contribute to clozapine's special efficacy or to its unique side effects.

mix of pharmacologic mechanisms. Awakenings have been observed on rare occasions in association with treatment with other atypical antipsychotics, but almost never in association with conventional antipsychotic treatment.

Clozapine is also the only antipsychotic that has been documented to reduce the risk of suicide in schizophrenia. Clozapine may actually reduce tardive dyskinesia severity in some patients with this problem, especially over long treatment intervals. Although certainly a $5HT_{2A}$–D_2 antagonist, the

mechanism of clozapine's apparently enhanced efficacy profile compared to other antipsychotics remains the topic of vigorous debate. Obviously, it is beyond just the $5HT_{2A}$–D_2 antagonism shared by many agents, but the question remains: is it the unique cluster of receptor binding properties of clozapine or some as yet unknown mechanism of clozapine that accounts for its robust efficacy?

Clozapine is also the antipsychotic associated with greatest risk of developing a life-threatening and occasionally fatal complication called agranulocytosis, in

0.5–2% of patients. Because of this, patients must have their blood counts monitored for as long as they are treated with clozapine. Clozapine also has an increased risk of seizures, especially at high doses. It can be very sedating, can cause excessive salivation, has an increased risk of myocarditis, and is associated with the greatest degree of weight gain and possibly the greatest cardiometabolic risk among the antipsychotics. Thus, clozapine may have the greatest efficacy but also the most side effects among the atypical antipsychotics.

Because of these side-effect risks, clozapine is not considered to be a first-line treatment, but is used when other antipsychotics fail. The mechanisms of clozapine's ability to cause agranulocytosis, myocarditis, and seizures are entirely unknown, although the weight gain may be associated with its blockade of both H_1-histamine and $5HT_{2C}$ receptors (Figures 5-29A, 5-36, 5-39A). Sedation is probably linked to clozapine's potent antagonism of M_1-muscarinic, H_1-histaminic, and α_1-adrenergic receptors (Figures 5-36, 5-39A, 5-40A). Profound muscarinic blockade can also cause excessive salivation, especially at higher doses, as well as severe constipation, even leading to bowel obstruction from paralytic ileus. Clozapine is among the antipsychotics most notable for increasing cardiometabolic risks, including increases in fasting plasma triglyceride levels and increases in insulin resistance by an unknown but postulated pharmacologic mechanism (receptor X in Figure 5-42). Because of these side effects and the hassle of arranging for blood counts, the use of clozapine is low in clinical practice, perhaps too low. It is important not to lose the art of how to prescribe clozapine and for whom, as clozapine remains a powerful therapeutic intervention for many patients.

Olanzapine

Although this agent has a chemical structure related to clozapine and is also an antagonist at both serotonin $5HT_{2A}$ and dopamine D_2 receptors, olanzapine is more potent than clozapine, and has several differentiating pharmacologic (Figure 5-46) and clinical features. Olanzapine is "atypical" in that it generally lacks EPS not only at moderate antipsychotic doses, but usually even at higher antipsychotic doses. Olanzapine lacks the extreme sedating properties of clozapine, but can be somewhat sedating in some patients, as it does have antagonist properties at M_1-muscarinic, H_1-histaminic, and α_1-adrenergic

receptors (Figures 5-36, 5-39A, 5-40A). Olanzapine does not often raise prolactin levels with long-term treatment. Olanzapine is consistently associated with weight gain, perhaps because of its antihistaminic and $5HT_{2C}$ antagonist properties (Figures 5-36 and 5-46). It ranks among the antipsychotics with the greatest known cardiometabolic risks, as it robustly increases fasting triglyceride levels and increases insulin resistance by an unknown pharmacologic mechanism postulated to be active for some atypical antipsychotics in at least some patients (receptor X in Figures 5-42 and 5-46).

Olanzapine tends to be used in most patients in clinical practice in higher doses (> 15 mg/day) than originally studied and approved for marketing (10–15 mg/day), since there is the sense that higher doses might be associated not only with greater efficacy (i.e., improvement of clinical symptoms) but also with greater effectiveness (i.e., clinical outcome based upon the balance of safety and efficacy), especially in institutional settings where the dose can exceed 40 mg/day off-label. Olanzapine improves mood not only in schizophrenia but also in bipolar disorder and in treatment-resistant depression, particularly when combined with antidepressants such as fluoxetine. Perhaps the $5HT_{2C}$ antagonist properties, with the weaker $5HT_7$ and α_2 antagonist properties of olanzapine (Figures 5-36 and 5-46), especially when combined with the $5HT_{2C}$ antagonist properties of the antidepressant fluoxetine (see Chapter 7), may explain some aspects of olanzapine's apparent efficacy for mood symptoms.

For patients with significant weight gain or who develop significant cardiometabolic risks, such as dyslipidemia (elevated fasting triglycerides) or diabetes, olanzapine may be considered a second-line agent. Olanzapine can, however, be considered an appropriate choice for patients when agents with lower propensity for weight gain or cardiometabolic disturbances fail to achieve sufficient efficacy, as olanzapine can often have greater efficacy than some other agents in some patients, particularly at higher doses and for patients seen in institutional settings. The decision to use any atypical antipsychotic requires monitoring not only of efficacy but also of risks, including cardiometabolic risks, and is a tradeoff between risks and benefits that must be determined for each individual patient and for each individual drug. Olanzapine is available as an oral disintegrating tablet, as an acute intramuscular injection, and as a long-acting 4-week intramuscular depot.

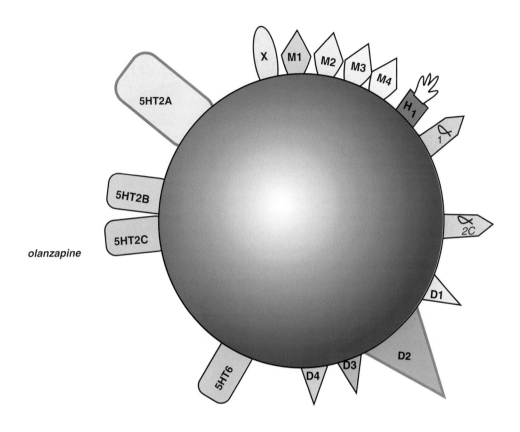

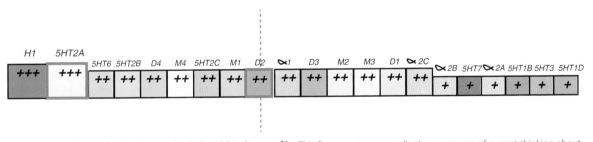

Figure 5-46. Olanzapine's pharmacological and binding profile. This figure portrays a qualitative consensus of current thinking about the binding properties of olanzapine. It has a complex pharmacology that somewhat overlaps with that of clozapine. Olanzapine binds at several receptors more potently than it does at the D_2 receptor; in fact, it has strongest potency for the histamine H_1 and serotonin $5HT_{2A}$ receptors. Olanzapine's $5HT_{2C}$ antagonist properties may contribute to its efficacy for mood and cognitive symptoms, although together with its H_1 antihistamine properties they could also contribute to its propensity to cause weight gain. As with all atypical antipsychotics discussed in this chapter, binding properties vary greatly with technique and from one laboratory to another; they are constantly being revised and updated.

Quetiapine

Quetiapine also has a chemical structure related to clozapine, and is an antagonist at both serotonin $5HT_{2A}$ and dopamine D_2 receptors, but has several differentiating pharmacologic properties, especially at different doses and with different oral formulations

(Figure 5-47). The net pharmacologic actions of quetiapine are actually due to the combined pharmacologic actions not only of quetiapine itself but also of its active metabolite, norquetiapine. Norquetiapine has unique pharmacologic properties compared to quetiapine, especially norepinephrine transporter

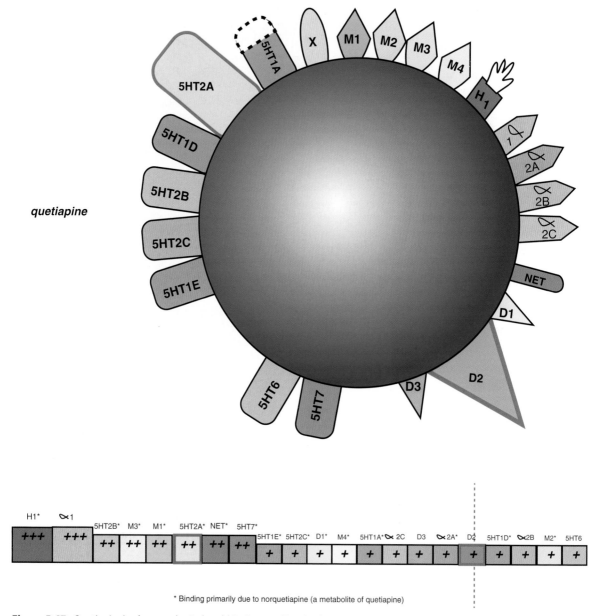

quetiapine

* Binding primarily due to norquetiapine (a metabolite of quetiapine)

Figure 5-47. Quetiapine's pharmacological and binding profile. This figure portrays a qualitative consensus of current thinking about the binding properties of quetiapine plus norquetiapine. Quetiapine does not actually have particularly potent binding at D_2 receptors. Quetiapine's prominent H_1 antagonist properties probably contribute to its ability to enhance sleep, and this may contribute as well to its ability to improve sleep disturbances in bipolar and unipolar depression as well as in anxiety disorders. However, this property can also contribute to daytime sedation, especially combined with M_1 antimuscarinic and α_1-adrenergic antagonist properties. Recently, a potentially important active metabolite of quetiapine, norquetiapine, has been identified; norquetiapine may contribute additional actions at receptors, as noted in the binding profile with an asterisk. $5HT_{1A}$ partial agonist actions, norepinephrine transporter (NET) inhibition, and $5HT_{2C}$ antagonist actions may all contribute to mood-improving properties as well as to cognitive enhancement by quetiapine. However, $5HT_{2C}$ antagonist actions combined with H_1 antagonist actions may contribute to weight gain. Muscarinic cholinergic antagonist actions cause anticholinergic side effects. As with all atypical antipsychotics discussed in this chapter, binding properties vary greatly with technique and from one laboratory to another; they are constantly being revised and updated.

(NET) inhibition (i.e., norepinephrine reuptake inhibition), but also $5HT_7$, $5HT_{2C}$, and α_2 antagonism as well as $5HT_{1A}$ partial agonist actions, all of which may contribute to quetiapine's overall clinical profile, especially its robust antidepressant effects (Figure 5-47). Quetiapine has an overall very complex set of binding properties to numerous neurotransmitter receptors, many of which have higher potency than to the D_2 receptor, and this may account for why this drug appears to be far more than simply an antipsychotic.

Different drug with different formulations? Quetiapine is a very interesting agent, since it acts like several different drugs, depending upon the dose and the formulation. Quetiapine comes in an immediate-release (IR) formulation and in an extended-release (XR) formulation. The IR formulation has a relatively rapid onset and short duration of action, although most patients only need to take it once a day, and they usually take it at night because quetiapine is most sedating at its peak delivery shortly after taking it, due in large part to its antihistamine properties. In some ways, this makes an ideal hypnotic but not an ideal antipsychotic.

At 300 mg per day, probably the lowest effective antipsychotic dose, quetiapine IR rapidly occupies more than 60% of D_2 receptors, sufficient for antipsychotic action, but then quickly falls below 60% D_2 receptor occupancy (Figure 5-48A). This means that the antipsychotic effect may wear off after a few hours, or require dosing more than once daily or very high doses to sustain adequate D_2 receptor occupancy above 60% for a full day, as its plasma drug levels fall off rapidly (Figure 5-48A). By contrast, at 300 mg per day, the XR formulation of quetiapine more slowly hits its peak, yet has a rapid enough onset of 60% D_2 occupancy to be effective without the same amount of sedation as quetiapine IR, and its duration of action above the 60% threshold is several hours longer than quetiapine IR (Figure 5-48A).

At the maximum dose of quetiapine generally used except for treatment-resistant cases, 800 mg of quetiapine IR still only occupies D_2 receptors for about 12 hours above the 60% threshold, risking breakthrough symptoms at the end of the day, but quetiapine XR maintains fully effective D_2 occupancy until the next dose 24 hours later (Figure 5-48B). The XR formulation is thus ideal for an antipsychotic, with less peak-dose sedation but duration of action lasting all day; however, the XR formulation is not ideal for a hypnotic, because the peak is much delayed from the time when the patient takes the pill, delaying sleep onset, with a good deal of residual drug present when the patient wakes up, increasing the chances of causing hangover effects.

Different drug at different doses? If the pharmacology of D_2 partial agonists such as aripiprazole is the tale of Goldilocks, as discussed above, then the story of quetiapine dosing is the story of the three bears (Figure 5-49). The antipsychotic quetiapine is an 800 mg Papa Bear, ideally in the XR formulation. The antidepressant quetiapine is a 300 mg Mama Bear, also ideally in the XR formulation. The sedative hypnotic quetiapine is a 50 mg Baby Bear, ideally in the IR formulation. Higher and higher doses not only occupy more and more D_2 receptors, but also recruit the blockade of additional receptors, moving to the right along the line of receptors at the bottom of Figure 5-47 as the dose goes up. The lowest doses act at the receptors that have the highest affinity for quetiapine (to the left in the line of receptors at the bottom of Figure 5-47).

Starting with Baby Bear, only the most potent binding properties of quetiapine to the far left in the strip at the bottom of Figure 5-47 are relevant, especially H_1 antihistaminic properties. With the IR formulation, almost all H_1 receptors are blocked within minutes of oral administration (Figure 5-50A), increasing the chances of rapid onset of sleep, whereas with the XR formulation (Figure 5-50B), this peak is not reached until it is almost time to wake up, assuming quetiapine is taken at bedtime. Also, with the IR formulation, quetiapine rapidly declines in terms of H_1 occupancy, diminishing the chances of a hangover (Figure 5-50A), but this is just the opposite for the XR formulation (Figure 5-50B). Baby Bear doses are not approved for use as a hypnotic, and this can be an expensive option with metabolic risks, so is not considered a first-line option for sleep. Note that with either formulation, only a very small number of the antidepressant-related receptors $5HT_{2C}$ and norepinephrine transporter are blocked, theoretically insufficient for antidepressant efficacy. Also, the amount of D_2 occupancy is far below the 60% threshold, so this is insufficient for antipsychotic efficacy as well.

Mama Bear is the surprise bear in many ways. Although developed as an antipsychotic, quetiapine was anecdotally observed to have antidepressant effects in bipolar and unipolar depressed patients,

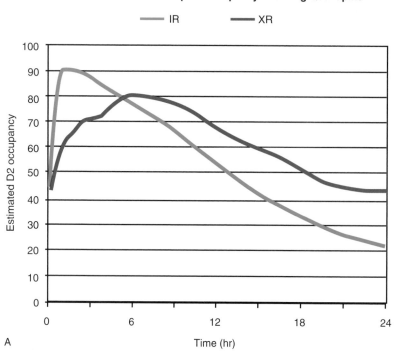

Estimated Striatal D2 Receptor Occupancy at 300mg Quetiapine

A

Figure 5-48. Estimated striatal D$_2$ receptor occupancy at different doses of quetiapine. The estimated striatal D$_2$ receptor occupancy binding for quetiapine differs with both the dose and the formulation. (A) At 300 mg of the immediate-release (IR) formulation, D$_2$ receptor occupancy peaks quickly at approximately 90% and then drops fairly rapidly. At 300 mg of the extended-release (XR) formulation, D$_2$ receptor occupancy peaks at approximately 80% after 6 hours, and then exhibits a more gradual decline of the next 18 hours. (B) At 800 mg of the IR formulation, D$_2$ receptor occupancy peaks early at nearly 100% and then drops fairly rapidly, although not as drastically as at the lower dose. At 800 mg of the XR formulation, D$_2$ receptor occupancy peaks above 90% after 6 hours and then exhibits a slow decline to approximately 70% over the next 18 hours.

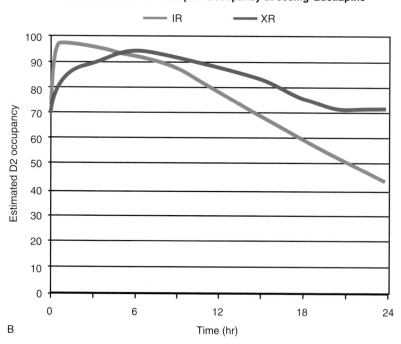

Estimated Striatal D2 Receptor Occupancy at 800mg Quetiapine

B

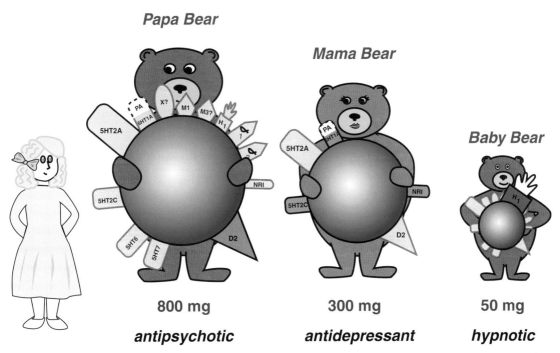

Figure 5-49. Binding profile of quetiapine at different doses. The binding properties of quetiapine vary depending on the dose used. At antipsychotic doses (i.e., up to 800 mg/day), quetiapine has a relatively wide binding profile, with actions at multiple serotonergic, muscarinic, and α-adrenergic receptors. Histamine 1 receptor blockade is also present. At antidepressant doses (i.e., approximately 300 mg/day), the binding profile of quetiapine is more selective and consists primarily of actions at D_2, $5HT_{2A}$, $5HT_{2C}$, and $5HT_{1A}$ receptors as well as inhibition of the norepinephrine transporter. At sedative-hypnotic doses (i.e., 50 mg/day), the most prominent pharmacological property of quetiapine is histamine 1 antagonism.

beyond helping them sleep, and in the absence of psychotic symptoms. Over time, clinical trials have repeatedly demonstrated that in the 300 mg range, quetiapine has some of the most robust antidepressant effects of any agent in bipolar depression. At first, this did not make any sense pharmacologically for a $5HT_{2A}$–D_2 antagonist with antihistaminic properties, but then the active metabolite norquetiapine was discovered with its norepinephrine reuptake blocking and $5HT_{2C}$ antagonist properties, much greater than for the parent quetiapine itself. These two mechanisms can individually increase the release of both dopamine and norepinephrine, and together appear to have synergistic actions at doses below those that cause 60% D_2 occupancy (Figure 5-50C and D). In addition, quetiapine has $5HT_{1A}$ partial agonist, $5HT_7$, α_2, and $5HT_{1B/D}$ antagonist properties, also theoretically linked to antidepressant actions. These multiple concomitant pharmacological actions theoretically have accounted for ushering in the arrival of antidepressant quetiapine, a 300 mg Mama Bear. This constitutes a big paradigm shift for a drug

originally developed as an antipsychotic for schizophrenia. Although both the IR (Figure 5-50C) and XR (Figure 5-50D) formulations appear to have antidepressant efficacy, the XR formulation has more consistent day-long receptor occupancy of both $5HT_{2C}$ receptors and norepinephrine transporters as well as other key receptors, and may thus be theoretically the preferred formulation for the treatment of depression. Quetiapine is approved both for bipolar depression and as an augmenting agent to SSRIs/SNRIs in unipolar depression that fails to respond sufficiently to SSRI/SNRI monotherapy. Thus, the combination of quetiapine with these other antidepressants in unipolar treatment-resistant depression would have the triple monoamine actions of increasing serotonin (via SSRI/SNRI actions), dopamine, and norepinephrine (the latter two neurotransmitters theoretically via quetiapine/norquetiapine $5HT_{2C}$ antagonist actions plus both quetiapine and SNRI prefrontal cortex NET blockade), while simultaneously treating symptoms of insomnia and anxiety by antihistaminic action (Figure 5-50C and D).

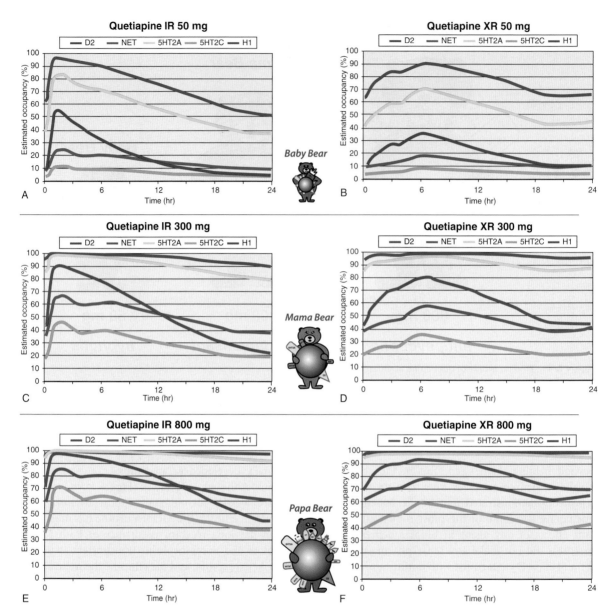

Figure 5-50. Binding profile of quetiapine with different doses and formulations. (A, B) The estimated receptor occupancy for quetiapine IR and XR at 50 mg/day is shown here. Although quetiapine binds to multiple receptors at this dose, its most prominent action is at histamine 1 receptors, thus explaining its use as a sedative-hypnotic at this dose. (C, D) At antidepressant doses, histamine 1 and $5HT_{2A}$ antagonism are the most prominent binding properties of both quetiapine IR and XR, with additional binding at D_2 receptors, the norepinephrine transporter, and $5HT_{2C}$ receptors. (E, F) At antipsychotic doses, the strongest binding properties of quetiapine IR and XR are also histamine 1 and $5HT_{2A}$ antagonism. However, occupancy at the D_2 receptor, norepinephrine transporter, and $5HT_{2C}$ receptor is greater than at lower doses.

Finally, Papa Bear is 800 mg quetiapine, which completely saturates both H_1-histamine and $5HT_{2A}$ receptors continuously in both cases, but has more consistent occupancy above 60% for D_2 receptors with the XR formulation (compare Figure 5-50E and F). Substantial occupancy of the antidepressant-

related receptors also occurs with either formulation, but this amount of $5HT_{2C}$ and norepinephrine transporter blockade is not necessary for antidepressant actions, since most studies show that even 300 mg once a day has the same antidepressant efficacy as 600 mg. The 800 mg dose (Figure 5-50E and F) is really an antipsychotic dose, and potentially excessive and less well tolerated for the treatment of depression.

No matter what the dose or the formulation, quetiapine is "very atypical" in that it causes virtually no EPS at any dose, nor prolactin elevations. Thus, quetiapine tends to be a preferred atypical antipsychotic for patients with Parkinson's disease who require treatment for psychosis (as is clozapine). Quetiapine can cause weight gain, particularly when given in moderate to high doses, as it blocks histamine 1 receptors (Figure 5-47); the $5HT_{2C}$ antagonist actions of its active metabolite norquetiapine may contribute to weight gain at moderate to high doses of quetiapine (Figure 5-47). Quetiapine can increase fasting triglyceride levels and insulin resistance, particularly at moderate to high doses, and with intermediate to high risk compared to other atypical antipsychotics, possibly via the same unknown pharmacologic mechanism postulated to be active for some other atypical antipsychotics (receptor X in Figures 5-42 and 5-47).

Asenapine

Asenapine is one of the newer atypical antipsychotics (Figure 5-51). It has a chemical structure related to the antidepressant mirtazapine and shares several of mirtazapine's pharmacological binding properties, especially $5HT_{2A}$, $5HT_{2C}$, H_1, and α_2 antagonism, plus many other properties that mirtazapine does not have, especially D_2 antagonism, as well as actions upon many additional serotonin receptor subtypes (Figure 5-51). This suggests that asenapine would be an antipsychotic with antidepressant actions, but only antipsychotic/antimanic actions have been proven.

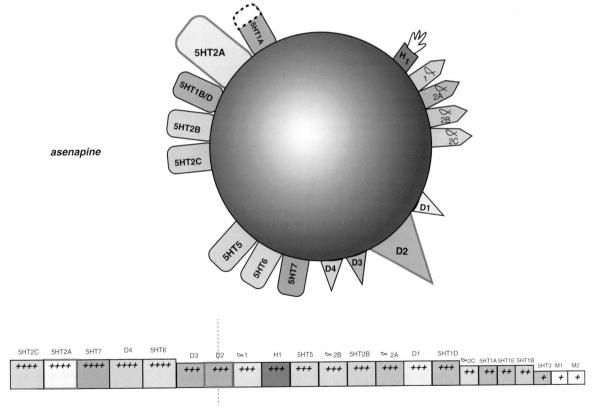

Figure 5-51. Asenapine's pharmacological and binding profile. This figure portrays a qualitative consensus of current thinking about the binding properties of asenapine. Asenapine has a complex binding profile, with more potent binding at multiple serotonergic and dopaminergic receptors than it has at D_2 receptors. In particular, $5HT_{2C}$ antagonist properties may contribute to its efficacy for mood and cognitive symptoms, while $5HT_7$ antagonist properties may contribute to its efficacy for mood, cognitive, and sleep symptoms. As with all atypical antipsychotics discussed in this chapter, binding properties vary greatly with technique and from one laboratory to another; they are constantly being revised and updated.

Asenapine is unusual in that it is given as a sublingual formulation, because active drug is very poorly bioavailable if asenapine is swallowed, due to extensive first-pass metabolism. The surface area of the oral cavity for oral absorption may limit the size of the dose and the extent of drug absorption at high doses, so asenapine is generally taken twice a day despite a long half-life. Since asenapine is rapidly absorbed sublingually with rapid peak drug levels, unlike similar oral formulations of other antipsychotics such as olanzapine that simply dissolve rapidly in the mouth but are followed by delayed absorption, theoretical considerations and anecdotal observations suggest that asenapine can be used as a rapid-acting oral PRN (as needed) antipsychotic to "top up" some psychotic and disturbed patients rapidly without resorting to an injection. One side effect of sublingual administration in some patients is oral hypoesthesia; also, patients may not eat or drink for 10 minutes following sublingual administration, to avoid the drug being washed out of oral absorption sites and into the stomach, where extensive first-pass metabolism will cause minimal active drug bioavailability. Asenapine can be sedating, especially upon first dosing, but does not have a high propensity either for EPS or for weight gain/dyslipidemia despite its $5HT_{2C}$ antagonist plus weaker antihistaminic properties.

The antagonist actions of asenapine at $5HT_{2C}$, $5HT_7$, $5HT_{1B/D}$, and α_2 receptors with partial agonist actions at $5HT_{1A}$ receptors, as well as anecdotal clinical reports, support the prospects of demonstrating antidepressant properties for asenapine. That is, antagonist action at $5HT_{2C}$ receptors releases dopamine and norepinephrine in prefrontal cortex, which would hypothetically improve depression. The mechanism of this is shown in Figures 5-52A and 5-52B. Serotonin input to $5HT_{2C}$ receptors on GABA interneurons – both in the brainstem and in the prefrontal cortex – normally causes GABA release onto norepinephrine and dopamine neurons, which then inhibits the release of norepinephrine and dopamine out of these neurons in prefrontal cortex. These $5HT_{2C}$ actions at the brainstem level are shown in Figure 5-52A. When these $5HT_{2C}$ receptors are blocked, norepinephrine and dopamine release is disinhibited in prefrontal cortex, which theoretically has an antidepressant effect (Figure 5-52B). Established antidepressants such as agomelatine and mirtazapine and others have $5HT_{2C}$ antagonist properties.

Not only does asenapine (like other atypical antipsychotics) have $5HT_{2C}$ antagonist actions (Figure 5-51), it also has numerous other potent pharmacologic actions linked theoretically to antidepressant actions that are predicted to raise norepinephrine, serotonin, and dopamine levels via α_2 antagonism (see Chapter 7) and to potentiate the elevation of serotonin levels in the presence of serotonin reuptake blockade by an SSRI/SNRI via $5HT_{1B/D}$ as well as $5HT_7$ antagonism (see Chapter 7). These same binding properties and actions on monoamines of asenapine in preclinical models also suggest theoretical utility for negative symptoms of schizophrenia, and an early study in fact suggested better efficacy than a comparator for treatment of negative symptoms, but this has not been replicated. The compelling theoretical antidepressant pharmacologic profile of asenapine also remains to be studied adequately in patients with either treatment-resistant depression or bipolar depression.

Zotepine

Zotepine is an atypical antipsychotic available in Japan and Europe, but not in the US. Zotepine has a chemical structure related to clozapine, but with some distinguishing pharmacologic (Figure 5-53) and clinical properties. Although classified usually as an atypical antipsychotic, some EPS have nevertheless been observed, as have prolactin elevations. Like clozapine, there is an increased risk of seizures, especially at high doses, as well as weight gain and sedation. Zotepine probably increases risk for insulin resistance, dyslipidemia, and diabetes, but it has not been extensively studied for these side effects. Unlike clozapine, however, there is no clear evidence yet that zotepine is as effective for patients who fail to respond to conventional antipsychotics. Zotepine dose dependently prolongs QTc interval and is generally administered three times daily. Zotepine is a $5HT_{2C}$ antagonist, an α_2 antagonist, a $5HT_7$ antagonist, and a weak partial agonist of $5HT_{1A}$ receptors as well as a weak inhibitor of norepinephrine reuptake (NET or norepinephrine transporter) (Figure 5-53), suggesting potential antidepressant effects that have not been well established yet in clinical trials.

The dones

Risperidone

This agent is a "done" and thus has a different chemical structure and a different pharmacologic profile than the "pines" (compare Figure 5-24A and B; see

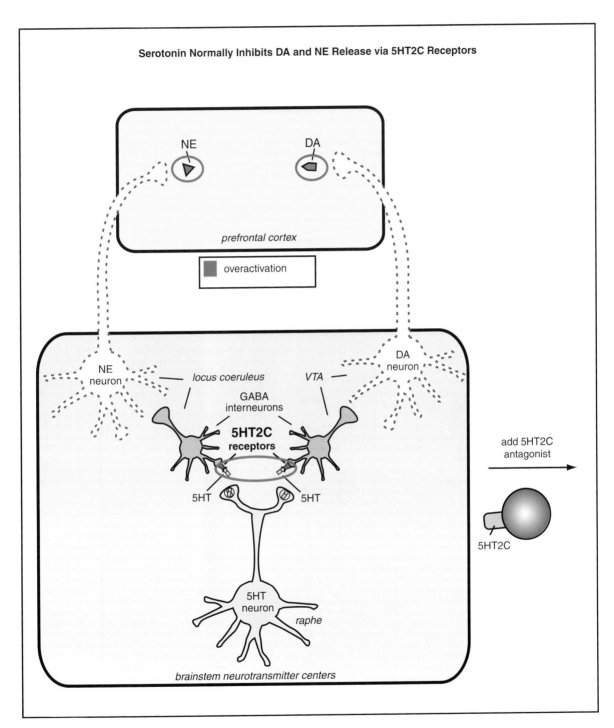

Figure 5-52A. Serotonin inhibits norepinephrine and dopamine release. Normally, serotonin binding at $5HT_{2C}$ receptors on γ-aminobutyric acid (GABA) interneurons (bottom red circle) inhibits norepinephrine and dopamine release in the prefrontal cortex (top red circles).

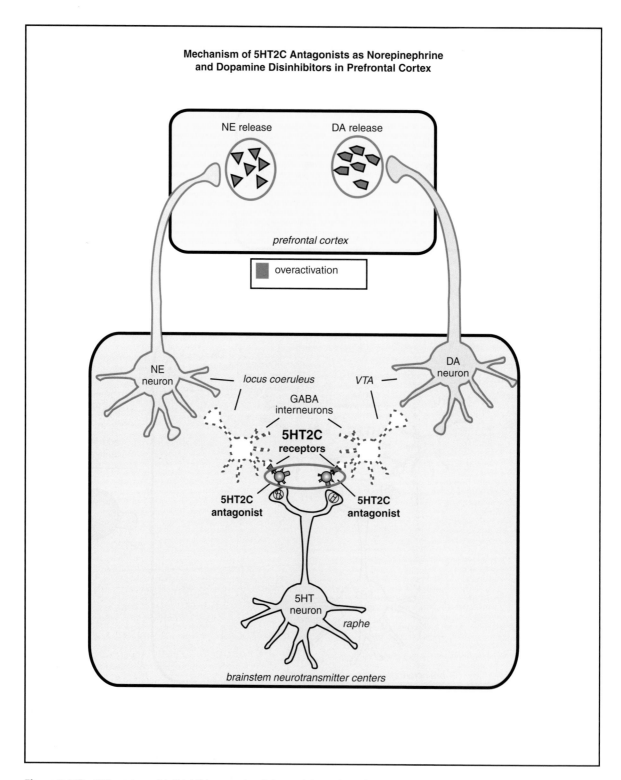

Figure 5-52B. 5HT$_{2C}$ antagonist disinhibits norepinephrine and dopamine release. When a 5HT$_{2C}$ antagonist binds to 5HT$_{2C}$ receptors on γ-aminobutyric acid (GABA) interneurons (bottom red circle), it prevents serotonin from binding there and thus prevents inhibition of norepinephrine and dopamine release in the prefrontal cortex; in other words, it disinhibits their release (top red circles).

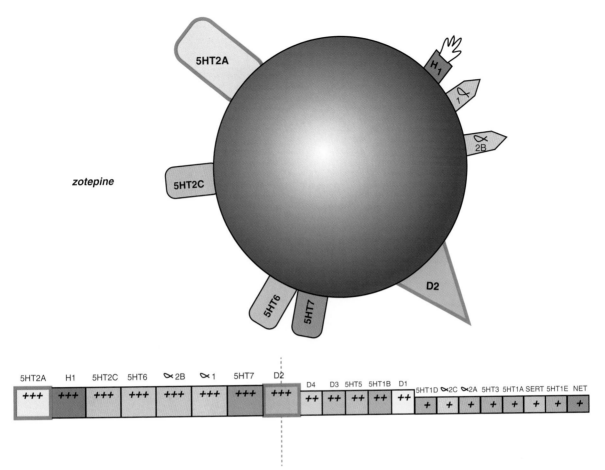

5HT2A	H1	5HT2C	5HT6	α2B	α1	5HT7	D2	D4	D3	5HT5	5HT1B	D1	5HT1D	α2C	α2A	5HT3	5HT1A	SERT	5HT1E	NET
+++	+++	+++	+++	+++	+++	+++	+++	++	++	++	++	++	+	+	+	+	+	+	+	+

Figure 5-53. Zotepine's pharmacological and binding profile. This figure portrays a qualitative consensus of current thinking about the binding properties of zotepine. $5HT_{2C}$ and histamine 1 antagonist properties can contribute to weight gain, H_1 and $α_1$-adrenergic antagonist properties can contribute to sedation, and $5HT_{2C}$ and $5HT_7$ antagonist properties suggest possible efficacy for mood symptoms. As with all atypical antipsychotics discussed in this chapter, binding properties vary greatly with technique and from one laboratory to another; they are constantly being revised and updated.

Figure 5-54). Risperidone has atypical antipsychotic properties especially at lower doses, but can become more "conventional" at high doses in that EPS can occur if the dose is too high. Risperidone thus has favored uses in schizophrenia and bipolar mania at moderate doses, but also for other conditions where lower or moderate doses of antipsychotics can be used, such as for children and adolescents with psychotic disorders. Risperidone is approved for treatment of irritability associated with autistic disorder in children and adolescents (ages 5–16), including symptoms of aggression towards others, deliberate self-injury, tantrums, and quickly changing moods, for bipolar disorder (ages 10–17), and for schizophrenia (ages 13–17). Low-dose risperidone is occasionally used

"off-label" for the controversial – due to a "black box" safety warning – treatment of agitation and psychosis associated with dementia. This occurs despite the fact that elderly patients with dementia-related psychosis treated with any atypical antipsychotic are at increased risk of death compared to placebo, even though that overall risk is low. Obviously, the risks versus benefits must be weighed for each patient carefully prior to prescribing an atypical antipsychotic for any use. Risperidone is available in a long-term depot injectable formulation lasting for 2 weeks. Such dosage formulations may improve treatment adherence, and if adherence is enhanced may lead to better long-term outcomes. There are also an orally disintegrating tablet and liquid formulation of risperidone.

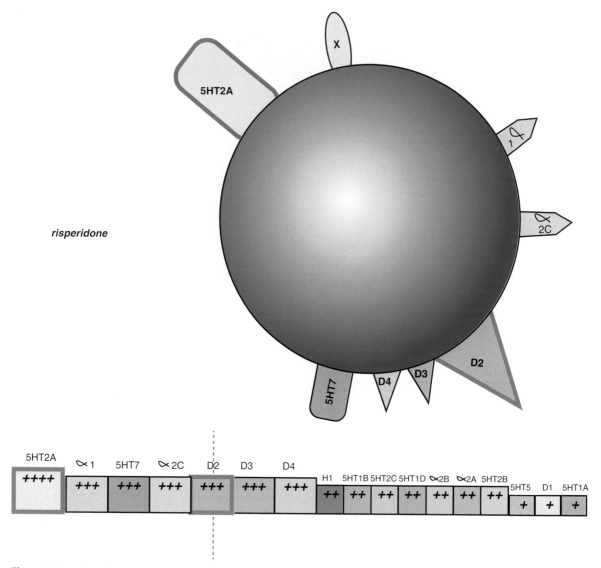

Figure 5-54. Risperidone's pharmacological and binding profile. This figure portrays a qualitative consensus of current thinking about the binding properties of risperidone. Alpha-2 (α_2) antagonist properties may contribute to efficacy for depression, but this can be diminished by simultaneous α_1 antagonist properties, which can also contribute to orthostatic hypotension and sedation. As with all atypical antipsychotics discussed in this chapter, binding properties vary greatly with technique and from one laboratory to another; they are constantly being revised and updated.

Although "atypical" in terms of reduced EPS at lower doses, risperidone does raise prolactin levels even at low doses. Risperidone has a moderate amount of risk for weight gain and dyslipidemia. Weight gain can be particularly a problem in children.

Paliperidone

Paliperidone, the active metabolite of risperidone, is also known as 9-hydroxy-risperidone, and it is an atypical antipsychotic with serotonin $5HT_{2A}$ and dopamine D_2 receptor antagonism (Figure 5-55). The binding profile of paliperidone (Figure 5-55) is similar to that of risperidone (Figure 5-54). One pharmacokinetic difference, however, between risperidone and paliperidone is that paliperidone is not hepatically metabolized; its elimination is based upon urinary excretion, and it thus has few pharmacokinetic drug interactions. Another pharmacokinetic difference is that the oral form of paliperidone is provided in a sustained-release

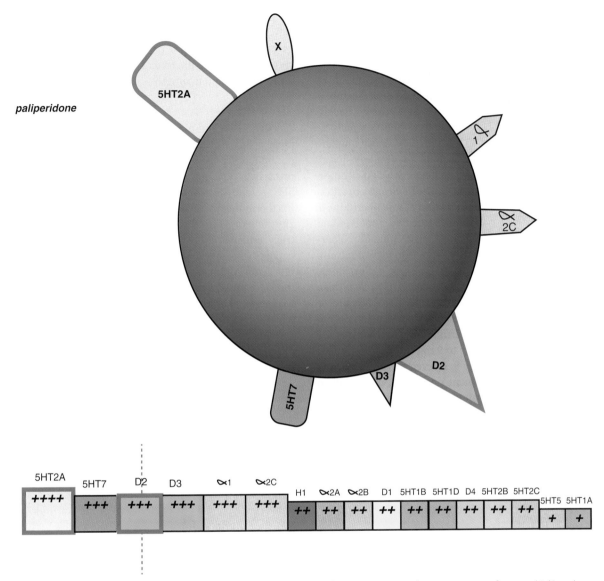

Figure 5-55. Paliperidone's pharmacological and binding profile. This figure portrays a qualitative consensus of current thinking about the binding properties of paliperidone, the active metabolite of risperidone. Paliperidone shares many pharmacological properties with risperidone. As with all atypical antipsychotics discussed in this chapter, binding properties vary greatly with technique and from one laboratory to another; they are constantly being revised and updated.

formulation, which risperidone is not, and this actually changes some of the clinical characteristics of paliperidone compared to risperidone, a fact that is not always well recognized and can lead to underdosing of oral paliperidone. Oral sustained-release means that paliperidone only needs to be administered once a day, whereas risperidone, especially when treatment is initiated, and especially in children or the elderly, may need to be given twice daily to avoid sedation and orthostasis. Side effects of

risperidone may be related in part to the rapid rate of absorption and higher peak doses with greater drug-level fluctuation leading to shorter duration of action, properties that are eliminated by the controlled-release formulation of paliperidone.

Despite the similar receptor binding characteristics of paliperidone and risperidone, paliperidone tends to be more tolerable, with less sedation, less orthostasis, and fewer EPS, although this is based upon anecdotal clinical experience and not head-to-head clinical studies. Paliperidone may have weight gain, insulin resistance, and diabetes associated with its use as well as elevations of plasma prolactin, much the same risk as risperidone.

The fact that paliperidone is an active metabolite of a known antipsychotic in a controlled-release formulation may lead some clinicians to erroneously believe that there are only trivial differences between paliperidone and risperidone, that they are essentially the same drugs, and that they should be similarly dosed, with the same mg dosing and the same up-titration when initiated. When this is done in clinical practice, this can lead to the false perception that paliperidone is not as effective as risperidone, but that problem can often be alleviated by recognizing that 1 mg of paliperidone is not equal to 1 mg of risperidone. A common mistake is to start patients on 3 mg of paliperidone, incorrectly assuming that it requires up-titration like risperidone and that 3 mg of paliperidone is more or less the same as 3 mg of risperidone. Actually, 6 mg paliperidone is a better starting dose and is generally well tolerated. An increase to 9 mg starting the second week of treatment on day 8, or even to 12 mg starting the third week of treatment on day 15, can result in optimal efficacy for paliperidone. Additional dosing tips are possibly to start a higher dose of paliperidone (9 mg) if the patient is at imminent risk of relapse, or if the patient has always needed higher doses of antipsychotics, or if the patient has persistent troublesome symptoms despite relatively high doses of the previous antipsychotic. On the other hand, lower doses (e.g., 3 mg daily) may be useful if the patient is very sensitive to side effects, at least at the start of dosing.

A depot palmitate formulation of paliperidone for long-term administration every 4 weeks is available and has become popular as the currently preferred depot atypical antipsychotic without the need to have oral treatment at the beginning of injections plus an injection every 2 weeks like long-acting risperidone injectable. The depot formulation of paliperidone also lacks the potential problems with severe sedation and monitoring recommended for long-acting olanzapine 4-week injectable. Although depot antipsychotics have always been more popular in some European countries than in the US, now that atypical antipsychotics such as paliperidone are becoming available as depot formulations, US clinicians are beginning not only to utilize them more, but to change their targeted patient types, from only administering depots to the most chaotic, least adherent patients, to using them

for patients early after the onset of psychosis. Assured adherence with a more tolerable depot atypical antipsychotic rather than a depot conventional antipsychotic early in the illness has the potential to lead to more favorable outcomes.

Ziprasidone

Ziprasidone is another atypical antipsychotic with a novel pharmacological profile (Figure 5-56). The major differentiating feature of ziprasidone is that it has little or no propensity for weight gain, despite its moderate $5HT_{2C}$ and H_1 antagonist actions (Figure 5-56). Furthermore, there seems to be little association of ziprasidone with dyslipidemia, elevation of fasting triglycerides, or insulin resistance. In fact, when patients who have developed weight gain and dyslipidemia from high-risk antipsychotics are switched from those antipsychotics to ziprasidone, there can be weight loss, and often lowering of fasting triglycerides, while continuing to receive treatment with ziprasidone. The pharmacologic properties that make ziprasidone different in terms of its lower cardiometabolic risk are unknown, but could be explained if ziprasidone lacks the ability to bind to receptors postulated to mediate insulin resistance and hypertriglyceridemia.

Ziprasidone is unusual as well because of the way it is dosed, namely twice a day and with food. Failure to give with about a 500 calorie meal can result in lowering oral absorption by half and inconsistent efficacy. Earlier concerns about dangerous QTc prolongation by ziprasidone now appear to be unjustified. Unlike iloperidone, zotepine, sertindole, and amisulpride, ziprasidone does not cause dose-dependent QTc prolongation, and few drugs have the potential to increase ziprasidone's plasma levels. Any antipsychotic that prolongs QTc interval – and this includes several conventional and atypical antipsychotics – should be given cautiously to patients receiving other drugs known to prolong QTc interval, but routine EKGs are generally not recommended. It is obviously prudent to be cautious when using any atypical antipsychotic or psychotropic drug in patients with cardiac problems, or in patients taking other drugs that affect cardiac function, or in those with a history of syncope or a family history of sudden death, and this is part of the routine risk–benefit calculation that is made for each individual patient prior to prescribing any of the atypical antipsychotic drugs. Ziprasidone has an intramuscular dosage formulation for rapid use in urgent circumstances.

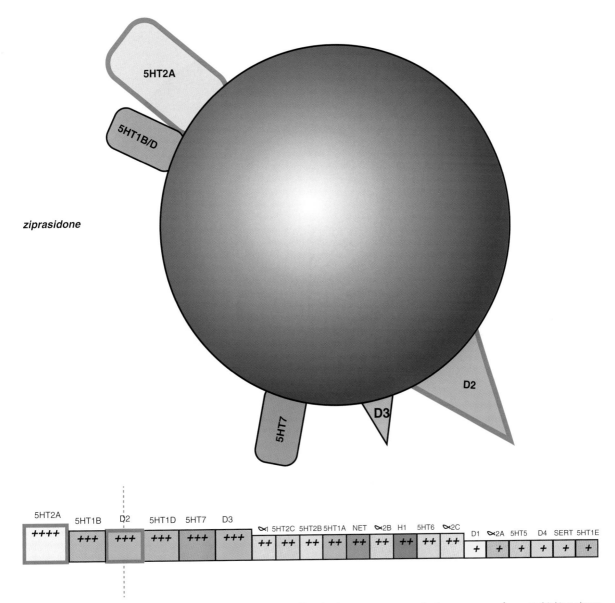

Figure 5-56. Ziprasidone's pharmacological and binding profile. This figure portrays a qualitative consensus of current thinking about the binding properties of ziprasidone. This compound seems to lack the pharmacological actions associated with weight gain and increased cardiometabolic risk such as increasing fasting plasma triglyceride levels or increasing insulin resistance. Ziprasidone also lacks many of the pharmacological properties associated with significant sedation. As with all atypical antipsychotics discussed in this chapter, binding properties vary greatly with technique and from one laboratory to another; they are constantly being revised and updated.

Ziprasidone has several pharmacologic properties suggesting it might have antidepressant actions, including $5HT_{2C}$, $5HT_7$, $5HT_{1B/D}$, and α_2 antagonism and $5HT_{1A}$ partial agonism, and weak norepinephrine and serotonin reuptake blockade (Figure 5-56), but has never been proven to have antidepressant actions in large clinical trials.

Iloperidone

Iloperidone is one of the newer atypical antipsychotics with $5HT_{2A}$–D_2 antagonist properties (Figure 5-57). Its most distinguishing clinical properties include a very low level of EPS, a low level of dyslipidemia, and a moderate level of weight gain associated with its use. Its most distinguishing pharmacology property is its

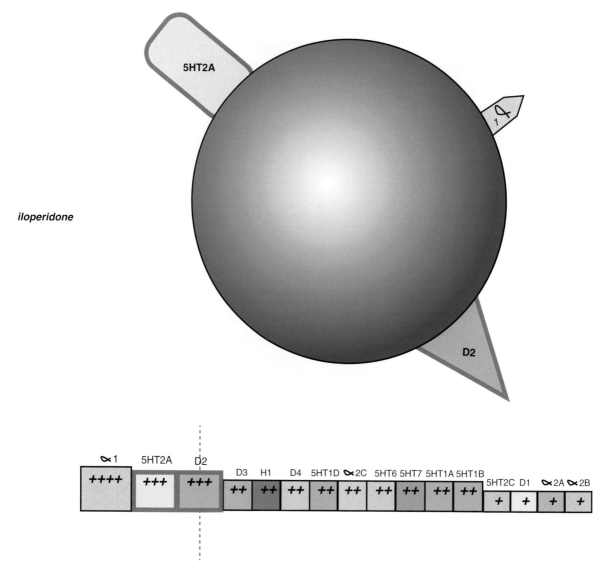

Figure 5-57. Iloperidone's pharmacological and binding profile. This figure portrays a qualitative consensus of current thinking about the binding properties of iloperidone. Among the atypical antipsychotics, iloperidone has one of the simplest pharmacological profiles and comes closest to a serotonin–dopamine antagonist (SDA). Its other prominent pharmacological property is potent α_1 antagonism, which may be responsible for the risk of orthostatic hypotension but also may contribute to its low risk of EPS. As with all atypical antipsychotics discussed in this chapter, binding properties vary greatly with technique and from one laboratory to another; they are constantly being revised and updated.

potent α_1 antagonism. As discussed earlier in this chapter, α_1 antagonism is generally associated with the potential for orthostatic hypotension and sedation, especially if rapidly dosed. Although iloperidone has an 18- to 33-hour half-life that theoretically supports once-daily dosing, it is generally dosed twice daily and titrated over several days when initiated in order to avoid both orthostasis and sedation. Slow dosing can delay onset of antipsychotic effects, so iloperidone is often used as a switch agent in non-urgent situations.

Although it is unknown why iloperidone, like quetiapine and clozapine, has such a low incidence of EPS, it may be in part due to the fact that all three of these agents have a high affinity for α_1 receptors as well as for $5HT_{2A}$ receptors (Figure 5-40). Theoretically, low EPS has been linked to high affinity for $5HT_{2A}$ (Figure 5-24), $5HT_{1A}$ (Figure 5-26), and muscarinic cholinergic receptors (Figure 5-39), as discussed earlier in this chapter. Actions at α_1 receptors are correlated mostly with side effects such as sedation and orthostasis (Figures 5-38 and 5-40). More recently, however, central α_1 receptors have been linked to potential therapeutic effects such as improvement in nightmares by the α_1 antagonist prazosin in posttraumatic stress disorder (PTSD) (discussed in Chapter 9 on anxiety) and maybe even reduction of EPS. The latter possibility is suggested by the fact that preclinical studies show that norepinephrine acting at postsynaptic α_1 receptors (Figure 5-58A) can stimulate the same pyramidal neurons in prefrontal cortex that serotonin acting at postsynaptic $5HT_{2A}$ receptors stimulates (Figure 5-15A). By analogy, therefore, if blocking $5HT_{2A}$ receptors reduces EPS by the downstream actions of such neurons (Figure 5-15B), it may be possible that blocking α_1 receptors on these same neurons would also reduce EPS (Figure 5-58B). This possibility is supported by the fact that clozapine (Figure 5-45) and iloperidone (Figure 5-57) both have the highest binding potencies of α_1 antagonism relative to D_2 antagonism among all the atypical antipsychotics; quetiapine (Figure 5-47) also has potent α_1 properties. All three of these agents exhibit few if any EPS in clinical use, although other atypical antipsychotics with higher EPS rates also have high α_1 receptor binding (Figure 5-40). Perhaps the combination of high $5HT_{2A}$ and α_1 affinities is a plausible explanation in particular for the low EPS of iloperidone and clozapine, but this is unproven and requires further research. Clinical use of atypical antipsychotics with high binding to α_1 receptors such as iloperidone for nightmares in PTSD is also theoretically appealing but requires much more clinical research.

In addition to potent α_1 antagonist properties, and very potent $5HT_{2A}$ antagonism relative to D_2 antagonism, iloperidone also has moderate α_2, $5HT_{1B/D}$, and $5HT_7$ antagonist and $5HT_{1A}$ partial agonist actions, suggesting potential antidepressant effects. However, there are no large-scale clinical studies of iloperidone yet in depression and it remains unproven as an antidepressant. Iloperidone exhibits dose-dependent QTc prolongation. There may be moderate weight gain with iloperidone but a low incidence of dyslipidemia. A 4-week depot preparation is in clinical testing.

Lurasidone

Lurasidone is one of the newer atypical antipsychotics with $5HT_{2A}$–D_2 antagonist properties (Figure 5-59). This compound exhibits high affinity for both $5HT_7$ and $5HT_{2A}$ receptors, as well as moderate affinity for $5HT_{1A}$ and α_2 receptors, yet minimal affinity for H_1-histamine and M_1-cholinergic receptors, properties that may explain some of lurasidone's clinical profile. It is an effective antipsychotic generally without sedation (especially if dosed at night), and along with ziprasidone and aripiprazole, has little or no weight gain or dyslipidemia. In fact, as with these other drugs, when a patient is switched to lurasidone from a previous agent associated with weight gain and dyslipidemia, such side effects may reverse. For the usual patient, there is little or no sedation, so the starting dose of 40 mg is an effective antipsychotic dose, although studies suggest that for maximum long-term efficacy, doses up to 160 mg per day may be useful in some patients, and in certain cases may possibly be more effective than some other antipsychotics. There may be moderate EPS with lurasidone, but this is reduced if lurasidone is given at night. As with ziprasidone, absorption of lurasidone is much greater when it is taken with 500 calories of food, which is recommended for consistent results. There is no QTc prolongation. Large-scale clinical trials show robust antidepressant efficacy in bipolar depression, and in addition trials are ongoing in mixed depression (depression with subsyndromal symptoms of mania). The receptor binding profile of lurasidone at $5HT_7$, $5HT_{1A}$, and α_2 receptors theoretically suggests why this drug has apparent antidepressant efficacy.

The potential antidepressant effects of $5HT_7$ antagonism (Figures 5-60 and 5-61) may be theoretically relevant to several atypical antipsychotics including lurasidone. It may also be relevant to the action of several known antidepressants, as discussed in Chapter 7. Briefly, $5HT_7$ receptors are located both on GABA neurons in the raphe and in the prefrontal cortex (Figures 5-60A and 5-61A). In both brain regions, *stimulation* of $5HT_7$ receptors by serotonin is thought to release GABA (Figures 5-60B and 5-61B). In the brainstem, $5HT_7$ receptor stimulation serves as a negative feedback loop and turns off further serotonin release (Figure 5-60B). In the cortex, stimulation of $5HT_7$ receptors excites the GABA interneurons, and this in turn inhibits pyramidal neurons in the cortex, reducing their release of glutamate downstream (Figure 5-61B).

On the other hand, *blocking* $5HT_7$ receptors in the brainstem raphe prevents their inhibition by GABA, and thus leads to increased release of serotonin from those raphe neurons, wherever they project, theoretically causing an antidepressant action (Figure 5-60C). This enhancement of serotonin release is

Cortical Alpha 1 Receptors May Decrease Dopamine Release

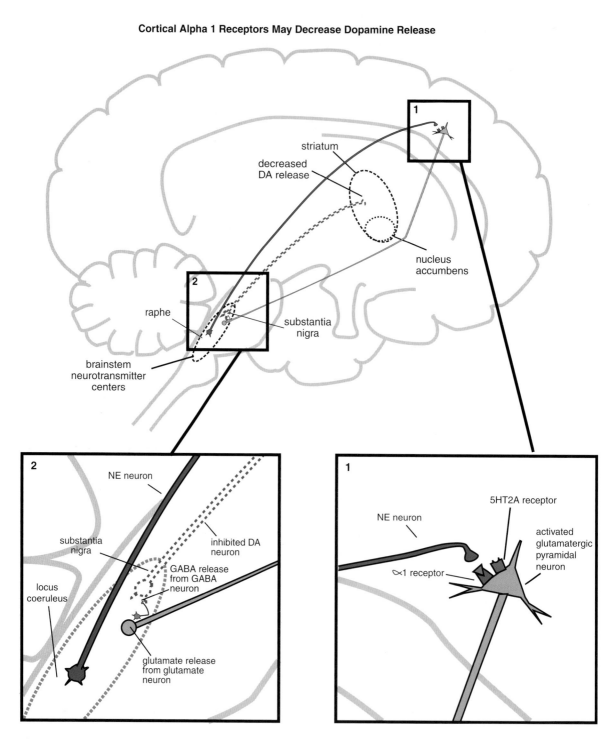

Figure 5-58A. Cortical α₁ receptor stimulation may decrease dopamine release. (1) Noradrenergic projections from the locus coeruleus to the cortex synapse with glutamatergic pyramidal neurons, where norepinephrine binds to α₁ receptors on the cortical glutamate neuron. (2) This causes glutamate release in the brainstem, which in turn causes GABA release in the substantia nigra, inhibiting dopaminergic neurons and therefore decreasing dopamine release into the striatum (indicated by the dotted outline of the dopaminergic neuron).

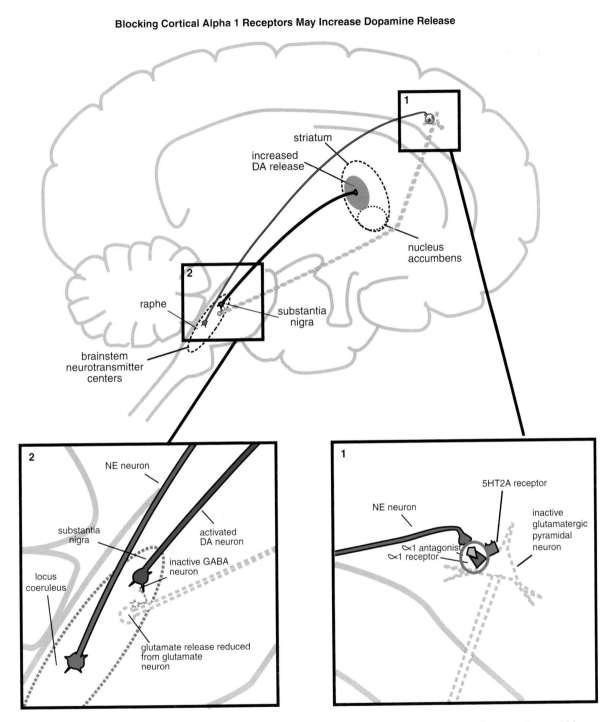

Figure 5-58B. Blocking cortical α₁ receptors may increase dopamine release. (1) When α_1 receptors on glutamatergic pyramidal neurons are blocked, this inactivates the glutamatergic neuron (indicated by the dotted outline of the glutamatergic neuron). (2) Glutamate release into the brainstem is therefore reduced and does not stimulate GABA release (indicated by the dotted outline of the GABA neuron). Without inhibitory input from GABA, dopaminergic neurons projecting from the substantia nigra to the striatum are activated and dopamine is released.

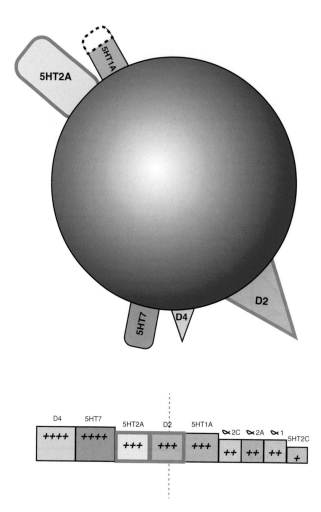

Figure 5-59. Lurasidone's pharmacological and binding profile. This figure portrays a qualitative consensus of current thinking about the binding properties of lurasidone. Among the atypical antipsychotics, lurasidone has a relatively simple pharmacological profile. It binds most potently to the D_4 receptor, the effects of which are not well understood, and to the $5HT_7$ receptor, which may contribute to efficacy for mood, cognitive, and sleep symptoms. As with all atypical antipsychotics discussed in this chapter, binding properties vary greatly with technique and from one laboratory to another; they are constantly being revised and updated.

increased in the presence of serotonin reuptake blockade in animals, suggesting a role for $5HT_7$ antagonists in augmenting SSRIs/SNRIs in depression/anxiety.

Blocking $5HT_7$ receptors in the prefrontal cortex causes less inhibition of certain populations of pyramidal neurons there and thus more downstream glutamate release from them (Figure 5-61C). There is potentially a wide variety of functional consequences of $5HT_7$ antagonism, which in experimental animals appear to be pro-cognitive, antidepressant, and synchronizing of circadian rhythms (Figure 5-61C). It is unknown yet whether these actions occur in human patients, as selective $5HT_7$ agents have not been widely tested in man, and the actions that many atypical antipsychotics with $5HT_7$ antagonist properties may have on mood and cognition in patients are only now being explored and are not yet proven. However, $5HT_7$ receptor antagonism remains a very plausible theoretical explanation for lurasidone's apparent antidepressant actions in bipolar depression, and suggests potential clinical efficacy in unipolar and treatment-resistant depression as well.

Two pips and a rip
Aripiprazole

This agent is a D_2 dopamine receptor partial agonist (DPA, D_2 partial agonist), a major differentiating pharmacologic feature compared to serotonin dopamine antagonists that are silent antagonists at D_2 receptors (Figures 5-35 and 5-62). Because of its D_2 partial agonist actions, aripiprazole is theoretically an atypical antipsychotic with reduced EPS and hyperprolactinemia despite not having $5HT_{2A}$ antagonist properties at higher affinity than its affinity

Baseline

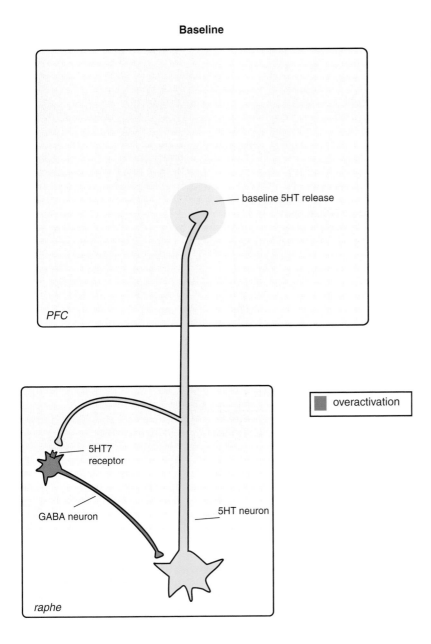

baseline 5HT release

PFC

overactivation

5HT7 receptor

GABA neuron

5HT neuron

raphe

Figure 5-60A. Function of 5HT₇ receptors in the raphe nucleus. Shown here is a serotonergic neuron projecting from the raphe nucleus to the prefrontal cortex (PFC), where it releases serotonin. The release of serotonin is regulated in part by GABAergic neurons within the raphe nucleus that contain 5HT₇ receptors.

for D_2 receptors (i.e., $5HT_{2A}$ lies to the right of D_2, unlike almost every other atypical antipsychotic in Figure 5-24). In addition, aripiprazole has $5HT_{1A}$ partial agonist actions that are more potent than its $5HT_{2A}$ antagonist actions, but less potent than its D_2 binding affinity (Figure 5-62), and this property hypothetically contributes to its atypical antipsychotic clinical properties, as discussed earlier in this chapter.

Aripiprazole is effective in treating schizophrenia and mania, and is also approved for use in various child and adolescent groups, including schizophrenia (age 13 and older), acute mania/mixed mania (age 10 and older), and autism-related irritability in children ages 6–17. Aripiprazole lacks the pharmacologic properties normally associated with sedation, namely, M_1-muscarinic cholinergic and H_1-histaminic antagonist properties, and thus is not generally sedating. A major differentiating feature of aripiprazole is that it has, like ziprasidone and lurasidone, little or no propensity for weight gain, although weight gain

Stimulation of 5HT7 Receptors in the Raphe Reduces Serotonin Release

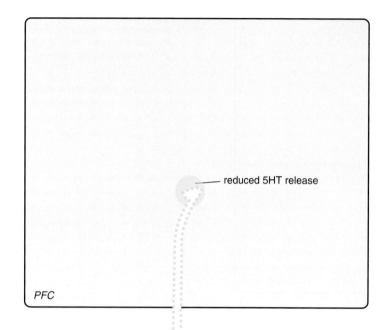

reduced 5HT release

PFC

Figure 5-60B. Stimulation of 5HT7 receptors in the raphe nucleus reduces serotonin release. When serotonin binds to 5HT7 receptors on GABAergic interneurons within the raphe nucleus, this activates the GABA neuron (indicated by the red color of the neuron) to release GABA. GABA then inhibits serotonergic projections from the raphe nucleus to the prefrontal cortex, thus reducing serotonin release there (indicated by the dotted outline of the serotonin neuron).

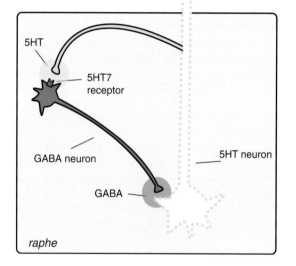

5HT

5HT7 receptor

GABA neuron

GABA

5HT neuron

raphe

▇ overactivation

without dyslipidemia can be a problem for some, including children and adolescents. Furthermore, there seems to be little association of aripiprazole with dyslipidemia, elevation of fasting triglycerides, or insulin resistance. In fact, as with ziprasidone and lurasidone, when patients with weight gain and dyslipidemia caused by other antipsychotics switch to aripiprazole, there can be weight loss and lowering of fasting triglyceride levels. The pharmacologic

properties that make aripiprazole different in terms of its lower metabolic risk are unknown, but could be explained if aripiprazole lacks the ability to bind to postulated receptors that mediate insulin resistance and hypertriglyceridemia (Figure 5-42).

Aripiprazole is approved as an antidepressant for augmenting SSRIs/SNRIs in treatment-resistant major depressive disorder, and although not specifically approved, is often used as well in bipolar depression.

Blockade of 5HT7 Receptors in the Raphe Increases Serotonin Release

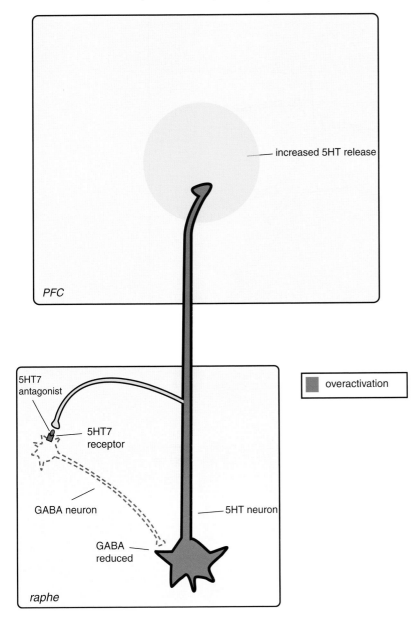

PFC

— increased 5HT release

overactivation

5HT7
antagonist

5HT7
receptor

GABA neuron

5HT neuron

GABA
reduced

raphe

Figure 5-60C. Blockade of 5HT$_7$ receptors in the raphe nucleus increases serotonin release. If 5HT$_7$ receptors on GABAergic interneurons in the raphe nucleus are blocked, then GABA release is inhibited (indicated by the dotted outline of the GABA neuron). Without the presence of GABA, the serotonergic projection from the raphe nucleus to the prefrontal cortex can become overactivated (indicated by the red color of the neuron), leading to increased serotonin release in the prefrontal cortex.

How aripiprazole works in depression as compared to how it works in schizophrenia is of course unknown, but its potent 5HT$_{1A}$ partial agonist and 5HT$_7$ antagonist properties are theoretical explanations for potential antidepressant actions, as these would be active at the low doses generally used to treat depression. It is also possible that partial agonist actions at both D$_2$ and D$_3$ receptors mean that aripiprazole could act more as an agonist than as an antagonist at dopamine receptors at low doses, in fact slightly boosting rather than blocking hypothetically deficient dopamine neurotransmission in depression, but this is unproven.

So, is aripiprazole the perfect "Goldilocks" D$_2$ partial agonist? Some believe it is "too hot," meaning that it is too much of an agonist and not enough of an antagonist, and that aripiprazole would thus be optimized if it were more of an antagonist, noting that aripiprazole can sometimes have dopamine

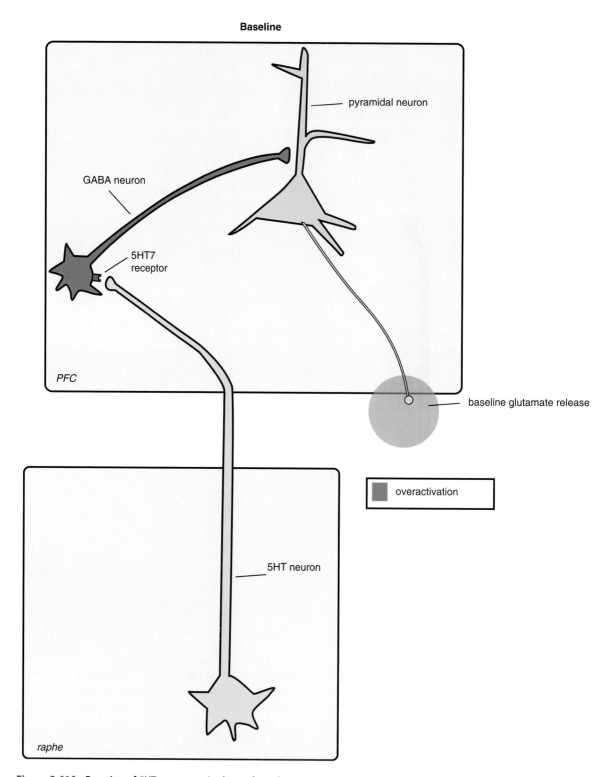

Figure 5-61A. Function of 5HT$_7$ receptors in the prefrontal cortex. A major function of 5HT$_7$ receptors may be to regulate serotonin–glutamate interactions. Serotonergic projections from the raphe nucleus to the prefrontal cortex synapse with GABAergic interneurons that contain 5HT$_7$ receptors. The GABAergic neurons, in turn, synapse with glutamatergic pyramidal neurons.

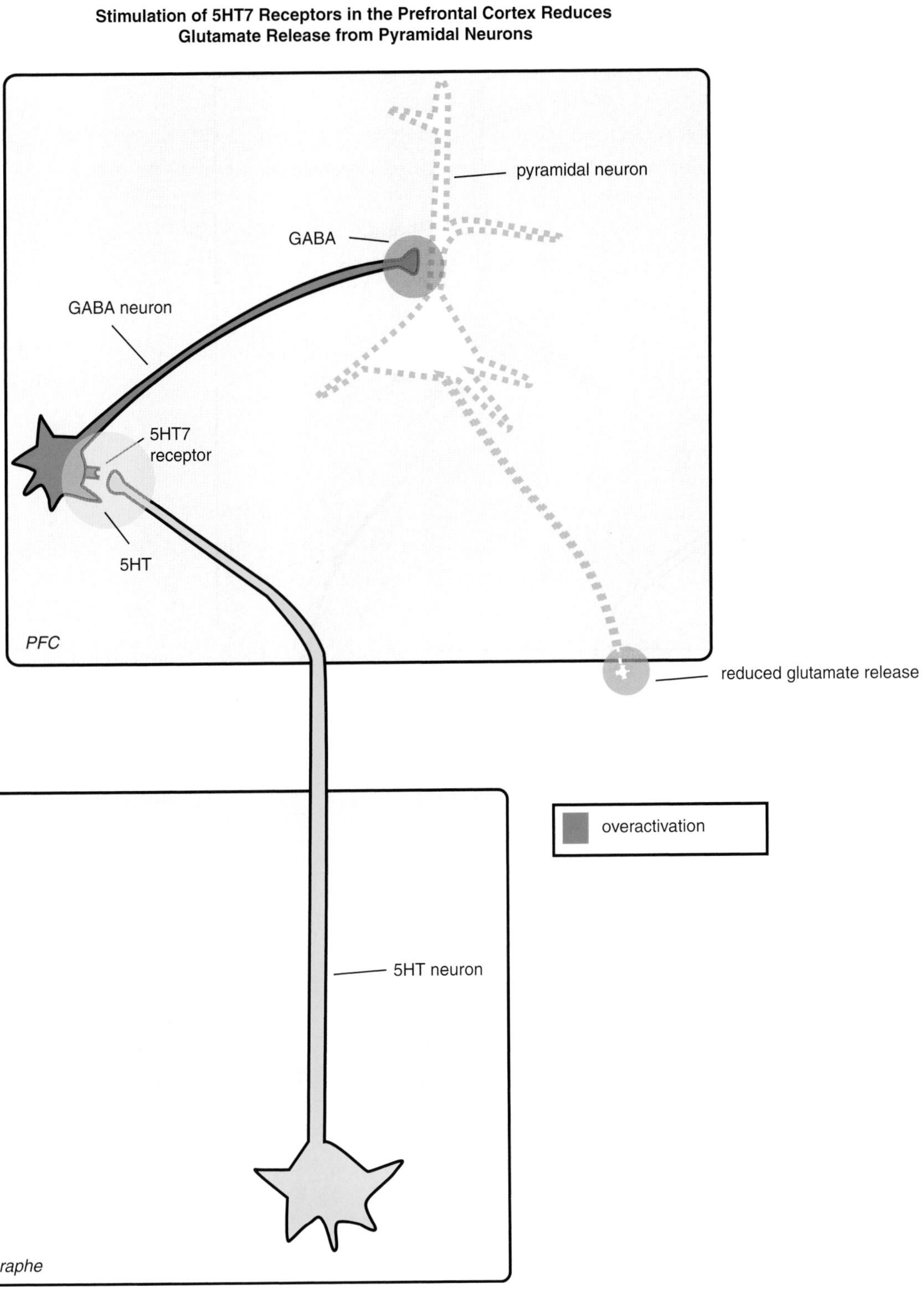

Figure 5-61B. Stimulation of 5HT$_7$ receptors in the prefrontal cortex reduces glutamate release from pyramidal neurons. Serotonin binds to 5HT$_7$ receptors on GABA interneurons in the prefrontal cortex. This stimulates GABA release (indicated by the red color of the neuron), which in turn inhibits glutamate release (indicated by the dotted outline of the glutamatergic neuron).

**Blockade of 5HT7 Receptors in the Prefrontal Cortex Enhances
Glutamate Release from Pyramidal Neurons**

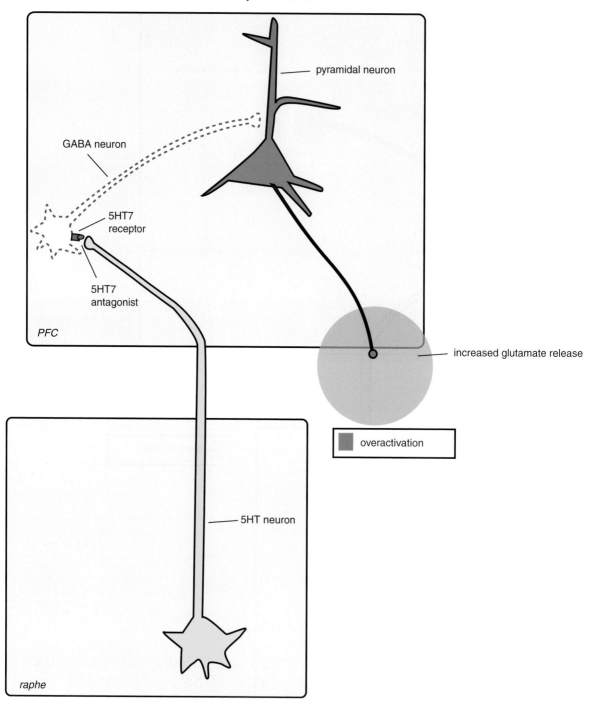

Figure 5-61C. Blockade of 5HT₇ receptors in the prefrontal cortex increases glutamate release from pyramidal neurons. If 5HT₇
receptors on GABAergic interneurons in the prefrontal cortex are blocked, then GABA release is inhibited (indicated by the dotted outline of
the GABA neuron). Without the presence of GABA, glutamatergic pyramidal neurons in the prefrontal cortex can become overactivated
(indicated by the red color of the neuron), leading to increased glutamate release.

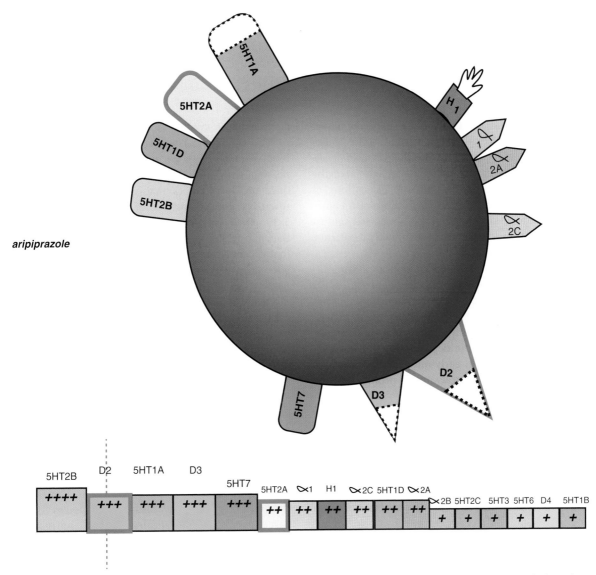

aripiprazole

Figure 5-62. Aripiprazole's pharmacological and binding profile. This figure portrays a qualitative consensus of current thinking about the binding properties of aripiprazole. Aripiprazole differs from most other antipsychotics in that it is a partial agonist at D_2 receptors rather than an antagonist. Additional important pharmacological properties that may contribute to its clinical profile include $5HT_{2A}$ antagonist actions, $5HT_{1A}$ partial agonist actions, and $5HT_7$ antagonist actions. Aripiprazole lacks or has weak binding potency at receptors usually associated with significant sedation. Aripiprazole also seems to lack the pharmacologic actions associated with weight gain and increased cardiometabolic risk, such as increasing fasting plasma triglyceride levels or increasing insulin resistance. As with all atypical antipsychotics discussed in this chapter, binding properties vary greatly with technique and from one laboratory to another; they are constantly being revised and updated.

agonist-like actions, such as being activating in some patients, causing mild agitation instead of tranquilization and antipsychotic actions, and can also cause nausea and occasionally vomiting. Also, high doses of aripiprazole sometimes do not seem to deliver sufficient antipsychotic efficacy in some very difficult-to-treat patients; in some psychotic cases,

higher doses beyond a certain point are no more effective or even slightly less effective than somewhat lower doses. Such observations suggest that aripiprazole could be improved in those patients by greater antagonist actions, with closer placement towards the full antagonist part of the left hand of the spectrum shown in Figure 5-35.

On the other hand, some believe that aripiprazole is "too cold," meaning that it is too much of an antagonist because it can have antagonist-like actions such as causing akathisia in some patients, which is often decreased by dose reduction or by administering an anticholinergic agent or a benzodiazepine. In this case, aripiprazole might be improved by closer placement towards the agonist part of the spectrum shown in Figure 5-35. The truth is that there is no Goldilocks drug that fits every patient. In late-stage clinical development are drugs that are both more antagonist on the spectrum than aripiprazole (see the discussions of brexpiprazole and cariprazine that follow, and Figure 5-35). Soon there may be a portfolio of partial agonist options to customize the needs of individual patients, since one size cannot fit all.

An intramuscular dosage formulation of aripiprazole for short-term use is available, as are an orally disintegrating tablet and a liquid formulation. A long-acting 4-week injectable is in the late stages of clinical development and is eagerly awaited as another potential atypical antipsychotic depot option for assuring adherence, especially in early-onset psychosis where aripiprazole's favorable tolerability profile may be particularly well received.

Brexpiprazole

Just as its name suggests, brexpiprazole is chemically related to aripiprazole. It differs from aripiprazole in several ways from a pharmacologic perspective (compare Figures 5-63 and 5-62). Brexpiprazole is still in late-stage clinical trials, so the clinical correlates of these pharmacological differences are only now being established. Firstly, brexpiprazole is more of a D_2 antagonist than aripiprazole, moving it to the left towards the full antagonist part of the spectrum in Figure 5-35. Secondly, brexpiprazole has more potent $5HT_{2A}$ antagonism, $5HT_{1A}$ partial agonism, and α_1 antagonism relative to its D_2 partial agonism (Figure 5-63) than aripiprazole (Figure 5-62), which should theoretically enhance its atypical antipsychotic properties and reduce EPS despite its being more of a D_2 antagonist than aripiprazole. Clinical trials in fact confirm this so far, as there is a very low incidence of EPS and only rare akathisia for brexpiprazole. This must be confirmed in large-scale trials now in progress. Brexpiprazole would be predicted to have antipsychotic and antimanic activity like aripiprazole, but with perhaps a more favorable tolerability profile. Its $5HT_{1A}$ partial agonist and $5HT_7$ antagonist properties (Figure 5-63) also suggest antidepressant

actions like aripiprazole. Finally, brexpiprazole is a potential treatment for agitation and psychosis in dementia, but a good deal of clinical testing will be necessary to confirm both its efficacy and its safety for this application.

Cariprazine

Cariprazine is another dopamine D_2 partial agonist in late-stage clinical testing for schizophrenia, acute bipolar mania, bipolar depression, and treatment-resistant depression. Cariprazine is more of an antagonist at D_2 receptors than aripiprazole, moving it towards the antagonist end of the spectrum in Figure 5-35. However, cariprazine is also less of an agonist than the related partial agonist bifeprunox, an agent that did not receive FDA approval as it had clinical effects consistent with being too much of an agonist – namely, less efficacy than comparator antipsychotics, too activating, too slow dose titration, and too much nausea and vomiting. In theory, cariprazine may be preferred at higher doses for mania and schizophrenia, to emphasize its antagonist actions, and at lower doses for depression, to emphasize its agonist actions and potentially its uniquely D_3-preferring properties. Dosing, efficacy, and side effects are still under investigation, but little weight gain or metabolic problems have been identified thus far. This compound has two very long-lasting active metabolites with the novel and interesting potential for development as a weekly, biweekly, or even monthly "oral depot."

Cariprazine so far shows a low incidence of EPS in clinical testing, perhaps because it has potent $5HT_{1A}$ partial agonist actions and lesser $5HT_{2A}$ antagonism (Figure 5-64). At higher doses cariprazine could potentially block $5HT_7$ and $5HT_{2C}$ receptors for hypothetical antidepressant actions. At very low doses there are interesting theoretical possibilities suggested by cariprazine's unique D_3-preferring over D_2 affinity, with both actions being partial agonist actions rather than antagonist actions (Figure 5-64). The role of D_3 receptors is largely unknown but may be linked to cognition, mood, emotions, and reward/substance abuse. It has been difficult to dissect the role of D_2 receptors from D_3 receptors, since essentially all antipsychotics act at both receptors, with the clinical effects attributed to their D_2 actions. However, with cariprazine, there is a window of selectivity for D_3 actions at low doses where D_3 receptors are preferentially occupied (Figure 5-64), and this creates the theoretical opportunity to determine whether D_3-preferring actions have a different

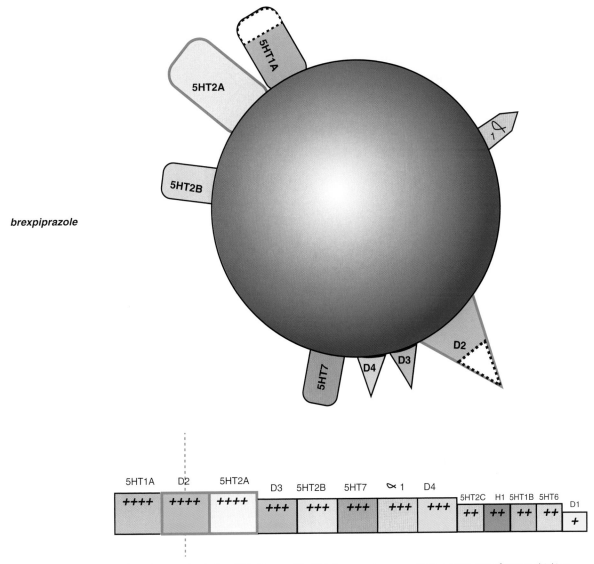

Figure 5-63. Brexpiprazole's pharmacological and binding profile. This figure portrays a qualitative consensus of current thinking about the binding properties of brexpiprazole. Brexpiprazole has a pharmacological profile similar to that of aripiprazole: it is a partial agonist at D_2 receptors rather than an antagonist, and also binds potently to $5HT_{2A}$, $5HT_{1A}$, and $5HT_7$ receptors. Brexpiprazole also seems to lack actions at receptors usually associated with significant sedation, weight gain, and increased cardiometabolic risk, although it is too early to evaluate the clinical profile of this medication. As with all atypical antipsychotics discussed in this chapter, binding properties vary greatly with technique and from one laboratory to another; they are constantly being revised and updated.

clinical profile than the D_2 (plus D_3) actions of all other antipsychotics.

The others

Sulpiride

Sulpiride is an earlier compound structurally related to amisulpride that was developed as a conventional antipsychotic (Figure 5-65). Although it generally causes EPS and prolactin elevation at usual antipsychotic doses, it may be activating and have efficacy for negative symptoms of schizophrenia and for depression at low doses, where it is D_3-preferring. This agent, if a D_2 partial agonist, is likely to have pharmacologic properties very, very close to those of a silent antagonist and may only function as a partial agonist at low doses and as a more conventional D_2 antagonist at higher, antipsychotic doses (Figure 5-35).

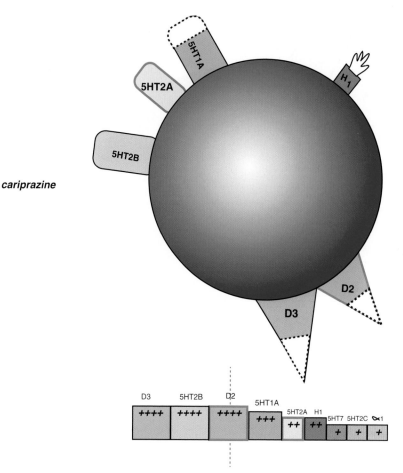

Figure 5-64. Cariprazine's pharmacological and binding profile. This figure portrays a qualitative consensus of current thinking about the binding properties of cariprazine. Cariprazine has potent actions at D_3, $5HT_{2B}$, D_2, and $5HT_{1A}$ receptors, with relatively weaker affinity for $5HT_{2A}$ and H_1 receptors. As with all atypical antipsychotics discussed in this chapter, binding properties vary greatly with technique and from one laboratory to another; they are constantly being revised and updated.

Amisulpride

Amisulpride, like sulpiride, was developed in Europe and elsewhere prior to full appreciation of the concept of dopamine partial agonism. Thus, it has not been tested in the same preclinical pharmacology systems as newer agents, but there are some clinical hints not only that amisulpride is an atypical antipsychotic, but that it has these clinical properties because it is a partial agonist very close to the full antagonist end of the D_2 spectrum (Figure 5-35). Amisulpride has no appreciable affinity for $5HT_{2A}$ or $5HT_{1A}$ receptors to explain its low propensity for EPS and its observations of improvement of negative symptoms in schizophrenia and of depression, particularly at low doses, but it is an antagonist at $5HT_7$ receptors (Figure 5-66). Like all antipsychotics, it is not known how amisulpride's actions at D_3 receptors may contribute to its clinical profile.

Amisulpride's ability to cause weight gain, dyslipidemia, and diabetes has not been extensively investigated. It causes dose-dependent QTc prolongation. Since amisulpride can cause prolactin elevation, if it is appropriately classifiable as a partial agonist at all, it is likely closer to a silent antagonist than aripiprazole on the partial agonist spectrum, and it may only function as a partial agonist at low doses and a more conventional D_2 antagonist at high doses (see Figure 5-35).

Sertindole

Sertindole is an atypical antipsychotic with serotonin $5HT_{2A}$–dopamine D_2 receptor antagonist properties (Figure 5-67), originally approved in some European countries, then withdrawn for further testing of its cardiac safety and QTc-prolonging potential, and then reintroduced into certain countries as a second-line agent. It may be useful for some patients in whom other antipsychotics have failed, and who can have close monitoring of their cardiac status and drug interactions.

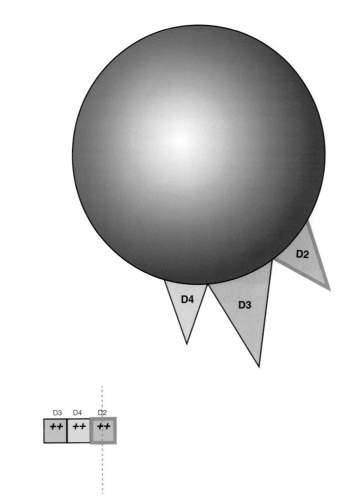

sulpiride

Figure 5-65. Sulpiride's pharmacological and binding profile. This figure portrays a qualitative consensus of current thinking about the binding properties of sulpiride. At usual doses, sulpiride has the profile of a conventional antipsychotic, but at low doses it may be a partial agonist at D₂ receptors, though likely still closer to the antagonist end of the spectrum. As with all atypical antipsychotics discussed in this chapter, binding properties vary greatly with technique and from one laboratory to another; they are constantly being revised and updated.

Perospirone

Perospirone is an atypical antipsychotic with $5HT_{2A}$ and D_2 antagonist properties available in Japan (Figure 5-68). $5HT_{1A}$ partial agonist actions may contribute to its efficacy. Its ability to cause weight gain, dyslipidemia, insulin resistance, and diabetes are not well investigated. It is generally administered three times a day, with more experience in the treatment of schizophrenia than in the treatment of mania.

Antipsychotics in clinical practice

Prescribing antipsychotics in clinical practice can be very different than studying them in clinical trials. Real patients are often more complicated, may have diagnoses that do not meet diagnostic criteria for the formally studied indications, and generally have much more comorbidity than patients studied in clinical trials. Thus, it is important for the practicing psychopharmacologist to appreciate that different atypical antipsychotics can have clinically distinctive effects in different patients in clinical practice and that these are not always well studied in randomized controlled trials. What this also means is that median clinical effects in clinical trials may not be the best indicator of the range of clinical responses possible for individual patients. Furthermore, optimal doses suggested from clinical trials often do not match optimal doses used in clinical practice (too high for some drugs, too low for others). Finally, although virtually all studies are head-to-head comparisons of monotherapies and/ or placebo, many patients receive two antipsychotics or antipsychotics plus other psychotropic drugs in clinical practice settings. Sometimes this is rational and justified, but sometimes it is not. Here we will briefly discuss some of the issues that arise

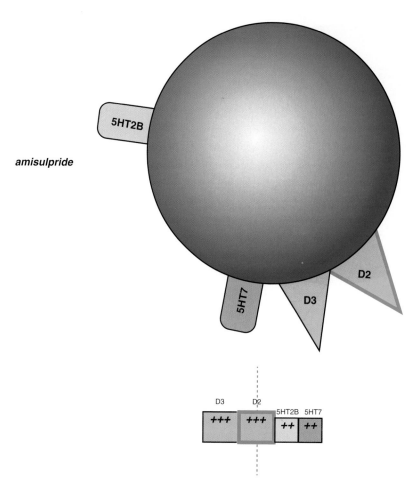

Figure 5-66. Amisulpride's pharmacological and binding profile. This figure portrays a qualitative consensus of current thinking about the binding properties of amisulpride. Amisulpride does not have affinity for $5HT_{2A}$ or $5HT_{1A}$ receptors, but it may be a partial agonist at D_2 receptors rather than an antagonist. As with all atypical antipsychotics discussed in this chapter, binding properties vary greatly with technique and from one laboratory to another; they are constantly being revised and updated.

when trying to apply knowledge about the pharmacological mechanisms of action discussed so far in this chapter to the clinical utilization of atypical antipsychotics in clinical practice.

The art of switching antipsychotics

It might seem that it would be easy to switch from one antipsychotic to another, but this has proven to be problematic for many patients. Switching antipsychotics actually requires skill to convert patients from one agent to another. Otherwise, patients can develop agitation, activation, insomnia, rebound psychosis, and withdrawal effects, especially anticholinergic rebound, if it is done too quickly or without finesse, especially if one tries to precipitously stop one antipsychotic and start the other at full dose (Figure 5-69). Of course, this must occasionally be done under urgent circumstances when there is not the time to more carefully transition from one drug to

another. Full doses can be given to patients who are not taking any antipsychotic at the time when one is started, but in a switch scenario, some form of transition is usually necessary in order for the clinical situation to stay stable or improve, and the best results are usually obtained by cross-titration over several days to weeks (Figure 5-70). This creates concomitant administration of two antipsychotics for a while as one goes up and the other goes down in dose, and this is acceptable and in fact desirable polypharmacy until the transition is complete (Figure 5-70).

Sometimes the transition between two similar agents can take a long time; nevertheless it is important to complete the transition and not get caught in cross-titration as shown in Figure 5-71. Sometimes as the dose of the second drug goes up and the dose of the first drug comes down, the patient begins to do better, and the clinician just stops without completing the transition to a full dose of the second agent and complete discontinuation of the first. That is not

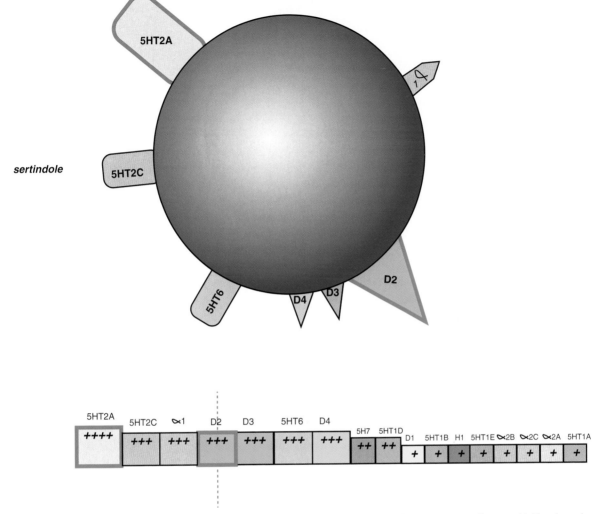

Figure 5-67. Sertindole's pharmacological and binding profile. This figure portrays a qualitative consensus of current thinking about the binding properties of sertindole. Potent antagonist actions at α_1 receptors may account for some of sertindole's side effects. As with all atypical antipsychotics discussed in this chapter, binding properties vary greatly with technique and from one laboratory to another; they are constantly being revised and updated.

generally recommended, since a full trial on the second agent is the goal, and long-term polypharmacy of two agents is not well studied and can be quite expensive. If the second agent is not satisfactory, it is generally preferable to try a third (Figure 5-70) rather than use two agents together indefinitely in what can be unacceptable polypharmacy (Figure 5-71).

Switching between two agents that have similar pharmacology is generally easiest, fastest, and has the fewest complications, namely a pine to a pine, or a done to a done, over as little as a week's time (Figure 5-72). However, problems can occur if the switch is too

fast from a pine to a done (Figure 5-73). As discussed extensively in this chapter, the binding characteristics of pines and dones are different, the most striking difference being that the pines in general have more anticholinergic and antihistaminic actions (Figure 5-39), and more α_1 antagonist actions (Figure 5-40), and thus are in general more sedating than the dones, which have less potent binding at these sites.

Therefore, when switching from a pine to a done, it is generally a good idea to stop the pine slowly – over at least 2 weeks – to allow the patient to readapt to the withdrawal of blocking cholinergic, histaminic, and α_1

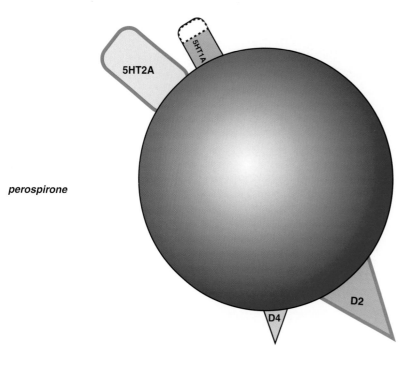

perospirone

Figure 5-68. Perospirone's pharmacological and binding profile. This figure portrays a qualitative consensus of current thinking about the binding properties of perospirone. 5HT$_{1A}$ partial agonist actions may contribute to efficacy for mood and cognitive symptoms. As with all atypical antipsychotics discussed in this chapter, binding properties vary greatly with technique and from one laboratory to another; they are constantly being revised and updated.

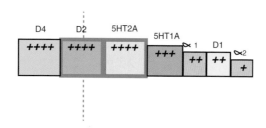

How Not to Switch Antipsychotics

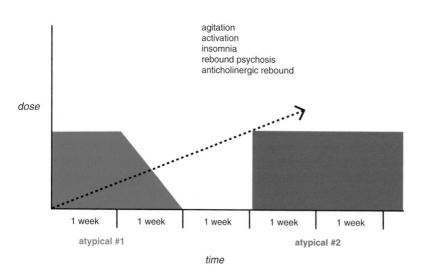

agitation
activation
insomnia
rebound psychosis
anticholinergic rebound

Figure 5-69. How not to switch antipsychotics. Converting patients from one antipsychotic to another requires great care in order to ensure that they do not develop withdrawal symptoms, rebound psychosis, or aggravation of side effects. Generally, this means not precipitously discontinuing the first antipsychotic, not allowing gaps between the administration of the two antipsychotics, and not starting the second antipsychotic at full dose.

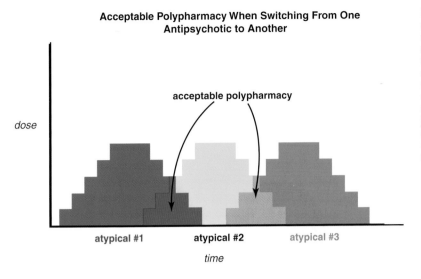

Acceptable Polypharmacy When Switching From One Antipsychotic to Another

acceptable polypharmacy

atypical #1   atypical #2   atypical #3

time

dose

Figure 5-70. Switching from one antipsychotic to another. When switching from one antipsychotic to another, it is frequently prudent to "cross-titrate" – that is, to build down the dose of the first drug while building up the dose of the other over a few days to a few weeks. This leads to transient administration of two drugs but is justified in order to reduce side effects and the risk of rebound symptoms, and to accelerate the successful transition to the second drug.

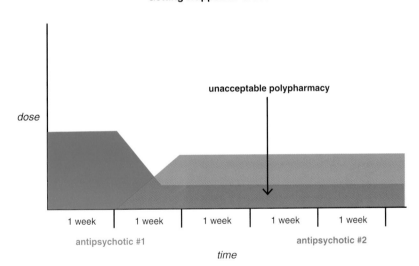

Getting Trapped in Cross-Titration

unacceptable polypharmacy

1 week   1 week   1 week   1 week   1 week

antipsychotic #1   antipsychotic #2

time

dose

Figure 5-71. Getting trapped in cross-titration. When switching from one atypical antipsychotic to another, the patient may improve in the middle of cross-titration. Polypharmacy results if cross-titration is stopped at this point and the patient continues both drugs indefinitely. It is generally better to complete the cross titration as shown in Figure 5-70, with discontinuation of the first agent and an adequate monotherapy trial of the second drug before trying long-term polypharmacy.

receptors, which makes the transition more tolerable without anticholinergic rebound, agitation, and insomnia (Figure 5-73). When stopping the specific pine clozapine, it should always be stopped very slowly, over 4 weeks or more if possible, to minimize the chances of rebound psychosis as well as anticholinergic rebound (Figure 5-74).

When switching in the other direction, namely, from a done to a pine, it is generally best to titrate up the pine over 2 weeks or more, although the done can usually be stopped as quickly as over 1 week. This allows the patient to become tolerant to the sedating effects of most pines (Figure 5-75).

Switching to and from aripiprazole is a special case, in part because it has different pharmacologic properties, and in part because it has higher potency for the D_2 receptor than many other drugs, meaning that its administration causes essentially immediate withdrawal of the first drug from D_2 receptors. These principles are likely to be applicable to the new "pip and a rip" (namely, brexpiprazole and cariprazine), as they both have similar binding characteristics and D_2 potencies, and are D_2 partial agonists, but there is little experience as yet with switching to or from either brexpiprazole or cariprazine.

Switching from One Pine or Done to Another: Pines to Pines or Dones to Dones

Pines

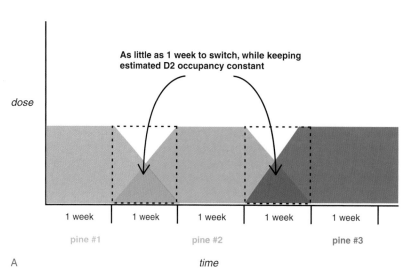

A

time

Dones

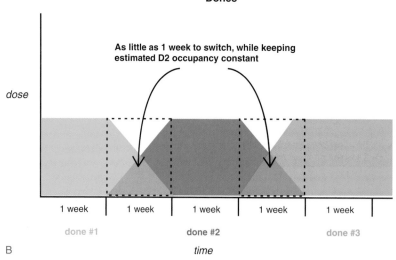

B

time

Figure 5-72. Switching from one pine or done to another. (A) When switching from one "pine" (clozapine, olanzapine, quetiapine, asenapine) to another, it is prudent to make the switch in as little as 1 week, while keeping estimated D_2 receptor occupancy constant. (B) Likewise, when switching from one "done" (risperidone, paliperidone, ziprasidone, iloperidone, lurasidone) to another, it is prudent to make the switch in as little as 1 week, while keeping estimated D_2 receptor occupancy constant.

Switching to aripiprazole

Specifically, when switching to aripiprazole from a pine, it can be a good idea in many patients to start a middle, and not a low, dose when adding aripiprazole, building the aripiprazole dose up rapidly over 3–7 days while taking 2 weeks to taper the pine (Figure 5-76). The recommendation for fast up-titration of aripiprazole arises from the fact that it essentially replaces the first drug at the D_2 receptor

immediately, and it can be helpful therefore to get aripiprazole to its therapeutic dose rapidly. The slower down-titration of the pine allows readaptation of cholinergic and histaminergic receptors to minimize withdrawal, and the taper also allows slower offset of any sedating actions while the full dose of aripiprazole is being established (Figure 5-76). When switching to aripiprazole from a done (Figure 5-77), it can also be helpful to start a middle, not a low,

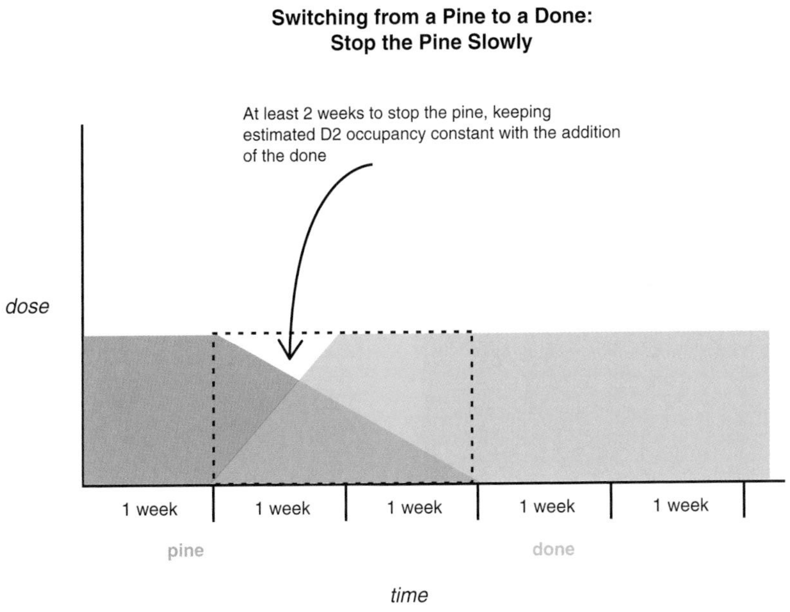

Switching from a Pine to a Done: Stop the Pine Slowly

At least 2 weeks to stop the pine, keeping estimated D2 occupancy constant with the addition of the done

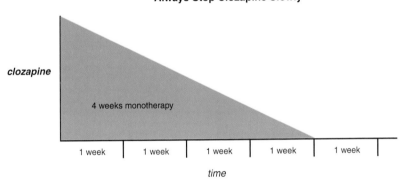

dose

1 week | 1 week | 1 week | 1 week | 1 week

pine   done

time

Figure 5-73. Switching from a pine to a done. When switching from a "pine" (clozapine, olanzapine, quetiapine, asenapine) to a done (risperidone, paliperidone, ziprasidone, iloperidone, lurasidone), it is prudent to take at least 2 weeks to stop the pine, while keeping the estimated D$_2$ receptor occupancy constant during the addition of the done.

Always Stop Clozapine Slowly

clozapine

4 weeks monotherapy

1 week | 1 week | 1 week | 1 week | 1 week

time

Figure 5-74. Stopping clozapine. When stopping clozapine, it is always necessary to do so slowly, with 4 weeks of down-titration prior to starting another antipsychotic.

Switching from a Done to a Pine: Start the Pine Slowly

For best tolerability unless clinically urgent, take 2 weeks to start the pine, keeping estimated D2 occupancy constant as done is stopped

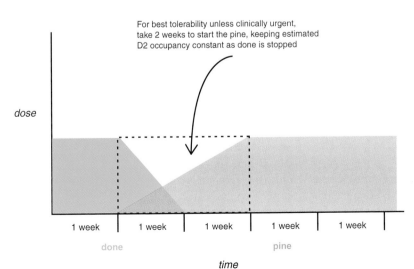

dose

1 week | 1 week | 1 week | 1 week | 1 week

done   pine

time

Figure 5-75. Switching from a done to a pine. When switching from a "done" (risperidone, paliperidone, ziprasidone, iloperidone, lurasidone) to a "pine" (clozapine, olanzapine, quetiapine, asenapine), tolerability may be best if the pine can be titrated up over the course of 2 weeks, while keeping the estimated D$_2$ receptor occupancy constant as the done is stopped.

Switching to Aripiprazole from a Pine

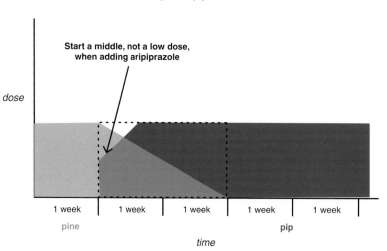

Start a middle, not a low dose, when adding aripiprazole

dose

| 1 week | 1 week | 1 week | 1 week | 1 week |

pine   pip

time

Figure 5-76. Switching to aripiprazole from a pine. Aripiprazole has higher affinity for D$_2$ receptors than most "pines" (clozapine, olanzapine, quetiapine, asenapine); thus, breakthrough symptoms may be more likely when switching from a pine to aripiprazole. A prudent approach, therefore, is to start aripiprazole at a middle dose, rather than a low dose, while down-titrating the pine slowly over 2 weeks.

Switching to Aripiprazole from a Done

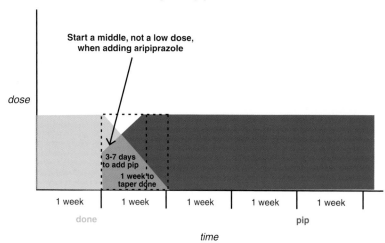

Start a middle, not a low dose, when adding aripiprazole

dose

3-7 days to add pip

1 week to taper done

| 1 week | 1 week | 1 week | 1 week | 1 week |

done   pip

time

Figure 5-77. Switching to aripiprazole from a done. When switching to aripiprazole from a "done" (risperidone, paliperidone, ziprasidone, iloperidone, lurasidone), it is recommended to start aripiprazole at a middle dose, rather than a low dose, while down-titrating the done over 1 week.

dose of the aripiprazole, and build it up rapidly over 3–7 days, but it is possible to taper the done over 1 week, since the dones are less likely to be associated with anticholinergic and antihistaminic withdrawal symptoms.

Switching from aripiprazole

In the other direction, when stopping aripiprazole and switching to a pine, consider immediately stopping the aripiprazole, which has not only high potency for D$_2$ receptors but a very long half-life (more than 2 days), while starting a middle, and not a low, dose of the pine,

tapered up over 2 weeks (Figure 5-78). When switching from aripiprazole to a done, also consider immediately stopping the aripiprazole, and starting a middle, and not a low, dose of the done, tapered up over 1 week (Figure 5-79).

These are very basic generalities that certainly do not apply in all situations for all antipsychotics discussed here, but may be useful guidelines based not only on receptor binding properties but also on empiric clinical experience. In many individual cases, switching may need to be even slower than illustrated here – but generally not faster, unless encountering clinically urgent circumstances.

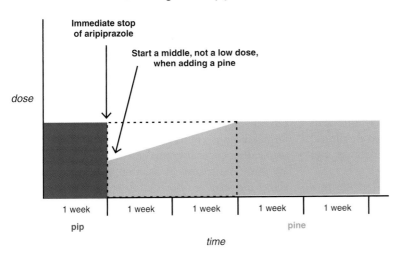

Switching from Aripiprazole to a Pine

Figure 5-78. Switching from aripiprazole to a pine. When switching from aripiprazole to a "pine" (clozapine, olanzapine, quetiapine, asenapine), it is recommended to stop aripiprazole immediately and start the pine at a middle, rather than a low, dose. The pine can be up-titrated over a period of 2 weeks.

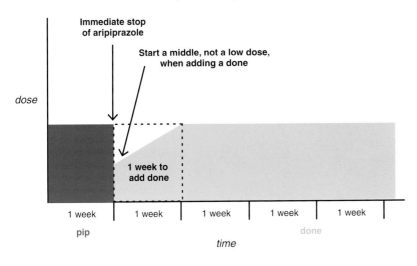

Switching from Aripiprazole to a Done

Figure 5-79. Switching from aripiprazole to a done. When switching from aripiprazole to a "done" (risperidone, paliperidone, ziprasidone, iloperidone, lurasidone), it is recommended to stop aripiprazole immediately and start the done at a middle, rather than a low, dose. The done can be up-titrated over a period of 1 week.

Treatment resistance and violence

Although this chapter has discussed the well-researched and approved uses of antipsychotics in schizophrenia, namely as monotherapies at extensively studied doses with documented safety and efficacy in standard patient populations participating in clinical trials, what do you do when the antipsychotic is not working? This is often called treatment-resistant psychosis, and it can be characterized by delusions and hallucinations and thought disorder; that is, predominantly positive symptoms that do not respond to standard doses of several trials of individual conventional or atypical antipsychotics. Treatment guidelines suggest the use of clozapine at this point. However, what if clozapine does not work or you cannot prescribe it for medical reasons, or if the patient refuses it?

And what if the problem is aggressive symptoms, hostility, impulsivity, and even violence unresponsive to standard doses of several different antipsychotics or even clozapine? This is a common problem in institutional and forensic settings, and treatment guidelines from large-scale multicenter trials do not provide specific recommendations for these clinical scenarios. Principles of psychopharmacology coupled with case-based evidence do provide some potential solutions for treatment resistance with or without violence; however, these solutions are controversial to some experts and not based on traditional evidence since such patients for ethical and practical reasons (formal legal incompetence and institutionalization, etc.) cannot be studied in randomized controlled trials. Nevertheless, high dosing, use of two concomitant antipsychotics, and augmentation of an antipsychotic with a mood stabilizer are all commonly used in clinical practice as solutions for treatment resistance and violence. Is this rational or justified?

The rationale for treating violence when antipsychotic monotherapies fail is shown in Figure 5-80, and is based upon the specific hypothetical etiology

of aggression and violence. Thus, violence that is linked to psychotic behavior despite standard antipsychotic dosing may be caused by inadequate occupancy of D_2 receptors due to pharmacokinetic failure (Figures 5-80 and 5-81). That is, ideal pharmacokinetics are assumed at standard doses to attain 60% or more striatal D_2 occupancy, but if drug is not adequately absorbed or is excessively metabolized, it can cause a pharmacokinetic failure (Figure 5-81). The formal diagnosis of this is possible by measuring therapeutic drug concentrations and documenting that they are low. The treatment solution is to raise the dose above the standard dose in order to compensate for the low amount of drug getting to D_2 receptors. One can also document that plasma drug levels are increased

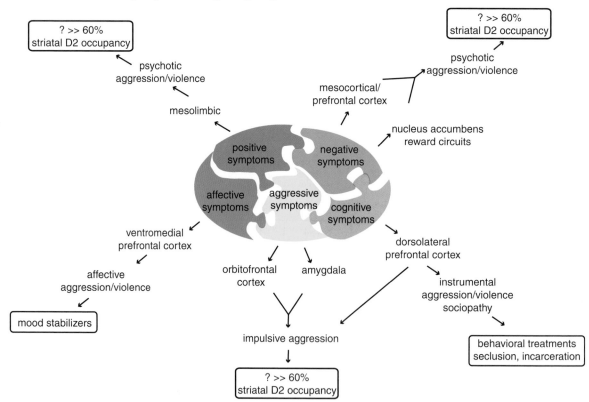

Psychopharmacologic Targeting of Circuits Associated with Violence

Figure 5-80. Psychopharmacologic targeting of circuits associated with violence. Violent behavior can be associated with circuits that are relevant to schizophrenia, and may therefore be targeted by psychopharmacologic strategies that target those circuits. The mesolimbic and mesocortical pathways, which are thought to be responsible for positive and negative symptoms, may also be involved in aggression and violence. It is possible that agents targeting much more than 60% D_2 receptor occupancy in these pathways could reduce these symptoms. Likewise, the orbitofrontal cortex and the amygdala may play a role in impulsive aggression, which could theoretically be alleviated by agents targeting much more than 60% D_2 receptor occupancy. Affective symptoms that may contribute to violent behavior may be mediated by the ventromedial prefrontal cortex and could potentially be treated with mood stabilizers. Finally, instrumental aggression and violent sociopathy may be mediated by the dorsolateral prefrontal cortex, and may best be managed with behavioral strategies, including seclusion and incarceration.

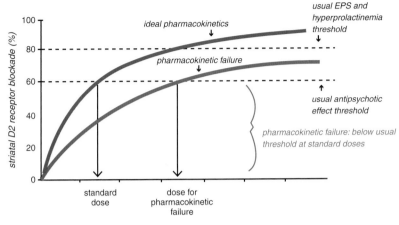

**Treatment Resistance:
Is Adequate Drug Getting to the Receptors for >60% Occupancy?
(Pharmacokinetic Failures)**

Figure 5-81. Treatment resistance or pharmacokinetic failure. In general, D2 receptor occupancy greater than 80% is needed in the mesolimbic pathway for antipsychotic effects, while D2 occupancy greater than 80% in the dorsal striatum is associated with extrapyramidal side effects (EPS) and D2 occupancy greater than 80% in the pituitary is associated with hyperprolactinemia. However, although the majority of patients may achieve 80% D2 receptor occupancy in the mesolimbic pathway and 60% D2 receptor occupancy in the striatum with standard doses of antipsychotics, this may not be true for all patients. That is, pharmacokinetic factors may influence how much drug reaches the target receptor. For instance, individuals with certain CYP450 variants may be rapid metabolizers of certain medications, and thus never get adequate D2 receptor occupancy from standard doses. Low drug levels may also occur due to poor drug absorption, which may be the case for patients with gastric bypass, lap bands, ileostomies, colectomies, or for unknown reasons. Food can also affect the absorption of certain antipsychotics. If standard dosing attains less than 80% D2 receptor occupancy in the mesolimbic region or 60% D2 receptor occupancy in the striatum, then such doses may not be effective no matter how many drugs one tries. To that end, pharmacokinetic failure may be suspected for patients who do not respond to a sequence of monotherapies and also do not have side effects. This can be confirmed by measurement of therapeutic drug levels; if confirmed, higher than usual doses would be justified.

to the normal range when this otherwise high dose is given (Figure 5-81). In the case of pharmacokinetic failures, a high dose is really a standard dose for such patients, as it just takes more peripherally administered oral antipsychotic to attain the standard amount of D_2 occupancy (Figure 5-81).

Although some patients have *pharmacokinetic* failures to explain their lack of treatment response, many have instead what can be called *pharmacodynamic* failures: that is, they fail to have adequate clinical responses despite attaining 60% or more striatal D_2 receptor occupancy. Many potential causes of this are illustrated in Figure 5-80. For example, one cause of antipsychotic treatment failure despite attaining 60% or more striatal D_2 occupancy can be that the patient has an affective disturbance that requires augmentation with a mood stabilizer, especially divalproex or lamotrigine, but even lithium or an antidepressant (Figure 5-80). Another cause of antipsychotic treatment failure in such cases can be that some patients

are slow responders to 60% striatal D_2 receptor occupancy (Figure 5-82). Evidence from long-term clinical trials is accumulating to show that many patients will respond with late onset of efficacy, particularly for remission of psychosis or for improvement of negative symptoms, and after many months of treatment (Figure 5-82). The solution for those patients able to wait for their clinical effects to "kick in" is to use "time as a drug" and treat for many weeks hoping to get a good outcome (Figure 5-83). There is no way to predict who will have such late-onset responses, so finding these patients is largely a matter of trial and error.

Another potential approach to pharmacodynamic antipsychotic treatment failures is to postulate that some patients require much more than 60% D_2 occupancy to have an adequate treatment response (Figures 5-84 through 5-87). Such patients may have psychotic symptoms and/or impulsive symptoms associated with aggression and violence that can require urgent management to prevent harm to others (Figure 5-80).

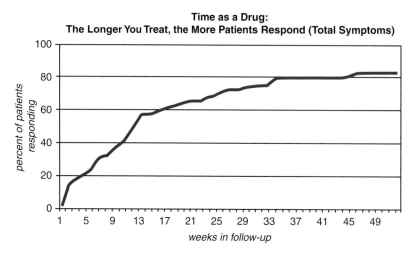

Figure 5-82. Time as a drug. It may be that maintaining a patient on the same medication over an extended period of time, rather than switching early, could lead to additional improvement in symptoms.

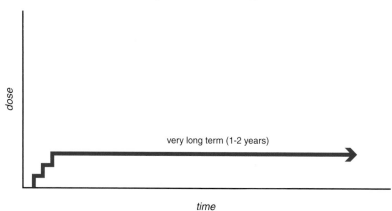

Figure 5-83. Nonresponse/violence: very long treatment using time as a drug. It is possible that some patients may experience pharmacodynamic failure. For such patients, it may be that the downstream effects of D_2 blockade take longer to manifest than the typical 6 weeks allotted for a drug trial. For these individuals, time itself may be a therapeutic treatment.

Empirically, patients like this can respond to very high doses associated with high plasma drug levels, and it can be assumed that drugs administered in high doses are occupying more than 60% of D_2 receptors (Figure 5-84). However, this has never been proven in randomized controlled trials nor quantitatively measured by PET scans. Usually these patients are too disturbed either to give informed consent or to cooperate with research studies, or to receive blinded treatments that may not work, so we only have case-based anecdotes to support this approach. To the extent that case-based evidence can be used to establish treatment recommendations in the absence of controlled trials, it does appear that some patients – those with psych-otic or impulsive violence – do indeed respond to high-dose monotherapy (Figure 5-85), and that the tradeoff between side effects and therapeutic actions can be surprisingly in favor of continued high-dose treatment (Figures 5-84 and 5-85).

Another way to target greater than 60% D_2 receptor occupancy is to use standard doses of two antipsychotics at the same time, sometimes called antipsychotic polypharmacy (Figures 5-86 and 5-87) rather than high doses of one antipsychotic (Figures 5-84 and 5-85). Because the curve of increasing D_2 occupancy is very flat at the upper range of monotherapy dosing (Figure 5-84), it can actually be a more effective approach to give standard doses of

Violence and Treatment-Resistant Psychosis: Are Hypothetical Thresholds for Atypical Antipsychotic Drug Effects Altered? (Pharmacodynamic Failure?)

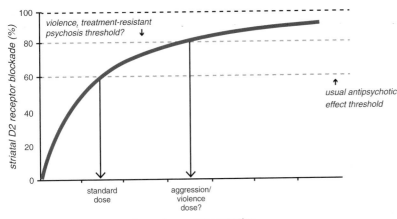

Figure 5-84. Nonresponse/violence: are hypothetical thresholds for drug effects altered? It is possible that some patients may experience pharmacodynamic failure. For such patients, it may be that they require more than 80% D2 receptor occupancy in the mesolimbic pathway in order to achieve therapeutic effects. This may be true particularly for patients who have failed to respond to multiple, adequately-dosed agents, and who still have aggression or violence. It is possible that, for these patients, using high doses that achieve 80–100% limbic D2 receptor occupancy may be necessary for therapeutic effects.

Novel Solution to Nonresponse/Violence: High to Very High Doses Beyond the Generally Recommended Range

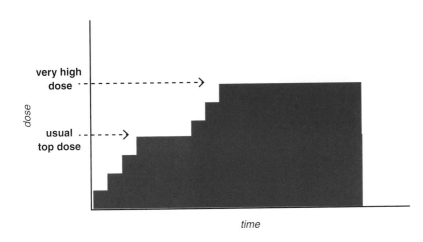

Figure 5-85. Nonresponse/violence: high to very high doses. Patients who have failed to respond to multiple, adequately dosed agents and who have aggression or violence may have pharmacodynamic failure and require doses that achieve 80–100% striatal D_2 receptor occupancy. They may therefore require higher doses beyond the generally recommended range. The evidence base for high-dose monotherapy varies for the different atypical antipsychotics, and there are certain agents for which it may not be appropriate.

two antipsychotics, as the receptor occupancy curve of the second antipsychotic may be steep (Figure 5-86). Some clinicians prefer augmenting clozapine for treatment-resistant cases, and this form of antipsychotic polypharmacy has been studied the most. Others try augmenting an atypical antipsychotic with a conventional antipsychotic, or giving two atypical antipsychotics together. All of these have empiric case-based evidence for improvement of psychosis, aggression, and violence in some patients with schizophrenia, but other patients can have intolerable side effects, most commonly sedation, EPS, and weight gain, but occasionally paralytic ileus (especially with very high-dose pines such as clozapine, quetiapine, and olanzapine), and cognitive dysfunction. Generally speaking, very-high-dose monotherapy or antipsychotic polypharmacy should be used sparingly and in selected cases of treatment resistance, violence,

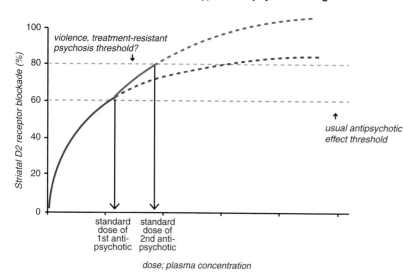

Hypothetical Thresholds for Atypical Antipsychotic Drug Effects

Striatal D2 receptor blockade (%)

violence, treatment-resistant psychosis threshold?

usual antipsychotic effect threshold

standard dose of 1st anti-psychotic

standard dose of 2nd anti-psychotic

dose; plasma concentration

Figure 5-86. Nonresponse/violence: hypothetical thresholds for drug effects. Patients who have failed to respond to multiple, adequately-dosed agents and who have aggression or violence may have pharmacodynamic failure and require 80–100% limbic D2 receptor occupancy. This can potentially be achieved by adding a standard dose of a second antipsychotic to a standard dose of the first antipsychotic.

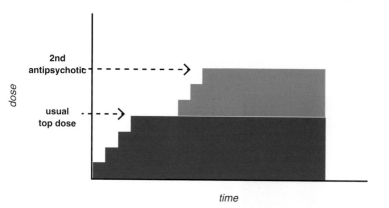

Novel Solution to Nonresponse/Violence: Add Second Antipsychotic (Polypharmacy) to a First Antipsychotic Given in the Generally Recommended Dosing Range

dose

2nd antipsychotic

usual top dose

time

Figure 5-87. Nonresponse/violence: polypharmacy. Patients who have failed to respond to multiple, adequately dosed agents and who have aggression or violence may have pharmacodynamic failure and require 80–100% striatal D_2 receptor occupancy. This can potentially be achieved by adding a standard dose of a second antipsychotic to a standard dose of the first antipsychotic. This strategy is not well studied and should truly be reserved for cases in which all else fails.

and aggression, and only "when all else fails" – and even in such cases only when demonstrated to be clearly beneficial. Another group of patients for whom pharmacodynamic antipsychotic treatment failures are a problem that should generally not be managed by high-dose monotherapy or antipsychotic polypharmacy consists of those with instrumental aggression related to sociopathy and antisocial personality disorder; no amount of D_2 antagonism is likely to help such patients, who may instead need behavioral treatments, seclusion, or even incarceration (Figure 5-80).

Psychotherapy and schizophrenia

Although this is a psychopharmacology textbook, it is increasingly clear that psychotherapies can be combined with antipsychotics to leverage the effectiveness of these agents. Integrating psychopharmacology and psychotherapy in psychotic disorders is an area of growing interest and increasing research and is included in many treatment guidelines for schizophrenia. This includes adding cognitive behavioral psychotherapy to antipsychotics in order to strengthen the patient's capacity for normal thinking using

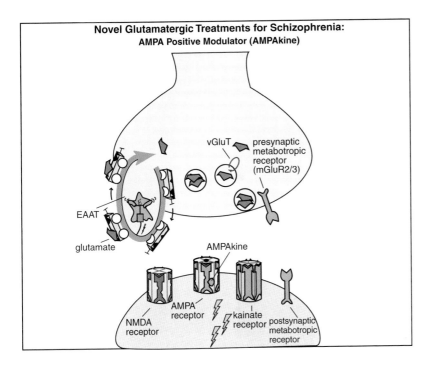

Novel Glutamatergic Treatments for Schizophrenia:
AMPA Positive Modulator (AMPAkine)

vGluT
presynaptic
metabotropic
receptor
(mGluR2/3)

EAAT

glutamate

AMPAkine

NMDA
receptor

AMPA
receptor

kainate
receptor

postsynaptic
metabotropic
receptor

Figure 5-88. Novel glutamatergic treatments for schizophrenia: AMPA positive modulator. Positive modulation at postsynaptic AMPA receptors could help regulate ion flow and neuronal depolarization in postsynaptic neurons, leading to appropriate NMDA receptor activation. Also shown postsynaptically are NMDA receptors, kainate receptors, and postsynaptic metabotropic receptors, all for glutamate. Shown presynaptically are the presynaptic reuptake pump for glutamate, the excitatory amino acid transporter (EAAT), the presynaptic metobotropic autoreceptor mGluR2/3, and the synaptic vesicle transporter for glutamate or vGluT.

mental exercises and self-observation. If patients can pay attention, learn, and remember, they are able to cope better with residual positive symptoms and are more likely to live an independent life. Patients who are stabilized on antipsychotics are often capable of being taught at that point in their illness to critically analyze hallucinations and examine any underlying beliefs in their hallucinations and delusions.

Family and outside support is critical to foster positive social interactions, which in turn may help to keep delusions under control. Family support is essential for encouraging patients to comply with their antipsychotics and to recognize early signs of relapse or side effects. It also helps family members understand the illness and reduce their own emotional reactions to the patient and this devastating illness, so that their own emotions do not trigger more acting-out by the patient.

Community treatment programs are highly beneficial, helping patients with vocational rehabilitation, finding paid work, enhancing self-esteem, and keeping a job if they have one, even though up to 90% of patients with severe symptoms are unemployed.

Motivational therapies, which assume that the mental health professional does not always know best and solicit active agreement and participation from the patient, have been shown to be effective in schizophrenia.

Cognitive remediation is a novel psychotherapy that is rapidly gaining popularity for the treatment of schizophrenia. It utilizes computerized therapies designed to improve neurocognition in such areas as attention, working memory, cognitive flexibility and planning, and executive capacity, which leads to improved social functioning.

Future treatments for schizophrenia
Glutamate-linked mechanisms and new treatments for schizophrenia
AMPAkines

AMPA (α-amino-3-hydroxy-5-methyl-4-isoxazole-propionic acid) receptors are one of the glutamate receptor subtypes, and they regulate ion flow and neuronal depolarization that can lead to NMDA (N-methyl-D-aspartate) receptor activation. A number of modulators of the AMPA receptor are under development, including those that do not act directly at the

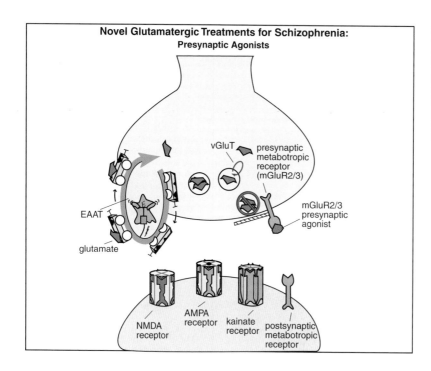

Novel Glutamatergic Treatments for Schizophrenia:
Presynaptic Agonists

Figure 5-89. Novel glutamatergic treatments for schizophrenia: presynaptic agonist. Presynaptic metabotropic glutamate receptors (mGluR2/3) act as autoreceptors to prevent glutamate release. Thus, stimulating these receptors could block glutamate release, and thereby decrease activity at postsynaptic glutamate receptors.

glutamate site of the AMPA receptor, but at positive allosteric modulating (i.e., PAM) sites on this receptor, e.g., CX 516 (Figure 5-88). Sometimes, these AMPA PAMs are also called AMPAkines. Preliminary evidence from animal studies suggests that AMPAkines might enhance cognition, but early results with CX516 in schizophrenia are somewhat disappointing. However, more potent AMPAkines are being developed (CX546, CX619/Org 24448, Org 25573, Org 25271, Org 24292, Org 25501, LY293558) and these might have more efficacy for cognitive symptoms in schizophrenia without showing activation of positive symptoms or neurotoxicity.

mGluR presynaptic antagonists/postsynaptic agonists

Another class of glutamate receptor, known as metabotropic glutamate receptors (mGluRs), regulates neurotransmission at glutamate synapses as well (discussed in Chapter 4 and illustrated in Figures 4-22 and 4-23). Normally, presynaptic mGluRs act as autoreceptors to prevent glutamate release (Figure 4-23B). Thus, an agent acting at this site as a presynaptic mGluR2/3 agonist (Figure 5-89) could potentially prevent excessive glutamate release from glutamate neurons (Figures 5-90B and 5-91B), as is postulated

to occur as the downstream consequence of NMDA hypoactivity (Figures 4-29B, 5-90A, 5-91A) and thereby improve the symptoms of schizophrenia. One such compound, LY2140023, has been tested with proof of concept of efficacy in schizophrenia but has been dropped from clinical development.

Glycine agonists

In Chapter 4 we discussed the actions of coagonists at the glycine site of NMDA receptors and illustrated them in Figures 4-20, 4-21, 4-25, and 4-26. Agonists at the glycine site of NMDA receptors include the naturally occurring amino acids glycine and D-serine as well as an analogue of D-serine, called D-cycloserine, which is also active at the glycine coagonist site of NMDA receptors. All of these agents have been tested in schizophrenia, with evidence that they can reduce negative and/or cognitive symptoms (Figure 5-92). Further testing is in progress, and synthetic agonists with greater potency are in discovery. Perhaps stimulating the glycine site will boost NMDA receptor activity in a manner that is sufficient to overcome its hypothetical hypofunction (Figures 4-29B, 5-90A, 5-91A) and thereby reduce negative and cognitive symptoms, but possibly even positive symptoms in schizophrenia (Figure 5-92).

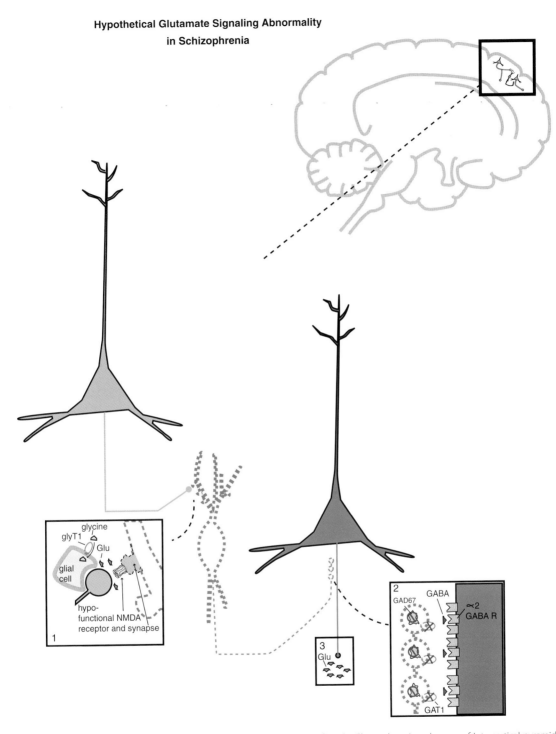

Hypothetical Glutamate Signaling Abnormality
in Schizophrenia

Figure 5-90A. Hypothetical glutamate signaling abnormality in schizophrenia. Shown here is a close-up of intracortical pyramidal neurons communicating via GABAergic interneurons in the presence of hypofunctional NMDA receptors. (1) Glutamate is released from an intracortical pyramidal neuron. However, the NMDA receptor that it would normally bind to is hypofunctional, preventing glutamate from exerting its effects at the receptor. (2) This prevents GABA release from the interneuron; thus, stimulation of α_2 GABA receptors on the axon of another glutamate neuron does not occur. (3) When GABA does not bind to the α_2 GABA receptors on its axon, the pyramidal neuron is no longer inhibited. Instead, it is disinhibited and overactive, releasing excessive glutamate into the cortex.

Hypothetical Mechanism of Action of mGluR2/3 Agonists in Schizophrenia: Reducing Excessive Downstream Glutamate Release

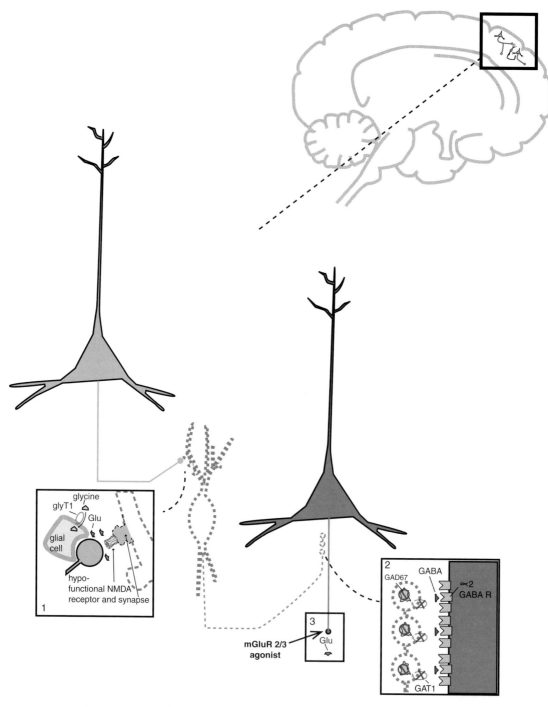

Figure 5-90B. Hypothetical mechanism of action of mGluR2/3 agonists in schizophrenia. Metabotropic glutamate 2/3 receptors (mGluR2/3) are presynaptic autoreceptors that act to prevent glutamate release. Thus, mGluR2/3 agonists may be able to reduce excessive downstream glutamate release (3) even in the presence of reduced GABA inhibition of glutamatergic neurons (2) due to hypothetical NMDA receptor activation on GABAergic interneurons (1).

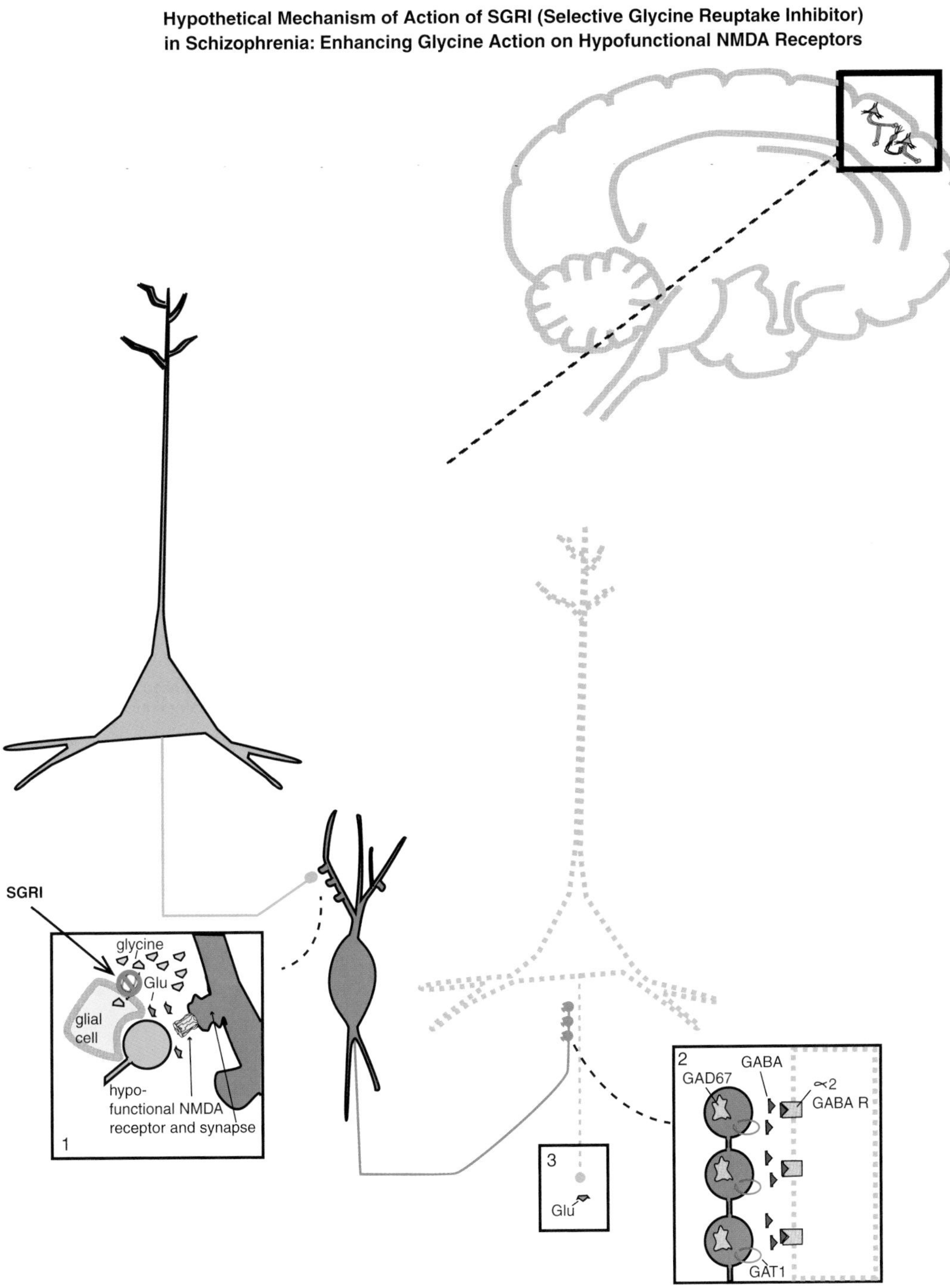

Hypothetical Mechanism of Action of SGRI (Selective Glycine Reuptake Inhibitor) in Schizophrenia: Enhancing Glycine Action on Hypofunctional NMDA Receptors

Figure 5-90C. Hypothetical mechanism of action of selective glycine reuptake inhibitors (SGRI) in schizophrenia. Another mechanism to reduce excessive glutamate neurotransmission may be to enhance glycine action at hypofunctional NMDA receptors. Glycine is needed, in addition to glutamate, in order to activate NMDA receptors. By blocking its reuptake, more glycine will be available in the synapse to bind to NMDA receptors, which could theoretically enhance their function.

231

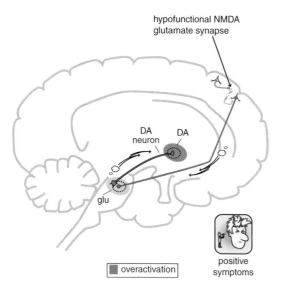

Figure 5-91A. Hypofunctional NMDA receptors and positive symptoms of schizophrenia. If NMDA receptors on cortical GABA interneurons are hypoactive, then the cortical brainstem glutamate pathway to the ventral tegmental area (VTA) will be overactivated, leading to excessive release of glutamate in the VTA. This will lead to excessive stimulation of the mesolimbic dopamine pathway and thus excessive dopamine release in the nucleus accumbens (indicated by the red color of the dopaminergic neuron). This is the theoretical biological basis for the mesolimbic dopamine hyperactivity thought to be associated with the positive symptoms of psychosis.

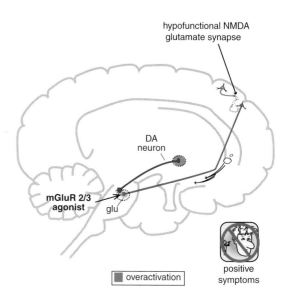

Figure 5-91B. Hypothetical mechanism of action of mGluR2/3 agonists in schizophrenia. Metabotropic glutamate 2/3 receptors (mGluR2/3) are presynaptic autoreceptors that act to prevent glutamate release. Thus, mGluR2/3 agonists may be able to reduce excessive glutamate release in the ventral tegmental area (VTA). This in turn would prevent excessive stimulation of the mesolimbic dopamine pathway.

GlyT1 inhibitors

In Chapter 4 we also discussed the role of glycine transporters on glial cells, known as GlyT1, in terminating the action of glycine released by glial cells into the synapses to act at the glycine site of NMDA receptors (Figure 4-20). Several GlyT1 inhibitors are now in clinical testing, including the natural agent *N*-methylglycine, also known as sarcosine, RG1678 (bitopertin), and Org 25935/SCH 900435, as well as others in preclinical testing such as SSR 504734, SSR 241586, and JNJ17305600. GlyT1 inhibitors, sometimes called selective glycine reuptake inhibitors or SGRIs, are analogous to drugs that inhibit reuptake of other neurotransmitters, such as the selective serotonin reuptake inhibitors (SSRIs) and their actions at the serotonin transporter or SERT. When GlyT1 pumps are blocked by a GlyT1 inhibitor, this increases the synaptic availability of glycine, and thus enhances NMDA neurotransmission (Figure 5-93). The downstream consequence of GlyT1 inhibition is to reverse the hypofunctional NMDA receptor (compare Figures 5-90A and 5-90C; also compare Figures 5-91A and 5-91C).

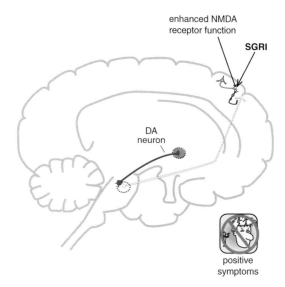

Figure 5-91C. Hypothetical mechanism of action of selective glycine reuptake inhibitors (SGRI) in schizophrenia. Another mechanism to reduce excessive glutamate neurotransmission may be to enhance glycine action at hypofunctional NMDA receptors. Glycine is needed, in addition to glutamate, in order to activate NMDA receptors. By blocking its reuptake, more glycine will be available in the synapse to bind to NMDA receptors, which could theoretically enhance their function. This would lead to enhanced GABAergic neurotransmission in the cortex, which in turn would reduce glutamatergic neurotransmission (indicated by the dotted outline of the glutamatergic neuron). Reduced glutamate release in the ventral tegmental area (VTA) would prevent excessive stimulation of the mesolimbic dopamine pathway.

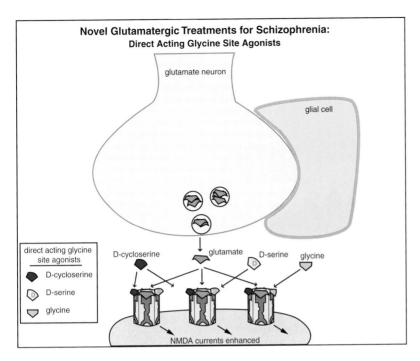

Figure 5-92. Novel glutamatergic treatments for schizophrenia: direct acting glycine site agonists. NMDA (*N*-methyl-D-aspartate) receptors require the presence of both glutamate and a coagonist at the glycine site in order to be fully active. Since schizophrenia may be linked to hypoactive NMDA receptors, agonists at the glycine coagonist site may enhance NMDA functioning. Several agonists at this coagonist site – including glycine, D-serine, and D-cycloserine – have been tested in schizophrenia and indeed show evidence that they can reduce negative and/or cognitive symptoms. Glycine agonists may thus be promising future treatments for negative and cognitive symptoms of schizophrenia without worsening positive symptoms.

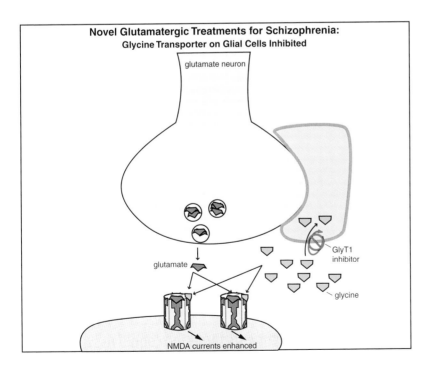

Figure 5-93. Novel glutamatergic treatments for schizophrenia: glycine transporter on glial cells inhibited. The glycine transporter 1 (GlyT1) normally terminates the actions of glycine at NMDA receptors in the glutamate synapse by transporting the glycine back up into glial cells as a reuptake pump. Thus, inhibitors at GlyT1 would increase availability of synaptic glycine, enhancing activity at NMDA receptors. This is analogous to the actions of an SSRI (selective serotonin reuptake inhibitor) at serotonin synapses. GlyT1 inhibition could potentially improve cognitive and negative symptoms of schizophrenia by enhancing the availability of glycine at hypofunctioning NMDA receptors. Preclinical evidence does suggest cognitive improvements with GlyT1 inhibition, and one such naturally occurring inhibitor, sarcosine, has been shown to improve the negative, cognitive, and depressive symptoms of schizophrenia, including symptoms such as alogia and blunted affect.

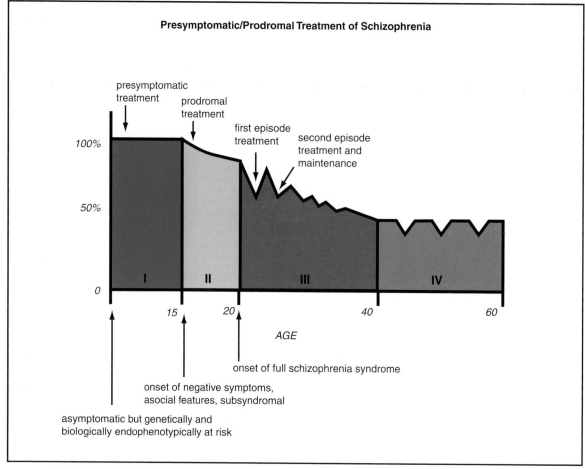

Figure 5-94. Presymptomatic/prodromal treatment of schizophrenia. The stages of schizophrenia are shown here over a lifetime. The patient often has full functioning (100%) early in life and is virtually asymptomatic (stage I). However, during a prodromal phase (stage II) starting in the teens, there may be odd behaviors and subtle negative symptoms. The acute phase of the illness usually announces itself fairly dramatically in the twenties (stage III), with positive symptoms, remissions, and relapses but never a complete return to previous levels of functioning. This is often a chaotic stage of the illness, with a progressive downhill course. The final phase of the illness (stage IV) may begin in the forties or later, with prominent negative and cognitive symptoms and some waxing and waning during its course, but often more of a burnout stage of continuing disability. There may not necessarily be a continuing and relentless downhill course, but the patient may become progressively resistant to treatment with antipsychotic medications during this stage. An emerging concept in psychopharmacology is that the treatments that reduce symptoms could also be disease-modifying. That is, perhaps these agents given to high-risk individuals either in a presymptomatic (stage I) or prodromal (stage II) state could prevent or delay progression through the subsequent stages of schizophrenia.

Sarcosine has been shown to improve negative, cognitive, and depressive symptoms, including symptoms such as alogia and blunted affect in schizophrenia. The SGRI RG1678 (bitopertin) also has reported proof of concept for reduction of both positive and negative symptoms in schizophrenia. The hope is that SGRI type GlyT1 inhibitors will be able to adequately reduce the hypofunctioning of NMDA receptors in order to lead to improvement, particularly in the negative and cognitive symptoms of schizophrenia, perhaps also augmenting the improvement in positive symptoms from treatment with atypical antipsychotics, and thus attain maximum overall efficacy in schizophrenia.

Treatments targeting cognitive symptoms in schizophrenia

Cognitive symptoms of course are not particularly amenable to treatment with the currently marketed antipsychotics, yet cognitive symptoms of schizophrenia are extremely important in determining long-term outcomes in this illness. Thus, a major unmet need in schizophrenia is for an agent that can improve cognitive symptoms and thereby improve functional outcome. There is a long list of agents with a wide variety of pharmacological mechanisms that have been added to antipsychotics in the hope that they would improve cognitive symptoms; to date the results have been largely disappointing. Nevertheless, the targeting of cognitive symptoms with novel therapeutics remains an area of considerable active investigation.

Presymptomatic and prodromal treatments for schizophrenia: putting the cart before the horse or preventing disease progression?

An emerging concept in psychopharmacology is the possibility that treatments that reduce symptoms could also be disease-modifying (Figure 5-94). In this chapter we have discussed almost entirely how atypical antipsychotics treat symptoms of schizophrenia after the illness has fully emerged. However, it is hypothesized that these same agents may also be able to prevent the emergence of schizophrenia when given to high-risk individuals who are either pre-symptomatic or in a state with only mild prodromal symptoms, and thus prevent or delay progression to schizophrenia.

Current concepts about the natural history of schizophrenia hypothesize that this illness progresses from a state of high risk without symptoms (presymptomatic), then to a prodrome with cognitive and negative but not psychotic symptoms, and ultimately to first-episode schizophrenia with psychotic symptoms (Figure 5-94). Throughout the field of psychiatry, it is being debated whether remission of symptoms of any psychiatric disorder with psychopharmacological treatments is able to prevent disease progression, possibly by preventing the plastic changes in brain circuits that fully establish and worsen psychiatric disorders. In schizophrenia, therefore the question is whether "prophylactic" antipsychotics can keep you from "catching" schizophrenia.

Pilot results from early intervention studies in first-episode cases of schizophrenia already suggest that treatment with atypical antipsychotics as soon as possible after the onset of first psychotic symptoms can improve outcomes (first-episode treatment in Figure 5-94). What if high-risk patients without any symptoms could be identified from genetic or neuroimaging techniques? How about patients with the prodromal cognitive and negative symptoms that frequently precede the onset of psychotic symptoms? Could treatment of patients at these points prevent the all-too-common long-term course of schizophrenia with waxing and waning positive symptoms and ever-worsening cognitive and negative symptoms (Figure 5-94)?

Early results with atypical antipsychotics are not definitive, although some suggest that treating prodromal symptoms with antipsychotics, antidepressants, or anxiolytics may delay onset of schizophrenia. Other studies do not confirm this, and of course treatments have costs in terms of both money and side effects and at this point cannot be recommended for either presymptomatic or prodromal treatment of psychosis. However, the promise of disease-modifying treatments for psychiatric disorders in general and for schizophrenia in particular is leading to studies that fully investigate this exciting possibility. The validation of diagnostic criteria for early-onset schizophrenia, prodromal schizophrenia, and ultra-high risk for schizophrenia could help determine not only who should be tested with novel potential therapeutic interventions, but also who should avoid high-risk behaviors such as use of marijuana and other drugs of abuse, sleep deprivation, and high-stress activities.

Summary

This chapter has reviewed the pharmacology of antipsychotic drugs, including conventional antipsychotics with dopamine D_2 antagonist properties and atypical antipsychotic drugs with dopamine D_2 antagonist, $5HT_{2A}$ antagonist, dopamine D_2 partial agonist, and/or $5HT_{1A}$ partial agonist properties. Multiple receptor binding properties are hypothesized to be linked to additional clinical actions of antipsychotics, from antimanic actions, to antidepressant effects, to cardiometabolic risk and sedation. The pharmacologic and clinical properties of more than a dozen specific atypical antipsychotics are discussed in detail. Use of these as a class in clinical practice settings is reviewed, including considerations on how to switch from one antipsychotic to another and how to use antipsychotics in difficult patients who are treatment-resistant or violent. Finally, several new treatments under development for schizophrenia are presented, particularly those targeting the glutamate system.

This chapter discusses disorders characterized by abnormalities of mood: namely, depression, mania, or both. Included here are descriptions of a wide variety of mood disorders that occur over a broad clinical spectrum. Also included in this chapter is an analysis of how monoamine neurotransmitter systems are hypothetically linked to the biological basis of mood disorders. The three principal monoamine neurotransmitters are norepinephrine (NE; also called noradrenaline or NA), discussed in this chapter, dopamine (DA), discussed in Chapter 4, and serotonin (also called 5-hydroxytryptamine or 5HT), discussed in Chapter 5.

The approach taken here is to deconstruct each mood disorder into its component symptoms, followed by matching each symptom to hypothetically malfunctioning brain circuits, each regulated by one or more of the monoamine neurotransmitters. Genetic regulation and neuroimaging of these hypothetically malfunctioning brain circuits are also discussed. Coverage of symptoms and circuits of mood disorders in this chapter is intended to set the stage for understanding the pharmacological concepts underlying the mechanisms of action and use of antidepressants and mood stabilizing drugs, which will be reviewed in the following two chapters (Chapters 7 and 8).

Clinical descriptions and criteria for how to diagnose disorders of mood will only be mentioned in passing. The reader should consult standard reference sources for this material.

Description of mood disorders

Disorders of mood are often called affective disorders, since affect is the external display of mood, an emotion that is felt internally. Depression and mania are often seen as opposite ends of an affective or mood spectrum. Classically, mania and depression are "poles" apart, thus generating the terms *unipolar* depression (i.e., patients who just experience the *down* or depressed pole) and *bipolar* (i.e., patients who at different times experience either the *up* [i.e., manic] pole or the *down* [i.e., depressed] pole). Depression and mania may even occur simultaneously, which is called a *mixed* mood state. Mania may also occur in lesser degrees, known as *hypomania*, or switch so

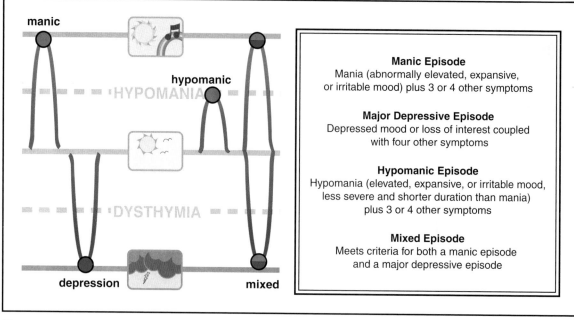

Manic Episode
Mania (abnormally elevated, expansive,
or irritable mood) plus 3 or 4 other symptoms

Major Depressive Episode
Depressed mood or loss of interest coupled
with four other symptoms

Hypomanic Episode
Hypomania (elevated, expansive, or irritable mood,
less severe and shorter duration than mania)
plus 3 or 4 other symptoms

Mixed Episode
Meets criteria for both a manic episode
and a major depressive episode

Figure 6-1. Mood episodes. Bipolar disorder is generally characterized by four types of illness episodes: manic, major depressive, hypomanic, and mixed. A patient may have any combination of these episodes over the course of illness; subsyndromal manic or depressive episodes also occur during the course of illness, in which case there are not enough symptoms or the symptoms are not severe enough to meet the diagnostic criteria for one of these episodes. Thus the presentation of mood disorders can vary widely.

fast between mania and depression that it is called *rapid cycling*.

Mood disorders can be usefully visualized not only to contrast different mood disorders from one another, but also to summarize the course of illness for individual patients by showing them mapped onto a mood chart. Thus, mood ranges from hypomania to mania at the top, to euthymia (or normal mood) in the middle, to dysthymia and depression at the bottom (Figure 6-1). The most common and readily recognized mood disorder is major depressive disorder (Figure 6-2), with single or recurrent episodes. Dysthymia is a less severe but long-lasting form of depression (Figure 6-3). Patients with a major depressive episode who have poor inter-episode recovery, only to the level of dysthymia, followed by another episode of major depression are sometimes said to have "double depression," alternating between major depression and dysthymia, but not remitting (Figure 6-4).

Patients with bipolar I disorder have full-blown manic episodes or mixed episodes of mania plus depression, often followed by a depressive episode (Figure 6-5). When mania recurs at least four times a year, it is called rapid cycling (Figure 6-6A). Patients

with bipolar I disorder can also have rapid switches from mania to depression and back (Figure 6-6B). By definition, this occurs at least four times a year, but can occur much more frequently than that.

Bipolar II disorder is characterized by at least one hypomanic episode that follows a depressive episode (Figure 6-7). Cyclothymic disorder is characterized by mood swings that are not as severe as full mania and full depression, but still wax and wane above and below the boundaries of normal mood (Figure 6-8). There may be lesser degrees of variation from normal mood that are stable and persistent, including both depressive temperament (below normal mood but not a mood disorder) and hyperthymic temperament (above normal mood but also not a mood disorder) (Figure 6-9). Temperaments are personality styles of responding to environmental stimuli that can be heritable patterns present early in life and persisting throughout a lifetime; temperaments include such independent personality dimensions as novelty seeking, harm avoidance, and conscientiousness. Some patients may have mood-related temperaments, and these may render them vulnerable to mood disorders, especially bipolar spectrum disorders, later in life.

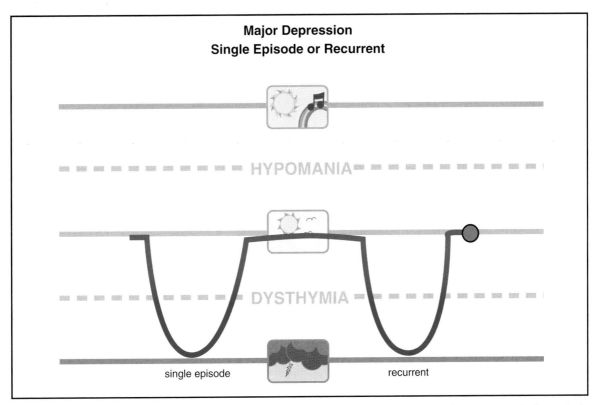

Figure 6-2. Major depression. Major depression is the most common mood disorder and is defined by the occurrence of at least a single major depressive episode, although most patients will experience recurrent episodes.

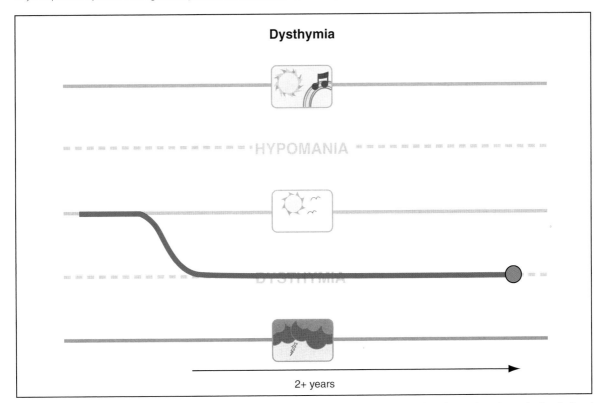

Figure 6-3. Dysthymia. Dysthymia is a less severe form of depression than major depression, but long-lasting (over 2 years in duration) and often unremitting.

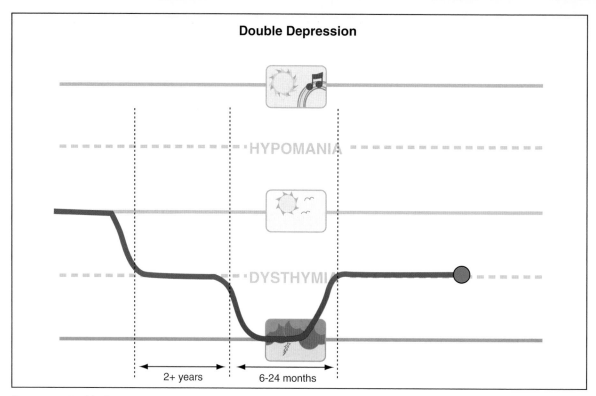

Figure 6-4. Double depression. Patients with unremitting dysthymia who also experience the superimposition of one or more major depressive episodes are described as having double depression. This is also a form of recurrent major depressive episodes with poor inter-episode recovery.

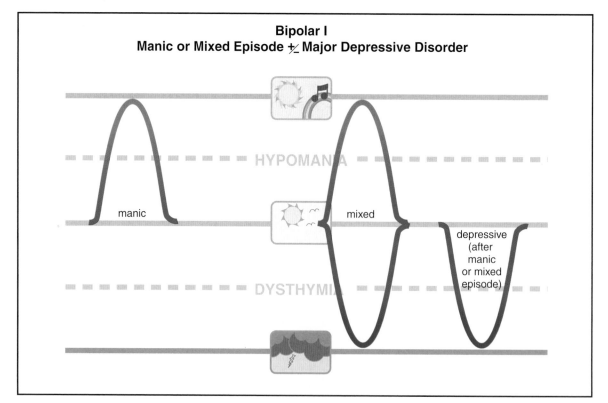

Figure 6-5. Bipolar I disorder. Bipolar I disorder is defined as the occurrence of at least one manic or mixed (full mania and full depression simultaneously) episode. Patients with bipolar I disorder typically experience major depressive episodes as well, although this is not necessary for the bipolar I diagnosis.

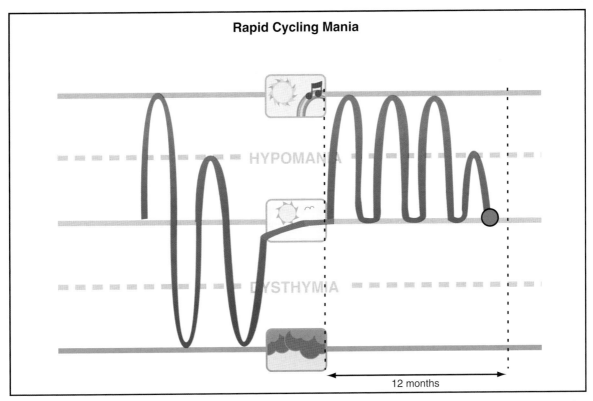

Figure 6-6A. Rapid cycling mania. The course of bipolar disorder can be rapid cycling, which means that at least four episodes occur within a 1-year period. This can manifest itself as four distinct manic episodes, as shown here. Many patients with this form of mood disorder experience switches much more frequently than four times a year.

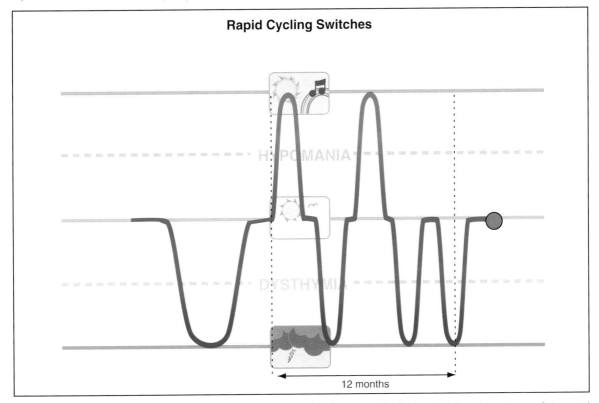

Figure 6-6B. Rapid cycling switches. A rapid cycling course (at least four distinct mood episodes within 1 year) can also manifest as rapid switches between manic and depressive episodes.

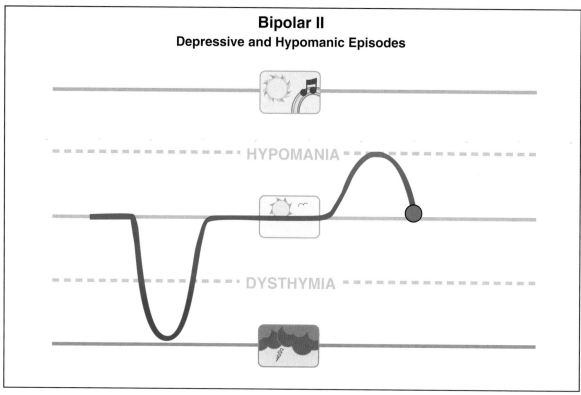

Figure 6-7. Bipolar II disorder. Bipolar II disorder is defined as an illness course consisting of one or more major depressive episodes and at least one hypomanic episode.

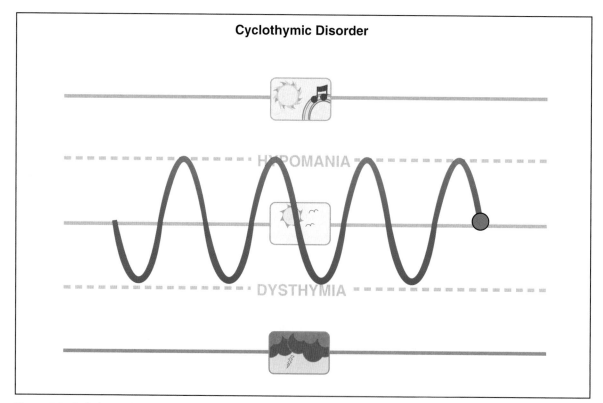

Figure 6-8. Cyclothymic disorder. Cyclothymic disorder is characterized by mood swings between hypomania and dysthymia but without any full manic or major depressive episodes.

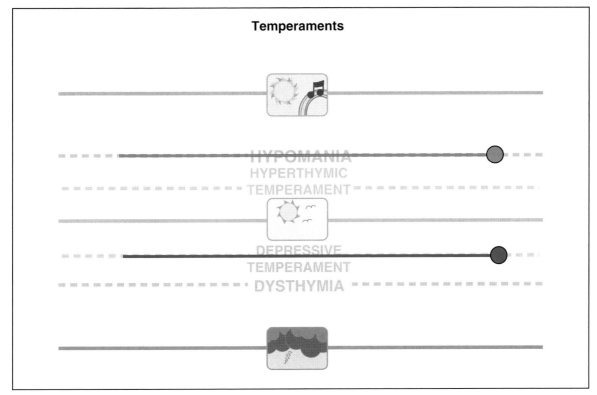

Figure 6-9. Temperaments. Not all mood variations are pathological. Individuals with depressive temperament may be consistently sad or apathetic but do not meet the criteria for dysthymia and do not necessarily experience any functional impairment. However, individuals with depressive temperament may be at greater risk for the development of a mood disorder later in life. Hyperthymic temperament, in which mood is above normal but not pathological, includes stable characteristics such as extroversion, optimism, exuberance, impulsiveness, overconfidence, grandiosity, and lack of inhibition. Individuals with hyperthymic temperament may be at greater risk for the development of a mood disorder later in life.

The bipolar spectrum

From a strict diagnostic point of view, our discussion of mood disorders could now be mostly complete. However, there is the growing recognition that many patients seen in clinical practice have a mood disorder not well described by the above categories. Formally, they would be called "not otherwise specified" or "NOS," but this creates a huge single category for many patients that belies the richness and complexity of their symptoms. Increasingly, such patients are seen as belonging in general to the "bipolar spectrum" (Figure 6-10), and in particular to one of several additional descriptive categories that have been proposed by experts such as Hagop Akiskal (Figures 6-10 through 6-20).

Bipolar ¼ (0.25)

One mood disorder often considered to be "not quite bipolar" and sometimes called bipolar ¼ (or 0.25) designates an unstable form of unipolar depression that responds sometimes rapidly but in an unsustained manner to antidepressants, the latter sometimes called antidepressant "poop-out" (Figure 6-11). These patients have unstable mood but not a formal bipolar disorder, yet can benefit from mood-stabilizing treatments added to robust antidepressant treatments.

Bipolar ½ (0.5) and schizoaffective disorder

Another type of mood disorder is called different things by different experts, from bipolar ½ (or 0.5) to "schizobipolar disorder" to "schizoaffective disorder" (Figure 6-12). For over a century, experts have debated whether psychotic disorders are dichotomous from mood disorders (Figure 6-13A) or are part of a continuous disease spectrum from psychosis to mood (Figure 6-13B).

The dichotomous disease model is in the tradition of Kraepelin and proposes that schizophrenia is a chronic unremitting illness with poor outcome and decline in

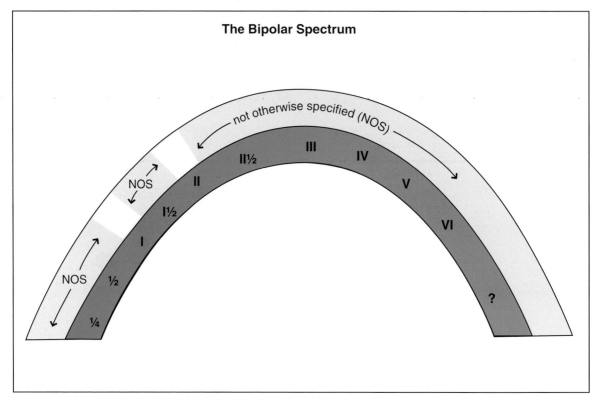

Figure 6-10. Bipolar spectrum. There is a huge variation in the presentation of patients with bipolar disorder. Historically, bipolar disorder has been categorized as I, II, or not otherwise specified (NOS). It may be more useful, instead, to think of these patients as belonging to a bipolar spectrum and to identify subcategories of presentations, as has been done by Akiskal and other experts and as illustrated in the next several figures.

function whereas bipolar disorder is a cyclical illness with a better outcome and good restoration of function between episodes. However, there is great debate as to how to define the borders between these two illnesses. One notion is that cases with overlapping symptoms and intermediate disease courses can be seen as a third illness, schizoaffective disorder. Today, many define this border with the idea that "even a trace of schizophrenia is schizophrenia." From this "schizophrenia-centered perspective," many overlapping cases of psychotic mania and psychotic depression might be considered either to be forms of schizophrenia, or to be schizoaffective disorder as a form of schizophrenia with affective symptoms. A competing point of view within the dichotomous model is that "even a trace of mood disturbance is a mood disorder." From this "mood-centered perspective," many overlapping cases of psychotic mania and psychotic depression might be considered either to be forms of a mood/bipolar disorder or to be schizoaffective disorder as a form of mood/bipolar disorder with psychotic symptoms. Where

patients have a mixture of mood symptoms and psychosis, it can obviously be very difficult to tell whether they have a psychotic disorder such as schizophrenia, a mood disorder such as bipolar disorder, or a third condition, schizoaffective disorder. Some even want to eliminate the diagnosis of schizoaffective disorder entirely.

Proponents of the dichotomous model point out that treatments for schizophrenia differ from those for bipolar disorder, since lithium is rarely helpful in schizophrenia, and anticonvulsant mood stabilizers have limited efficacy for psychotic symptoms in schizophrenia, and perhaps only as augmenting agents. Treatments for schizoaffective disorder can include both treatments for schizophrenia and treatments for bipolar disorder. The current debate within the dichotomous model is: If you have bipolar disorder, do you have a good outcome? – but if you have schizophrenia, do you have a poor outcome? – and what genetic and biological markers rather than clinical symptoms can distinguish one dichotomous entity from the other?

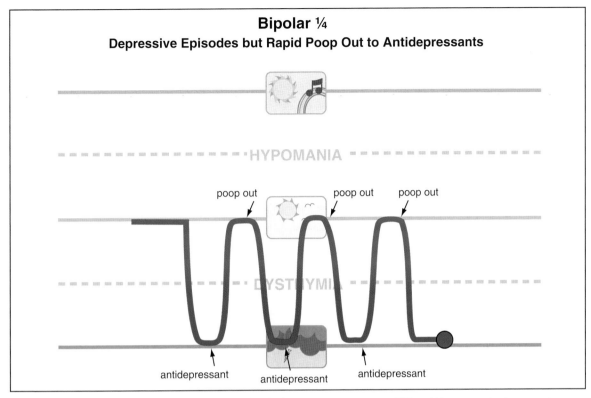

Figure 6-11. Bipolar ¼. Some patients may present only with depressive symptoms yet exhibit rapid but unsustained response to antidepressant treatment (sometimes called rapid "poop out"). Although such patients may have no spontaneous mood symptoms above normal, they potentially could benefit from mood-stabilizing treatment. This presentation may be termed bipolar ¼ (or bipolar 0.25).

The continuum disease model proposes that psychotic and mood disorders are both manifestations of one complex set of disorders that is expressed across a spectrum, at one end schizophrenia (plus schizophreniform disorder, brief psychotic disorder, delusional disorder, shared psychotic disorder, subsyndromal/ultra-high-risk psychosis prodrome, schizotypal, paranoid, schizoid, and even avoidant personality disorders), and at the other end bipolar/mood disorders (mania, depression, mixed states, melancholic depression, atypical depression, catatonic depression, postpartum depression, psychotic depression, seasonal affective disorder), with schizoaffective disorder in the middle, combining features of positive symptoms of psychosis with manic, hypomanic, or depressive episodes (Figure 6-13B).

Modern genomics suggests that the spectrum is not a single disease, but a complex of hundreds if not thousands of different diseases, with overlapping genetic, epigenetic, and biomarkers as well as overlapping clinical symptoms and functional outcomes. Proponents of the continuum model point out that treatments for schizophrenia overlap greatly now with those for bipolar disorder, since second-generation atypical antipsychotics are effective in the positive symptoms of schizophrenia and in psychotic mania and psychotic depression, and are also effective in nonpsychotic mania and in bipolar depression and unipolar depression. These same second-generation atypical antipsychotics are effective for the spectrum of symptoms in schizoaffective disorder. From the continuum disease perspective, failure to give mood-stabilizing medications may lead to suboptimal symptom relief in patients with psychosis, even those whose prominent or eye-catching psychotic symptoms mask or distract clinicians from seeing underlying and perhaps more subtle mood symptoms. In the continuum disease model, schizophrenia can be seen as the extreme end of a spectrum of severity of mood disorders and not a disease unrelated to a mood disorder. Schizophrenia can therefore share with schizoaffective disorder severe psychotic symptoms that obscure mood symptoms, a chronic course that eliminates cycling, resistance to antipsychotic treatments, and prominent

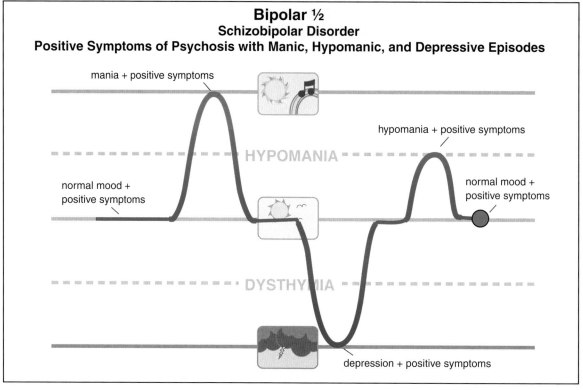

Bipolar ½
Schizobipolar Disorder
Positive Symptoms of Psychosis with Manic, Hypomanic, and Depressive Episodes

mania + positive symptoms

HYPOMANIA

hypomania + positive symptoms

normal mood + positive symptoms

normal mood + positive symptoms

DYSTHYMIA

depression + positive symptoms

Figure 6-12. Bipolar ½. Bipolar ½ (0.5) has been described as schizobipolar disorder, which combines positive symptoms of psychosis with manic, hypomanic, and depressive episodes.

Schizophrenia and Bipolar Disorder

Dichotomous Disease Model

Schizophrenia	Schizoaffective Disorder	Bipolar Disorder
• psychosis	• psychosis	• mania
• chronic, unremitting	and	• mood disorder
• poor outcome	• mania	• cyclical
• "even a trace of schizophrenia is schizophrenia"	• mood disorder	• good outcome
		• "even a trace of a mood disturbance is a mood disorder"

Figure 6-13A. Schizophrenia and bipolar disorder: dichotomous disease model. Schizophrenia and bipolar disorder have been conceptualized both as dichotomous disorders and as belonging to a continuum. In the dichotomous disease model, schizophrenia consists of chronic, unremitting psychosis, with poor outcomes expected. Bipolar disorder consists of cyclical manic and other mood episodes and has better expected outcomes than schizophrenia. A third distinct disorder is schizoaffective disorder, characterized by psychosis and mania as well as other mood symptoms.

Schizophrenia and Bipolar Disorder
Continuum Disease Model

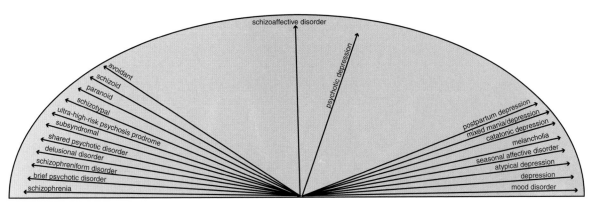

Figure 6-13B. Schizophrenia and bipolar disorder: continuum disease model. Schizophrenia and bipolar disorder have been conceptualized both as dichotomous disorders and as belonging to a continuum. In the continuum disease model, schizophrenia and mood disorders fall along a continuum in which psychosis, delusions, and paranoid avoidant behavior are on one extreme and depression and other mood symptoms are on the other extreme. Falling in the middle are psychotic depression and schizoaffective disorder.

negative symptoms, yet be just a severe form of the same illness. In the continuum disease model, schizoaffective disorder would be a milder form of the illness with less severe psychotic features and more severe mood features.

The debate rages on . . .

Bipolar I½ (1.5)

Although patients with protracted or recurrent hypomania without depression are not formally diagnosed as bipolar II disorder, they are definitely part of the bipolar spectrum, and may benefit from mood stabilizers that have been studied mostly in bipolar I disorder (Figure 6-14). Eventually, such patients will often develop a major depressive episode and their diagnosis will then change to bipolar II disorder, but in the meantime they can be treated for hypomania while being vigilant to the future onset of a major depressive episode.

Bipolar II½ (2.5)

Bipolar II½ is the designation for cyclothymic patients who develop major depressive episodes (Figure 6-15). Many patients with cyclothymia are just considered "moody" and do not consult professionals until experiencing full depressive episodes. It is important to recognize patients in this part of the bipolar spectrum, because treatment of their major

depressive episodes with antidepressant monotherapy may actually cause increased mood cycling or even induction of a full manic episode, just as can happen in patients with bipolar I or II depressive episodes.

Bipolar III (3.0)

Patients who develop a manic or hypomanic episode on an antidepressant are sometimes called bipolar III (Figure 6-16). According to formal diagnostic criteria, however, when an antidepressant causes mania or hypomania, the diagnosis is not bipolar disorder, but rather, "substance-induced mood disorder." Many experts disagree with this designation and feel that patients who have a hypomanic or manic response to an antidepressant do so because they have a bipolar spectrum disorder, and can be more appropriately diagnosed as bipolar III disorder (Figure 6-16) until they experience a spontaneous manic or hypomanic episode while taking no drugs, at which point their diagnosis would be bipolar I or II, respectively. The bipolar III designation is helpful in the meantime, reminding clinicians that such patients are not good candidates for antidepressant monotherapy.

Bipolar III½ (3.5)

A variant of this bipolar III disorder has been called bipolar III½, to designate a type of bipolar disorder associated with substance abuse (Figure 6-17).

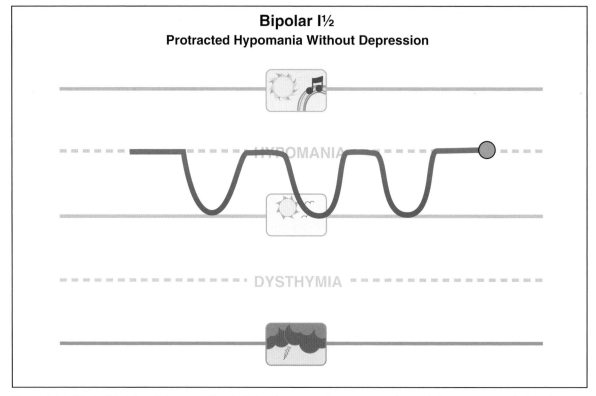

Figure 6-14. Bipolar I½. A formal diagnosis of bipolar II disorder requires the occurrence of not only hypomanic episodes but also depressive episodes. However, some patients may experience recurrent hypomania without having experienced a depressive episode – a presentation that may be termed bipolar I½. These patients may be at risk of eventually developing a depressive episode and are candidates for mood-stabilizing treatment, although no treatment is formally approved for this condition.

Although some of these patients can utilize substances of abuse to treat depressive episodes, others have previously experienced natural or drug-induced mania and take substances of abuse to induce mania. This combination of a bipolar disorder with substance abuse is a formula for chaos, and can often be the story of a patient prior to seeking treatment from a mental health professional.

Bipolar IV (4.0)

Bipolar IV disorder is the association of depressive episodes with a pre-existing hyperthymic temperament (Figure 6-18). Patients with hyperthymia are often sunny, optimistic, high-output, successful individuals with stable temperament for years and then suddenly collapse into a severe depression. In such cases, it may be useful to be vigilant to the need for more than antidepressant monotherapy if the patient is unresponsive to such treatment, or if the patient develops rapid cycling or hypomanic or mixed states in response to antidepressants. Despite not having a

formal bipolar disorder, such patients may respond best to mood stabilizers.

Bipolar V (5.0)

Bipolar V disorder is depression with mixed hypomania (Figure 6-19). Formal diagnostic criteria for mixed states require full expression of both depression and mania simultaneously, but in the real world, many depressed patients can have additional symptoms that only qualify as hypomania or subsyndromal hypomania, or even just a few manic symptoms or only mild manic symptoms. Depression simultaneous with full hypomania is represented in Figure 6-1 and Figure 6-5 and requires mood stabilizer treatment, not antidepressant monotherapy. Under debate is whether there should be a separate diagnostic category for depression with subthreshold hypomania; some experts believe that up to half of patients with major depression also have a lifetime history of subsyndromal hypomania, and that these patients are much more likely to progress to a formal bipolar

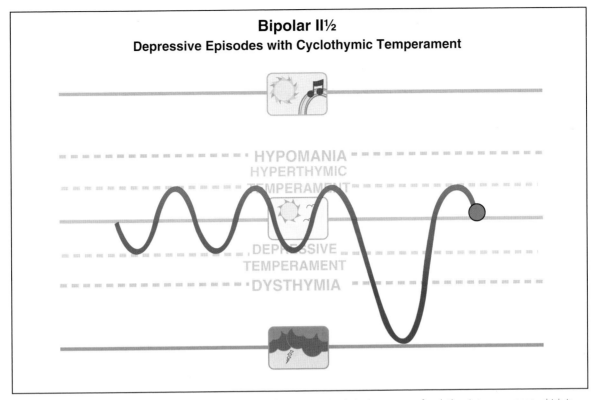

Figure 6-15. Bipolar II½. Patients may present with a major depressive episode in the context of cyclothymic temperament, which is characterized by oscillations between hyperthymic or hypomanic states (above normal) and depressive or dysthymic states (below normal) upon which a major depressive episode intrudes (bipolar II½). Individuals with cyclothymic temperament who are treated for the major depressive episodes may be at increased risk for antidepressant-induced mood cycling.

diagnosis. Patients with depression and subthreshold hypomania generally have a worse outcome, more mood episodes, more work impairment, are more likely to have a family member with mania or other bipolar disorder, and to have an early onset of depression. For depression with subsyndromal hypomania it may be more important to emphasize overactivity rather than just mood elevation, and a duration of only 2 days as opposed to the 4 days required in most diagnostic systems for hypomania. Whether these patients can be treated with antidepressant monotherapy without precipitating mania, or instead require agents with potentially greater side effects such as mood stabilizers, lithium, and/or atypical antipsychotics, is still under investigation.

Related conditions to depression mixed with subsyndromal hypomania include other mood states where full diagnostic criteria are not reached, ranging from full mixed states (both full mania diagnostic criteria [M] and full depression diagnostic criteria [D]) to depression with hypomania or only a few hypomanic symptoms (mD) as already discussed. In addition, other combinations of mania and depression range from full mania with only a few depressive symptoms (Md, sometimes also called "dysphoric" mania), to subsyndromal but unstable states characterized by some symptoms of both mania and depression, but not diagnostic of either (md) (Table 6-1). All of these states differ from unipolar depression and belong in the bipolar spectrum; they may require treatment with the same agents that are used to treat bipolar I or II disorder, with appropriate caution for antidepressant monotherapy. Just because a patient is depressed, it does not mean he or she should start with an antidepressant for treatment. Patients with mixed states of depression and mania may be particularly vulnerable to the induction of activation, agitation, rapid cycling, dysphoria, hypomania, mania, or suicidality when treated with antidepressants, particularly without the concomitant use of a mood stabilizer or an atypical antipsychotic.

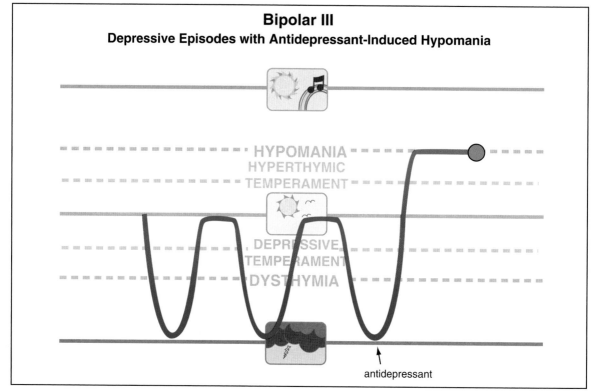

Figure 6-16. Bipolar III. Although the *Diagnostic and Statistical Manual of Mental Disorders*, fourth edition (DSM-IV), defines antidepressant-induced (hypo)mania as a substance-induced mood disorder, some experts believe that individuals who experience substance-induced (hypo)mania are actually predisposed to these mood states and thus belong to the bipolar spectrum (bipolar III).

Bipolar VI (6.0)

Finally, bipolar VI disorder (Figure 6-20) represents bipolarity in the setting of dementia, where it can be incorrectly attributed to the behavioral symptoms of dementia rather than recognized and treated as a comorbid mood state with mood stabilizers and even with atypical antipsychotics.

Many more subtypes of mood disorders can be described within the bipolar spectrum. The important thing to take away from this discussion is that not all patients with depression have major depressive disorder requiring treatment with antidepressant monotherapy, and that there are many states of mood disorder within the bipolar spectrum beyond just bipolar I and II disorders.

Can unipolar depression be distinguished from bipolar depression?

One of the important developments in the field of mood disorders in recent years in fact is the recognition that many patients once considered to have major depressive disorder actually have a form of bipolar disorder, especially bipolar II disorder or one of the conditions within the bipolar spectrum (Figure 6-21). Since symptomatic patients with bipolar disorder spend much more of their time in the depressed state rather than in the manic, hypomanic, or mixed state, this means that many depressed patients in the past were incorrectly diagnosed with unipolar major depression, and treated with antidepressant monotherapy instead of being diagnosed as a bipolar spectrum disorder and treated first with lithium, anticonvulsant mood stabilizers, and/or atypical antipsychotics prior to adding an antidepressant, if an antidepressant is even used at all.

Up to half of patients once considered to have a unipolar depression are now considered to have a bipolar spectrum disorder (Figure 6-21), and although they would not necessarily be good candidates for antidepressant monotherapy, this is often the treatment that they receive when the bipolar nature of their condition is not recognized. Antidepressant treatment of unrecognized bipolar patients

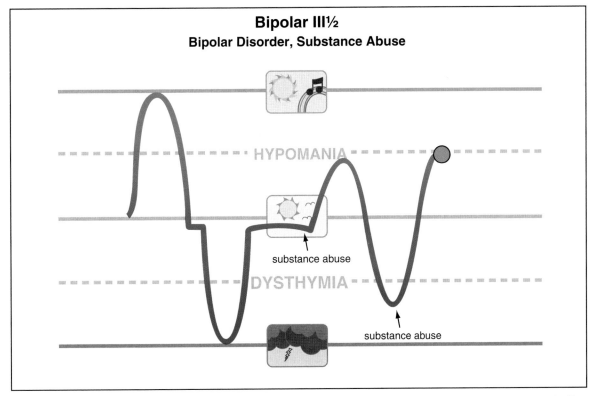

Figure 6-17. Bipolar III½. Bipolar III½ (3.5) is bipolar disorder with substance abuse, in which the substance abuse is associated with efforts to achieve hypomania. Such patients should be evaluated closely to determine if (hypo)mania has ever occurred in the absence of substance abuse.

may not only increase mood cycling, mixed states, and conversion to hypomania and mania, as mentioned above, but may also contribute to the increase in suicidality in younger patients treated with antidepressants, i.e., children and adults younger than 25.

Thus it becomes important to recognize whether a depressed patient has a bipolar spectrum disorder or a unipolar major depressive disorder. How can this be done? In reality, patients with either unipolar or bipolar depression often have identical current symptoms, so obtaining the profile of current symptomatology is obviously not sufficient for distinguishing unipolar from bipolar depression. The answer may be in part to ask the two questions shown in Table 6-2, namely, "Who's your daddy?" and "Where's your mama?"

"Who's your daddy?" can mean "what is your family history?" since a first-degree relative with a bipolar spectrum disorder can give a strong hint that the patient also has a bipolar spectrum disorder rather than unipolar depression. "Where's your mama?" can mean "I need to get additional history from someone

else close to you," since patients tend to under-report their manic symptoms, and the insight and observations of an outside informant such as a mother or spouse can describe a history quite different from the one the patient is reporting, and thus help establish a bipolar spectrum diagnosis that patients themselves do not perceive, or deny. Some hints, but not sufficient for diagnostic certainty, can even come from current symptoms to suggest a bipolar spectrum depression, such as more time sleeping, overeating, comorbid anxiety, motor retardation, mood lability, psychotic symptoms or suicidal thoughts (Figure 6-22). Hints that the depression may be in the bipolar spectrum can also come from the course of the untreated illness prior to the current symptoms, such as early age of onset, high frequency of depressive symptoms, high proportion of time spent ill, and acute abatement or onset of symptoms. Prior response to antidepressants that suggests bipolar depression can be multiple antidepressant failures, rapid recovery, and activating side effects such as

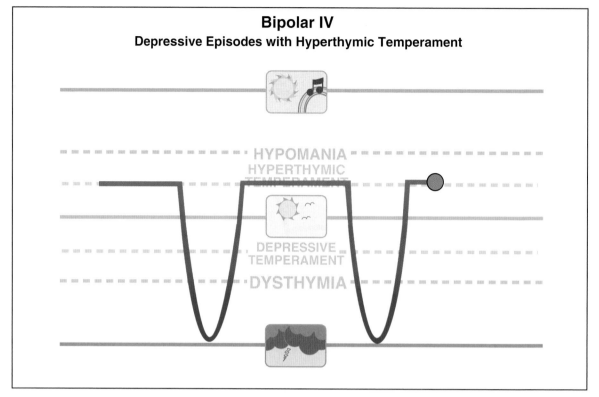

Figure 6-18. Bipolar IV. Bipolar IV is seen in individuals with longstanding and stable hyperthymic temperament into which a major depressive episode intrudes. Individuals with hyperthymic temperament who are treated for depressive episodes may be at increased risk for antidepressant-induced mood cycling, and may instead respond better to mood stabilizers.

insomnia, agitation, and anxiety. Although none of these features can discriminate bipolar depression from unipolar depression with certainty, the point is to be vigilant to the possibility that what looks like a unipolar depression might actually be a bipolar spectrum depression when investigated more carefully, and when response to treatment is monitored.

Are mood disorders progressive?

One of the major unanswered questions about the natural history of depressive illnesses is whether they are progressive (Figures 6-23 and 6-24). Some observers believe that there is an increasing number of patients in mental health practices who have bipolar spectrum illnesses rather than unipolar illnesses, especially compared to a few decades ago. Is this merely the product of changing diagnostic criteria, or does unipolar depression progress to bipolar depression (Figure 6-23)? A corollary of this question is whether chronic and widespread undertreatment of unipolar depression,

allowing residual symptoms to persist and relapses and recurrences to occur, results first in more rapidly recurring episodes of major depression, then in poor inter-episode recovery, then progression to a bipolar spectrum condition, and finally to treatment resistance (Figure 6-23). Many treatment-resistant mood disorders in psychiatric practices have elements of bipolar spectrum disorder that can be identified, and many of these patients require treatment with more than antidepressants, or with mood stabilizers and atypical antipsychotics instead of antidepressants. For patients already diagnosed with bipolar disorder, there is similar concern that the disorder may be progressive, especially without adequate treatment. Thus, discrete manic and depressive episodes may progress to mixed and dysphoric episodes, and finally to rapid cycling, instability, and treatment resistance (Figure 6-24). The hope is that recognition and treatment of both unipolar and bipolar depressions, causing all symptoms to remit for long periods of time, might prevent progression to more difficult states. This is not proven, but is a major

Table 6-1 Mixed states of mania and depression

Description	Designation	Comment
DSM-IV mixed	MD	Full diagnostic criteria for both mania and depression
Depression with hypomania	mD	Bipolar V
Depression with some manic symptoms	mD	Bipolar NOS
Mania with some depressive symptoms	Md	Dysphoric mania
Subsyndromal mania and subsyndromal depression	md	Prodrome or presymptomatic state of incomplete remission

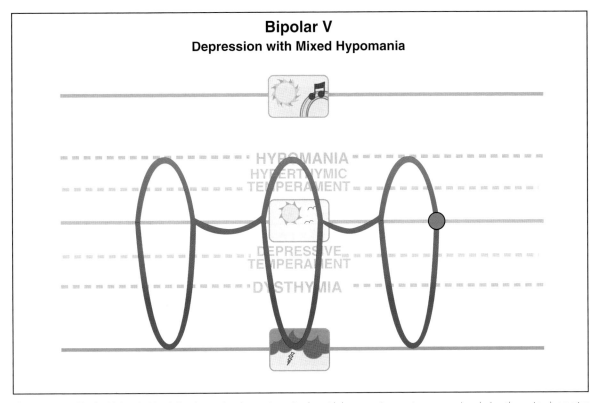

Figure 6-19. Bipolar V. Bipolar V is defined as major depressive episodes with hypomanic symptoms occurring during the major depressive episode but without the presence of discrete hypomanic episodes. Because the symptoms do not meet the full criteria for mania, these patients would not be considered to have a full mixed episode, but they nonetheless exhibit a mixed presentation and may require mood stabilizer treatment as opposed to antidepressant monotherapy.

hypothesis in the field at the present time. In the meantime, practitioners must decide whether to commit "sins of omission," and be conservative with the diagnosis of bipolar spectrum disorder, and err on the side of undertreatment of mood disorders, or "sins of commission," and overdiagnose and overtreat symptoms in the hope that this will prevent disease progression.

Neurotransmitters and circuits in mood disorders

Three principal neurotransmitters have long been implicated in both the pathophysiology and treatment of mood disorders. They are norepinephrine, dopamine, and serotonin, and comprise what is sometimes called

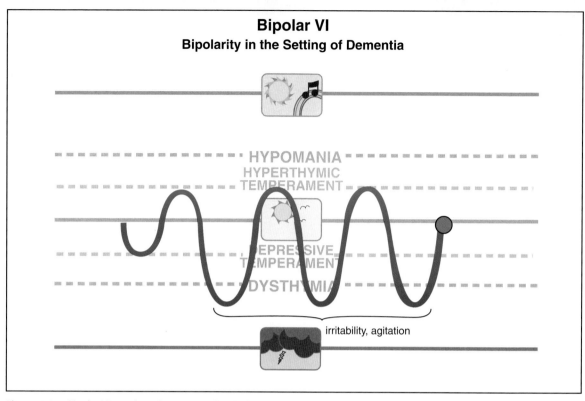

Figure 6-20. Bipolar VI. Another subcategory within the bipolar spectrum may be "bipolarity in the setting of dementia," termed bipolar VI. Mood instability here begins late in life, followed by impaired attention, irritability, reduced drive, and disrupted sleep. The presentation may initially appear to be attributable to dementia or be considered unipolar depression, but it is likely to be exacerbated by antidepressants and may respond to mood stabilizers.

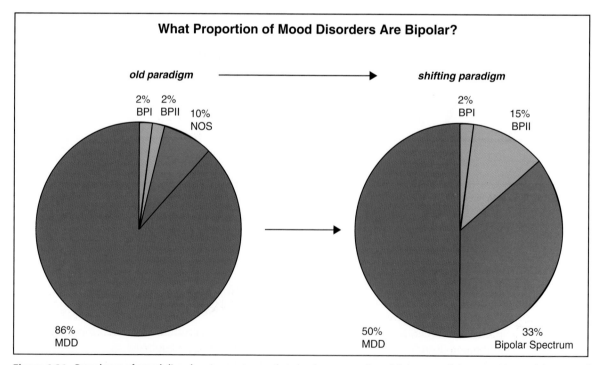

Figure 6-21. Prevalence of mood disorders. In recent years there has been a paradigm shift in terms of the recognition and diagnosis of patients with mood disorders. That is, many patients once considered to have major depressive disorder (old paradigm, left) are now recognized as having bipolar II disorder or another form of bipolar illness within the bipolar spectrum (shifting paradigm, right).

254

Table 6-2 Is it unipolar or bipolar depression? Questions to ask

Who's your daddy?

What is your family history of:

- mood disorder?
- psychiatric hospitalizations?
- suicide?
- anyone who took lithium, mood stabilizers, antipsychotics, antidepressants?
- anyone who received ECT?

These can be indications of a unipolar or bipolar spectrum disorder in relatives.

Where's your mama?

I need to get additional history about you from someone close to you, such as your mother or your spouse.

Patients may especially lack insight about their manic symptoms and under-report them.

the monoamine neurotransmitter system. These three monoamines often work in concert. Many of the symptoms of mood disorders are hypothesized to involve dysfunction of various combinations of these three systems. Essentially all known treatments for mood disorders act upon one or more of these three systems.

We have extensively discussed the dopamine system in Chapter 4 and illustrated it in Figures 4-5 through 4-11. We have extensively discussed the serotonin system in Chapter 5 and illustrated it in Figures 5-13, 5-14, 5-25, and 5-27. Here we introduce the reader to the norepinephrine system, and also show some interactions among these three monoaminergic neurotransmitter systems.

Noradrenergic neurons

The noradrenergic neuron utilizes norepinephrine (noradrenaline) as its neurotransmitter. Norepinephrine (NE) is synthesized, or produced, from the precursor

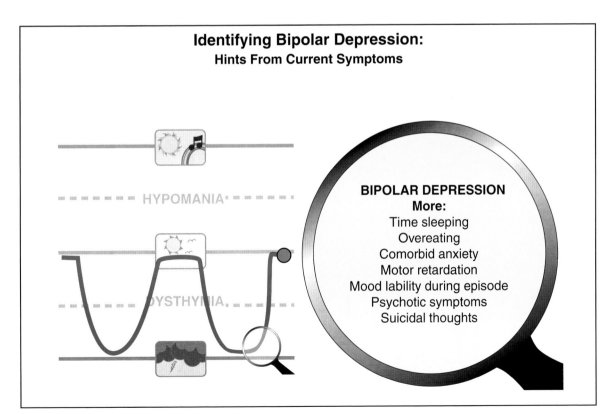

Figure 6-22. Bipolar depression symptoms. Although all symptoms of a major depressive episode can occur in either unipolar or bipolar depression, some symptoms may present more often in bipolar versus unipolar depression, providing hints if not diagnostic certainty that the patient has a bipolar spectrum disorder. These symptoms include increased time sleeping, overeating, comorbid anxiety, psychomotor retardation, mood lability during episodes, psychotic symptoms, and suicidal thoughts.

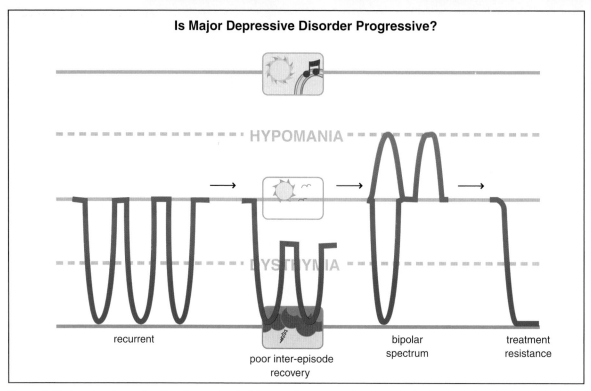

Figure 6-23. Is major depressive disorder progressive? A currently unanswered question is whether mood disorders are progressive. Does undertreatment of unipolar depression, in which residual symptoms persist and relapses occur, lead to progressive worsening of illness, such as more frequent recurrences and poor inter-episode recovery? And can this ultimately progress to a bipolar spectrum condition and finally treatment resistance?

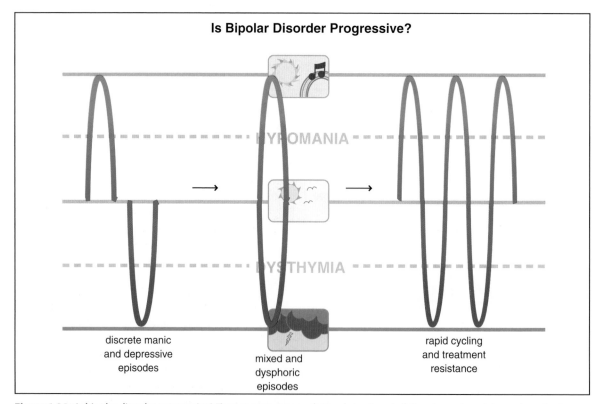

Figure 6-24. Is bipolar disorder progressive? There is some concern that undertreatment of discrete manic and depressive episodes may progress to mixed and dysphoric episodes and finally to rapid cycling and treatment resistance.

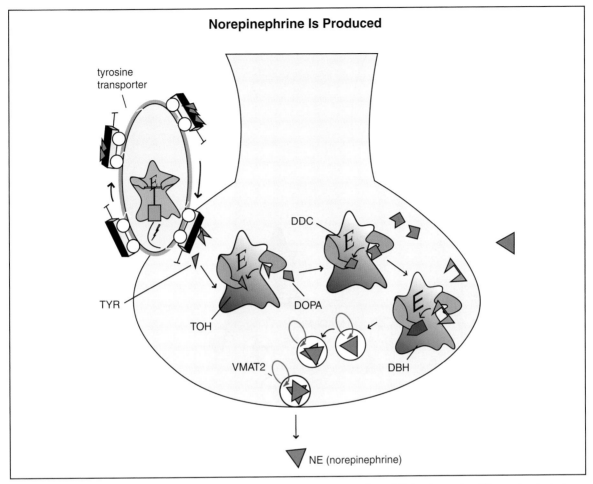

Figure 6-25. Norepinephrine is produced. Tyrosine (TYR) a precursor to norepinephrine (NE), is taken up into NE nerve terminals via a tyrosine transporter and converted into DOPA by the enzyme tyrosine hydroxylase (TOH). DOPA is then converted into dopamine (DA) by the enzyme DOPA decarboxylase (DDC). Finally, DA is converted into NE by dopamine β-hydroxylase (DBH). After synthesis, NE is packaged into synaptic vesicles via the vesicular monoamine transporter (VMAT2) and stored there until its release into the synapse during neurotransmission.

amino acid tyrosine, which is transported into the nervous system from the blood by means of an active transport pump (Figure 6-25). Once inside the neuron, the tyrosine is acted upon by three enzymes in sequence. First, tyrosine hydroxylase (TOH), the rate-limiting and most important enzyme in the regulation of NE synthesis. Tyrosine hydroxylase converts the amino acid tyrosine into DOPA. The second enzyme then acts, namely, DOPA decarboxylase (DDC), which converts DOPA into dopamine (DA). DA itself is a neurotransmitter in dopamine neurons, as discussed in Chapter 4 and illustrated in Figure 4-5. However, for NE neurons, DA is just a precursor of NE. In fact the third and final NE synthetic enzyme, dopamine β-hydroxylase (DBH), converts DA into NE. NE is then stored in synaptic

packages called vesicles until released by a nerve impulse (Figure 6-25).

NE action is terminated by two principal destructive or catabolic enzymes that turn NE into inactive metabolites. The first is monoamine oxidase (MAO) A or B, which is located in mitochondria in the presynaptic neuron and elsewhere (Figure 6-26). The second is catechol-O-methyl-transferase (COMT), which is thought to be located largely outside of the presynaptic nerve terminal (Figure 6-26).

The action of NE can be terminated not only by enzymes that destroy NE, but also by a transport pump for NE that removes NE from acting in the synapse without destroying it (Figure 6-27). In fact, such inactivated NE can be restored for reuse in a later

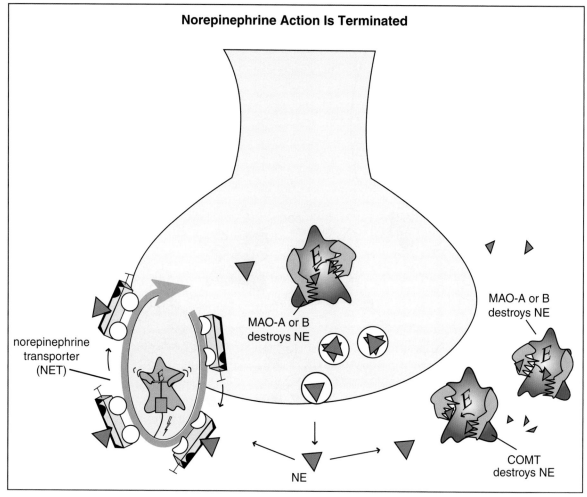

Figure 6-26. Norepinephrine's action is terminated. Norepinephrine's action can be terminated through multiple mechanisms. Dopamine can be transported out of the synaptic cleft and back into the presynaptic neuron via the norepinephrine transporter (NET), where it may be repackaged for future use. Alternatively, norepinephrine may be broken down extracellularly via the enzyme catechol-O-methyltransferase (COMT). Other enzymes that break down norepinephrine are monoamine oxidase A (MAO-A) and monoamine oxidase B (MAO-B), which are present in mitochondria both within the presynaptic neuron and in other cells, including neurons and glia.

neurotransmitting nerve impulse. The transport pump that terminates synaptic action of NE is sometimes called the "NE transporter" or NET and sometimes the "NE reuptake pump." This NE reuptake pump is located on the presynaptic noradrenergic nerve terminal as part of the presynaptic machinery of the neuron, where it acts as a vacuum cleaner whisking NE out of the synapse, off the synaptic receptors, and stopping its synaptic actions. Once inside the presynaptic nerve terminal, NE can either be stored again for subsequent reuse when another nerve impulse arrives, or destroyed by NE-destroying enzymes (Figure 6-26).

The noradrenergic neuron is regulated by a multiplicity of receptors for NE (Figure 6-27). The norepinephrine transporter or NET is one type of receptor, as is the vesicular monoamine transporter (VMAT2) that transports NE in the cytoplasm of the presynaptic neuron into storage vesicles (Figure 6-27). NE receptors are classified as α_1 or α_{2A}, α_{2B}, or α_{2C}, or as β_1, β_2, or β_3. All can be postsynaptic, but only α_2 receptors can act as presynaptic autoreceptors (Figures 6-27 through 6-29). Postsynaptic receptors convert their occupancy by norepinephrine at α_1, α_{2A}, α_{2B}, α_{2C}, β_1, β_2, or β_3 receptors into physiological functions, and ultimately into

Norepinephrine Receptors

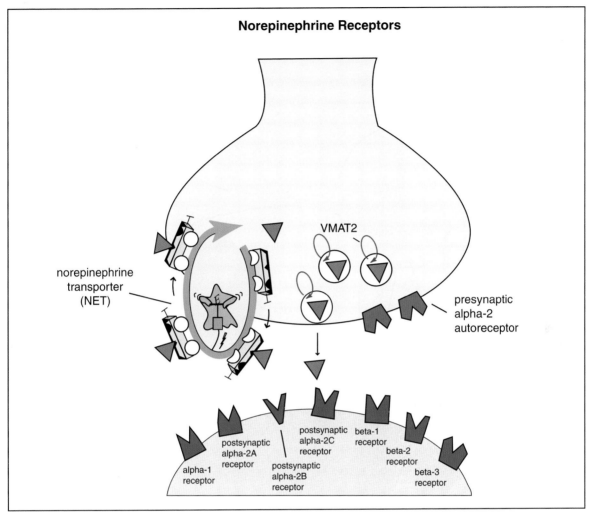

Figure 6-27. Norepinephrine receptors. Shown here are receptors for norepinephrine that regulate its neurotransmission. The norepinephrine transporter (NET) exists presynaptically and is responsible for clearing excess norepinephrine out of the synapse. The vesicular monoamine transporter (VMAT2) takes norepinephrine up into synaptic vesicles and stores it for future neurotransmission. There is also a presynaptic α_2 autoreceptor, which regulates release of norepinephrine from the presynaptic neuron. In addition, there are several postsynaptic receptors. These include α_1, α_{2A}, α_{2B}, α_{2C}, β_1, β_2, and β_3 receptors.

changes in signal transduction and gene expression in the postsynaptic neuron (Figure 6-27).

Presynaptic α_2 receptors regulate norepinephrine release, so they are called *autoreceptors* (Figures 6-27 and 6-28). Presynaptic α_2 autoreceptors are located both on the axon terminal (i.e., terminal α_2 receptors: Figures 6-27 and 6-28) and at cell body (soma) and nearby dendrites; thus, these latter α_2 presynaptic receptors are called *somatodendritic* α_2 receptors (Figure 6-29). Presynaptic α_2 receptors are important because both the terminal and the somatodendritic α_2 receptors are autoreceptors. That is, when presynaptic α_2

receptors recognize NE, they turn off further release of NE (Figures 6-27 and 6-28). Thus, presynaptic α_2 autoreceptors act as a brake for the NE neuron, and also cause what is known as a negative-feedback regulatory signal. Stimulating this receptor (i.e., stepping on the brake) stops the neuron from firing. This probably occurs physiologically to prevent over-firing of the NE neuron, since it can shut itself off once the firing rate gets too high and the autoreceptor becomes stimulated. It is worthy to note that drugs can not only mimic the natural functioning of the NE neuron by stimulating the presynaptic α_2 neuron, but drugs that antagonize this

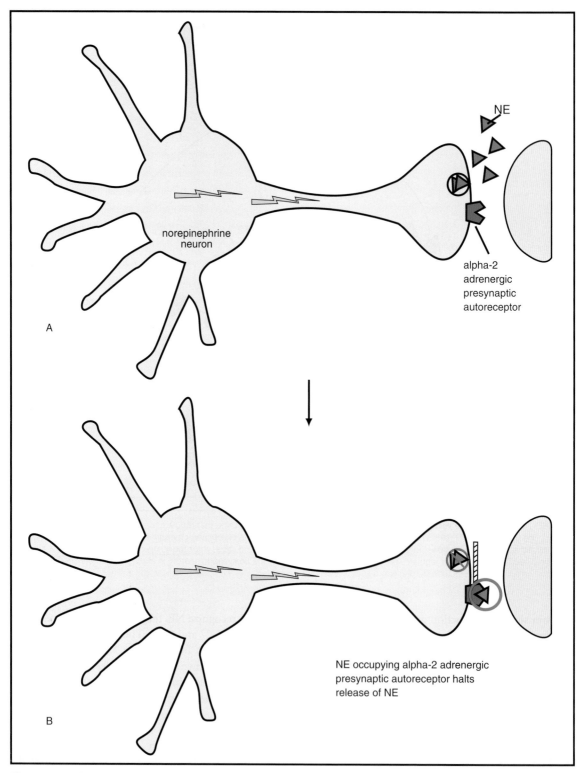

Figure 6-28. Alpha-2 receptors on axon terminal. Shown here are presynaptic α_2-adrenergic autoreceptors located on the axon terminal of the norepinephrine neuron. These autoreceptors are "gatekeepers" for norepinephrine. That is, when they are not bound by norepinephrine, they are open, allowing norepinephrine release (A). However, when norepinephrine binds to the gatekeeping receptors, they close the molecular gate and prevent norepinephrine from being released (B).

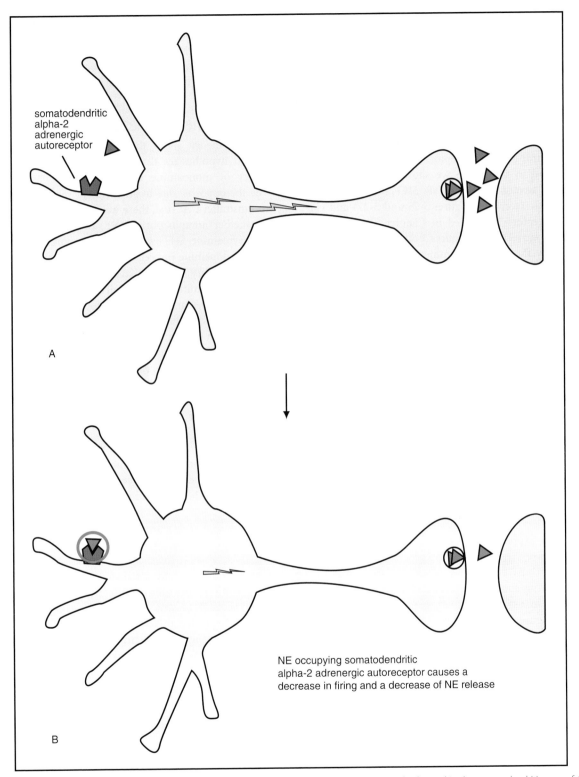

A

B

somatodendritic
alpha-2
adrenergic
autoreceptor

NE occupying somatodendritic
alpha-2 adrenergic autoreceptor causes a
decrease in firing and a decrease of NE release

Figure 6-29. Somatodendritic α₂ receptors. Presynaptic α₂-adrenergic autoreceptors are also located in the somatodendritic area of the norepinephrine neuron, as shown here. When norepinephrine binds to these α₂ receptors, it shuts off neuronal impulse flow in the norepinephrine neuron (see loss of lightning bolts in the neuron in the lower figure), and this stops further norepinephrine release.

same receptor will have the effect of cutting the brake cable, thus enhancing release of NE.

Monoamine interactions: NE regulation of 5HT release

Norepinephrine clearly regulates norepinephrine neurons via α_2 receptors (Figures 6-28 and 6-29); in Chapter 4, we showed that dopamine regulates dopamine neurons via D_2 receptors (Figures 4-8 through 4-10); and in Chapter 5 we showed that serotonin regulates serotonin neurons via $5HT_{1A}$ and $5HT_{1B/D}$ presynaptic receptors (Figures 5-25 and 5-27) and via $5HT_3$ receptors (illustrated in Chapter 7) and $5HT_7$ postsynaptic receptors (Figures 5-60A through 5-60C). Obviously, the three monoamines are all able to regulate their own release.

There are also numerous ways in which these three monoamines interact to regulate each other. For example, in Chapter 5 we showed that serotonin regulates dopamine release via $5HT_{1A}$ receptors (Figures 5-15C and 5-16C), $5HT_{2A}$ receptors (Figures 5-15A, 5-16A, 5-17) and $5HT_{2C}$ receptors (Figure 5-52A); we also showed that serotonin regulates norepinephrine release via $5HT_{2C}$ receptors (Figure 5-52A) and mentioned that serotonin regulates dopamine and norepinephrine via $5HT_3$ receptors, which is illustrated in Chapter 7 on antidepressants.

We now show that NE reciprocally regulates 5HT neurons via both α_1 and α_2 receptors (Figures 6-30A through 6-30C): α_1 receptors are the accelerator (Figure 6-30B), and α_2 receptors the brake (Figure 6-30C) on 5HT release. That is, NE neurons from the locus coeruleus travel a short distance to the midbrain raphe (Figure 6-30B, box 2) and there they release NE onto postsynaptic α_1 receptors on 5HT neuronal cell bodies. That directly stimulates 5HT neurons and acts as an accelerator for 5HT release, causing release of 5HT from their downstream axons (Figure 6-30B, box 1). Norepinephrine neurons also innervate the axon terminals of 5HT neurons (Figure 6-30C). Here NE is released directly onto postsynaptic α_2 receptors that inhibit 5HT neurons, acting as a brake on 5HT, thus inhibiting 5HT release (Figure 6-30C, box 1). Which action of NE predominates will depend upon which end of the 5HT neuron receives more noradrenergic input at any given time.

There are many brain areas where 5HT, NE, and DA projections overlap, creating opportunities for monoamine interactions throughout the brain and at many different receptor subtypes (Figures 6-31 through 6-33).

Numerous known inter-regulatory pathways and receptor interactions exist among the three monoaminergic neurotransmitter systems in order for them to influence each other and change the release not only of their own neurotransmitters, but also of other monoamines.

The monoamine hypothesis of depression

The classic theory about the biological etiology of depression hypothesizes that depression is due to a deficiency of monoamine neurotransmitters. Mania may be the opposite, due to an excess of monoamine neurotransmitters. At first, there was a great argument about whether norepinephrine (NE) or serotonin (5-hydroxytryptamine, 5HT) was the more important deficiency, and dopamine was relatively neglected. Now the monoamine theory suggests that the entire monoaminergic neurotransmitter system of all three monoamines NE, 5HT, and DA may be malfunctioning in various brain circuits, with different neurotransmitters involved depending upon the symptom profile of the patient.

The original conceptualization was rather simplistic and based upon observations that certain drugs that depleted these neurotransmitters could induce depression, and that all effective antidepressants act by boosting one or more of these three monoamine neurotransmitters. Thus, the idea was that the "normal" amount of monoamine neurotransmitters (Figure 6-34A) somehow became depleted, perhaps by an unknown disease process, by stress, or by drugs (Figure 6-34B), leading to the symptoms of depression.

Direct evidence for the monoamine hypothesis is still largely lacking. A good deal of effort was expended especially in the 1960s and 1970s to identify the theoretically predicted deficiencies of the monoamine neurotransmitters in depression and an excess in mania. This effort to date has unfortunately yielded mixed and sometimes confusing results, causing a search for better explanations of the potential link between monoamines and mood disorders.

The monoamine receptor hypothesis and gene expression

Because of these and other difficulties with the monoamine hypothesis, the focus of hypotheses for the etiology of mood disorders has shifted from the monoamine neurotransmitters themselves to their receptors

**Raphe Alpha 1 Receptors and Cortical Alpha 2 Receptors
Mediate Norepinephrine Regulation of 5HT Release**

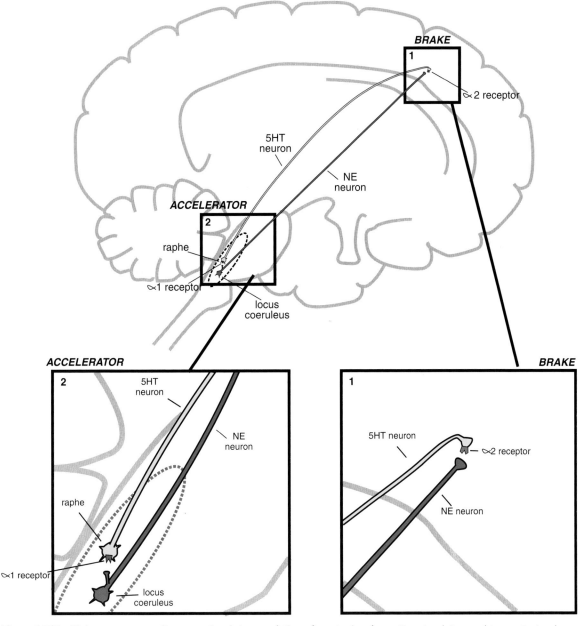

Figure 6-30A. Alpha receptors mediate norepinephrine regulation of serotonin release. Norepinephrine regulates serotonin release. It does this by acting as a brake on serotonin release at cortical α_2 receptors on axon terminals (1) and as an accelerator of serotonin release at α_1 receptors at the somatodendritic area (2).

Raphe Alpha 1 Receptors Stimulate Serotonin Release

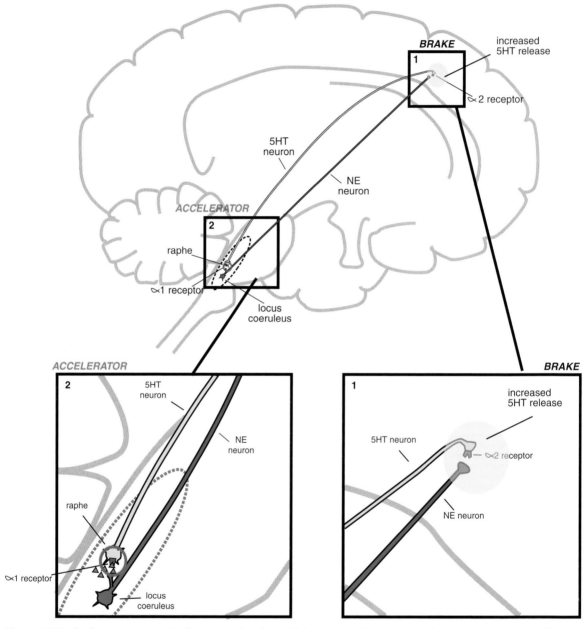

Figure 6-30B. Raphe α₁ receptors stimulate serotonin release. Alpha-1-adrenergic receptors are located in the somatodendritic regions of serotonin neurons. When these receptors are unoccupied by norepinephrine, some serotonin is released from the serotonin neuron. However, when norepinephrine binds to the α₁ receptor (2), this stimulates the serotonin neuron, accelerating release of serotonin (1).

Cortical Alpha 2 Receptors Inhibit Serotonin Release

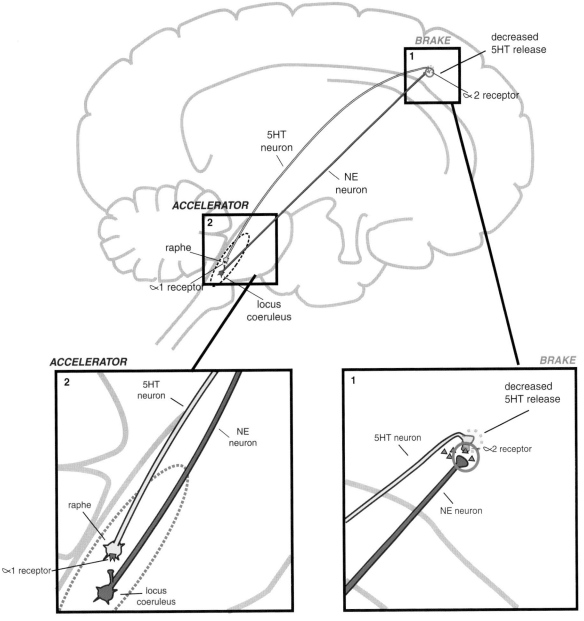

Figure 6-30C. Cortical α₂ receptors inhibit serotonin release. Alpha-2-adrenergic heteroreceptors are located on the axon terminals of serotonin neurons. When norepinephrine binds to the α₂ receptor this prevents serotonin from being released (1).

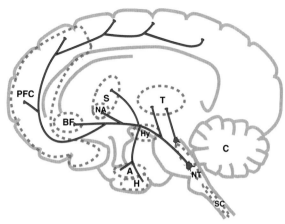

Figure 6-31. Major dopamine projections. Dopamine has widespread ascending projections that originate predominantly in the brainstem (particularly the ventral tegmental area and substantia nigra) and extend via the hypothalamus to the prefrontal cortex, basal forebrain, striatum, nucleus accumbens, and other regions. Dopaminergic neurotransmission is associated with movement, pleasure and reward, cognition, psychosis, and other functions. In addition, there are direct projections from other sites to the thalamus, creating the "thalamic dopamine system," which may be involved in arousal and sleep. PFC, prefrontal cortex; BF, basal forebrain; S, striatum; NA, nucleus accumbens; T, thalamus; Hy, hypothalamus; A, amygdala; H, hippocampus; NT, brainstem neurotransmitter centers; SC, spinal cord; C, cerebellum.

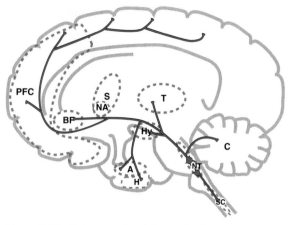

Figure 6-32. Major norepinephrine projections. Norepinephrine has both ascending and descending projections. Ascending noradrenergic projections originate mainly in the locus coeruleus of the brainstem; they extend to multiple brain regions, as shown here, and regulate mood, arousal, cognition, and other functions. Descending noradrenergic projections extend down the spinal cord and regulate pain pathways. PFC, prefrontal cortex; BF, basal forebrain; S, striatum; NA, nucleus accumbens; T, thalamus; Hy, hypothalamus; A, amygdala; H, hippocampus; NT, brainstem neurotransmitter centers; SC, spinal cord; C, cerebellum.

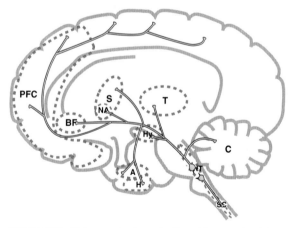

Figure 6-33. Major serotonin projections. Like norepinephrine, serotonin has both ascending and descending projections. Ascending serotonergic projections originate in the brainstem and extend to many of the same regions as noradrenergic projections, with additional projections to the striatum and nucleus accumbens. These ascending projections may regulate mood, anxiety, sleep, and other functions. Descending serotonergic projections extend down the brainstem and through the spinal cord; they may regulate pain. PFC, prefrontal cortex; BF, basal forebrain; S, striatum; NA, nucleus accumbens; T, thalamus; Hy, hypothalamus; A, amygdala; H, hippocampus; NT, brainstem neurotransmitter centers; SC, spinal cord; C, cerebellum.

and the downstream molecular events that these receptors trigger, including the regulation of gene expression and the role of growth factors. There is also great interest in the influence of nature and nurture on brain circuits regulated by monoamines, especially what happens when epigenetic changes from stressful life experiences are combined with the inheritance of various risk genes that can make an individual vulnerable to those environmental stressors.

The neurotransmitter receptor hypothesis of depression posits that an abnormality in the receptors for monoamine neurotransmitters leads to depression (Figure 6-35). Thus, if depletion of monoamine neurotransmitters is the central theme of the monoamine hypothesis of depression (Figure 6-34B), the neurotransmitter receptor hypothesis of depression takes this theme one step further: namely, that the depletion of neurotransmitter causes compensatory upregulation of postsynaptic neurotransmitter receptors (Figure 6-35). Direct evidence for this hypothesis is also generally lacking. Postmortem studies do consistently show increased numbers of serotonin 2 receptors in the frontal cortex of patients who commit suicide. Also, some neuroimaging studies have identified abnormalities in serotonin receptors of depressed patients, but this approach has not yet been successful in identifying consistent and replicable molecular lesions in receptors

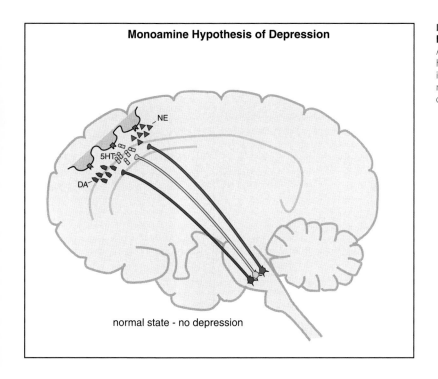

Monoamine Hypothesis of Depression

NE

5HT

DA

normal state - no depression

Figure 6-34A. Classic monoamine hypothesis of depression, part 1. According to the classic monoamine hypothesis of depression, when there is a "normal" amount of monoamine neurotransmitter activity, there is no depression present.

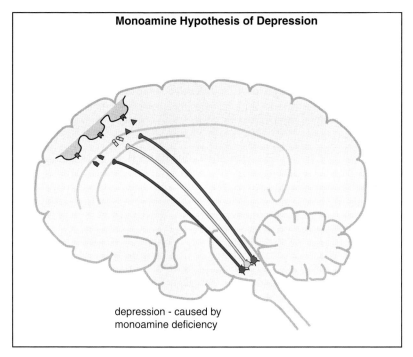

Monoamine Hypothesis of Depression

depression - caused by monoamine deficiency

Figure 6-34B. Classic monoamine hypothesis of depression, part 2. The monoamine hypothesis of depression posits that if the "normal" amount of monoamine neurotransmitter activity becomes reduced, depleted, or dysfunctional for some reason, depression may ensue.

for monoamines in depression. Thus, there is no clear and convincing evidence that monoamine deficiency accounts for depression – i.e., there is no "real" monoamine deficit. Likewise, there is no clear and convincing evidence that abnormalities in monoamine receptors account for depression. Although the monoamine hypothesis is obviously an overly simplified notion about mood disorders, it has been very valuable in

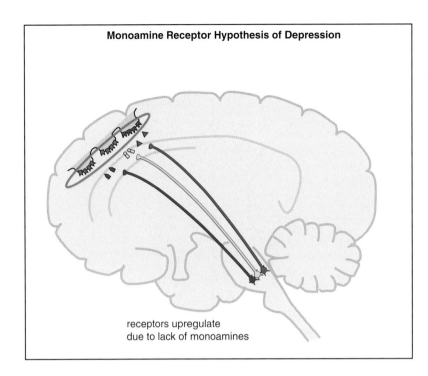

Monoamine Receptor Hypothesis of Depression

receptors upregulate
due to lack of monoamines

Figure 6-35. Monoamine receptor hypothesis of depression. The monoamine receptor hypothesis of depression extends the classic monoamine hypothesis of depression, positing that deficient activity of monoamine neurotransmitters causes upregulation of postsynaptic monoamine neurotransmitter receptors, and that this leads to depression.

focusing attention upon the three monoamine neurotransmitter systems norepinephrine, dopamine, and serotonin. This has led to a much better understanding of the physiological functioning of these three neurotransmitters, and especially the various mechanisms by which all known antidepressants act to boost neurotransmission at one or more of these three monoamine neurotransmitter systems, and how certain mood-stabilizing drugs may also act on the monoamines. Research is now turning to the possibility that in depression there may be a deficiency in downstream signal transduction of the monoamine neurotransmitter and its postsynaptic neuron that is occurring in the presence of normal amounts of neurotransmitter and receptor. Thus, the hypothesized molecular problem in depression could lie within the molecular events distal to the receptor, in the signal transduction cascade system, and in appropriate gene expression (Figure 6-36). Different molecular problems may account for mania and bipolar disorder.

Stress and depression

Stress, BDNF, and brain atrophy in depression

One candidate mechanism that has been proposed as the site of a possible flaw in signal transduction from monoamine receptors in depression is the target gene for brain-derived neurotrophic factor (BDNF) (Figures 6-36, 6-37, 6-38). Normally, BDNF sustains the viability of brain neurons (Figure 6-37), but under stress, the gene for BDNF may be repressed (Figure 6-38). Stress can lower 5HT levels and can acutely increase, then chronically deplete, both NE and DA. These monoamine neurotransmitter changes together with deficient amounts of BDNF may lead to atrophy and possible apoptosis of vulnerable neurons in the hippocampus and other brain areas such as prefrontal cortex (Figure 6-37). An artist's concept of the hippocampal atrophy that has been reported in association with chronic stress and with both major depression and various anxiety disorders, especially PTSD, is shown in Figures 6-39A and 6-39B. Fortunately, some of this neuronal loss may be reversible. That is, restoration of monoamine-related signal transduction cascades by antidepressants (Figure 6-36) can increase BDNF and other trophic factors (Figure 6-37) and potentially restore lost synapses. In some brain areas such as the hippocampus, not only can synapses potentially be restored, but it is possible that some lost neurons might even be replaced by neurogenesis.

Neurons from the hippocampal area and amygdala normally suppress the hypothalamic–pituitary–adrenal (HPA) axis (Figure 6-39A), so if stress causes hippocampal and amygdala neurons to atrophy, with loss of

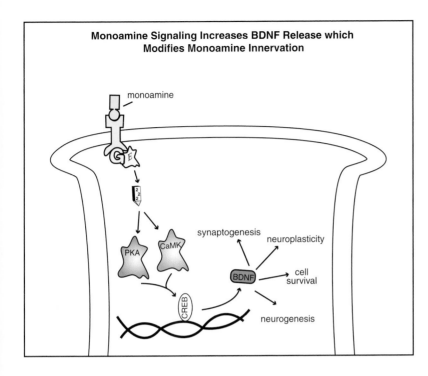

Monoamine Signaling Increases BDNF Release which Modifies Monoamine Innervation

Figure 6-36. Monoamine signaling and brain-derived neurotrophic factor (BDNF) release. The neurotrophic hypothesis of depression states that depression may be caused by reduced synthesis of proteins involved in neurogenesis and synaptic plasticity. BDNF promotes the growth and development of immature neurons, including monoaminergic neurons, enhances the survival and function of adult neurons, and helps maintain synaptic connections. Because BDNF is important for neuronal survival, decreased levels may contribute to cell atrophy. In some cases, low levels of BDNF may even cause cell loss. Monoamines can increase the availability of BDNF by initiating signal transduction cascades that lead to its release. Thus, if monoamine levels are low, then BDNF levels may correspondingly be low. CaMK, calcium/calmodulin-dependent protein kinase; CREB, cAMP response element-binding protein; PKA, protein kinase A.

their inhibitory input to the hypothalamus, this could lead to overactivity of the HPA axis (Figure 6-39B). In depression, abnormalities of the HPA axis have long been reported, including elevated glucocorticoid levels and insensitivity of the HPA axis to feedback inhibition (Figure 6-39B). Some evidence suggests that glucocorticoids at high levels could even be toxic to neurons and contribute to their atrophy under chronic stress (Figure 6-39B). Novel antidepressant treatments are in testing that target corticotropin-releasing factor 1 (CRF-1) receptors, vasopressin 1B receptors, and glucocorticoid receptors (Figure 6-39B), in an attempt to halt and even reverse these HPA abnormalities in depression and other stress-related psychiatric illnesses.

Stress and the environment: how much stress is too much stress?

In many ways the body is built for the purpose of handling stress, and in fact a certain amount of "stress load" on bones, muscles, and brain is necessary for growth and optimal functioning and can even be associated with developing resilience to future stressors (Figure 6-40). However, certain types of stress such as child abuse can sensitize brain circuits and render them vulnerable rather than resilient to future stressors (Figure 6-41).

For patients with such vulnerable brain circuits who then become exposed to multiple life stressors as adults, the result can be the development of depression (Figure 6-42). Thus, the same amount of stress that would be handled without developing depression in someone who has not experienced child abuse could hypothetically cause depression in someone with a prior history of child abuse. This demonstrates the potential impact of the environment upon brain circuits. Many studies in fact confirm that in women abused as children, depression can be found up to four times more often than in never-abused women. Hypothetically, epigenetic changes caused by environmental stress create relatively permanent molecular alterations in the brain circuits at the time of the child abuse that do not cause depression per se, but make brain circuits vulnerable to breakdown into depression upon exposure to future stressors as an adult.

Stress and vulnerability genes: born fearful?

Modern theories of mood disorders do not propose that any single gene can cause depression or mania, but as discussed for schizophrenia in Chapter 4

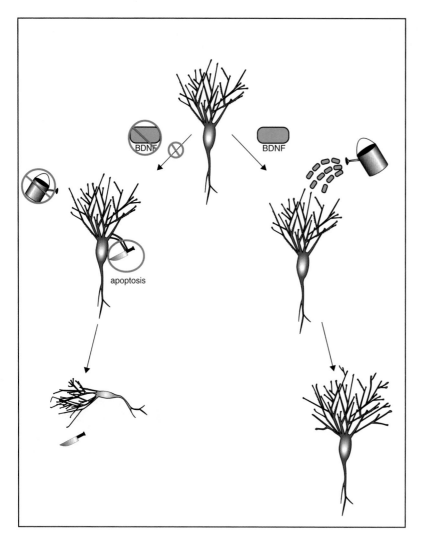

apoptosis

Figure 6-37. Suppression of brain-derived neurotrophic factor (BDNF) production. BDNF plays a role in the proper growth and maintenance of neurons and neuronal connections (right). If the genes for BDNF are turned off (left), the resultant decrease in BDNF could compromise the brain's ability to create and maintain neurons and their connections. This could lead to loss of synapses or even whole neurons by apoptosis.

(see also Figure 4-33), mood disorders are theoretically caused by a "conspiracy" among many vulnerability genes and many environmental stressors leading to breakdown of information processing in specific brain circuits and thus the various symptoms of a major depressive or manic episode. There is a great overlap between those genes thought to be vulnerability genes for schizophrenia and those thought to be vulnerability genes for bipolar disorder. A comprehensive discussion of genes for bipolar disorder or for major depression is beyond the scope of this book, but one of the vulnerability genes for depression is the gene coding for the serotonin transporter or SERT (i.e., the serotonin reuptake pump), which is the site of action of SSRI and SNRI antidepressants. The type of serotonin transporter (SERT)

with which you are born determines in part whether your amygdala is more likely to over-react to fearful faces (Figure 6-43), whether you are more likely to develop depression when exposed to multiple life stressors, and how likely your depression is to respond to an SSRI/SNRI or whether you can even tolerate an SSRI/SNRI (Figure 6-43).

Specifically, an excessive reaction of the amygdala to fearful faces for carriers of the s variant of the gene for SERT is shown in Figure 6-43. Fearful faces can be considered a stressful load on the amygdala and its circuitry, and can be visualized using modern neuroimaging techniques. For those with the s genotype of SERT, they are more likely to develop an affective disorder when exposed to multiple life stressors and may have more hippocampal

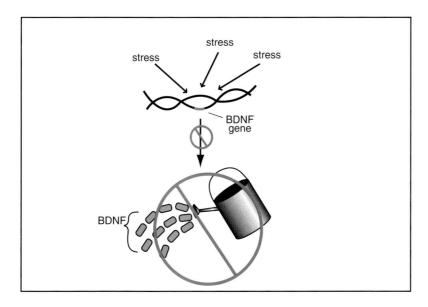

Figure 6-38. Stress and brain-derived neurotrophic factor (BDNF). One factor that could contribute to potential brain atrophy is the impact that chronic stress can have on BDNF, which plays a role in the proper growth and maintenance of neurons and neuronal connections. During chronic stress, the genes for BDNF may be turned off, potentially reducing its production.

The Hypothalamic - Pituitary - Adrenal (HPA) Axis

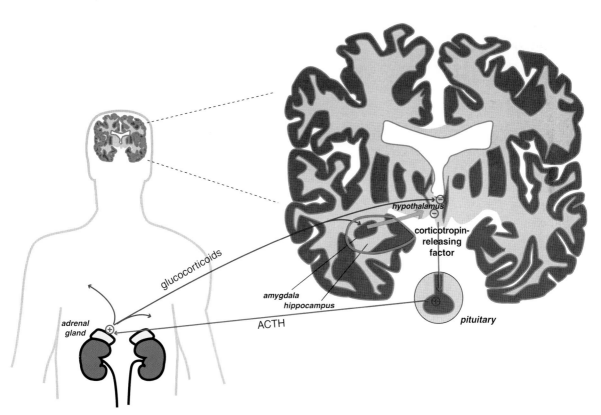

Figure 6-39A. Hypothalamic–pituitary–adrenal (HPA) axis. The normal stress response involves activation of the hypothalamus and a resultant increase in corticotropin-releasing factor (CRF), which in turn stimulates the release of adrenocorticotropic hormone (ACTH) from the pituitary. ACTH causes glucocorticoid release from the adrenal gland, which feeds back to the hypothalamus and inhibits CRF release, terminating the stress response.

Hippocampal Atrophy and Hyperactive HPA in Depression

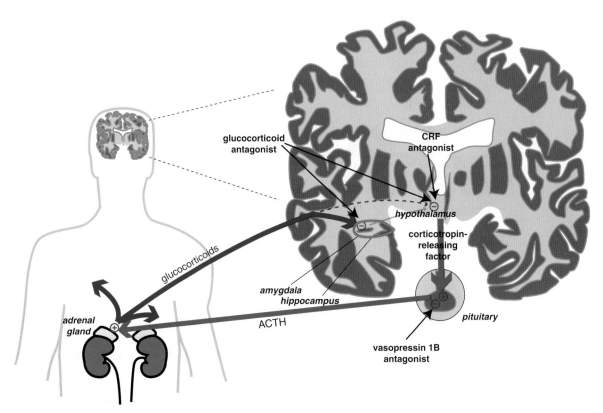

Figure 6-39B. Hippocampal atrophy and hyperactive HPA axis in depression. In situations of chronic stress, excessive glucocorticoid release may eventually cause hippocampal atrophy. Because the hippocampus inhibits the HPA axis, atrophy in this region may lead to chronic activation of the HPA axis, which may increase risk of developing a psychiatric illness. Because the HPA axis is central to stress processing, it may be that novel targets for treating stress-induced disorders lie within the axis. Mechanisms being examined include antagonism of glucocorticoid receptors, corticotropin-releasing factor 1 (CRF-1) receptors, and vasopressin 1B receptors.

atrophy, more cognitive symptoms, and less responsiveness or tolerance to SSRI/SNRI treatment. Exposure to multiple life stressors may cause the otherwise silent overactivity and inefficient information processing of affective loads in the amygdala to become an overt major depressive episode (Figure 6-43), an interaction of their genes with the environment (nature plus nurture). The point is that the specific gene that you have for the serotonin transporter can alter the efficiency of affective information processing by your amygdala and, consequently, your risk for developing major depression if you experience multiple life stressors as an adult (Figure 6-43). On the other hand, the l genotype of SERT is a more resilient genotype, with less amygdala reactivity to fearful faces, less likelihood of breaking down into a major depressive episode when exposed to multiple life stressors, as well as more likelihood of responding to or tolerating SSRIs/SNRIs if you do develop a depressive episode (Figure 6-43).

Whether you have the l or the s genotype of SERT accounts for only a small amount of the variance for whether or not you will develop major depression after experiencing multiple life stressors, and thus cannot predict who will get major depression and who will not. However, this example does prove the importance of genes in general and those for serotonin neurons in particular in the regulation of the amygdala and in determining the odds of developing major depression under stress. Thus, perhaps one is not born fearful, but born vulnerable or resilient to

Development of Stress Resilience

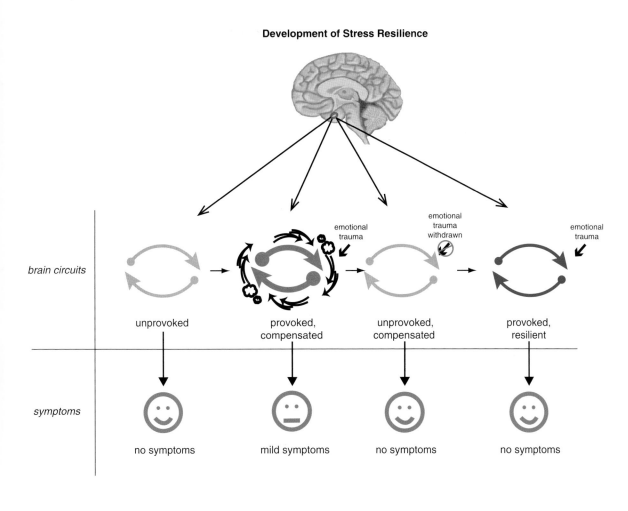

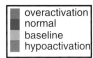

Figure 6-40. Development of stress resilience. In a healthy individual, stress can cause a temporary activation of circuits which is resolved when the stressor is removed. As shown here, when the circuit is unprovoked, no symptoms are produced. In the presence of a stressor such as emotional trauma, the circuit is provoked yet able to compensate for the effects of the stressor. By its ability to process the information load from the environment, it can avoid producing symptoms. When the stressor is withdrawn, the circuit returns to baseline functioning. Individuals exposed to this type of short-term stress may even develop resilience to stress, whereby exposure to future stressors provokes the circuit but does not result in symptoms.

developing major depression in response to future adult stressors, especially if they are chronic, multiple, and severe.

Symptoms and circuits in depression

Currently, the monoamine hypothesis of depression is now being applied to understanding how monoamines regulate the efficiency of information processing in a wide variety of neuronal circuits that may be responsible for mediating the various symptoms of depression. Obviously, there are numerous symptoms required for the diagnosis of a major depressive episode (Figure 6-44). Each symptom is hypothetically associated with inefficient information processing in various brain circuits, with different symptoms topographically localized to specific brain regions (Figure 6-45).

Development of Stress Sensitization

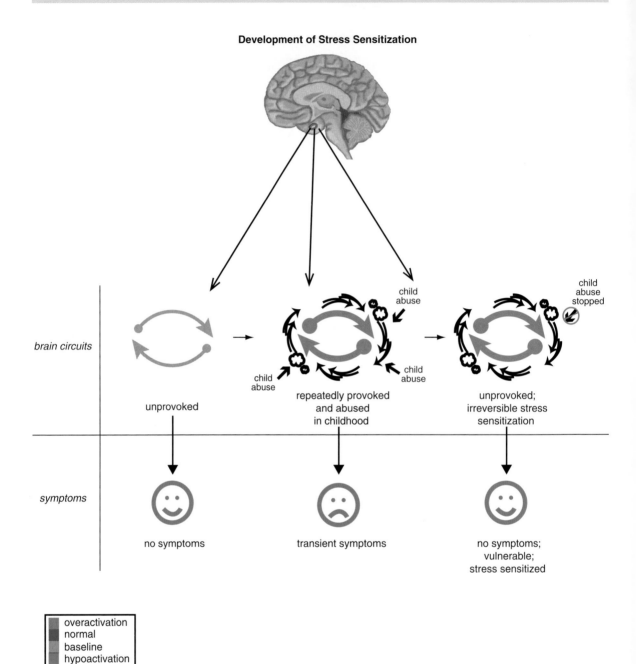

Figure 6-41. Development of stress sensitization. Prolonged activation of circuits due to repeated exposure to stressors can lead to a condition known as "stress sensitization," in which circuits not only become overly activated but remain overly activated even when the stressor is withdrawn. Thus, an individual with severe stress in childhood will exhibit transient symptoms during stress exposure, with resolution of the symptoms when the stressor is removed. The circuits remain overly activated in this model, but the individual exhibits no symptoms because these circuits can somehow still compensate for this additional load. However, the individual with "stress-sensitized" circuits is now vulnerable to the effects of future stressors, so that the risk for developing psychiatric symptoms is increased. Stress sensitization may therefore constitute a "presymptomatic" state for some psychiatric symptoms. This state might be detectable with functional brain scans of circuits but not from psychiatric interviews or patient complaints.

Progression from Stress Sensitization to Depression

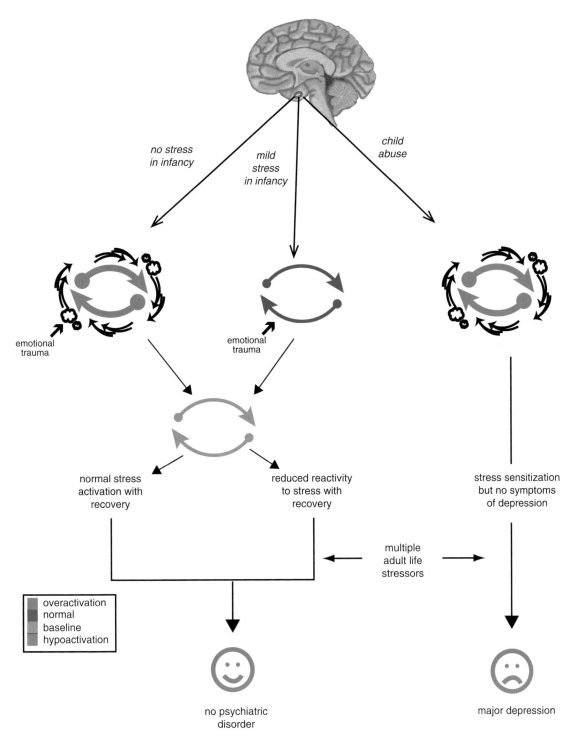

Figure 6-42. Progression from stress sensitization to depression. It may be that the degree of stress one experiences during early life affects how the circuits develop and therefore how a given individual responds to stress in later life. No stress during infancy may lead to a circuit that exhibits "normal" activation during stress and confers no increased risk of developing a psychiatric disorder. Interestingly, mild stress during infancy may actually cause the circuits to exhibit reduced reactivity to stress in later life and provide some resilience to adult stressors. Overwhelming and/or chronic stress from child abuse, however, may lead to stress-sensitized circuits that may become activated even in the absence of a stressor. Individuals with stress sensitization may not exhibit phenotypic symptoms but may be at increased risk of developing a mental illness if exposed to future stressors.

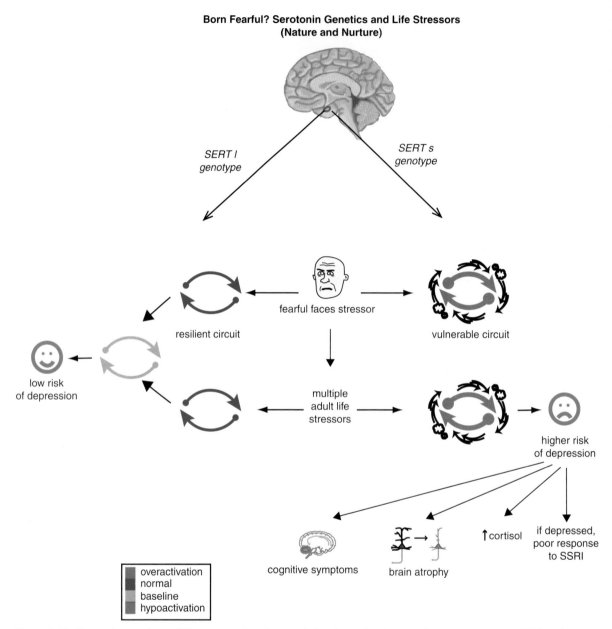

Figure 6-43. Serotonin genetics and life stressors. Genetic research has shown that the type of serotonin transporter (SERT) with which you are born can affect how you process fearful stimuli and perhaps also how you respond to stress. Specifically, individuals who are carriers of the s variant of the gene for SERT appear to be more vulnerable to the effects of stress or anxiety, whereas those who carry the l variant appear to be more resilient. Thus, s carriers exhibit increased amygdala activity in response to fearful faces and may also be more likely to develop a mood or anxiety disorder after suffering multiple life stressors. The higher risk of depression may also be related to increased likelihood of cognitive symptoms, brain atrophy, increased cortisol, and, if depressed, poor response to selective serotonin reuptake inhibitors (SSRIs).

Not only can each of the nine symptoms listed for the diagnosis of a major depressive episode be mapped onto brain circuits whose inefficient information processing theoretically mediates these symptoms (Figure 6-45), but the hypothetical monoaminergic regulation of each of these various brain areas can also be mapped onto each brain region they innervate (Figures 6-31 through 6-33). This creates a set of monoamine neurotransmitters that regulates each specific hypothetically malfunctioning brain region. Targeting each region with

Symptom Dimensions of a Major Depressive Episode

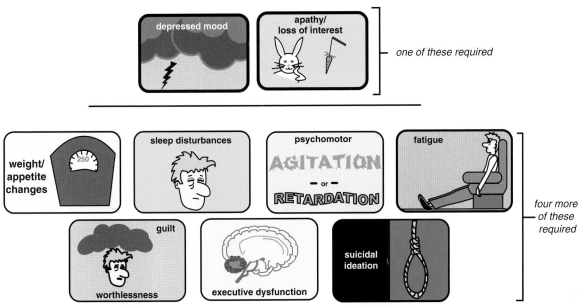

one of these required

four more of these required

Figure 6-44. Symptoms of depression. According to the *Diagnostic and Statistical Manual of Mental Disorders*, a major depressive episode consists of either depressed mood or loss of interest and at least four of the following: weight/appetite changes, insomnia or hypersomnia, psychomotor agitation or retardation, fatigue, feelings of guilt or worthlessness, executive dysfunction, and suicidal ideation.

Match Each Diagnostic Symptom for a Major Depressive Episode to Hypothetically Malfunctioning Brain Circuits

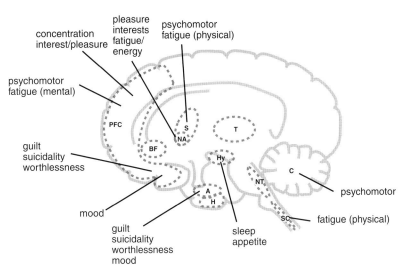

Figure 6-45. Matching depression symptoms to circuits. Alterations in neuronal activity and in the efficiency of information processing within each of the eleven brain regions shown here can lead to symptoms of a major depressive episode. Functionality in each brain region is hypothetically associated with a different constellation of symptoms. PFC, prefrontal cortex; BF, basal forebrain; S, striatum; NA, nucleus accumbens; T, thalamus; Hy, hypothalamus; A, amygdala; H, hippocampus; NT, brainstem neurotransmitter centers; SC, spinal cord; C, cerebellum.

drugs that act on the relevant monoamine(s) that innervate those brain regions potentially leads to reduction of each individual symptom experienced by a specific patient by enhancing the efficiency of information processing in malfunctioning circuits for each specific symptom. If successful, this targeting of monoamines in specific brain areas could even eliminate symptoms, and cause a major depressive episode to go into remission.

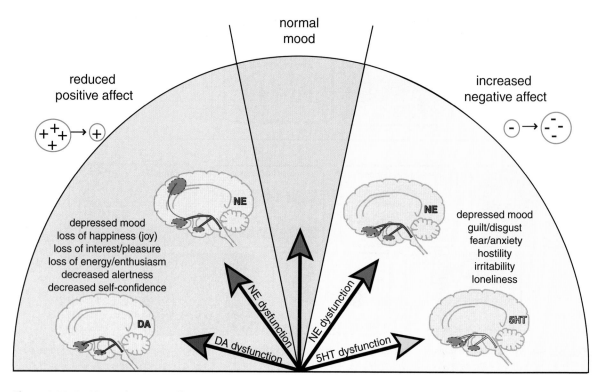

Figure 6-46. Positive and negative affect. Mood-related symptoms of depression can be characterized by their affective expression – that is, whether they cause a reduction in positive affect or an increase in negative affect. Symptoms related to reduced positive affect include depressed mood; loss of happiness, interest, or pleasure; loss of energy or enthusiasm; decreased alertness; and decreased self-confidence. Reduced positive affect may be hypothetically related to dopaminergic dysfunction, with a possible role of noradrenergic dysfunction as well. Symptoms associated with increased negative affect include depressed mood, guilt, disgust, fear, anxiety, hostility, irritability, and loneliness. Increased negative affect may be linked hypothetically to serotonergic dysfunction and perhaps also noradrenergic dysfunction.

Many of the mood-related symptoms of depression can be categorized as having either too little positive affect, or too much negative affect (Figure 6-46). This idea is linked to the fact that there are diffuse anatomic connections of monoamines throughout the brain, with diffuse dopamine dysfunction in this system driving predominantly the reduction of positive affect, diffuse serotonin dysfunction driving predominantly the increase in negative affect, and norepinephrine dysfunction being involved in both. Thus, reduced positive affect includes such symptoms as depressed mood but also loss of happiness, joy, interest, pleasure, alertness, energy, enthusiasm, and self-confidence (Figure 6-46, left). Enhancing dopamine function, and possibly also norepinephrine function may improve information processing in the circuits mediating this cluster of symptoms. On the other hand, increased negative affect includes not only depressed mood but guilt, disgust, fear, anxiety, hostility, irritability and loneliness (Figure 6-46, right). Enhancing serotonin function, and possibly also

norepinephrine function, may improve information processing in the circuits that hypothetically mediate this cluster of symptoms. For patients with symptoms of both clusters, they may require triple-action treatments that boost all three of the monoamines.

Symptoms and circuits in mania

The same general paradigm of monoamine regulation of the efficiency of information processing in specific brain circuits can be applied to mania as well as depression, although this is frequently thought to be in the opposite direction and in some overlapping but also some different brain regions compared to depression. The numerous symptoms required for the diagnosis of a manic episode are shown in Figure 6-47. Like major depression, each symptom of mania is also hypothetically associated with inefficient information processing in various brain circuits, with different symptoms topographically localized to specific brain regions (Figure 6-48).

Symptom Dimensions of a Manic Episode

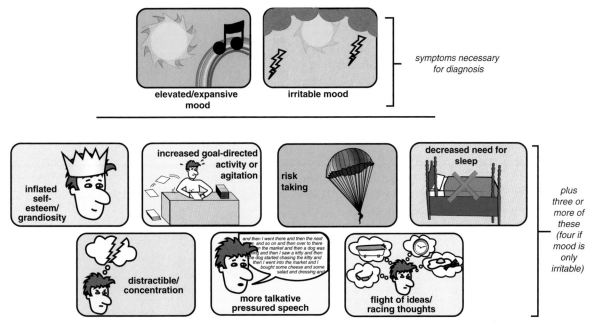

Figure 6-47. Symptoms of mania. According to the *Diagnostic and Statistical Manual of Mental Disorders*, a manic episode consists of either elevated/expansive mood or irritable mood. In addition, at least three of the following must be present (four if mood is irritable): inflated self-esteem/grandiosity, increased goal-directed activity or agitation, risk taking, decreased need for sleep, distractibility, pressured speech, and racing thoughts.

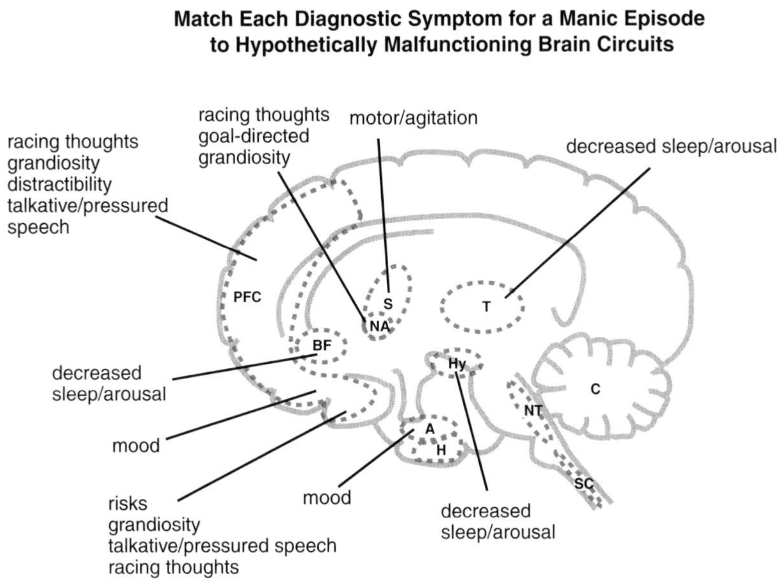

Match Each Diagnostic Symptom for a Manic Episode to Hypothetically Malfunctioning Brain Circuits

racing thoughts
grandiosity
distractibility
talkative/pressured
speech

racing thoughts
goal-directed
grandiosity

motor/agitation

decreased sleep/arousal

PFC

S
NA

T

BF

Hy

A
H

NT

C

SC

decreased
sleep/arousal

mood

risks
grandiosity
talkative/pressured speech
racing thoughts

mood

decreased
sleep/arousal

Figure 6-48. Matching mania symptoms to circuits. Alterations in neurotransmission within each of the eleven brain regions shown here can be hypothetically linked to the various symptoms of a manic episode. Functionality in each brain region may be associated with a different constellation of symptoms. PFC, prefrontal cortex; BF, basal forebrain; S, striatum; NA, nucleus accumbens; T, thalamus; Hy, hypothalamus; A, amygdala; H, hippocampus; NT, brainstem neurotransmitter centers; SC, spinal cord; C, cerebellum.

Generally, the inefficient functioning in these circuits in mania may be essentially the opposite of the malfunctioning hypothesized for depression, but may be more accurately portrayed as "out of tune" rather than simply excessive or deficient, especially since some patients can simultaneously have both manic and depressed symptoms. Generally, treatments for mania either reduce or stabilize monoaminergic regulation of circuits associated with symptoms of mania.

Neuroimaging in mood disorders

It is not currently possible to diagnose depression or bipolar disorder with any neuroimaging technique. However, some progress is being made in mapping inefficient information processing in various circuits in mood disorders. In depression, the dorsolateral prefrontal cortex, associated with cognitive symp-

toms, may have reduced activity, and the amygdala, associated with various emotional symptoms including depressed mood, may have increased activity (Figure 6-49). Furthermore, provocative testing of patients with mood disorders may provide some insight into malfunctioning of brain circuits exposed to environmental input, and thus required to process that information. For example, some studies of

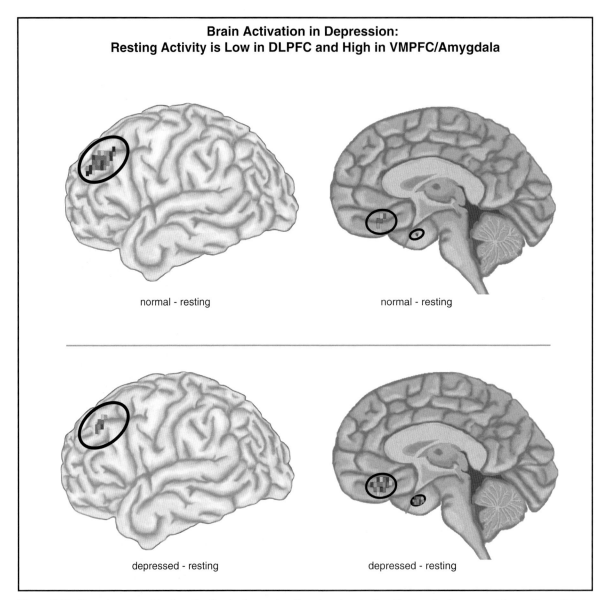

Figure 6-49. Neuroimaging of brain activation in depression. Neuroimaging studies of brain activation suggest that resting activity in the dorsolateral prefrontal cortex (DLPFC) of depressed patients is low compared to that in nondepressed individuals (left, top and bottom), whereas resting activity in the amygdala and ventromedial prefrontal cortex (VMPFC) of depressed patients is high compared to that in nondepressed individuals (right, top and bottom).

**Depressed Patients May Be More Responsive to
Induction of Sadness Than to Induction of Happiness**

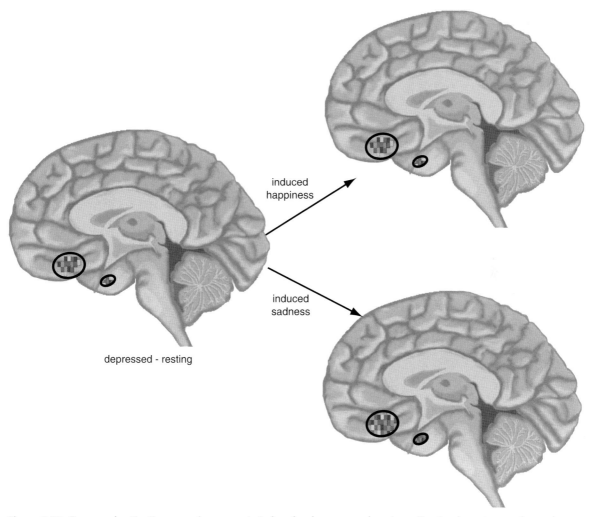

induced
happiness

induced
sadness

depressed - resting

Figure 6-50. Depressed patient's neuronal response to induced sadness versus happiness. Emotional symptoms such as sadness or happiness are regulated by the ventromedial prefrontal cortex (VMPFC) and the amygdala, two regions in which activity is high in the resting state of depressed patients (left). Interestingly, provocative tests in which these emotions are induced show that neuronal activity in the amygdala is over-reactive to induced sadness (bottom right) but under-reactive to induced happiness (top right).

depressed patients show that their neuronal circuits at the level of the amygdala are over-reactive to induced sadness but under-reactive to induced happiness (Figure 6-50). On the other hand, imaging of the orbitofrontal cortex of manic patients shows that they fail to appropriately activate this brain region in a test that requires them to suppress a response, suggesting problems with impulsivity associated with mania and with this specific brain region (Figure 6-51). In general, these neuroimaging findings support the mapping of symptoms to brain regions discussed earlier in this chapter, but much further work is currently in progress and must be completed before the results of neuroimaging can be applied to diagnostic or therapeutic decision making in clinical practice.

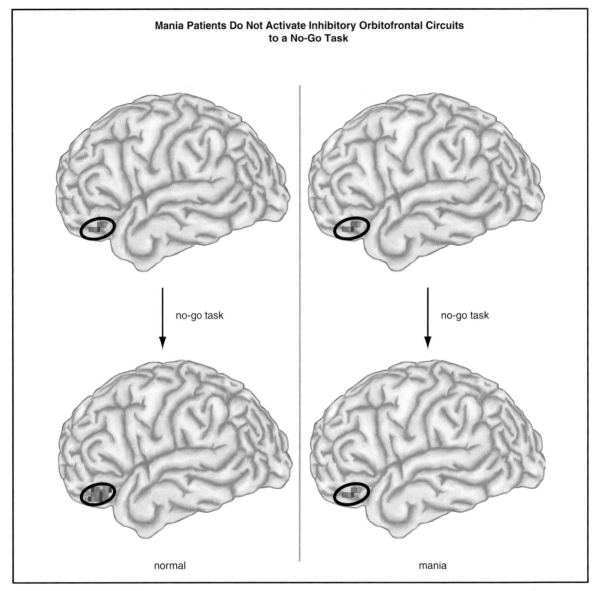

Figure 6-51. Mania patient's neuronal response to no-go task. Impulsive symptoms of mania, such as risk taking and pressured speech, are related to activity in the orbitofrontal cortex (OFC). Neuroimaging data show that this brain region is hypoactive in mania (bottom right) versus healthy (bottom left) individuals during the no-go task, which is designed to test response inhibition.

Summary

This chapter has described the mood disorders, including those across the bipolar spectrum. For prognostic and treatment purposes, it is increasingly important to be able to distinguish unipolar depression from bipolar spectrum depression. Although mood disorders are indeed disorders of mood, they are much more, and several different symptoms in addition to a mood symptom are required to make a diagnosis of a major depressive episode or a manic episode. Each symptom can be matched to a hypothetically malfunctioning neuronal circuit. The monoamine hypothesis of depression suggests that dysfunction, generally due to underactivity, of one or more of the three monoamines DA, NE, or 5HT may be linked to symptoms in major depression. Boosting one or more of the monoamines in specific brain regions may improve the efficiency of information processing there, and reduce the symptom caused by that area's malfunctioning. Other brain areas associated with the symptoms of a manic episode can similarly be mapped to various hypothetically malfunctioning brain circuits. Understanding the localization of symptoms in circuits, as well as the neurotransmitters that regulate these circuits in different brain regions, can set the stage for choosing and combining treatments for each individual symptom of a mood disorder, with the goal being to reduce all symptoms and lead to remission.

In this chapter, we will review pharmacological concepts underlying the use of antidepressant drugs. There are many different classes of antidepressants and dozens of individual drugs. The goal of this chapter is to acquaint the reader with current ideas about how the various antidepressants work. We will explain the mechanisms of action of these drugs by building upon general pharmacological concepts introduced in earlier chapters. We will also discuss concepts about how to use these drugs in clinical practice, including strategies for what to do if initial treatments fail and how to rationally combine one antidepressant with another, or with a modulating agent. Finally, we will introduce the reader to several new antidepressants in clinical development.

Our discussion of antidepressants in this chapter is at the conceptual level, and not at the pragmatic level. The reader should consult standard drug handbooks (such as the companion *Stahl's Essential Psychopharmacology: the Prescriber's Guide*) for details of doses, side effects, drug interactions, and other issues relevant to the prescribing of these drugs in clinical practice. Here we will discuss putting together an antidepressant "portfolio" of two or more mechanisms of action, often requiring more than one drug, as a strategy for patients who have not responded to a single pharmacological mechanism. This treatment strategy for depression is very different than that for schizophrenia, where single antipsychotic drugs as treatments are the rule and the expected improvement in symptomatology may be only a 20–30% reduction of symptoms with few if any patients with schizophrenia becoming truly asymptomatic and in remission. Thus, the chance to reach a genuine state of sustained and asymptomatic remission in major depression is the challenge for those who treat this disorder; this is the reason for learning the mechanisms of action of so many drugs, the complex biological rationale for combining specific sets of drugs, and the practical tactics for tailoring a unique drug treatment portfolio to fit the needs of an individual patient.

General principles of antidepressant action

Patients who have a major depressive episode and who receive treatment with any antidepressant often experience improvement in their symptoms, and when this improvement reaches the level of 50% reduction of symptoms or more, it is called a response (Figure 7-1). This used to be the goal of treatment with antidepressants: namely, reduce symptoms substantially, and at least by 50%. However, the paradigm for antidepressant treatment has shifted dramatically in recent years so that now the goal of treatment is complete remission of symptoms (Figure 7-2), while maintaining that level of improvement so that the patient's major depressive episode does not relapse shortly after remission, nor does the patient have a recurrent episode in the future (Figure 7-3). Given the known limits to the efficacy of available antidepressants, especially when multiple antidepressant

treatment options are not deployed aggressively and early in the course of this illness, the goal of sustained remission can be difficult to reach. In fact, remission is usually not even reached with the first antidepressant treatment choice.

Do antidepressants work anymore in clinical trials?

Although remission (Figure 7-2) without relapse or recurrence (Figure 7-3) is the widely accepted goal of antidepressant treatment, it is becoming more and more difficult to prove that antidepressants – even well-established antidepressants – work any better than placebo in clinical trials. This is generally due to the fact that in modern clinical trials, the placebo effect has inflated so much over recent decades that placebo now seems to work as well as antidepressants in some trials and nearly as well as antidepressants in other trials. Why this is occurring is the subject of vigorous debate. Some experts propose that it is due to problems conducting clinical ratings in a clinical trial setting that is now unlike a clinical practice setting since patients are seen weekly, often for hours, whether they receive an antidepressant or not; other experts point out that subjects in trials may really be "symptomatic volunteers" who are less ill and less complicated than "real" patients. Critics of psychiatry and psychopharmacology proclaim from clinical trial evidence that antidepressants don't even work and that their side effects and costs do not justify their use at all. This phenomenon of shrinking and erratic efficacy of long-established antidepressants as well as new antidepressants in clinical trials has also caused

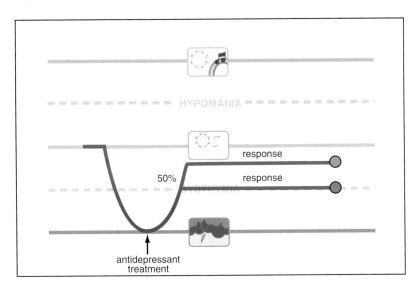

Figure 7-1. Response. When treatment of depression results in at least 50% improvement in symptoms, it is called a response. Such patients are better but not well. Previously, this was considered the goal of depression treatment.

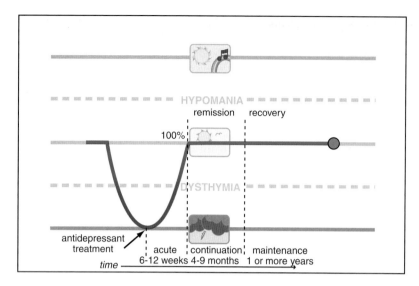

Figure 7-2. Remission. When treatment of depression results in removal of essentially all symptoms, it is called remission for the first several months and then recovery if it is sustained for longer than 6 months. Such patients are not just better – they are well. However, they are not cured, since depression can still recur. Remission and recovery are now the goals when treating patients with depression.

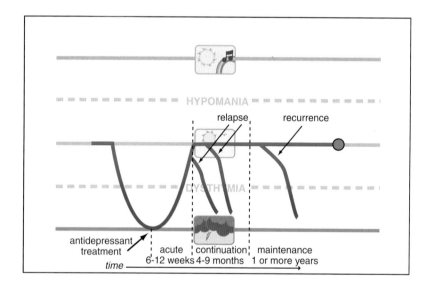

Figure 7-3. Relapse and recurrence. When depression returns before there is a full remission of symptoms or within the first several months following remission of symptoms, it is called a relapse. When depression returns after a patient has recovered, it is called a recurrence.

the pharmaceutical industry to increasingly abandon the development of new antidepressants. Even patients seem to be affected by this debate, perhaps losing their confidence in the efficacy of antidepressants, since up to a third of patients in a real clinical practice setting never fill their first antidepressant prescription, and for those who do, perhaps less than half get a second month of treatment and maybe less than a quarter get an adequate trial of 3 months or longer. One thing is for sure about antidepressants, and that is that they don't work if you don't take them. Thus, the clinical effectiveness of antidepressants in clinical practice

settings is reduced by this failure of "persistency" of treatment for a long enough period of time to give the drug a chance to work.

Whatever the cause of this controversy over the efficacy of antidepressants in clinical trials, one only needs to spend a short time in a clinical practice setting to be convinced that antidepressants are powerful therapeutic agents in many patients. Nevertheless, there have been some useful consequences of the debate on the efficacy of antidepressants, such as re-energizing the integration of psychotherapies with antidepressants, searching for new non-medication

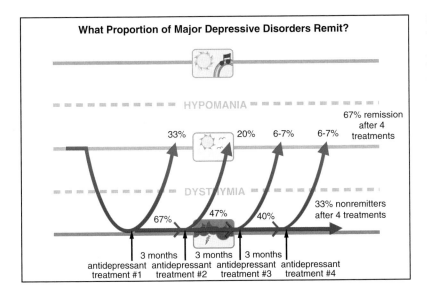

What Proportion of Major Depressive Disorders Remit?

67% remission after 4 treatments

33% | 20% | 6-7% | 6-7%

67% | 47% | 40% | 33% nonremitters after 4 treatments

3 months | 3 months | 3 months
antidepressant treatment #1 | antidepressant treatment #2 | antidepressant treatment #3 | antidepressant treatment #4

HYPOMANIA

DYSTHYMIA

Figure 7-4. Remission rates in MDD. Approximately one-third of depressed patients will remit during treatment with any antidepressant initially. Unfortunately, for those who fail to remit, the likelihood of remission with another antidepressant monotherapy goes down with each successive trial. Thus, after a year of treatment with four sequential antidepressants taken for 12 weeks each, only two-thirds of patients will have achieved remission.

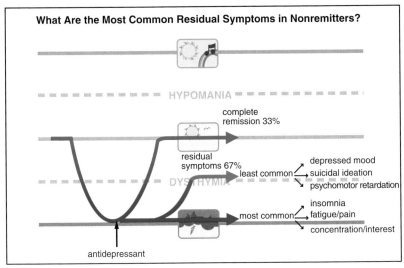

What Are the Most Common Residual Symptoms in Nonremitters?

HYPOMANIA

complete remission 33%

residual symptoms 67%

least common — depressed mood / suicidal ideation / psychomotor retardation

DYSTHYMIA

most common — insomnia / fatigue/pain / concentration/interest

antidepressant

Figure 7-5. Common residual symptoms. In patients who do not achieve remission, the most common residual symptoms are insomnia, fatigue, painful physical complaints, problems concentrating, and lack of interest. The least common residual symptoms are depressed mood, suicidal ideation, and psychomotor retardation.

neurostimulation therapeutics, and studying the combination of currently available antidepressants in order to gain better outcomes, all of which will be discussed in this chapter.

How well do antidepressants work in the real world?

"Real world" trials of antidepressants tested in clinical practice settings that include patients normally excluded from marketing trials, such as the STAR*D trial of antidepressants (Sequenced Treatment Alternatives to Relieve Depression), have recently provided sobering results. Only a third of such patients remit on their first antidepressant treatment, and even after a year of treatment with a sequence of four different

antidepressants given for 12 weeks each, only about two-thirds of depressed patients achieve remission of their symptoms (Figure 7-4).

What are the most common symptoms that persist after antidepressant treatment, causing this disorder not to go into remission? The answer is shown in Figure 7-5, and the symptoms include insomnia, fatigue, multiple painful physical complaints (even though these are not part of the formal diagnostic criteria for depression), as well as problems concentrating, and lack of interest or motivation. Antidepressants appear to work fairly well in improving depressed mood, suicidal ideation, and psychomotor retardation (Figure 7-5).

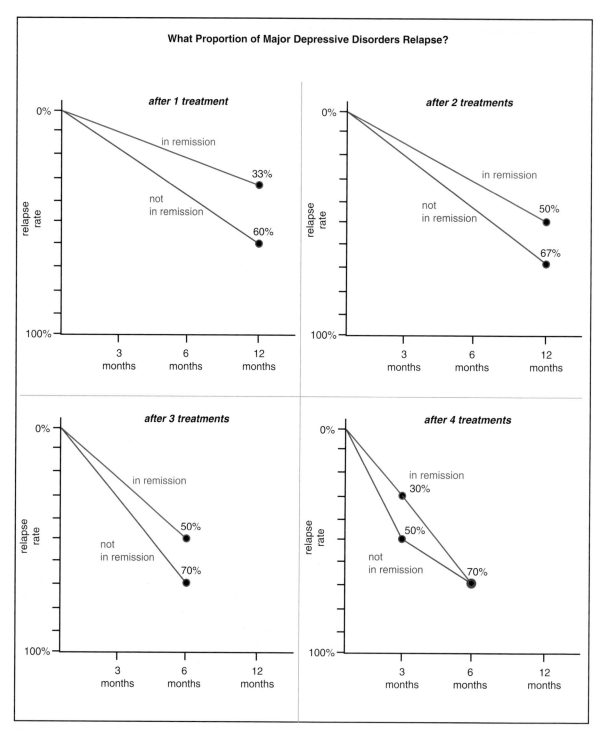

Figure 7-6. Relapse rates. The rate of relapse of major depression is significantly less for patients who achieve remission. However, there is still risk of relapse even in remitters, and the likelihood increases with the number of treatments it takes to get the patient to remit. Thus the relapse rate for patients who do not remit ranges from 60% at 12 months after one treatment to 70% at 6 months after four treatments; but for those who do remit, it ranges from only 33% at 12 months after one treatment all the way to 70% at 6 months after four treatments. In other words, the protective nature of remission virtually disappears once it takes four treatments to achieve remission.

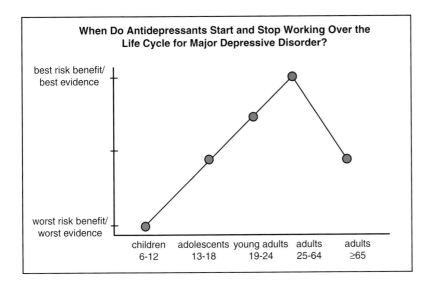

When Do Antidepressants Start and Stop Working Over the Life Cycle for Major Depressive Disorder?

best risk benefit/
best evidence

worst risk benefit/
worst evidence

| children 6-12 | adolescents 13-18 | young adults 19-24 | adults 25-64 | adults ≥65 |

Figure 7-7. Antidepressants over the life cycle. The efficacy, tolerability, and safety of antidepressants have been studied mostly in individuals between the ages of 25 and 64. Existing data across all age groups suggest that the risk–benefit ratio is most favorable for adults between the ages of 25 and 64 and somewhat less so for adults between the ages of 19 and 24, due to a possibly increased risk of suicidality in younger adults. Limited data in children and adolescents also suggest increased risk of suicidality; this, coupled with a lack of data demonstrating clear antidepressant efficacy, gives children between the ages of 6 and 12 the worst risk–benefit ratio, with adolescents intermediate between young adults and children. Elderly patients, 65 years of age and older, may not respond as well or as quickly to antidepressants as other adults and may also experience more side effects than younger adults.

Why should we care whether a patient is in remission from major depression or has just a few persistent symptoms? The answer can be found in Figure 7-6, which shows both good news and bad news about antidepressant treatment over the long run. The good news is that if an antidepressant gets your patient into remission, that patient has a significantly lower relapse rate. The bad news is that there are still very frequent relapses in the remitters, and these relapse rates get worse the more treatments the patient needs to take in order to get into remission (Figure 7-6).

Data like these have galvanized researchers and clinicians alike to treat patients to the point of remission of all symptoms whenever possible, and to try to intervene as early as possible in this illness of major depression, not only to be merciful in trying to relieve current suffering from depressive symptoms, but also because of the possibility that aggressive treatment may prevent disease progression. The concept of disease progression in major depression is controversial, unproven, and provocative, but makes a good deal of sense intuitively for many clinicians and investigators (Figure 6-23). The idea is that chronicity of major depression, development of treatment resistance, and likelihood of relapse could all be reduced, with a better overall outcome, with aggressive treatment of major depressive episodes that leads to remission of all symptoms, thus potentially modifiying the course of this illness. This may pose an especially difficult challenge for treatment of younger patients, where

risks versus benefits of antidepressants are currently debated (Figure 7-7).

Antidepressants over the life cycle

Adults between the ages of 25 and 64 might have the best chance of getting a good response and with the best tolerability to an antidepressant (Figure 7-7). Adults aged 65 or older may not respond as quickly or as robustly to antidepressants, especially if their first episode starts at this age, and especially when their presenting symptoms are lack of interest and cognitive dysfunction rather than depressed mood, but do not have increased suicidality from taking an antidepressant. At the other end of the adult age range, those younger than 25 may benefit from antidepressant efficacy but with a slightly but statistically greater risk of suicidality (but not completed suicide) (Figure 7-7). Age is thus an important consideration for whether, when, and how to treat a patient with antidepressants throughout the life cycle, and with what potential risk versus benefit.

Antidepressant classes
Blocking monoamine transporters

Classic antidepressant action is to block one or more of the transporters for serotonin, norepinephrine, and/or dopamine. This pharmacologic action is entirely consistent with the monoamine hypothesis of depression, which states that monoamines are

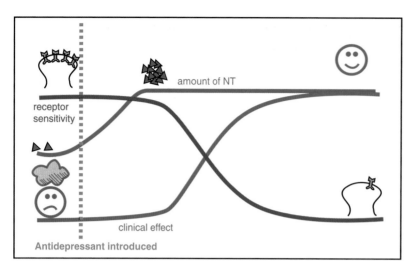

amount of NT

receptor
sensitivity

clinical effect

Antidepressant introduced

Figure 7-8. Time course of antidepressant effects. This figure depicts the different time courses for three effects of antidepressant drugs – namely, clinical changes, neurotransmitter (NT) changes, and receptor sensitivity changes. Specifically, the amount of NT changes relatively rapidly after an antidepressant is introduced. However, the clinical effect is delayed, as is the desensitization, or downregulation, of neurotransmitter receptors. This temporal correlation of clinical effects with changes in receptor sensitivity has given rise to the hypothesis that changes in neurotransmitter receptor sensitivity may actually mediate the clinical effects of antidepressant drugs. These clinical effects include not only antidepressant and anxiolytic actions but also the development of tolerance to the acute side effects of antidepressant drugs.

somehow depleted (Figure 6-34B), and when boosted with effective antidepressants relieve depression (Figure 7-8). One problem for the monoamine hypothesis, however, is that the action of antidepressants at monoamine transporters can raise monoamine levels quite rapidly in some brain areas, and certainly sooner than the antidepressant clinical effects occur in patients weeks later (Figure 7-8). How could immediate changes in neurotransmitter levels caused by antidepressants be linked to clinical actions that are much later in time? The answer may be that the acute increases in neurotransmitter levels cause adaptive changes in neurotransmitter *receptor sensitivity* in a delayed time course consistent with the onset of clinical antidepressant actions (Figure 7-8). Specifically, acutely enhanced synaptic levels of neurotransmitter (Figure 7-9A) could lead to adaptive downregulation and desensitization of postsynaptic neurotransmitter receptors over time (Figure 7-9B).

This concept of antidepressants causing changes in neurotransmitter receptor sensitivity is also consistent with the neurotransmitter receptor hypothesis of depression causing upregulation of neurotransmitter receptors in the first place (Figure 7-9A). Thus, antidepressants theoretically reverse this pathological upregulation of receptors over time (Figure 7-9B). Furthermore, the time course of receptor adaptation fits both with the onset of therapeutic effects and with the onset of tolerance to many side effects. Different receptors likely mediate these different actions, but both the onset of therapeutic action and the onset of

tolerance to side effects may occur with the same delayed time course.

Adaptive changes in receptor number or sensitivity are likely the result of alterations in gene expression (Figure 7-10). This may include not only turning off the synthesis of neurotransmitter receptors, but also increasing the synthesis of various neurotrophic factors such as BDNF (brain-derived neurotrophic factor) (Figure 7-10), as also discussed in Chapter 6 and illustrated in Figures 6-36 through 6-38. Such mechanisms may apply broadly to all effective antidepressants, and may provide a final common pathway for the action of antidepressants.

Selective serotonin reuptake inhibitors (SSRIs)

Rarely has a class of drugs transformed a field as dramatically as have the SSRIs transformed clinical psychopharmacology. Some estimate that SSRI prescriptions in the US alone occur at the rate of six prescriptions per second, 24/7, year round. Already prominent in Europe, SSRIs are now entering Japan and all across Asia, with increasing use throughout the entire world. Clinical indications for the use of SSRIs range far beyond major depressive disorder, especially to a number of anxiety disorders, and also to premenstrual dysphoric disorder, eating disorders, and beyond. There are six principal agents in this group that all share the common property of serotonin reuptake inhibition, and thus they all belong to

Neurotransmitter Receptor Hypothesis of Antidepressant Action

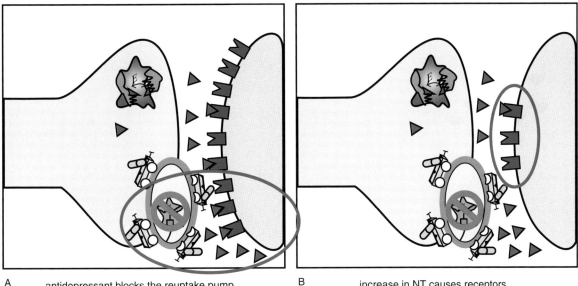

A antidepressant blocks the reuptake pump, causing more NT to be in the synapse

B increase in NT causes receptors to downregulate

Figure 7-9. Neurotransmitter receptor hypothesis of antidepressant action. Although antidepressants cause an immediate increase in monoamines, they do not have immediate therapeutic effects. This may be explained by the monoamine receptor hypothesis of depression, which states that depression is caused by upregulation of monoamine receptors; thus antidepressant efficacy would be related to downregulation of those receptors, as shown here. (A) When an antidepressant blocks a monoamine reuptake pump, this causes more neurotransmitter (NT) (in this case, norepinephrine) to accumulate in the synapse. (B) The increased availability of NT ultimately causes receptors to downregulate. The time course of receptor adaptation is consistent both with the delayed clinical effects of antidepressants and with development of tolerance to antidepressant side effects.

the same drug class, known as SSRIs. However, each of these six drugs also has unique pharmacological properties that allow them to be distinguished from each other. First, we will discuss what these six drugs share in common, and then we will explore their distinctive individual properties that allow sophisticated prescribers to match specific drug profiles to individual patient symptom profiles.

What the six SSRIs have in common

All six SSRIs have the same major pharmacologic feature in common: selective and potent inhibition of serotonin reuptake, also known as inhibition of the serotonin transporter or SERT (Figure 7-11). This simple concept was introduced in Chapter 5 and illustrated in Figure 5-14 and is shown here in Figure 7-12. Although the action of SSRIs at the *presynaptic axon terminal* has classically been emphasized (Figure 7-12), it now appears that events occurring at the *somatodendritic* end of the serotonin neuron (near the cell body) may be more important in explaining the therapeutic actions of the SSRIs (Figures 7-13 through 7-17). That

is, in the depressed state, the monoamine hypothesis of depression states that serotonin may be deficient, both at presynaptic somatodendritic areas near the cell body (on the left in Figure 7-13) and in the synapse itself near the axon terminal (on the right in Figure 7-13). The neurotransmitter receptor hypothesis proposes that monoamine receptors may be upregulated as shown in Figure 7-13, representing the depressed state before treatment. Neuronal firing rates may also be dysregulated in depression, contributing to regional abnormalities in information processing, and the development of specific symptoms depending upon the region affected, as discussed in Chapter 6 and shown in Figures 6-33 and 6-45.

When an SSRI is given acutely, it is well known that 5HT rises due to blockade of SERT. What is somewhat surprising, however, is that blocking the presynaptic SERT does *not* immediately lead to a great deal of serotonin in many synapses. In fact, when SSRI treatment is initiated, 5HT rises to much greater levels at the somatodendritic area located in the midbrain raphe (on the left in Figure 7-14) due to

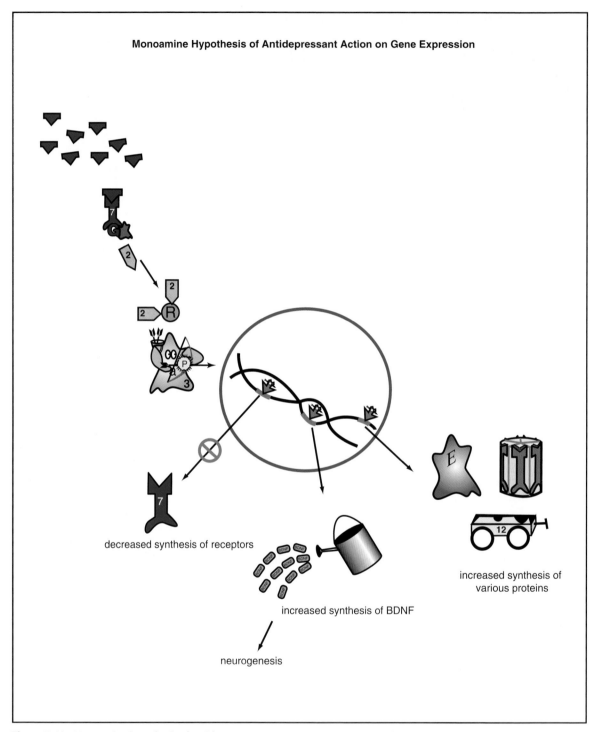

Figure 7-10. Monoamine hypothesis of antidepressant action on gene expression. Adaptations in receptor number or sensitivity are likely due to alterations in gene expression, as shown here. The neurotransmitter at the top is presumably increased by an antidepressant. The cascading consequence of this is ultimately to change the expression of critical genes in order to effect an antidepressant response. This includes downregulating some genes so that there is decreased synthesis of receptors as well as upregulating other genes so that there is increased synthesis of critical proteins, such as brain-derived neurotrophic factor (BDNF).

SSRI

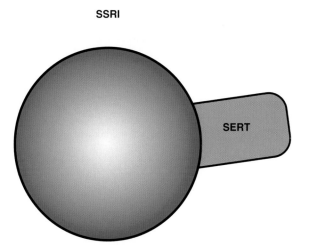

SERT

Figure 7-11. Selective serotonin reuptake inhibitors. Shown here is an icon depicting the core feature of selective serotonin reuptake inhibitors (SSRIs), namely serotonin reuptake inhibition. Although the agents in this class have unique pharmacological profiles, they all share the common property of serotonin transporter (SERT) inhibition.

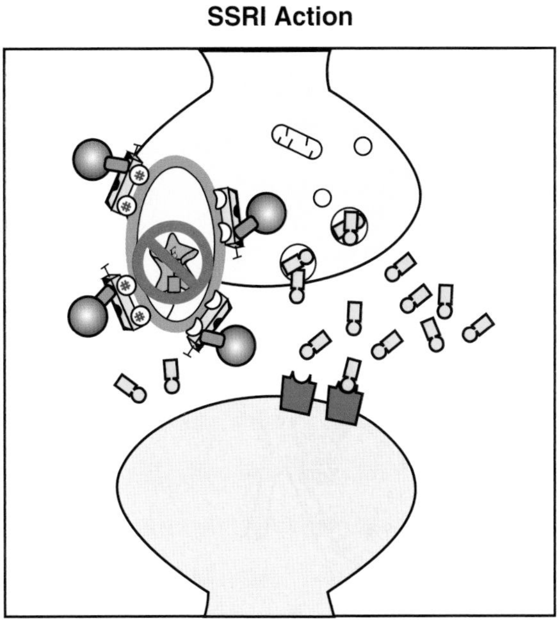

SSRI Action

Figure 7-12. SSRI action. In this figure, the serotonin reuptake inhibitor (SRI) portion of the SSRI molecule is shown inserted into the serotonin reuptake pump (the serotonin transporter, or SERT), blocking it and causing an antidepressant effect.

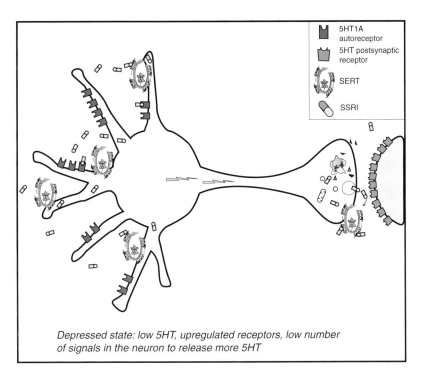

5HT1A
autoreceptor

5HT postsynaptic
receptor

SERT

SSRI

Depressed state: low 5HT, upregulated receptors, low number of signals in the neuron to release more 5HT

Figure 7-13. Mechanism of action of selective serotonin reuptake inhibitors (SSRIs), part 1. Depicted here is a serotonin (5HT) neuron in a depressed patient. In depression, the 5HT neuron is conceptualized as having a relative deficiency of the neurotransmitter 5HT. Also, the number of 5HT receptors is upregulated, including presynaptic 5HT$_{1A}$ autoreceptors as well as postsynaptic 5HT receptors.

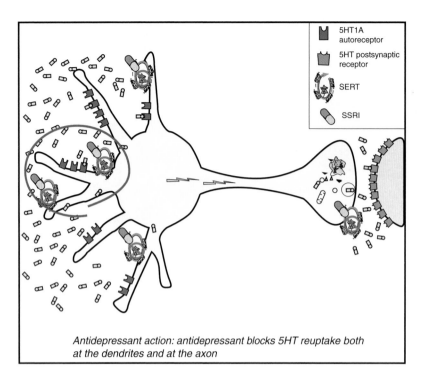

Figure 7-14. Mechanism of action of selective serotonin reuptake inhibitors (SSRIs), part 2. When an SSRI is administered, it immediately blocks the serotonin reuptake pump (see icon of an SSRI drug capsule blocking the reuptake pump, or serotonin transporter [SERT]). However, this causes serotonin to increase initially only in the somatodendritic area of the serotonin neuron (left) and not very much in the axon terminals (right).

5HT1A autoreceptor

5HT postsynaptic receptor

SERT

SSRI

Antidepressant action: antidepressant blocks 5HT reuptake both at the dendrites and at the axon

blockade of SERTs there, rather than in the areas of the brain where the axons terminate (on the right in Figure 7-14).

The somatodendritic area of the serotonin neuron is therefore where 5HT increases first (on the left in Figure 7-14). Serotonin receptors in this brain area have $5HT_{1A}$ pharmacology as discussed in Chapter 5 and illustrated in Figure 5-25. When serotonin levels rise in the somatodendritic area, they stimulate nearby $5HT_{1A}$ autoreceptors (also on the left in Figure 7-14). These immediate pharmacologic actions obviously cannot explain the delayed therapeutic actions of the SSRIs. However, these immediate actions may explain the side effects that are caused by the SSRIs when treatment is initiated.

Over time, the increased 5HT acting at the somatodendritic $5HT_{1A}$ autoreceptors causes them to downregulate and become desensitized (on the left in Figure 7-15). This desensitization occurs because the increase in serotonin is recognized by these presynaptic $5HT_{1A}$ receptors, and this information is sent to the cell nucleus of the serotonin neuron. The genome's reaction to this information is to issue instructions that cause these same receptors to become desensitized over time. The time course of

this desensitization correlates with the onset of therapeutic actions of the SSRIs.

Once the $5HT_{1A}$ somatodendritic autoreceptors are desensitized, 5HT can no longer effectively turn off its own release. Since 5HT is no longer inhibiting its own release, the serotonin neuron is therefore disinhibited (Figure 7-16). This results in a flurry of 5HT release from axons and an increase in neuronal impulse flow (shown as lightning in Figure 7-16 and release of serotonin from the axon terminal on the right). This is just another way of saying the serotonin release is "turned on" at the axon terminals. The serotonin that now pours out of the various projections of serotonin pathways in the brain is what theoretically mediates the various therapeutic actions of the SSRIs.

While the presynaptic somatodendritic $5HT_{1A}$ autoreceptors are desensitizing (Figure 7-15), serotonin is building up in synapses (Figure 7-16), and causes the postsynaptic serotonin receptors to desensitize as well (on the right in Figure 7-17). These various postsynaptic serotonin receptors in turn send information to the cell nucleus of the *postsynaptic* neuron that serotonin is targeting (on the far right of Figure 7-17). The reaction of the genome in the

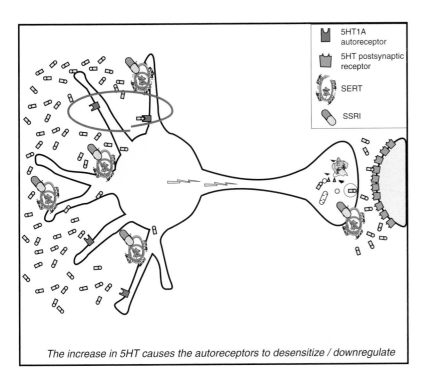

The increase in 5HT causes the autoreceptors to desensitize / downregulate

Figure 7-15. Mechanism of action of selective serotonin reuptake inhibitors (SSRIs), part 3. The consequence of serotonin increasing in the somatodendritic area of the serotonin (5HT) neuron, as depicted in Figure 7-14, is that the somatodendritic 5HT$_{1A}$ autoreceptors desensitize or downregulate (red circle).

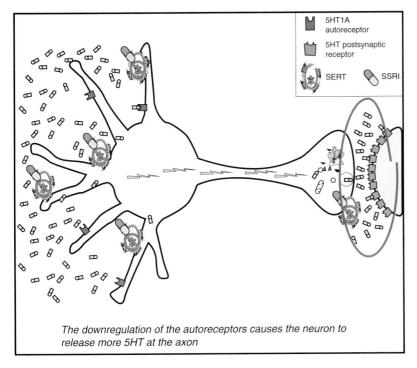

The downregulation of the autoreceptors causes the neuron to release more 5HT at the axon

Figure 7-16. Mechanism of action of selective serotonin reuptake inhibitors (SSRIs), part 4. Once the somatodendritic receptors downregulate, as depicted in Figure 7-15, there is no longer inhibition of impulse flow in the serotonin (5HT) neuron. Thus, neuronal impulse flow is turned on. The consequence of this is release of 5HT in the axon terminal (red circle). However, this increase is delayed as compared with the increase of 5HT in the somatodendritic areas of the 5HT neuron, depicted in Figure 7-14. This delay is the result of the time it takes for somatodendritic 5HT to downregulate the 5HT$_{1A}$ autoreceptors and turn on neuronal impulse flow in the 5HT neuron. This delay may explain why antidepressants do not relieve depression immediately. It is also the reason why the mechanism of action of antidepressants may be linked to increasing neuronal impulse flow in 5HT neurons, with 5HT levels increasing at axon terminals before an SSRI can exert its antidepressant effects.

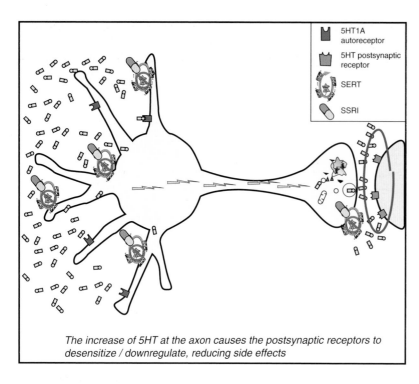

The increase of 5HT at the axon causes the postsynaptic receptors to desensitize / downregulate, reducing side effects

Legend:

5HT1A autoreceptor

5HT postsynaptic receptor

SERT

SSRI

Figure 7-17. Mechanism of action of selective serotonin reuptake inhibitors (SSRIs), part 5. Finally, once the SSRIs have blocked the reuptake pump (or serotonin transporter [SERT] in Figure 7-14), increased somatodendritic serotonin (5HT) (Figure 7-14), desensitized somatodendritic 5HT$_{1A}$ autoreceptors (Figure 7-15), turned on neuronal impulse flow (Figure 7-16), and increased release of 5HT from axon terminals (Figure 7-16), the final step (shown here) may be the desensitization of postsynaptic 5HT receptors. This desensitization may mediate the reduction of side effects of SSRIs as tolerance develops.

postsynaptic neuron is also to issue instructions to downregulate or desensitize these receptors as well. The time course of this desensitization correlates with the onset of tolerance to the side effects of the SSRIs (Figure 7-17).

This theory thus suggests a pharmacological cascading mechanism whereby the SSRIs exert their therapeutic actions: namely, powerful but delayed disinhibition of serotonin release in key pathways throughout the brain. Furthermore, side effects are hypothetically caused by the acute actions of serotonin at undesirable receptors in undesirable pathways. Finally, side effects may attenuate over time by desensitization of the very receptors that mediate them.

Unique properties of each SSRI: the not-so-selective serotonin reuptake inhibitors

Although the six SSRIs clearly share the same mechanism of action, individual patients often react very differently to one SSRI versus another. This is not generally observed in large clinical trials, where mean group differences between two SSRIs either in efficacy or in side effects are very difficult to document. Rather, such differences are seen by prescribers treating patients one at a time, with some patients

experiencing a therapeutic response to one SSRI and not another, and other patients tolerating one SSRI and not another.

If blockade of SERT explains the shared clinical and pharmacological actions of SSRIs, what explains their differences? Although there is no generally accepted explanation that accounts for the commonly observed clinical phenomena of different efficacy and tolerability of various SSRIs in individual patients, it makes sense to consider those pharmacologic characteristics of the six SSRIs that are not shared with each other as candidates to explain the broad range of individual patient reactions to different SSRIs (Figures 7-18 through 7-23). Each SSRI has secondary pharmacologic actions other than SERT blockade, and no two SSRIs have identical secondary pharmacological characteristics. Whether these secondary binding profiles can account for the differences in efficacy and tolerability in individual patients remains to be proven. However, it does lead to provocative hypothesis generation and gives a rational basis for psychopharmacologists trying more than one of these agents rather than thinking "they are all the same." Sometimes only an empiric trial of different SSRIs will lead to the best match of drug to an individual patient.

Fluoxetine: an SSRI with 5HT$_{2C}$ antagonist properties

This SSRI also has 5HT$_{2C}$ antagonist actions that may explain many of its unique clinical properties (Figure 7-18). 5HT$_{2C}$ antagonism is explained in Chapter 5 and illustrated in Figures 5-52A and 5-52B. Other antidepressants with 5HT$_{2C}$ antagonist properties include mirtazapine and agomelatine; several atypical antipsychotics including quetiapine with proven antidepressant properties, as well as olanzapine, asenapine, and clozapine, also have potent 5HT$_{2C}$ antagonist actions. Blocking serotonin action at 5HT$_{2C}$ receptors disinhibits (i.e., enhances) release of both NE and DA (Figure 5-52B). 5HT$_{2C}$ antagonism may contribute not only to fluoxetine's therapeutic actions but also to its tolerability profile.

The good news about 5HT$_{2C}$ antagonism may be that it is generally activating, and many patients, even from the first dose, detect an energizing and fatigue-reducing effect of fluoxetine, with improvement in concentration and attention as well. This mechanism is perhaps best matched to depressed patients with reduced positive affect, hypersomnia, psychomotor retardation, apathy, and fatigue (Figure 6-46). Fluoxetine is also approved in some countries in combination with olanzapine for treatment-resistant unipolar depression and for bipolar depression. Since olanzapine

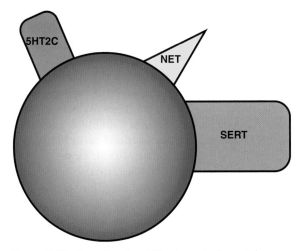

fluoxetine

Figure 7-18. Fluoxetine. In addition to serotonin reuptake inhibition, fluoxetine has norepinephrine reuptake inhibition (NRI) and serotonin 2C (5HT$_{2C}$) antagonist actions. Fluoxetine's activating effects may be due to its actions at 5HT$_{2C}$ receptors. Norepinephrine reuptake inhibition may be clinically relevant only at very high doses. Fluoxetine is also an inhibitor at CYP 2D6 and 3A4.

also has 5HT$_{2C}$ antagonist actions (Figure 5-46), it may be that adding together the 5HT$_{2C}$ antagonist actions of both drugs could theoretically lead to further enhanced DA and NE release in cortex to mediate the antidepressant actions of this combination. 5HT$_{2C}$ antagonism may also contribute to the anti-bulimia effect of higher doses of fluoxetine, the only SSRI approved for the treatment of this eating disorder.

The bad news about 5HT$_{2C}$ antagonism is that it can be activating, so the 5HT$_{2C}$ antagonist actions of fluoxetine may contribute to this agent being sometimes less well matched to patients with agitation, insomnia, and anxiety, who may experience unwanted activation and even a panic attack if given an agent that further activates them.

Other unique properties of fluoxetine (Figure 7-18) are weak NE reuptake blocking properties that may become clinically relevant at very high doses. Fluoxetine has a long half-life (2–3 days), and its active metabolite an even longer half-life (2 weeks). The long half-life is advantageous in that it seems to reduce the withdrawal reactions that are characteristic of sudden discontinuation of some SSRIs, but it also means that it takes a long time to clear the drug and its active metabolite after discontinuing fluoxetine, and prior to starting another agent such as a monoamine oxidase inhibitor (MAOI). Fluoxetine is available not only as a once-daily formulation, but also as a once-weekly oral dosage formulation.

Sertraline: an SSRI with dopamine transporter (DAT) inhibition and σ$_1$ binding

This SSRI has two candidate mechanisms that distinguish it: dopamine transporter (DAT) inhibition and sigma-1 (σ$_1$) receptor binding (Figure 7-19). The DAT inhibitory actions are controversial since they are weaker than the SERT inhibitory actions, thus leading some experts to suggest that there is not sufficient DAT occupancy by sertraline to be clinically relevant. However, as will be discussed later in the section on norepinephrine–dopamine reuptake inhibitors (NDRIs), it is not clear that high degrees of DAT occupancy are necessary or even desirable in order to contribute to antidepressant actions. That is, perhaps only a small amount of DAT inhibition is sufficient to cause improvement in energy, motivation, and concentration, especially when added to another action such as SERT inhibition. In fact,

sertraline

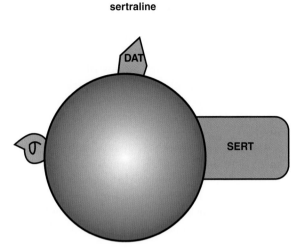

Figure 7-19. Sertraline. Sertraline has dopamine reuptake inhibition (DRI) and σ_1 receptor binding in addition to serotonin reuptake inhibition (SRI). The clinical relevance of sertraline's DRI is unknown, although it may improve energy, motivation, and concentration. Its σ properties may contribute to anxiolytic actions and may also be helpful in patients with psychotic depression.

paroxetine

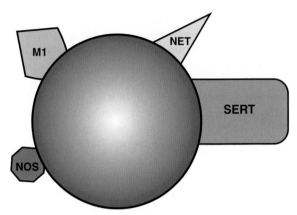

Figure 7-20. Paroxetine. In addition to serotonin reuptake inhibition (SRI), paroxetine has mild anticholinergic actions (M_1), which can be calming or possibly sedating, weak norepinephrine reuptake inhibition (NRI), which may contribute to further antidepressant actions, and inhibition of the enzyme nitric oxide synthetase (NOS), which may contribute to sexual dysfunction. Paroxetine is also a potent inhibitor of CYP 2D6.

high-impact DAT inhibition is the property of reinforcing stimulants, including cocaine and methylphenidate, and would not generally be desired in an antidepressant.

Anecdotally, clinicians have observed the mild and desirable activating actions of sertraline in some patients with "atypical depression," improving symptoms of hypersomnia, low energy, and mood reactivity. A favorite combination of some clinicians for depressed patients is to add bupropion to sertraline (i.e., Wellbutrin to Zoloft, sometimes called "Welloft"), adding together the weak DAT inhibitory properties of each agent. Clinicians have also observed the over-activation of some patients with panic disorder by sertraline, thus requiring slower dose titration in some patients with anxiety symptoms. All of these actions of sertraline are consistent with weak DAT inhibitory actions of sertraline contributing to its clinical portfolio of actions.

The σ_1 actions of sertraline are not well understood, but might contribute to its anxiolytic effects and especially to its effects in psychotic and delusional depression, where sertraline may have advantageous therapeutic effects compared to some other SSRIs. These σ_1 actions could theoretically contribute both to anxiolytic actions and to antipsychotic actions, as will be discussed further in the section on fluvoxamine below.

Paroxetine: an SSRI with muscarinic anticholinergic and norepinephrine transporter (NET) inhibitory actions

This SSRI is preferred by many clinicians for patients with anxiety symptoms. It tends to be more calming, even sedating, early in treatment compared to the more activating actions of both fluoxetine and sertraline discussed above. Perhaps the mild anticholinergic actions of paroxetine contribute to this clinical profile (Figure 7-20). Paroxetine also has weak NET (norepinephrine transporter) inhibitory properties, which could contribute to its efficacy in depression, especially at high doses. The advantages of dual serotonin plus norepinephrine reuptake inhibiting properties, or SNRI actions, are discussed below in the section on SNRIs. It is possible that weak to moderate NET inhibition of paroxetine may contribute importantly to its antidepressant actions.

Paroxetine inhibits the enzyme nitric oxide synthetase, which could theoretically contribute to sexual dysfunction especially in men. Paroxetine is also notorious for causing withdrawal reactions upon sudden discontinuation with symptoms such as akathisia, restlessness, gastrointestinal symptoms, dizziness, and tingling, especially when suddenly discontinued from long-term high-dose treatment. This is possibly due not only to

fluvoxamine

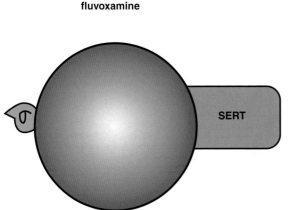

Figure 7-21. Fluvoxamine. Fluvoxamine's secondary properties include actions at σ₁ receptors, which may be anxiolytic as well as beneficial for psychotic depression, and inhibition of CYP 1A2 and 3A4.

citalopram

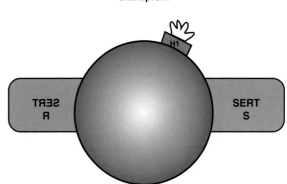

Figure 7-22. Citalopram. Citalopram consists of two enantiomers, R and S. The R enantiomer has weak antihistamine properties and is a weak inhibitor of CYP 2D6.

SERT inhibition properties, since all SSRIs can cause discontinuation reactions, but also to additional contributions from anticholinergic rebound when paroxetine is rapidly discontinued. Paroxetine is available in a controlled-release formulation, which may mitigate some of its side effects, including discontinuation reactions.

Fluvoxamine: an SSRI with σ₁ receptor binding properties

This SSRI was among the first to be launched for the treatment of depression worldwide, but was never officially approved for depression in the US, so has been considered more of an agent for the treatment of obsessive–compulsive disorder and anxiety in the US. A unique binding property of fluvoxamine, like sertraline, is its interaction at σ₁ sites, but this action is more potent for fluvoxamine than for sertraline (Figure 7-21). The physiological function of σ₁ sites is still a mystery, and thus sometimes called the "sigma enigma," but has been linked to both anxiety and psychosis. Although it is not entirely clear how to define an agonist or antagonist at σ₁ sites, recent studies suggest that fluvoxamine may be an agonist at σ₁ receptors, and that this property may contribute an additional pharmacologic action to help explain fluvoxamine's well-known anxiolytic properties. Fluvoxamine also has shown therapeutic activity in both psychotic and delusional depression, where it, like sertraline, may have advantages over other SSRIs.

Fluvoxamine is now available as a controlled-release formulation which makes once-a-day administration

possible, unlike immediate-release fluvoxamine, whose shorter half-life often requires twice-daily administration. In addition, recent trials of controlled-release fluvoxamine show impressive remission rates in both obsessive–compulsive disorder and social anxiety disorder, as well as possibly less peak dose sedation.

Citalopram: an SSRI with a "good" and a "bad" enantiomer

This SSRI is comprised of two enantiomers, R and S, one of which is the mirror image of the other (Figure 7-22). The mixture of these enantiomers is known as racemic citalopram, or commonly just as citalopram, and it has mild antihistaminic properties that reside in the R enantiomer (Figure 7-22). Racemic citalopram is generally one of the better-tolerated SSRIs, and has favorable findings in the treatment of depression in the elderly, but has a somewhat inconsistent therapeutic action at the lowest dose, often requiring dose increase to optimize treatment. However, dose increase is limited due to the potential for QTc prolongation. These findings all suggest that it is not favorable for citalopram to contain the R enantiomer. In fact, some pharmacologic evidence suggests that the R enantiomer may be pharmacologically active at SERT in a manner that does not inhibit SERT but actually interferes with the ability of the active S enantiomer to inhibit SERT. This could lead to reduced inhibition of SERT, reduced synaptic 5HT, and possibly reduced net therapeutic actions, especially at low doses.

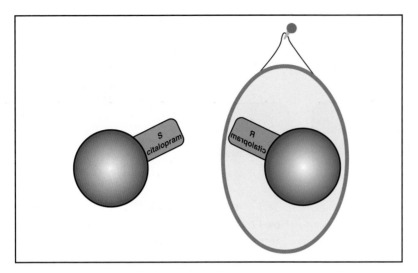

Figure 7-23. Escitalopram. The R and S enantiomers of citalopram are mirror images of each other but have slightly different clinical properties. The R enantiomer is the one with weak antihistamine properties and weak inhibition of CYP 2D6, while the S enantiomer does not have these properties. The R and S enantiomers may also differ in their effects at the serotonin transporter. The S enantiomer of citalopram has been developed and marketed as the antidepressant escitalopram.

Escitalopram: the quintessential SSRI

The solution to improving the properties of racemic citalopram is to remove the unwanted R enantiomer. The resulting drug is known as escitalopram, as it is composed of only the pure active S enantiomer (Figure 7-23). This maneuver appears to remove the antihistaminic properties, and there are no higher dose restrictions to avoid QTc prolongation. In addition, removal of the potentially interfering R isomer makes the lowest dose of escitalopram more predictably efficacious. Escitalopram is therefore the SSRI for which pure SERT inhibition is most likely to explain almost all of its pharmacologic actions. Escitalopram is considered perhaps the best-tolerated SSRI, with the fewest CYP-mediated drug interactions.

Serotonin partial agonist/reuptake inhibitors (SPARIs)

A new antidepressant introduced in the US is vilazodone, which combines SERT inhibition with a second property: $5HT_{1A}$ partial agonism. For this reason, vilazodone is called a SPARI (serotonin partial agonist/reuptake inhibitor) (Figure 7-24). The combination of serotonin reuptake inhibition with $5HT_{1A}$ partial agonism has long been known by clinicians to enhance the antidepressant properties and tolerability of SSRIs/SNRIs in some patients. Although vilazodone is the only approved agent selective for just these two actions, SERT inhibition combined

vilazodone

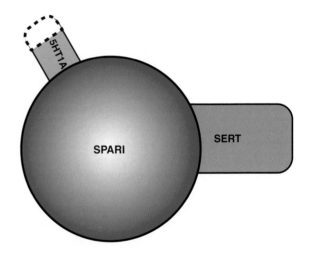

serotonin partial agonist/reuptake inhibitor

Figure 7-24. Vilazodone. Vilazodone is a partial agonist at the $5HT_{1A}$ receptor and also inhibits serotonin reuptake; thus, it is referred to as a serotonin partial agonist/reuptake inhibitor (SPARI). Its effects at $5HT_{1A}$ receptors are equal to or more potent than its effects at serotonin transporters.

with $5HT_{1A}$ partial agonism has been achieved in the past by adding atypical antipsychotics with $5HT_{1A}$ partial agonist actions such as quetiapine or aripiprazole to SSRIs/SNRIs (discussed in Chapter 5: see Figures 5-47 and 5-62). Vilazodone administration, however, is not completely identical to this option since atypical antipsychotics have many additional pharmacologic actions, some desirable and others not (Figures 5-47 and 5-62).

$5HT_{1A}$ partial agonist actions plus SERT inhibition can also be attained by augmenting SSRIs/SNRIs with the $5HT_{1A}$ partial agonist buspirone. However, this is not identical to the actions of vilazodone since buspirone and its active metabolite 6-hydroxybuspirone are weaker $5HT_{1A}$ partial agonists than vilazodone and are estimated to occupy fewer $5HT_{1A}$ receptors for a shorter time at clinically administered doses than does vilazodone. Buspirone and 6-hydroxybuspirone also bind to $5HT_{1A}$ receptors with lower affinity than 5HT itself, whereas vilazodone binds to $5HT_{1A}$ receptors with higher affinity than 5HT. This suggests that administration of buspirone as an augmenting agent to an SSRI/SNRI likely results in $5HT_{1A}$ receptor occupancy that occurs more robustly in states of low 5HT levels and not as robustly in states of high 5HT levels, whereas administration of vilazodone results in binding to $5HT_{1A}$ receptors even in the presence of 5HT. Another difference between buspirone plus an SSRI/SNRI versus vilazodone is that when buspirone augments an SSRI, the buspirone is generally dosed so that about 10–20% of $5HT_{1A}$ receptors are occupied

and the SSRI is dosed so that about 80% of SERTs are blocked. On the other hand, human neuroimaging studies suggest that vilazodone is dosed so that about 50% of both SERTs and $5HT_{1A}$ receptors are occupied. Whether this accounts for clinically significant differences between the administration of vilazodone monotherapy and the augmentation of SSRIs/SNRIs with buspirone is not known, but it could account for the apparent lesser incidence of sexual dysfunction with vilazodone than with either SSRIs alone or with the augmentation of SSRIs with buspirone. It is not known whether the enhanced efficacy of buspirone combined with SSRIs for depression demonstrated in clinical trials for patients who fail SSRI monotherapy also applies to vilazodone, as appropriate clinical trials to determine this have not yet been conducted. In animal models, adding $5HT_{1A}$ partial agonism to SSRIs causes more immediate and robust elevations of brain 5HT levels than SSRIs do alone. This is thought to be due to the fact that $5HT_{1A}$ partial agonists are a type of "artificial serotonin" selective especially for presynaptic somatodendritic $5HT_{1A}$ autoreceptors, and that $5HT_{1A}$ partial agonist action occurs immediately after drug is given (Figure 7-25). Thus, $5HT_{1A}$ immediate partial agonist actions are theoretically additive or

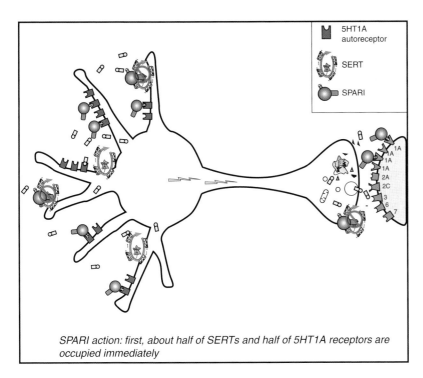

Figure 7-25. Mechanism of action of serotonin partial agonist/reuptake inhibitors (SPARIs), part 1. When a SPARI is administered, about half of serotonin transporters (SERTs) and half of serotonin 1A ($5HT_{1A}$) receptors are occupied immediately.

5HT1A autoreceptor

SERT

SPARI

SPARI action: first, about half of SERTs and half of 5HT1A receptors are occupied immediately

301

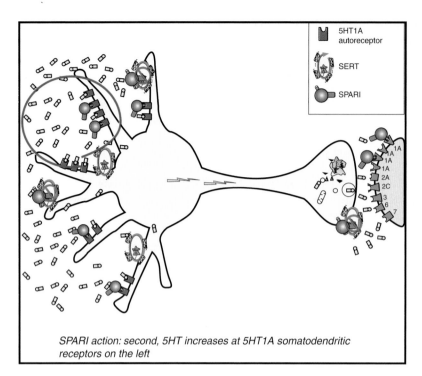

Figure 7-26. Mechanism of action of serotonin partial agonist/reuptake inhibitors (SPARIs), part 2. Blockade of the serotonin transporter (SERT) causes serotonin to increase initially in the somatodendritic area of the serotonin neuron (left).

5HT1A autoreceptor

SERT

SPARI

SPARI action: second, 5HT increases at 5HT1A somatodendritic receptors on the left

synergistic with simultaneous SERT inhibition, since this leads to faster and more robust actions at $5HT_{1A}$ somatodendritic autoreceptors (Figure 7-26) than with SERT inhibition alone (Figure 7-14), including their downregulation (Figure 7-27). This hypothetically causes faster and more robust elevation of synaptic 5HT (Figure 7-28) than is possible with SSRIs alone (Figure 7-16). In addition, $5HT_{1A}$ partial agonism with vilazodone's SPARI mechanism occurs immediately at postsynaptic $5HT_{1A}$ receptors (Figure 7-26), with actions at these receptors that are thus faster and with a different type of stimulation compared to the delayed full agonist actions of serotonin itself when increased by SERT inhibition alone (Figure 7-16). The down-stream actions of $5HT_{1A}$ receptors that lead to enhanced dopamine release (Figure 7-29), discussed in Chapter 5 and illustrated in Figures 5-15C and 5-16C, may be hypothetically responsible for the observed reduction in sexual dysfunction seen in patients with the combination of SERT inhibition plus $5HT_{1A}$ partial agonist actions compared to SERT inhibition alone.

Theoretically, SPARI actions could lead to faster antidepressant onset, if rapid elevation of 5HT is linked to rapid antidepressant onset. However,

clinical studies do not support this, because the rapid increase in serotonin is not well tolerated, due especially to gastrointestinal side effects, and dose titration must be slowed down in order to attain full dosing, also slowing down any potential rapid antidepressant onset. SPARI actions could hypothetically lead to more antidepressant efficacy than selective SERT inhibition, as suggested by buspirone augmentation of SSRIs, but this has not been demonstrated yet in head-to-head trials of vilazodone against an SSRI. Finally, SPARI actions could theoretically lead to less sexual dysfunction, due to lesser degrees of SERT inhibition than SSRIs plus favorable downstream dopaminergic actions. Low sexual dysfunction is shown for vilazodone in placebo-controlled trials but not yet proven to be less than that associated with SSRIs in head-to-head trials.

Serotonin–norepinephrine reuptake inhibitors (SNRIs)

SNRIs combine the robust SERT inhibition of the SSRIs with various degrees of inhibition of the nor-epinephrine transporter (or NET) (Figures 7-30

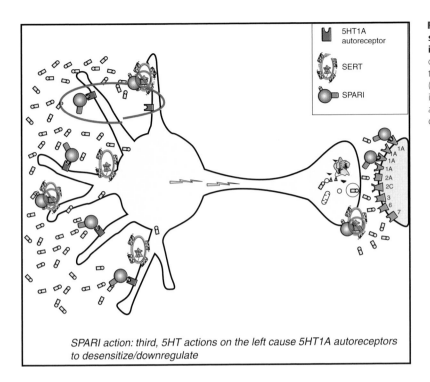

SPARI action: third, 5HT actions on the left cause 5HT1A autoreceptors to desensitize/downregulate

Figure 7-27. Mechanism of action of serotonin partial agonist/reuptake inhibitors (SPARIs), part 3. The consequence of serotonin increasing in the somatodendritic area of the serotonin (5HT) neuron, as depicted in Figure 7-26, is that the somatodendritic 5HT$_{1A}$ autoreceptors desensitize or downregulate (red circle).

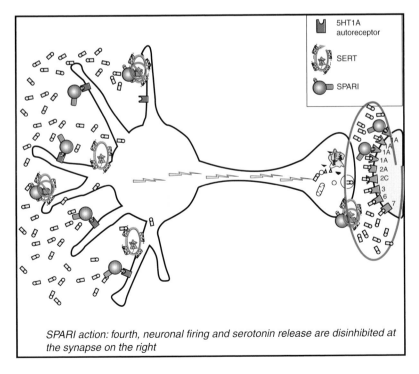

SPARI action: fourth, neuronal firing and serotonin release are disinhibited at the synapse on the right

Figure 7-28. Mechanism of action of serotonin partial agonist/reuptake inhibitors (SPARIs), part 4. Once the somatodendritic receptors downregulate, as depicted in Figure 7-27, there is no longer inhibition of impulse flow in the serotonin (5HT) neuron. Thus, neuronal impulse flow is turned on. The consequence of this is release of 5HT in the axon terminal (red circle).

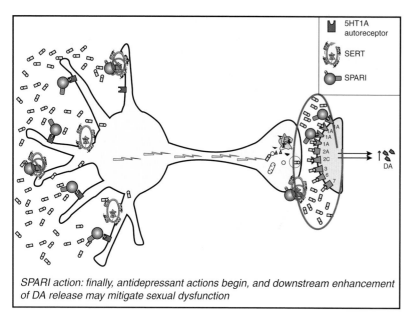

Figure 7-29. Mechanism of action of serotonin partial agonist/reuptake inhibitors (SPARIs), part 5. Finally, once the SPARIs have blocked the serotonin transporter (SERT) (Figure 7-25], increased somatodendritic serotonin (5HT) (Figure 7-26), desensitized somatodendritic 5HT$_{1A}$ autoreceptors (Figure 7-27), turned on neuronal impulse flow (Figure 7-28), and increased release of 5HT from axon terminals (Figure 7-28), the final step (shown here, red circle) may be the desensitization of postsynaptic 5HT receptors. This timeframe correlates with antidepressant action. In addition, the predominance of 5HT$_{1A}$ actions may lead to downstream enhancement of dopamine (DA) release, which may mitigate sexual dysfunction.

SPARI action: finally, antidepressant actions begin, and downstream enhancement of DA release may mitigate sexual dysfunction

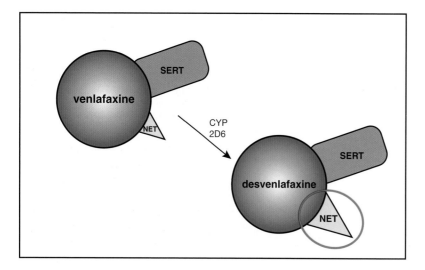

Figure 7-30. Venlafaxine and desvenlafaxine. Venlafaxine inhibits reuptake of both serotonin (SRI) and norepinephrine (NRI), thus combining two therapeutic mechanisms in one agent. Venlafaxine's serotonergic actions are present at low doses, while its noradrenergic actions are progressively enhanced as dose increases. Venlafaxine is converted to its active metabolite, desvenlafaxine, by CYP 2D6. Like venlafaxine, desvenlafaxine inhibits reuptake of serotonin (SRI) and norepinephrine (NRI), but its NRI actions are greater relative to its SRI actions compared to venlafaxine. Venlafaxine administration usually results in plasma levels of venlafaxine that are about half those of desvenlafaxine; however, this can vary depending on genetic polymorphisms of CYP 2D6 and whether patients are taking drugs that are inhibitors or inducers of CYP 2D6. Thus the degree of NET inhibition with venlafaxine administration may be unpredictable. Desvenlafaxine has now been developed as a separate drug. It has relatively greater norepinephrine reuptake inhibition (NRI) than venlafaxine but is still more potent at the serotonin transporter.

through 7-33). Theoretically, there should be some therapeutic advantage of adding NET inhibition to SERT inhibition, since one mechanism may add efficacy to the other mechanism by widening the reach of these antidepressants to the monoamine neurotransmitter systems throughout more brain regions. A practical indication that dual monoamine mechanisms may lead to more efficacy is the finding that the SNRI venlafaxine frequently seems to have greater antidepressant efficacy as the dose increases,

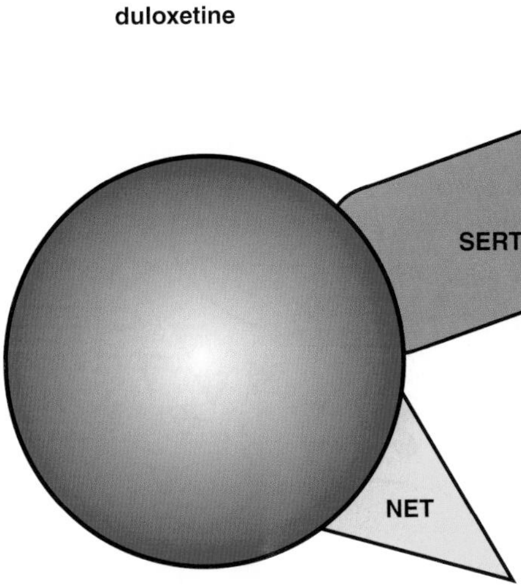

duloxetine

milnacipran

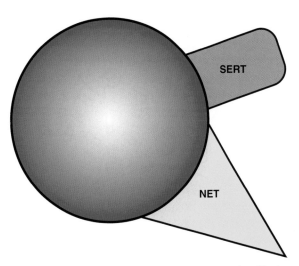

Figure 7-31. Duloxetine. Duloxetine inhibits reuptake of both serotonin (SRI) and norepinephrine (NRI). Its noradrenergic actions may contribute to efficacy for painful physical symptoms. Duloxetine is also an inhibitor of CYP 2D6.

Figure 7-32. Milnacipran. Milnacipran inhibits reuptake of both serotonin (SRI) and norepinephrine (NRI) but is a more potent inhibitor of the norepinephrine transporter (NET) than the serotonin transporter (SERT). Its robust NET inhibition may contribute to efficacy for painful physical symptoms.

theoretically due to recruiting more and more NET inhibition as the dose is raised (i.e., the noradrenergic "boost"). Clinicians and experts currently debate whether remission rates are higher with SNRIs compared to SSRIs or whether SNRIs are more helpful than other options in depressed patients who fail to respond to SSRIs. One area where SNRIs have established clear efficacy but SSRIs have not is in the treatment of multiple pain syndromes. SNRIs also may have greater efficacy than SSRIs in the treatment of vasomotor symptoms associated with perimenopause, although this is not as well established.

NET inhibition increases DA in prefrontal cortex

Although SNRIs are commonly called "dual action" serotonin–norepinephrine agents, they actually have a third action on dopamine in the prefrontal cortex, but not elsewhere in the brain. Thus, they are not "full" triple action agents since they do not inhibit the dopamine transporter (DAT), but SNRIs can perhaps be considered to have "two-and-a-half" actions, rather than just two. That is, SNRIs not only boost serotonin and norepinephrine throughout the brain (Figure 7-33), but they also boost dopamine specifically in prefrontal cortex (Figure 7-34). This third mechanism of boosting dopamine in an important area of the brain associated with several symptoms of depression should add another theoretical advantage to the pharmacology of SNRIs and to their efficacy in the treatment of major depression.

How does NET inhibition boost DA in prefrontal cortex? The answer is illustrated in Figure 7-34. In prefrontal cortex, SERTs and NETs are present in abundance on serotonin and norepinephrine nerve terminals, respectively, but there are very few DATs on dopamine nerve terminals in this part of the brain (Figure 7-34). The consequence of this is that once DA is released, it is free to cruise away from the synapse (Figure 7-34A). The diffusion radius of DA is thus wider (Figure 7-34A) than is the diffusion radius of NE in prefrontal cortex (Figure 7-34B), since there is NET at the NE synapse (Figure 7-34B) but no DAT at the DA synapse (Figure 7-34A). This arrangement may enhance the regulatory importance of dopamine in prefrontal cortex functioning, since DA in this part of the brain can interact with DA receptors not only at its own synapse but at a distance, perhaps enhancing the ability of DA to regulate cognition in an entire area within its diffusion radius, not just at a single synapse. This was discussed in Chapter 1 and illustrated in Figure 1-7.

Dopamine action is therefore not terminated by DAT in prefrontal cortex, but by two other mechanisms. That is, DA diffuses away from the DA synapse until it either encounters the enzyme COMT (catchol-O-methyl-transferase), which degrades it

SNRI Action

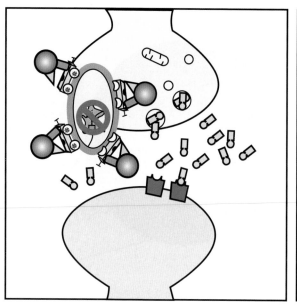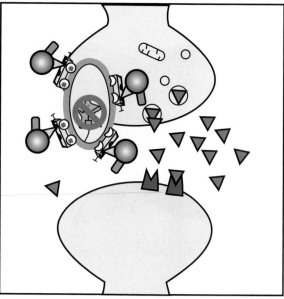

Figure 7-33. SNRI actions. In this figure, the dual actions of the serotonin–norepinephrine reuptake inhibitors (SNRIs) are shown. Both the serotonin reuptake inhibitor (SRI) portion of the SNRI molecule (left panel) and the norepinephrine reuptake inhibitor (NRI) portion of the SNRI molecule (right panel) are inserted into their respective reuptake pumps. Consequently, both pumps are blocked, and the drug mediates an antidepressant effect.

(see Figure 4-6), or until it encounters a norepinephrine reuptake pump, or NET, which transports it into the NE neuron (Figure 7-34A). NETs in fact have a greater affinity for DA than they do for NE, so they will pump DA as well as NE into NE nerve terminals, halting the action of either.

What is interesting is to see what happens when NET is inhibited in prefrontal cortex. As expected, NET inhibition enhances synaptic NE levels and increases the diffusion radius of NE (Figure 7-34B). Somewhat surprising may be that NET inhibition also enhances DA levels and increases DA's diffusion radius (Figure 7-34C). The bottom line is that NET inhibition increases both NE and DA in prefrontal cortex. Thus, SNRIs have "two-and-a-half" mechanisms: boosting serotonin throughout the brain, boosting norepinephrine throughout the brain and boosting dopamine in prefrontal cortex (but not in other DA projection areas).

Venlafaxine

Depending upon the dose, venlafaxine has different degrees of inhibition of 5HT reuptake (most potent and robust even at low doses), versus NE reuptake (moderate potency and robust only at higher doses) (Figure 7-30). However, there are no significant actions on other receptors. It remains controversial whether venlafaxine or other SNRIs have greater efficacy in major depression than SSRIs, either in terms of enhanced remission rates, more robust sustained remission over long-term treatment, or greater efficacy for treatment-resistant depression – but it seems plausible, given the two mechanisms and the boosting of two monoamines. Venlafaxine is approved and widely used for several anxiety disorders as well. Adding NET inhibition likely accounts for two side effects of venlafaxine in some patients, sweating and elevated blood pressure.

Venlafaxine is available as an extended-release formulation (venlafaxine XR), which not only allows for once-daily administration, but also significantly reduces side effects, especially nausea. In contrast to several other psychotropic drugs available in controlled-release formulations, venlafaxine XR is a considerable improvement over the immediate-release formulation. The immediate-release formulation of venlafaxine has actually fallen into little or no use because of unacceptable nausea and other side effects associated with this formulation, especially when venlafaxine immediate-release is started or when it is stopped. However, venlafaxine even in controlled-release formulation can cause

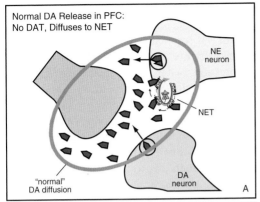

Normal DA Release in PFC:
No DAT, Diffuses to NET

NE
neuron

NET

"normal"
DA diffusion

DA
neuron

A

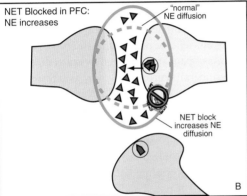

NET Blocked in PFC:
NE increases

"normal"
NE diffusion

NET block
increases NE
diffusion

B

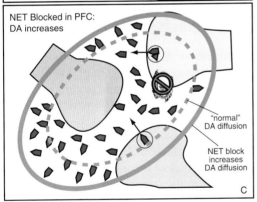

NET Blocked in PFC:
DA increases

"normal"
DA diffusion

NET block
increases
DA diffusion

C

Figure 7-34. Norepinephrine transporter blockade and dopamine in the prefrontal cortex. (A) Although there are abundant serotonin transporters (SERTs) and norepinephrine transporters (NETs) in the prefrontal cortex (PFC), there are very few dopamine transporters (DATs). This means that dopamine can diffuse away from the synapse and therefore exert its actions within a larger radius. Dopamine's actions are terminated at norepinephrine axon terminals, because DA is taken up by NET. (B) NET blockade in the prefrontal cortex leads to an increase in synaptic norepinephrine, thus increasing norepinephrine's diffusion radius. (C) Because NET takes up dopamine as well as norepinephrine, NET blockade also leads to an increase in synaptic dopamine, further increasing its diffusion radius. Thus, agents that block NET increase norepinephrine throughout the brain and both norepinephrine and dopamine in the prefrontal cortex.

withdrawal reactions, sometimes quite bothersome, especially after sudden discontinuation from high-dose long-term treatment. Nevertheless, the controlled-release formulation is highly preferred because of enhanced tolerability.

Desvenlafaxine

Venlafaxine is a substrate for CYP 2D6, which converts it to an active metabolite desvenlafaxine (Figure 7-30). Desvenlafaxine has greater NET inhibition relative to SERT inhibition compared to venlafaxine. Normally, after venlafaxine administration, the plasma levels of venlafaxine are about half of those for desvenlafaxine. However, this is highly variable, depending upon whether the patient is taking another drug that is a CYP 2D6 inhibitor, which shifts the plasma levels towards more venlafaxine and less desvenlafaxine, also reducing the relative amount of NET inhibition. Variability in plasma levels of venlafaxine versus desvenlafaxine is also due to genetic polymorphisms for CYP 2D6, such that poor metabolizers will shift the ratio of these two drugs towards more parent venlafaxine and away from the active metabolite desvenlafaxine, and thus reduce the relative amount of NET inhibition. As a result of these considerations, is can be somewhat unpredictable how much NET inhibition a given dose of venlafaxine will have in a given patient at a given time, whereas this is more predictable for desvenlafaxine. Expert clinicians have learned to solve this problem with skilled dose titration of venlafaxine, but the recent development of desvenlafaxine as a separate drug may also solve this problem with less need for dose titration and more consistent NET inhibition at a given dose across all patients.

Studies of desvenlafaxine have reported efficacy in reducing vasomotor symptoms (VMS) in perimenopausal women, whether they are depressed or not. Early studies have shown promising, if inconsistent, results for VMS with some SSRIs, as well as with the α_2 agonist clonidine and even the anticonvulsant/chronic pain agent gabapentin. However, the most promising results to date seem to be with SNRIs, especially the SNRI desvenlafaxine.

Many perimenopausal women develop hot flushes and other VMS, including night sweats, insomnia, and even depression, but do not wish to undergo estrogen replacement therapy (ERT). Desvenlafaxine appears to have efficacy in reducing VMS in such women and may provide an alternative to ERT for these women. However, it is not formally approved for this use despite several positive studies. It may be important to treat VMS not only because they are distressing in and of themselves, but also because they may be a harbinger of onset or relapse of major depression. Hypothetically, fluctuating estrogen levels not only can cause VMS, but also can be a physiological trigger for major depressive episodes during perimenopause. Dysregulation of neurotransmitter systems within hypothalamic thermoregulatory centers by irregular fluctuation of estrogen levels could lead to neurotransmitter deficiencies that trigger both VMS and depression. It is thus not surprising that other symptoms related to dysregulation of neurotransmitters within the hypothalamus can occur in both perimenopause and in depression, namely insomnia, weight gain, and decreased libido.

Postmenopausally, despite the lack of chaotic estrogen fluctuations, many women continue to experience VMS. This may be due to the loss of expression of sufficient numbers of brain glucose transporters due to low concentrations of estrogen. Theoretically, this would cause inefficient CNS transport of glucose, which would be detected in hypothalamic centers that would react by triggering a noradrenergic alarm, with vasomotor response, increase blood flow to the brain, and compensatory increase in brain glucose transport. Presumably, SNRI treatment could reduce an over-reactive hypothalamus and reduce consequent vasomotor symptoms. One issue of note relates to the observation that SSRIs seem to work better in women in the presence of estrogen than in the absence of estrogen. Thus, SSRIs may have more reliable efficacy in premenopausal women (who have normal cycling estrogen levels) and in postmenopausal women who are undergoing ERT than in postmenopausal women who are not taking ERT. By contrast, SNRIs seem to have consistent efficacy in both pre- and postmenopausal women, and in postmenopausal women whether they are undergoing ERT or not. Thus, the treatment of depression in postmenopausal women should take into consideration whether they have vasomotor symptoms, and whether they are taking ERT, before deciding whether to prescribe an SSRI or an SNRI.

Duloxetine

This SNRI, characterized pharmacologically by slightly more potent SERT than NET inhibition (Figure 7-31), has transformed how we think about depression and pain. Classic teaching was that depression caused pain that was psychic (as in "I feel your pain") and not somatic (as in "ouch"), and that psychic pain was secondary to emotional suffering in depression; therefore, it was thought, anything that made depression better would make psychic pain better nonspecifically. Somatic pain was conceptualized classically as different from psychic pain in depression, due to something wrong with the body and not due to something wrong with emotions. Somatic pain was thus not thought to be caused by depression, although depression could supposedly make it worse, and classically somatic pain was not treated with antidepressants.

Studies with duloxetine have changed all this. Not only does this SNRI relieve depression in the absence of pain, but it also relieves pain in the absence of depression. All sorts of pain are improved by duloxetine, from diabetic peripheral neuropathic pain, to fibromyalgia, to chronic musculoskeletal pain such as that associated with osteoarthritis and low back problems. These findings of the efficacy of duloxetine for multiple pain syndromes have also validated that painful physical (somatic) symptoms are a legitimate set of symptoms that accompany depression, and are not just a form of emotional pain. The use of SNRIs such as duloxetine in pain syndromes is discussed in Chapter 10. So, duloxetine has established efficacy not only in depression and in chronic pain, but also in patients with chronic painful physical symptoms of depression. Painful physical symptoms are frequently ignored or missed by patients and clinicians alike in the setting of major depression, and until recently the link of these symptoms to major depression was not well appreciated, in part because painful physical symptoms are not included in the list of symptoms for the formal diagnostic criteria for depression. Nevertheless, it is now widely appreciated that painful physical symptoms are frequently associated with a major depressive episode, and are also one of the leading residual symptoms after treatment with an antidepressant (Figure 7-5). It appears that the dual SNRI actions of duloxetine and other SNRIs are superior to the selective serotonergic actions of SSRIs for treatment of conditions such as neuropathic pain of diabetes and chronic painful physical symptoms associated with depression. The role of NET inhibition seems to be critical not only for the treatment of painful conditions without depression, but also for painful physical symptoms associated with depression. Duloxetine has also shown efficacy in the treatment of cognitive symptoms of depression that are prominent in geriatric depression, possibly exploiting the pro-noradrenergic and pro-dopaminergic consequences of NET inhibition in prefrontal cortex (Figure 7-34).

Duloxetine can be given once a day, but this is usually only a good idea after the patient has had a chance to become tolerant to it after initiating it at twice-daily dosing, especially during titration to higher doses. Duloxetine may have a lower incidence of hypertension and milder withdrawal reactions than venlafaxine.

Milnacipran

Milnacipran is the first SNRI marketed in Japan and many European countries such as France, where it is currently marketed as an antidepressant. In the US, milnacipran is not approved for depression, but is approved for fibromyalgia. Interestingly, milnacipran is not approved for the treatment of fibromyalgia in Europe. Milnacipran is a bit different from other SNRIs in that it is a relatively more potent NET than SERT inhibitor (Figure 7-32), whereas the others are more potent SERT than NET inhibitors (Figures 7-30 and 7-31). This unique pharmacologic profile may explain milnacipran's somewhat different clinical profile compared to other SNRIs. Since noradrenergic actions may be equally or more important for treatment of pain-related conditions compared to serotonergic actions, the robust NET inhibition of milnacipran suggests that it may be particularly useful in chronic pain-related conditions, not just fibromyalgia where it is approved, but possibly as well for the painful physical symptoms associated with depression and chronic neuropathic pain.

Milnacipran's potent NET inhibition also suggests a potentially favorable pharmacologic profile for the treatment of cognitive symptoms, including cognitive symptoms of depression as well as cognitive symptoms frequently associated with fibromyalgia, sometimes called "fibro-fog." Other clinical observations possibly linked to milnacipran's robust NET inhibition are that it can be more energizing and activating than other SNRIs. Common residual symptoms after treatment with an SSRI include not only cognitive symptoms, but also fatigue, lack of energy, and lack of interest, among other symptoms (Figure 7-5). An active enantiomer, levo-milnacipran, is in clinical development as an antidepressant, and is targeting fatigue and lack of energy as a potential clinical advantage due to its more potent NET inhibition.

NET inhibition may be related to observations that milnacipran may cause more sweating and urinary hesitancy than some other SNRIs. For patients with urinary hesitancy, generally due theoretically to robust pro-noradrenergic actions at bladder α_1 receptors, an α_1 antagonist can reduce these symptoms. Milnacipran must generally be given twice daily, because of its shorter half-life.

Norepinephrine–dopamine reuptake inhibitors (NDRIs): bupropion

For many years, the mechanism of action of bupropion has been somewhat unclear, and it still remains controversial among some experts. The leading hypothesis for bupropion's mechanism of action is that it inhibits the reuptake of both dopamine (i.e., dopamine transporter or DAT inhibitor) and norepinephrine (i.e., norepinephrine transporter or NET inhibitor) (Figures 7-35 and 7-36). No other specific or potent pharmacologic actions have been consistently identified for this agent.

Bupropion is metabolized to a number of active metabolites, some of which are not only more potent NET inhibitors than bupropion itself and equally potent DAT inhibitors, but are also concentrated in the brain. In some ways, therefore, bupropion is both an active

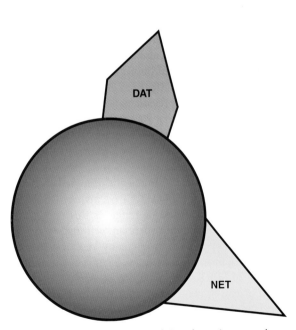

Figure 7-35. Icon of a norepinephrine–dopamine reuptake inhibitor (NDRI). Another class of antidepressant consists of norepinephrine–dopamine reuptake inhibitors (NDRIs), for which the prototypical agent is bupropion. Bupropion has weak reuptake blocking properties for dopamine (DRI) and norepinephrine (NRI) but is an efficacious antidepressant, which may be explained in part by the more potent inhibitory properties of its metabolites.

NDRI Action

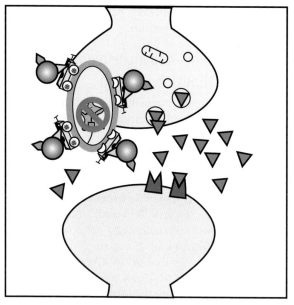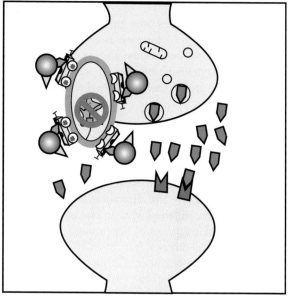

Figure 7-36. NDRI actions. In this figure the norepinephrine reuptake inhibitor (NRI) portion of the NDRI molecule (left panel) and the dopamine reuptake inhibitor (DRI) portion of the NDRI molecule (right panel) are inserted into their respective reuptake pumps. Consequently both pumps are blocked, and the drug mediates an antidepressant effect.

drug and a precursor for other active drugs (i.e., a prodrug for multiple active metabolites). The most potent of these is the + enantiomer of the 6-hydroxy metabolite of bupropion, also known as radafaxine.

Can the net effects of bupropion on NET (Figure 7-37A and B) and DAT (Figure 7-37C) account for its clinical actions in depressed patients at therapeutic doses? If one believes that 90% transporter occupancy of DAT and NET are required for antidepressant actions, the answer would be "no." Human PET scans suggest that no more than 20–30% and perhaps as little as 10–15% of striatal DATs may be occupied at therapeutic doses of bupropion. NET occupancy would be expected to be in this same range. Is this enough to explain bupropion's antidepressant actions?

Whereas it is clear from many research studies that SSRIs must be dosed to occupy a substantial fraction of SERT, perhaps up to 80 or 90% of these transporters, in order to be effective antidepressants, this is far less clear for NET or DAT occupancy, particularly in the case of drugs with an additional pharmacologic mechanism that may be synergistic with NET or DAT inhibition. That is, when most SNRIs are given in doses that occupy 80–90% of SERT, substantially fewer NETs are occupied, yet there is evidence of both additional therapeutic

actions and NE-mediated side effects of these agents with perhaps as little as 50% NET occupancy.

Furthermore, there appears to be such a thing as "too much DAT occupancy." That is, when 50% or more of DATs are occupied rapidly and briefly, this can lead to unwanted clinical actions, such as euphoria and reinforcement. In fact, rapid, short-lasting and high degrees of DAT occupancy is the pharmacologic characteristic of abusable stimulants such as cocaine and is discussed in Chapter 14 on drug abuse and reward. The link of DAT occupancy to substance abuse is also discussed in Chapter 14. When 50% or more of DATs are occupied more slowly and in a more long-lasting manner, especially with controlled-release formulations, stimulants are less abusable and more useful for attention deficit hyperactivity disorder (ADHD), discussed in more detail in Chapter 12. The issue to be considered here is whether a low level of slow-onset and long-lasting DAT occupancy is the desirable solution for the DAT mechanism to be useful as an antidepressant: thus, not too much or too fast DAT inhibition and therefore abusable; not too little DAT inhibition and therefore ineffective; but just enough DAT inhibition with slow enough onset and long enough duration of action to make it an antidepressant.

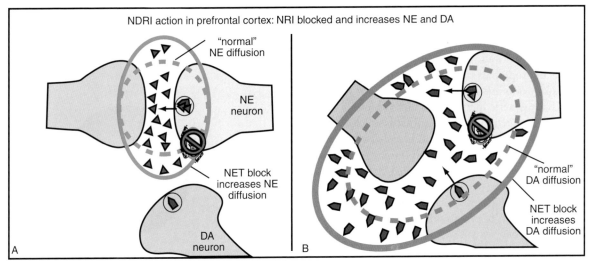

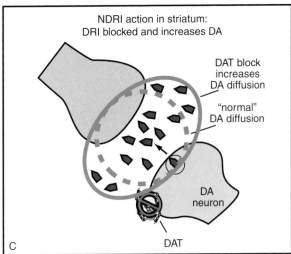

Figure 7-37. NDRI actions in prefrontal cortex and striatum. Norepinephrine–dopamine reuptake inhibitors (NDRIs) block the transporters for both norepinephrine (NET) and dopamine (DAT). (A) NET blockade in the prefrontal cortex leads to an increase in synaptic norepinephrine, thus increasing norepinephrine's diffusion radius. (B) Because the prefrontal cortex lacks DATs, and NETs transport dopamine as well as norepinephrine, NET blockade also leads to an increase in synaptic dopamine as well as NE in the prefrontal cortex, further increasing DA's diffusion radius. Thus, despite the absence of DAT in the prefrontal cortex, NDRIs still increase dopamine in the prefrontal cortex. (C) DAT is present in the striatum, and thus DAT inhibition increases dopamine diffusion there.

The fact that bupropion is not known to be particularly abusable, is not a scheduled substance, yet is proven effective for treating nicotine addiction, is consistent with the possibility that it is occupying DATs in the striatum and nucleus accumbens in a manner sufficient to mitigate craving but not sufficient to cause abuse (Figure 7-37C). This is discussed further in Chapter 14 on drug abuse and reward. Perhaps this is also how bupropion works in depression, combined with an equal action on NETs (Figure 7-37A and B). Clinical observations of depressed patients are also consistent with DAT and

NET inhibition as the mechanism of bupropion, since this agent appears especially useful in targeting the symptoms of "reduced positive affect" within the affective spectrum (see Figure 6-46), including improvement in the symptoms of loss of happiness, joy, interest, pleasure, energy, enthusiasm, alertness, and self-confidence.

Bupropion was originally marketed only in the US as an immediate-release dosage formulation with three-times-daily administration as an anti-depressant. Development of a twice-a-day formulation (bupropion SR) and more recently a once-a-day formulation (bupropion XL) have not only reduced the frequency of seizures at peak plasma drug levels, but have also increased convenience and enhanced compliance as well. Thus, the use of immediate-release bupropion is all but abandoned in favor of once-a-day administration. Now that bupropion SR and XL are generic in the US, some controversy exists over whether generic controlled-release technologies are as consistent as the original branded controlled-release technologies, and possibly might dose dump rather than deliver like the branded drugs, and be ineffective in some patients.

Bupropion is generally activating or even stimulating. Interestingly, bupropion does not appear to cause the bothersome sexual dysfunction that frequently occurs with antidepressants that act by SERT inhibition, probably because bupropion lacks a significant serotonergic component to its mechanism of action. Thus, bupropion has proven to be a useful antidepressant not only for patients who cannot tolerate the serotonergic side effects of SSRIs, but also for patients whose depression does not respond to serotonergic boosting by SSRIs. As discussed above, given its pharmacologic profile, bupropion is especially targeted at the symptoms of the "dopamine deficiency syndrome" and "reduced positive affect" (Figure 6-46). Almost every active clinician knows that patients who have residual symptoms of reduced positive affect following treatment with an SSRI or an SNRI, or who develop these symptoms as a side effect of an SSRI or SNRI, frequently benefit from switching to bupropion or from augmenting their SSRI or SNRI treatment with bupropion. The combination of bupropion with an SSRI or an SNRI has a theoretical rationale as a strategy for covering the entire symptom portfolio from symptoms of reduced positive affect to symptoms of increased negative affect (Figure 6-46).

Selective norepinephrine reuptake inhibitors (NRIs)

Although some tricyclic antidepressants (e.g., desipramine, maprotiline) block norepinephrine reuptake more potently than serotonin reuptake, even these tricyclics are not really selective, since they still block many other receptors such as α_1-adrenergic, H_1-histaminic, and muscarinic cholinergic receptors, as all tricyclics do. Tricyclic antidepressants are discussed later in this chapter.

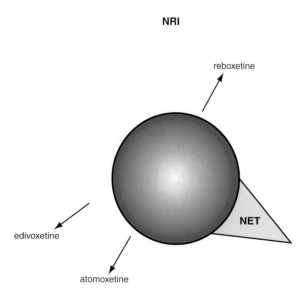

Figure 7-38. Icon of a selective norepinephrine reuptake inhibitor. Reboxetine, atomoxetine, and edivoxetine are antidepressants that have selective actions at the norepinephrine transporter (NET).

The first truly selective noradrenergic reuptake inhibitor marketed in Europe and other countries is reboxetine; the first in the US is atomoxetine (Figure 7-38). Both of these compounds are selective NRIs and lack the additional undesirable binding properties of tricyclic antidepressants. Reboxetine is approved as an antidepressant in Europe, but not in the US. Extensive testing in the US suggested inconsistent efficacy in major depression with the possibility of being less effective than SSRIs, so reboxetine was dropped from further development as an antidepressant in the US. Atomoxetine was never developed as an antidepressant but is marketed for the treatment of attention deficit hyperactivity disorder (ADHD) in the US and other countries. ADHD treatments are discussed in Chapter 12.

Many of the important concepts about NET inhibition have already been covered in the section on SNRIs above. This includes the observations that NET inhibition not only raises NE diffusely throughout all NE neuronal projections, but also raises DA levels in prefrontal cortex (Figure 7-34). It also includes both the therapeutic and side-effect profile of NET inhibition. There is some question about whether selective NET inhibition has any different clinical profile than when NET inhibition occurs simultaneously with SERT inhibition, such as when administering an SNRI or when giving a selective NRI with an SSRI. One thing that may be different is that NET inhibitors that are selective tend to be dosed so that there is a greater proportion of NET occupancy, close to saturation, compared to NET occupancy when dosed as an SNRI or as an NDRI, which as mentioned above may occupy substantially fewer NETs at clinically effective antidepressant doses. This higher degree of NET occupancy of selective NET inhibitors may be necessary for optimal efficacy for either depression or ADHD if there is no simultaneous SERT or DAT inhibition with which to add or synergize. One of the interesting observations is that high degrees of selective NET inhibition, although often activating, can also be sedating in some patients. Perhaps this is due to "over-tuning" noradrenergic input to cortical pyramidal neurons, which is discussed in Chapter 12 on ADHD.

There is less documentation that NET inhibition is as helpful for anxiety disorders as SERT inhibition, and neither of the selective NRIs discussed above is approved for anxiety disorders, although atomoxetine is approved for adult ADHD, which is frequently comorbid with anxiety disorders. A new selective NET inhibitor, sometimes called a NERI (norepinephrine reuptake inhibitor) and known as edivoxetine, is in testing as an augmenting agent to SSRIs in depression (Figure 7-38).

Agomelatine

Depression can alter circadian rhythms, causing a phase delay in the sleep/wake cycle (Figure 7-39). The degree of this phase delay correlates with the severity of depression. Numerous physiological measurements of circadian rhythms are also altered in depression, from flattening of the daily body temperature cycle to

elevation of cortisol secretion throughout the day, and also reducing the melatonin secretion that normally peaks at night and in the dark (Figure 7-40). Elevations of cortisol secretion and abnormalities of the HPA (hypothalamic–pituitary–adrenal) axis in depression are also discussed in Chapter 6 (see Figures 6-39A and 6-39B). Other normal circadian rhythms that may be disrupted in depression include a reduction in BDNF (brain-derived neurotrophic factor) and the neurogenesis that normally peaks at night (also discussed in Chapter 6: see Figures 6-36 through 6-38). Desynchronization of biological processes is so pervasive in depression that it is plausible to characterize depression as fundamentally a circadian illness. It is possible that depression is due to a "broken" circadian clock. Numerous genes operate in a circadian manner, sensitive to light–dark rhythms and called clock genes. Abnormalities in various clock genes have been linked to mood disorders. Also supporting the notion that depression is an illness with a broken circadian clock is the recent demonstration that specific pharmacological mechanisms – namely, melatonergic actions combined with monoaminergic actions – can resynchronize circadian rhythms in depression, essentially fixing the broken circadian clock and thereby exerting an antidepressant effect.

Agomelatine is an antidepressant approved in many countries outside of the US; it has agonist actions at melatonin 1 (MT_1) and melatonin 2 (MT_2) receptors and antagonist actions at $5HT_{2C}$ receptors (Figure 7-41). $5HT_{2C}$ antagonist actions are discussed in Chapter 5, and are a property of the antidepressants fluoxetine and mirtazapine and the atypical antipsychotics with antidepressant actions quetiapine and olanzapine. $5HT_{2C}$ receptors are not

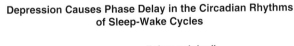

Depression Causes Phase Delay in the Circadian Rhythms of Sleep-Wake Cycles

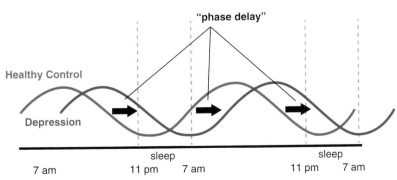

Figure 7-39. Depression causes phase delay in circadian rhythms of sleep/wake cycles. Circadian rhythms describe events that occur on a 24-hour cycle. Many biological systems follow a circadian rhythm; in particular, circadian rhythms are key to the regulation of sleep/wake cycles. In patients with depression, the circadian rhythm is often "phase delayed," which means that because wakefulness is not promoted in the morning, such patients tend to sleep later. They also have trouble falling asleep at night, which further promotes feelings of sleepiness during the day.

Physiological Measurements of Circadian Rhythms are Altered in Depression

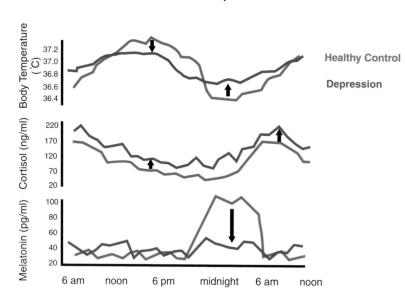

Healthy Control

Depression

Figure 7-40. Physiological measurements of circadian rhythms are altered in depression. Circadian rhythms are evident in multiple biological functions, including body temperature, hormone levels, blood pressure, metabolism, cellular regeneration, sleep/wake cycles, and DNA transcription and translation. The internal coordination ordered by the circadian rhythm is essential to optimal health. In depression, there are altered physiological measurements of circadian rhythms, including less fluctuation in body temperature over the course of a 24-hour cycle, the same pattern but elevated cortisol levels over 24 hours, and the absence of a spike in melatonin levels at night.

agomelatine

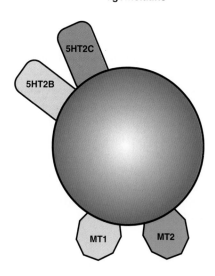

Figure 7-41. Agomelatine. Endogenous melatonin is secreted by the pineal gland and mainly acts in the suprachiasmatic nucleus to regulate circadian rhythms. There are three types of receptors for melatonin: MT_1 and MT_2, which are both involved in sleep, and MT_3, which is actually the enzyme NRH:quinine oxidoreductase 2 and not thought to be involved in sleep physiology. Agomelatine is not only an MT_1 and MT_2 receptor agonist, but is also a $5HT_{2C}$ and $5HT_{2B}$ receptor antagonist and is available as an antidepressant in Europe.

only located in the midbrain raphe and prefrontal cortex where they regulate the release of dopamine and norepinephrine (see Figures 5-52A and 5-52B); $5HT_{2C}$ receptors are also localized in the

suprachiasmatic nucleus (SCN) of the hypothalamus, the brain's "pacemaker," where they interact with melatonin receptors (Figures 7-42A through 7-42D). Light is detected by the retina during the day, and this information travels to the SCN via the retinohypothalamic tract (Figure 7-42A), which normally synchronizes many circadian rhythms downstream from the SCN. For example, both melatonin receptors and $5HT_{2C}$ receptors fluctuate in a circadian manner in the SCN, with high receptor expression at night/dark and low receptor expression in the day/light. That makes sense, since melatonin is only secreted at night in the dark (Figure 7-42B). In depression, however, circadian rhythms are "out of synch" including low melatonin secretion at night among numerous other changes (Figures 7-39, 7-40, 7-42C). Agomelatine, by stimulating melatonin receptors in the SCN and simultaneously blocking $5HT_{2C}$ receptors there as well, appears to resynchronize circadian rhythms, reverse the phase delay of depression, and thereby exert an antidepressant effect (Figure 7-42D).

Melatonergic actions are not sufficient for this antidepressant effect, as melatonin itself and selective melatonergic MT_1 and MT_2 receptor agonists do not have proven antidepressant action. $5HT_{2C}$ antagonism has been shown to interact with melatonin MT_1/MT_2 agonism by affecting the secretion of melatonin by the pineal gland, especially by regulating the suppression of melatonin secretion by light. The combination of $5HT_{2C}$ antagonism plus MT_1/MT_2 agonism creates numerous

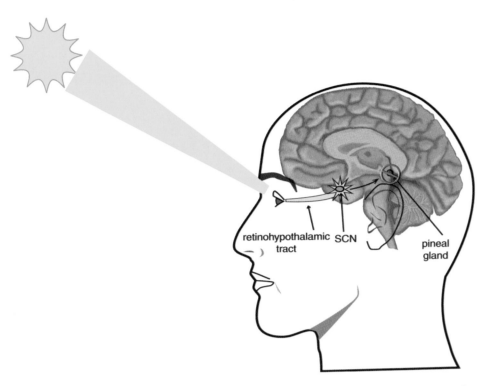

Figure 7-42A. The setting of circadian rhythms, part 1. Although various factors can affect the setting of circadian rhythms, light is the most powerful synchronizer. When light enters through the eye it is translated via the retinohypothalamic tract to the suprachiasmatic nucleus (or SCN) within the hypothalamus. The SCN, in turn, signals the pineal gland to turn off melatonin production.

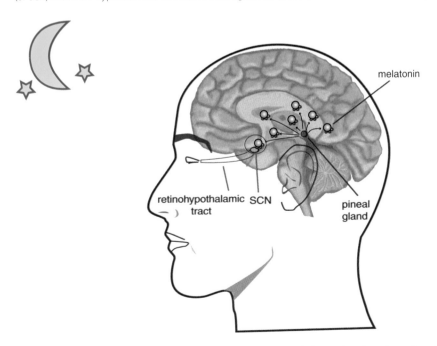

Figure 7-42B. The setting of circadian rhythms, part 2. During darkness, there is no input from the retinohypothalamic tract to the suprachiasmatic nucleus (SCN) within the hypothalamus. Thus, darkness signals the pineal gland to produce melatonin. Melatonin, in turn, can act on the SCN to reset circadian rhythms.

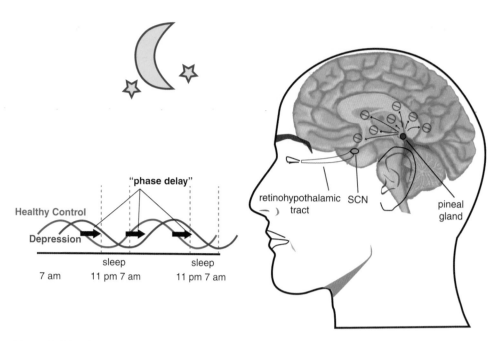

Figure 7-42C. The setting of circadian rhythms, part 3. In patients with depression, circadian rhythms are often "phase delayed," which means that because wakefulness is not promoted in the morning, such patients tend to sleep later. They also have trouble falling asleep at night, which further promotes feelings of sleepiness during the day. The phase delay observed in depression may be related to the fact that, even in darkness, there seems to be lack of melatonin production in the brains of patients with depression.

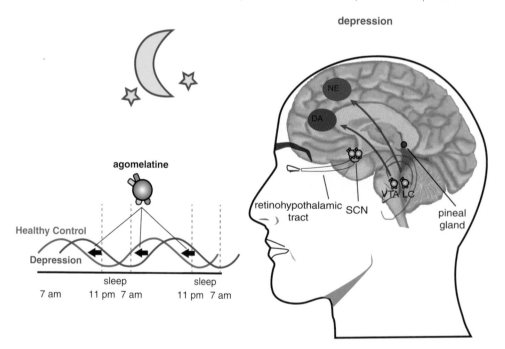

Figure 7-42D. The setting of circadian rhythms, part 4. Agomelatine, which acts as an agonist at melatonin 1 and 2 receptors, may resynchronize circadian rhythms by acting as "substitute melatonin." Thus, even in the absence of melatonin production in the pineal gland, agomelatine can bind to melatonin 1 and 2 receptors in the suprachiasmatic nucleus (SCN) to reset circadian rhythms. In addition, by blocking serotonin 2C receptors in the ventral tegmental area (VTA) and locus coeruleus (LC), agomelatine promotes dopamine (DA) and norepinephrine (NE) release in the prefrontal cortex (see Figures 5-52A, 5-52B, 7-43).

Agomelatine Releases Norepinephrine and Dopamine in the Frontal Cortex

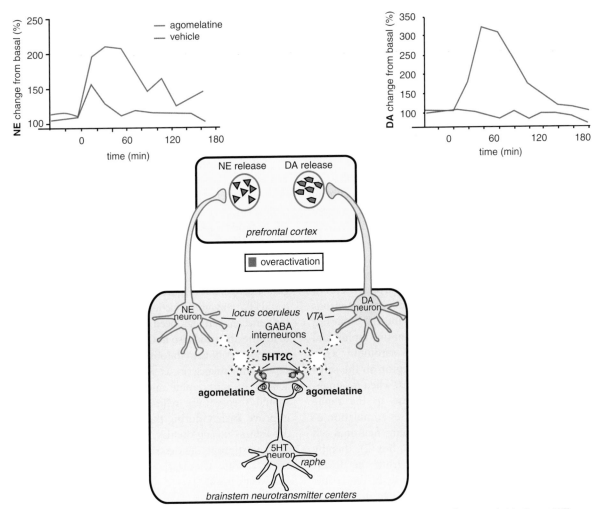

Figure 7-43. Agomelatine releases norepinephrine and dopamine in the prefrontal cortex. Normally, serotonin binding at 5HT$_{2C}$ receptors on γ-aminobutyric acid (GABA) interneurons in the brainstem inhibits norepinephrine and dopamine release in the prefrontal cortex. When a 5HT$_{2C}$ antagonist such as agomelatine binds to 5HT$_{2C}$ receptors on GABA interneurons (bottom red circle), it prevents serotonin from binding there and thus prevents inhibition of norepinephrine and dopamine release in the prefrontal cortex; in other words, it disinhibits their release (top red circles).

biological effects that are not triggered by either mechanism alone: namely, enhancing neurogenesis and BDNF; resetting sleep/wake and dark/light phases; decreasing stress-induced glutamate release; regulating downstream signal transduction cascades and clock genes; resynchronizing circadian rhythms and, most critically, antidepressant actions. Not only does 5HT$_{2C}$ antagonism raise norepinephrine and dopamine in prefrontal cortex, but with simultaneous stimulation of MT$_1$ and MT$_2$ receptors, agomelatine apparently resynchronizes circadian rhythms which potentially can optimize these changes in monoamines (Figure 7-43).

Alpha-2 antagonist actions and mirtazapine

Alpha-2 (α$_2$) antagonism is another way to enhance the release of monoamines and exert an antidepressant action. Recall that norepinephrine turns off its own release by interacting with presynaptic α$_2$ auto-receptors on noradrenergic neurons, as discussed in

Chapter 6 and illustrated in Figures 6-28 and 6-29. Therefore, when an α_2 antagonist is administered, norepinephrine can no longer turn off its own release and noradrenergic neurons are thus disinhibited from their axon terminals, such as those in the raphe and in the cortex (Figure 7-44A).

Recall also that norepinephrine turns off serotonin release by interacting with presynaptic α_2 heteroreceptors on serotonergic neurons (Figure 6-30C). Alpha-2 antagonists block norepinephrine from turning off serotonin release because α_2 heteroreceptors on serotonin axon terminals are blocked even in the presence of norepinephrine (Figure 7-44B). Therefore, serotonergic neurons become disinhibited and serotonin release is enhanced (Figure 7-44B). It is as though α_2 antagonists acting at serotonin axon terminals "cut the brake cable" of noradrenergic inhibition (NE stepping on the brake to prevent 5HT release, shown in Figure 6-30C, is blocked in Figure 7-44B).

A second mechanism to increase serotonin release after an α_2 antagonist is administered may be even more important. Recall that norepinephrine neurons from the locus coeruleus innervate the cell bodies of serotonergic neurons in the midbrain raphe and stimulate serotonin release from serotonin axon terminals via a postsynaptic α_1 receptor on the serotonin cell body (Figure 6-30B). Thus, when α_2 antagonists cause norepinephrine release in the raphe (Figure 7-44A, box 2), this also causes stimulation of postsynaptic α_1 receptors on serotonin neuronal cell bodies in the raphe (Figure 7-44B, box 2), thereby provoking more serotonin release from the downstream axon terminals, such as those in the cortex shown in Figure 7-44C box 1. This is like stepping on the serotonin accelerator. Thus, α_2 antagonists both "cut the brake cable" (Figure 7-44B) and "step on the accelerator" (Figure 7-44C) to facilitate serotonin release. Alpha-2 antagonist actions therefore yield dual enhancement of both 5HT and NE release, but unlike SNRIs they have this effect by a mechanism independent of blockade of monoamine transporters. These two mechanisms, monoamine transport blockade and α_2 antagonism, are synergistic, so that blocking them simultaneously gives a much more powerful disinhibitory signal to these two neurotransmitters than if only one mechanism is blocked. For this reason, the α_2 antagonist mirtazapine is often combined with SNRIs for treatment of cases that do not respond to an SNRI alone. This combination is sometimes called "California rocket fuel" because of the potentially powerful antidepressant action blasting the patient out of the depths of depression.

Although no selective α_2 antagonist is available for use as an antidepressant, there are several drugs with prominent α_2 properties, including mirtazapine, mianserin, and some of the atypical antipsychotics discussed in Chapter 5 (see Figure 5-37). Mirtazapine does not block any monoamine transporter; however, it not only blocks α_2 receptors, but has additional potent antagonist actions upon $5HT_{2A}$ receptors, $5HT_{2C}$ receptors, $5HT_3$ receptors, and H_1 histamine receptors (Figure 7-45). Two other α_2 antagonists are marketed as antidepressants in some countries (but not the US), namely mianserin (worldwide except US) and setiptiline (Japan). Unlike mirtazapine, mianserin also has potent α_1 antagonist properties which tend to mitigate its ability to enhance serotonergic neurotransmission, so that this drug enhances predominantly noradrenergic neurotransmission, yet with associated $5HT_{2A}$, $5HT_{2C}$, $5HT_3$, and H_1 antagonist properties (Figure 7-45).

$5HT_{2C}$ antagonist action as a potential antidepressant mechanism has been discussed above in regard to agomelatine and also in Chapter 5, and should theoretically contribute to the antidepressant effects of mirtazapine and mianserin as well. The H_1 antihistaminic actions of mirtazapine and mianserin (Figure 7-45) should theoretically relieve insomnia at night, and improve anxiety during the day, but could also cause drowsiness during the day. Combined with the $5HT_{2C}$ antagonist properties described above, the H_1 antihistaminic actions of mirtazapine could also cause weight gain (Figure 7-45).

$5HT_3$ antagonist action

$5HT_3$ receptors are localized in the chemoreceptor trigger zone of the brainstem, where they mediate nausea and vomiting, and in the gastrointestinal tract, where they mediate nausea, vomiting, and diarrhea/bowel motility when stimulated. Blocking these receptors can therefore protect against serotonin-induced gastrointestinal side effects that often accompany agents that increase 5HT release.

$5HT_3$ receptors in the brain also regulate the release of various neurotransmitters, especially norepinephrine and acetylcholine (Figure 7-46A), but also possibly serotonin, dopamine, and histamine as well. Serotonin acting at $5HT_3$ receptors reduces the release of these neurotransmitters (Figure 7-46B), so blocking $5HT_3$ receptors causes disinhibition of these

Alpha-2 Antagonism Increases NE Release in Raphe and Cortex

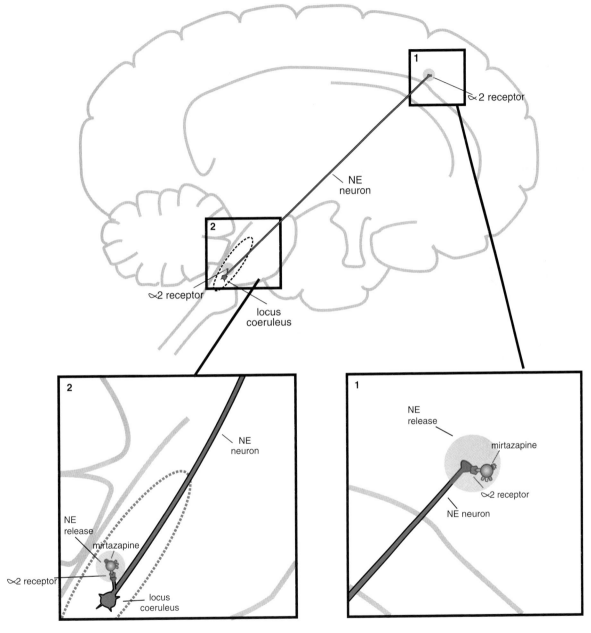

Figure 7-44A. Alpha-2 antagonism increases norepinephrine release in raphe and cortex. α_2-Adrenergic receptors are presynaptic autoreceptors and thus are the "brakes" on noradrenergic neurons. An α_2 antagonist (e.g., mirtazapine) can therefore increase norepinephrine release by binding to these receptors in the locus coeruleus (2) and in the cortex (1).

Alpha-2 Antagonism Increases 5HT and NE Release in Cortex

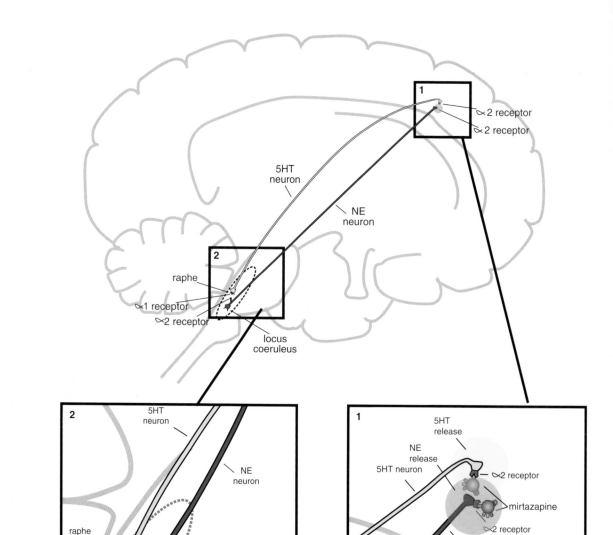

Figure 7-44B. Alpha-2 antagonism increases serotonin and norepinephrine release in the cortex. This figure shows how both noradrenergic and serotonergic neurotransmission are enhanced by α₂ antagonists. The noradrenergic neuron is disinhibited in the cortex because an α₂ antagonist is blocking its presynaptic α₂ autoreceptors. This has the effect of "cutting the brake cables" for norepinephrine (NE) release. In addition, α₂ antagonists "cut the 5HT brake cable" when α₂ presynaptic heteroreceptors are blocked on the 5HT axon terminal, thus leading to enhanced serotonin release.

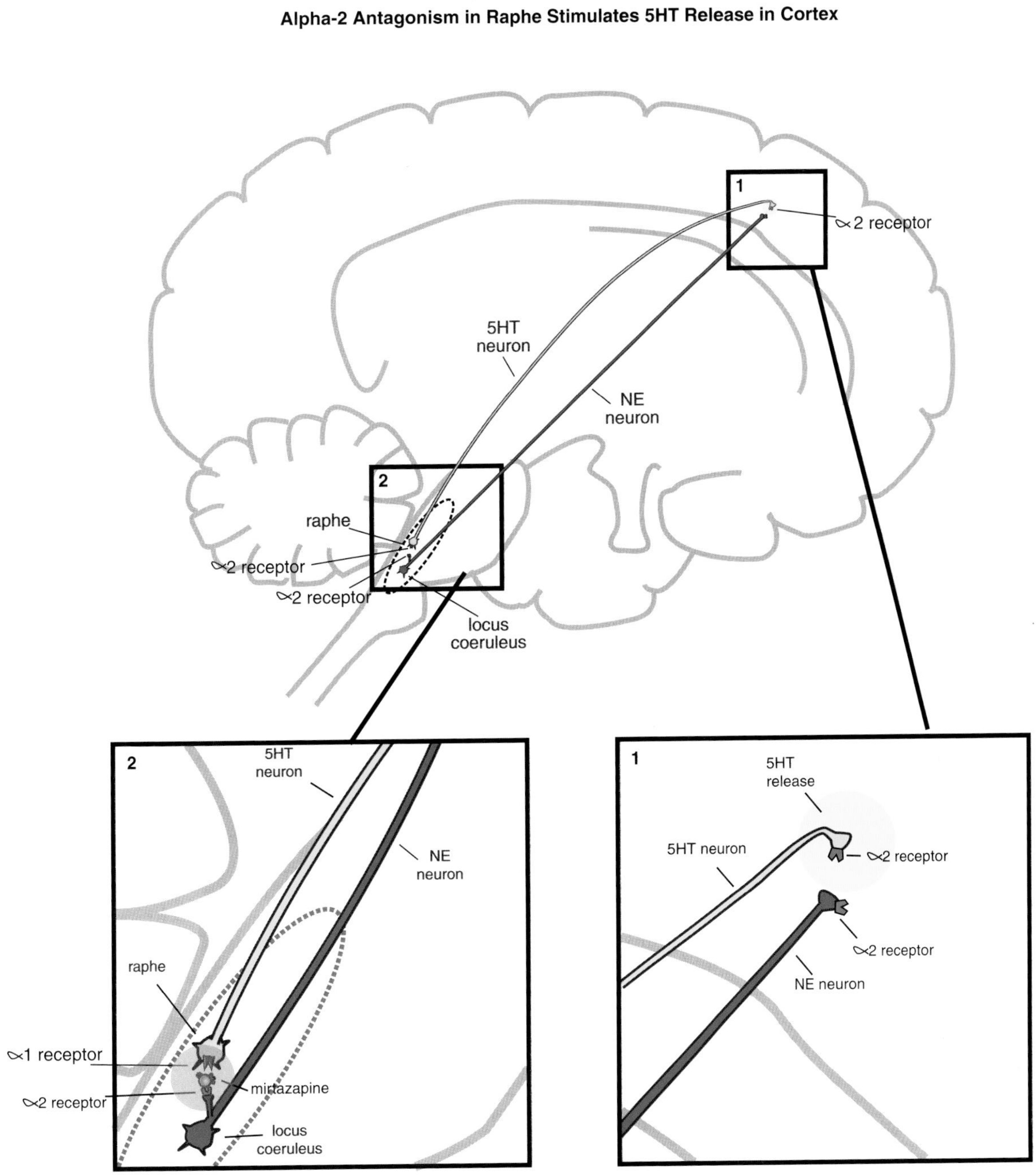

Alpha-2 Antagonism in Raphe Stimulates 5HT Release in Cortex

Figure 7-44C. Alpha-2 antagonism in raphe stimulates serotonin release in cortex. The noradrenergic neuron is disinhibited at its axon terminals in the brainstem because an α_2 antagonist is blocking its presynaptic α_2 autoreceptors (2). This has the effect of "cutting the brake cables" for norepinephrine (NE) release. Norepinephrine can then stimulate α_1 receptors on the serotonergic neuron, leading to serotonin release in the cortex (1).

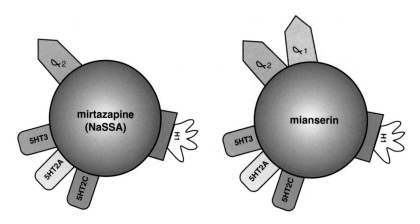

Figure 7-45. Mirtazapine and mianserin. Mirtazapine is sometimes called a noradrenergic and specific serotonergic antidepressant (NaSSA). Its primary therapeutic action is α_2 antagonism, as shown in Figures 7-44A through 7-44C. It also blocks three serotonin (5HT) receptors: $5HT_{2A}$, $5HT_{2C}$, and $5HT_3$. Finally, it blocks histamine 1 (H_1) receptors. Mianserin is also a NaSSA and has a similar binding profile to mirtazapine, the only difference being additional effects at α_1 receptors.

same neurotransmitters and thus enhances their release (Figure 7-46C). Thus, agents such as mirtazapine with $5HT_3$ antagonist properties should enhance the release of various neurotransmitters and this could contribute to antidepressant actions. Mianserin has $5HT_3$ antagonist properties, and so do some atypical antipsychotics. Potent $5HT_3$ antagonism is also one of the five multimodal pharmacologic actions of an experimental antidepressant vortioxetine, in late-stage clinical trials.

Serotonin antagonist/reuptake inhibitors (SARIs)

The prototype drug that blocks serotonin 2A and 2C ($5HT_{2A}$ and $5HT_{2C}$) receptors as well as serotonin reuptake is trazodone, classified as a serotonin antagonist/reuptake inhibitor (SARI), or, more fully, as a serotonin 2A/2C antagonist and serotonin reuptake inhibitor (Figure 7-47). Nefazodone is another SARI with robust $5HT_{2A}$ antagonist actions and weaker $5HT_{2C}$ antagonist and SERT inhibition, but is no longer commonly used because of rare liver toxicity (Figure 7-47). Trazodone is a very interesting agent, since it acts like two different drugs, depending upon the dose and the formulation. We discussed a very similar situation in Chapter 5 for quetiapine, and illustrated this in Figures 5-47 through 5-50.

Different drug at different doses?

The combined actions of $5HT_{2A}/5HT_{2C}$ antagonism with SERT inhibition only occur at moderate to high doses of trazodone (Figure 7-48). Doses of trazodone lower than those effective for antidepressant action are frequently used for the effective treatment of insomnia. Low doses exploit trazodone's potent actions as a $5HT_{2A}$ antagonist, and also its properties as an antagonist of H_1-histaminic and α_1-adrenergic receptors, but do not adequately exploit its SERT or $5HT_{2C}$ inhibition properties, which are weaker (Figure 7-48). As discussed in Chapter 5 and illustrated in Figure 5-38, blocking the brain's arousal system with H_1 and α_1 antagonism can cause sedation or sleep, and along with $5HT_{2A}$ antagonist properties this may explain the mechanism of how low doses of trazodone work as a hypnotic (Figure 7-48). Since insomnia is one of the most frequent residual symptoms of depression after treatment with an SSRI (discussed earlier in this chapter and illustrated in Figure 7-5), a hypnotic is often necessary for patients with a major depressive episode. Not only can a hypnotic potentially relieve the insomnia itself, but treating insomnia in patients with major depression may also increase remission rates due to improvement of other symptoms such as loss of energy and depressed mood. This may be the case not only for low-dose trazodone but also for the combination of antidepressants with sedative hypnotics (such as eszopiclone and others) in general, as long as insomnia is relieved. Thus, the ability of low doses of trazodone to improve sleep in depressed patients may be an important mechanism whereby trazodone can augment the efficacy of other antidepressants.

Trazodone inhibits $5HT_{2A}$ receptors at essentially any clinical dose, but to get an antidepressant action the dose must be raised to recruit SERT inhibition and thus to raise serotonin levels (Figure 7-48). However, what happens when trazodone raises serotonin levels is different than what happens when an SSRI/SNRI does this. Namely, the SSRI/SNRI raises

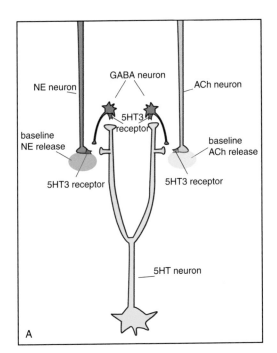

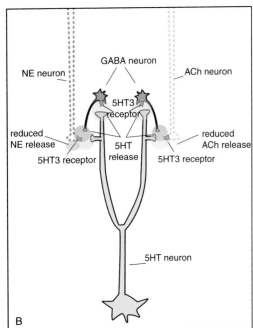

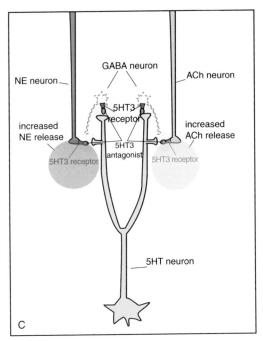

Figure 7-46. 5HT$_3$ antagonists increase norepinephrine and acetylcholine release. (A) Serotonergic neurons synapse with noradrenergic neurons, cholinergic neurons, and GABAergic interneurons, all of which contain serotonin 3 (5HT$_3$) receptors. (B) When serotonin is released, it binds to 5HT$_3$ receptors on GABAergic neurons, which release GABA onto noradrenergic and cholinergic neurons, thus reducing release of norepinephrine (NE) and acetylcholine (ACh), respectively. In addition, serotonin may bind to 5HT$_3$ receptors on noradrenergic and cholinergic neurons, further reducing release of those neurotransmitters. (C) A 5HT$_3$ antagonist binding at GABAergic neurons inhibits GABA release, which in turn disinhibits (or turns on) noradrenergic and cholinergic neurons, leading to release of norepinephrine and acetylcholine, respectively. Likewise, a 5HT$_3$ antagonist binding directly at noradrenergic and cholinergic neurons prevents serotonin from binding there and inhibiting release of their neurotransmitters.

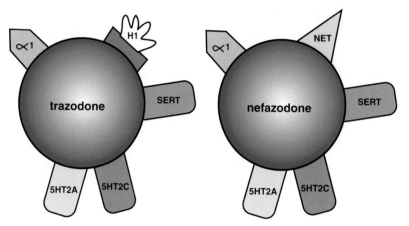

Figure 7-47. Serotonin antagonist/ reuptake inhibitors. Shown here are icons for two serotonin 2A (5HT$_{2A}$) antagonist/reuptake inhibitors (SARIs): trazodone and nefazodone. These agents have a dual action, but the two mechanisms are different from the dual action of the serotonin–norepinephrine reuptake inhibitors (SNRIs). The SARIs act by potent blockade of 5HT$_{2A}$ receptors as well as dose-dependent blockade of 5HT$_{2C}$ receptors and the serotonin transporter (SRI). SARIs also block α$_1$-adrenergic receptors. In addition, trazodone has the unique property of histamine 1 (H$_1$) receptor antagonism and nefazodone has the unique property of norepinephrine reuptake inhibition (NRI).

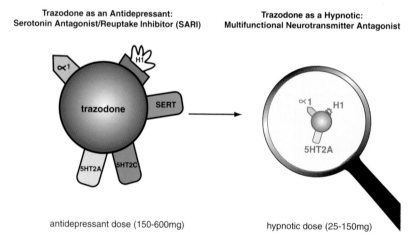

Trazodone as an Antidepressant:
Serotonin Antagonist/Reuptake Inhibitor (SARI)

Trazodone as a Hypnotic:
Multifunctional Neurotransmitter Antagonist

antidepressant dose (150-600mg)

hypnotic dose (25-150mg)

Figure 7-48. Trazodone at different doses. High doses that recruit saturation of the serotonin transporter (i.e., 150–600 mg) are required for trazodone to have antidepressant actions (icon on left). At this high antidepressant dose, trazodone is a multifunctional serotonergic agent with antagonist actions at 5HT$_{2A}$ and 5HT$_{2C}$ receptors as well. Thus, its antidepressant actions are attributed to these serotonergic properties. Trazodone is also an α$_1$ and H$_1$ antagonist at these doses. At lower doses of trazodone (i.e., 25–150 mg), it does not saturate the serotonin transporter; thus it loses its antidepressant actions while retaining antagonist actions at 5HT$_{2A}$, α$_1$, and H$_1$ receptors, and corresponding hypnotic efficacy (icon on right). Relative selectivities of trazodone for four key binding sites are shown in the chart at the bottom of the figure.

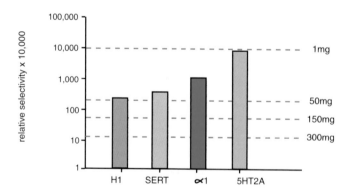

Relative Selectivities of Trazodone at Different Doses

SSRI Action

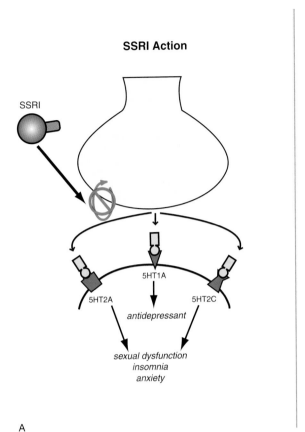

SARI Action at 5HT Synapses

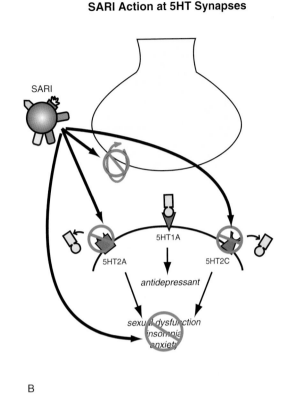

A

B

Figure 7-49. SSRI versus SARI. (A) Inhibition of the serotonin transporter (SERT) by a selective serotonin reuptake inhibitor (SSRI) at the presynaptic neuron increases serotonin at all receptors, with $5HT_{1A}$-mediated antidepressant actions but also $5HT_{2A}$- and $5HT_{2C}$-mediated sexual dysfunction, insomnia, and anxiety. (B) SERT inhibition by a serotonin 2A ($5HT_{2A}$) antagonist/reuptake inhibitor (SARI) at the presynaptic neuron increases serotonin at $5HT_{1A}$ receptors, where it leads to antidepressant actions. However, SARI action also blocks serotonin actions at $5HT_{2A}$ and $5HT_{2C}$ receptors, thus failing to cause sexual dysfunction, insomnia, or anxiety. In fact, these blocking actions at $5HT_{2A}$ and $5HT_{2C}$ receptors can improve insomnia and anxiety, and theoretically can exert antidepressant actions of their own.

serotonin levels to act at all serotonin receptors, both theoretically with therapeutic actions by stimulating $5HT_{1A}$ receptors, and with side effects as the "cost of doing business" by concomitantly stimulating $5HT_{2A}$ and $5HT_{2C}$ receptors that theoretically cause sexual dysfunction, insomnia, and activation/anxiety, as well as other 5HT receptors (Figure 7-49A). However, with trazodone, $5HT_{1A}$ receptors are stimulated by rising serotonin levels when SERT is inhibited, but $5HT_{2A}$ and $5HT_{2C}$ receptors are blocked by trazodone (Figure 7-49B). This pharmacologic profile alters the clinical profile of trazodone, and explains why trazodone is not associated with sexual dysfunction or insomnia/anxiety and is in fact a treatment for insomnia/anxiety. The same clinical profile applies to other agents with $5HT_{2A}$ antagonist properties such as atypical antipsychotics and mirtazapine, when added to SSRIs/SNRIs, which changes the clinical profile of SSRIs/SNRIs given as monotherapies (Figure 7-49). Also, the combination of $5HT_{2A}$ antagonism with $5HT_{1A}$ stimulation causes enhancement of both glutamate and dopamine release downstream, as discussed in Chapter 5 and illustrated in Figures 5-15 and 5-16, which may also contribute to the antidepressant profile of agents that simultaneously block $5HT_{2A}$ receptors and stimulate $5HT_{1A}$ receptors, such as trazodone, mirtazapine, some atypical antipsychotics, and the combination of SSRIs/SNRIs with these various drugs that are $5HT_{2A}$ antagonists.

325

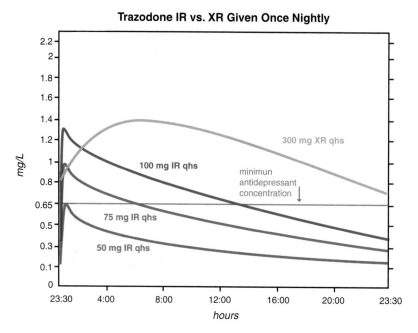

Figure 7-50. Trazodone IR versus XR given once nightly. Shown here are steady-state estimates of the plasma trazodone levels from the hypnotic dosing of 50, 75, or 100 mg once nightly of trazodone immediate-release (IR) over 9 days. Peak drug concentrations are reached rapidly with a similarly rapid fall-off over night. The minimum levels estimated for antidepressant actions of trazodone are reached transiently, if at all, by hypnotic dosing. By contrast, 300 mg of trazodone extended-release (XR) given once nightly generates plasma levels that rise slowly and never fall below minimum antidepressant concentrations. Peak levels of trazodone XR at 300 mg are about the same as the peak levels of trazodone IR at 100 mg.

Different drug in different formulations?

Trazodone is not commonly used at high doses as an antidepressant because it has a short half-life requiring multiple daily doses, and can be very sedating at antidepressant dosing levels. Trazodone comes in an immediate-release (IR) formulation and in various controlled-release formulations in different countries (Figure 7-50). The immediate-release formulation of trazodone has a relatively rapid onset and short duration of action, and in low doses as a hypnotic, patients only need to take it once a day at night (Figure 7-50). Trazodone levels rise rapidly and then fall from their peaks quickly after causing peak dose sedation, making the hypnotic actions rapid in onset, but wearing off before morning so there is no hangover effect (Figure 7-50). These pharmacologic properties make trazodone at low doses an ideal hypnotic but not an ideal antidepressant.

At higher antidepressant doses administered once a day at night, there can be a hangover effect the next morning; splitting the antidepressant dose into two or three times a day still leads to accumulation of trazodone levels and unacceptable daytime sedation (Figure 7-50). By contrast, high doses of controlled-release formulations given once daily at night do not attain the sedating peak levels of the immediate-release during the day, and thus are antidepressant without sedation, which is ideal for an antidepressant (Figure 7-50). For unclear reasons, high-dose trazodone in controlled-release formulations is not as extensively used in clinical practice as is the combination of low-dose trazodone with SSRIs/SNRIs, which is pharmacologically similar. Perhaps clinicians are not aware that the additional properties of trazodone added to SSRIs/SNRIs are likely not only to boost the efficacy of SSRIs/SNRIs in depression and anxiety, but also to have more than a hypnotic effect. These therapeutic effects might also be possible with the more tolerable controlled-release formulations of trazodone as a high-dose monotherapy.

Classic antidepressants: MAO inhibitors

The first clinically effective antidepressants to be discovered were inhibitors of the enzyme monoamine oxidase (MAO). They were discovered by accident when an anti-tuberculosis drug was observed to help depression that coexisted in some of the patients who had tuberculosis. This anti-tuberculosis drug, iproniazid, was eventually found to work in depression by inhibiting the enzyme MAO. However, inhibition of MAO was unrelated to its anti-tubercular actions. Although best known as powerful antidepressants, the monoamine oxidase inhibitors (MAOIs) are also highly effective therapeutic agents for certain anxiety disorders such as panic disorder and social phobia. MAOIs tend to be under-utilized in clinical practice, both because of the availability of many other options, and because of several prevailing myths and misinformation about MAOIs that prevent most modern-day clinicians from gaining familiarity with them.

The MAOIs phenelzine, tranylcypromine, and isocarboxazid are all irreversible enzyme inhibitors, and thus enzyme activity returns only after new enzyme is synthesized about 2–3 weeks later. Amphetamine is also a weak but reversible MAO inhibitor, and some MAOIs have properties related to amphetamine. For example, tranylcypromine has a chemical structure modeled on amphetamine, and thus in addition to MAO inhibitor properties, also has amphetamine-like dopamine-releasing properties. The MAOI selegiline itself does not have amphetamine-like properties, but is metabolized to both *l*-amphetamine and *l*-methamphetamine. Thus, there is a close mechanistic link between some MAOIs and additional amphetamine-like dopamine-releasing actions. It is therefore not surprising that one of the augmenting agents utilized to boost MAOIs in treatment-resistant patients is amphetamine, administered by experts with great caution while monitoring blood pressure.

MAO subtypes

MAO exists in two subtypes, A and B (Table 7-1). The A form preferentially metabolizes the monoamines most closely linked to depression (i.e., serotonin and norepinephrine) whereas the B form preferentially metabolizes trace amines such as

Table 7-1 MAO subtypes

	MAO-A	**MAO-B**
Substrates	Serotonin Norepinephrine Dopamine Tyramine	Dopamine Tyramine Phenylethylamine
Tissue distribution	Brain, gut, liver, placenta, skin	Brain, platelets, lymphocytes

phenylethylamine. Both MAO-A and MAO-B metabolize dopamine and tyramine. Both MAO-A and MAO-B are found in the brain. Noradrenergic neurons (Figure 6-26) and dopaminergic neurons (Figure 4-6) are thought to contain both MAO-A and MAO-B, with perhaps MAO-A activity predominant, whereas serotonergic neurons are thought to contain only MAO-B (Figure 5-14). MAO-A is the major form of this enzyme outside of the brain, with the exception of platelets and lymphocytes, which have MAO-B (Table 7-1).

Brain MAO-A must be inhibited for antidepressant efficacy to occur with MAOI treatment (Figure 7-51). This is not surprising, since this is the form of MAO that preferentially metabolizes serotonin and norepinephrine, two of the three monoamines linked to depression and to antidepressant actions, both of which demonstrate increased brain levels after MAO-A inhibition (Figure 7-51). MAO-A, along with MAO-B, also metabolizes dopamine, but inhibition of MAO-A alone does not appear to lead to robust increases in brain dopamine levels, since MAO-B can still metabolize dopamine (Figure 7-51).

Inhibition of MAO-B is not effective as an antidepressant, as there is no direct effect on either serotonin or norepinephrine metabolism, and little or no dopamine accumulates due to the continued action of MAO-A (Figure 7-52). What therefore is the therapeutic value of MAO-B inhibition? When this enzyme is selectively inhibited, it can boost the action of concomitantly administered levodopa in Parkinson's disease. MAO-B is also thought to convert some environmentally derived amine substrates, called protoxins, into toxins that may cause damage to neurons and possibly contribute to the cause or decline of function in Parkinson's disease. Inhibiting MAO-B could theoretically halt this process, and there is speculation that this might slow the degenerative course of various neurodegenerative disorders including Parkinson's disease, but this has not been proven. Two MAOIs, selegiline and rasagiline, when administered orally in doses selective for inhibition of MAO-B, are approved for use in patients with Parkinson's disease, but are not effective at these selective MAO-B doses as antidepressants.

When MAO-B is inhibited simultaneously with MAO-A, there is robust elevation of dopamine as well as serotonin and norepinephrine (Figure 7-53). This would theoretically provide the most powerful

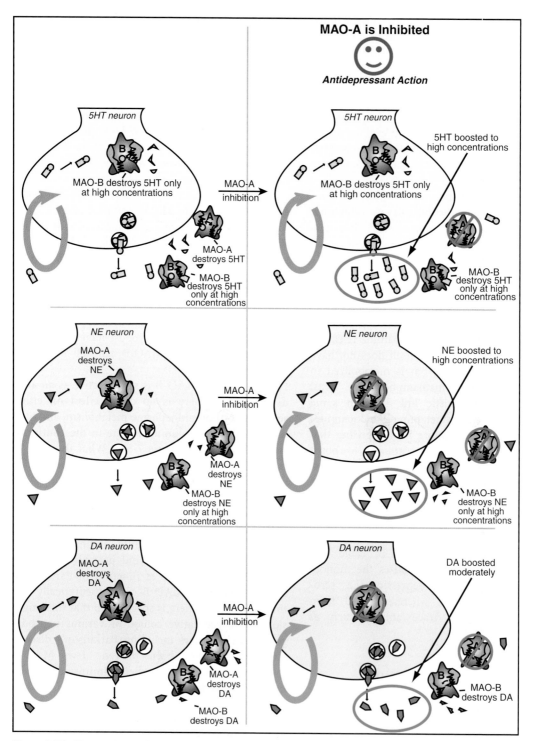

Figure 7-51. Monoamine oxidase A (MAO-A) inhibition. The enzyme MAO-A metabolizes serotonin (5HT) and norepinephrine (NE) as well as dopamine (DA) (left panels). Monoamine oxidase B (MAO-B) also metabolizes DA, but it metabolizes 5HT and NE only at high concentrations (left panels). This means that MAO-A inhibition increases 5HT, NE, and DA (right panels) but that the increase in DA is not as great as that of 5HT and NE because MAO-B can continue to destroy DA (bottom right panel). Inhibition of MAO-A is an efficacious antidepressant strategy.

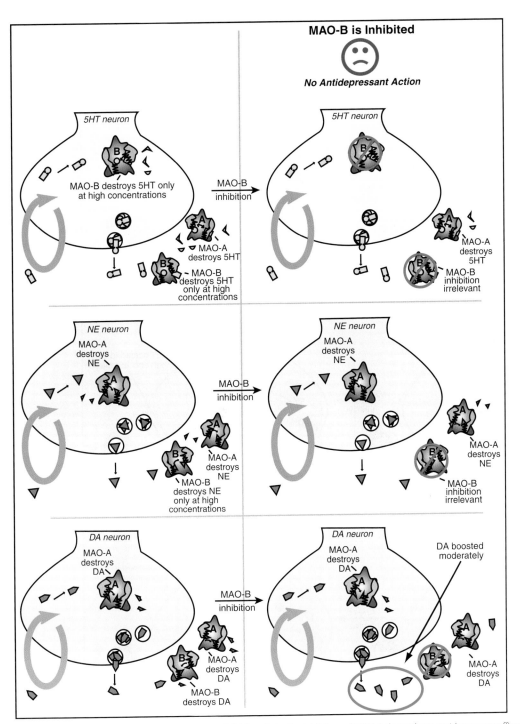

Figure 7-52. Monoamine oxidase B (MAO-B) inhibition. Selective inhibitors of MAO-B do not have antidepressant efficacy. This is because MAO-B metabolizes serotonin (5HT) and norepinephrine (NE) only at high concentrations (top two left panels). Since MAO-B's role in destroying 5HT and NE is small, its inhibition is not likely to be relevant to the concentrations of these neurotransmitters (top two right panels). Selective inhibition of MAO-B also has somewhat limited effects on dopamine (DA) concentrations, because MAO-A continues to destroy DA. However, inhibition of MAO-B does increase DA to some extent, which can be therapeutic in other disease states, such as Parkinson's disease.

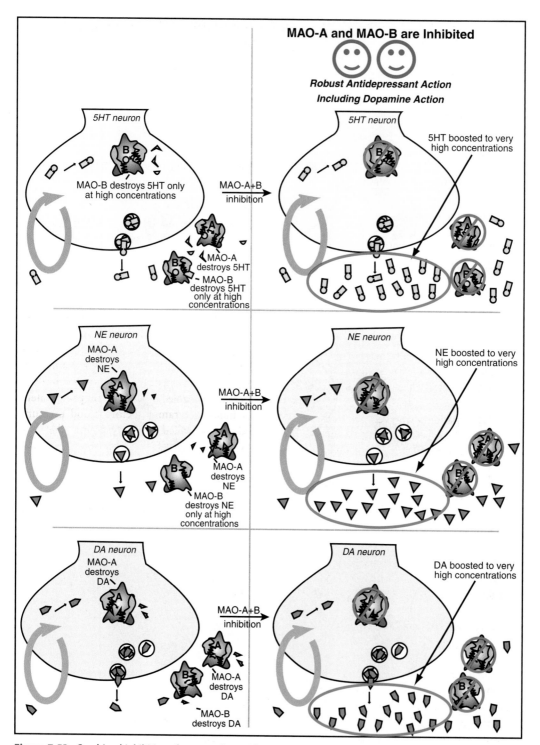

Figure 7-53. Combined inhibition of monoamine oxidase A (MAO-A) and monoamine oxidase B (MAO-B). Combined inhibition of MAO-A and MAO-B may have robust antidepressant actions owing to increases not only in serotonin (5HT) and norepinephrine (NE) but also dopamine (DA). Inhibition of both MAO-A, which metabolizes 5HT, NE, and DA, and MAO-B, which metabolizes primarily DA (left panels), leads to greater increases in each of these neurotransmitters than inhibition of either enzyme alone.

antidepressant efficacy across the range of depressive symptoms, from diminished positive affect to increased negative affect (Figure 6-46). Thus, MAO-A plus MAO-B inhibition is one of the few therapeutic strategies available to increase dopamine in depression, and therefore to treat refractory symptoms of diminished positive affect. This is a good reason for specialists in psychopharmacology to become adept at administering MAOIs, so that they can have an additional strategy within their armamentarium for cases with treatment-resistant symptoms of diminished positive affect, a very common problem in a referral practice.

Is increased MAO-A activity the cause of monoamine deficiency in some patients with depression?

One hypothesis for low levels of monoamines in depression comes from recent brain imaging studies of MAO-A, showing elevated levels of MAO-A activity in depressed patients. This would be predicted to lower the functional availability of monoamine neurotransmitters. MAO-A levels are not decreased by SSRIs, but of course are decreased by MAOIs. Some studies suggest that patients who recover from their depression with SSRI treatment, but do not simultaneously recover normal levels of MAO-A, have continuing vulnerability to relapse. Treatment with MAO-A inhibitors of course will uniquely lower the elevations in MAO-A activity compared to any other antidepressant, and thus may be preferable for some patients with depression. It is even possible that high levels of MAO-A may be linked to some types of treatment resistance. Supporting the potential role of abnormal MAO-A activity as a potential cause of depression or of some forms of treatment resistance is the discovery of a protein called R1 (repressor 1) that controls the expression of MAO-A. R1 may be depleted in both treated and untreated depression, causing a lack of repression of MAO-A synthesis and thus an increase in MAO-A activity in depression, with consequential decrease in monoamines. It is not currently possible to identify in advance those patients who might benefit from MAOI treatment, and these tests are not yet available in clinical practice, but it does point to the potential importance of knowing how to use MAOIs for the treatment of depression.

Myths, misinformation, and a manual for MAOIs

To prescribe MAOIs in clinical practice, it is necessary to understand how to manage two issues: diet and drug interactions. A series of tables that follows organizes these issues into several charts that address myths and misinformation about MAOIs, providing the truth about these myths and proposing clinical management solutions that we will call your MAOI "owner's manual."

The dietary tyramine interaction

One of the biggest barriers to using MAOIs has traditionally been the concern that a patient taking one of these drugs may develop a hypertensive crisis (Table 7-2) after ingesting tyramine in the diet. Normally, the release of norepinephrine by tyramine is inconsequential because MAO-A safely destroys this released norepinephrine (Figure 7-54). However, tyramine in the presence of MAO-A inhibition can elevate blood pressure because norepinephrine is not safely destroyed (Figure 7-55). The body normally has a huge capacity for processing tyramine, and the average person is able to handle approximately 400 mg of ingested tyramine before blood pressure is elevated. A so-called "high-tyramine diet" is unlikely to contain more than about 40 mg of tyramine. When MAO-A is inhibited, it may take as little as 10 mg of dietary tyramine to increase blood pressure (Figure 7-55). Because of the potential danger of a hypertensive crisis from a tyramine reaction in

Table 7-2 Hypertensive crisis

Defined by diastolic blood pressure > 120 mmHg **Potentially fatal reaction characterized by:**
Occipital headache that may radiate frontally
Palpitation
Neck stiffness or soreness
Nausea
Vomiting
Sweating (sometimes with fever)
Dilated pupils, photophobia
Tachycardia or bradycardia, which can be associated with constricting chest pain

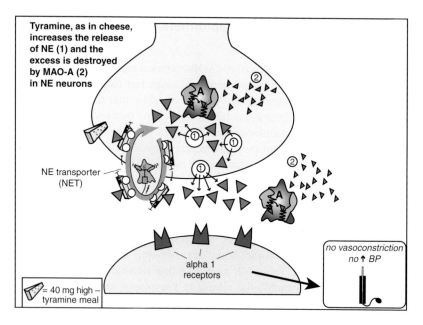

Figure 7-54. Tyramine increases norepinephrine release. Tyramine is an amine present in various foods, including cheese. Indicated in this figure is how a high-tyramine meal (40 mg, depicted here as cheese) acts to increase the release of norepinephrine (NE) (1). However, in normal circumstances the enzyme monoamine oxidase A (MAO-A) readily destroys the excess NE released by tyramine (2), and no harm is done (i.e., no vasoconstriction or elevation in blood pressure).

Labels in figure: Tyramine, as in cheese, increases the release of NE (1) and the excess is destroyed by MAO-A (2) in NE neurons; NE transporter (NET); alpha 1 receptors; = 40 mg high tyramine meal; no vasoconstriction no ↑ BP

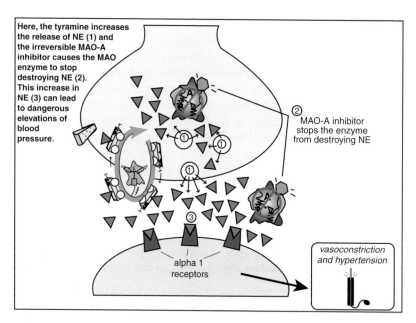

Figure 7-55. Inhibition of monoamine oxidase A (MAO-A) and tyramine. Here tyramine is releasing norepinephrine (NE) just as shown in Figure 7-54 (1). However, this time MAO-A is also being inhibited by an irreversible MAO-A inhibitor. This results in MAO-A stopping its destruction of NE (2). As indicated in Figure 7-51, such MAO-A inhibition in itself causes accumulation of NE. When MAO-A inhibition is taking place in the presence of tyramine, the combination can lead to a very large accumulation of NE (3). Such a great NE accumulation can lead to excessive stimulation of postsynaptic adrenergic receptors (3) and therefore dangerous vasoconstriction and elevation of blood pressure.

Labels in figure: Here, the tyramine increases the release of NE (1) and the irreversible MAO-A inhibitor causes the MAO enzyme to stop destroying NE (2). This increase in NE (3) can lead to dangerous elevations of blood pressure.; MAO-A inhibitor stops the enzyme from destroying NE; alpha 1 receptors; vasoconstriction and hypertension

patients taking irreversible MAOIs, a certain mythology has grown up around how much tyramine is in various foods and therefore what dietary restrictions are necessary (Table 7-3). Since the tyramine reaction is sometimes called a "cheese reaction," there is a myth that all cheese must be restricted for a patient taking an MAOI. However, that is true only for aged cheeses, but not for most processed cheese or for most cheese utilized in most commercial chain pizzas. Also, it is not true that patients taking an MAOI must avoid all wine and beer. Canned and bottled beer are low in tyramine; generally only tap and nonpasteurized beers must be avoided, and many wines are actually quite low in tyramine. Of course, all prescribers should counsel patients taking the classic MAOIs about diet and keep up to date with the tyramine content of the foods their patients wish to eat (Table 7-3).

Table 7-3 Dietary guidelines for patients taking MAO inhibitors

The myth
If you're taking an MAOI, you can't eat cheese, drink wine or beer, or have many other foods that contain tyramine, or else you will develop hypertensive crisis.

The truth
There are a few things to avoid (which are easy to remember), but in practice diet is not really a problem …   … unless you plan to drink a gallon of blue cheese.

The Owner's Manual	
Foods to avoid[a]	**Foods allowed**
Dried, aged, smoked, fermented, spoiled or improperly stored meat, poultry or fish	Fresh or processed meat, poultry and fish; properly stored pickled or smoked fish
Broad bean pods	All other vegetables
Aged cheeses	Processed cheese slices, cottage cheese, ricotta cheese, yogurt, cream cheese
Tap and unpasteurized beer	Canned or bottled beer and alcohol
Marmite	Brewer's and baker's yeast
Sauerkraut, kimchee	
Soy products/tofu	Peanuts
Banana peel	Bananas, avocados, raspberries
Tyramine-containing nutritional supplement	

[a] Not necessary for 6 mg transdermal or low-dose oral selegiline.

In fact, there are two MAOIs that do not require any dietary restrictions. Selegiline is a selective MAO-B inhibitor at low oral doses; administering low oral doses of selegiline does not have any dietary restrictions but also does not inhibit MAO-A in the brain and is therefore not an antidepressant. At high oral doses selegiline does inhibit MAO-A and therefore has antidepressant effects, but requires the need to restrict dietary tyramine. However, delivering selegiline through a transdermal patch allows inhibition of both MAO-A and MAO-B in the brain while largely bypassing inhibition of MAO-A in the gut (Figure 7-56). That is, transdermal delivery is like an intravenous infusion without the needle, delivering drug directly into the systemic circulation, hitting the brain in high doses, and avoiding a first pass through the liver (Figure 7-56). By the time the drug recirculates to the intestine and liver, it has much decreased levels and significantly inhibits only MAO-B in these tissues. This action is sufficiently robust and selective at low doses of transdermal selegiline, and thus no

dietary tyramine restrictions are necessary. At high doses of transdermal selegiline, there is likely some MAO-A inhibition in the gut, and thus some dietary tyramine restrictions may be prudent.

Another mechanism to theoretically reduce risk of tyramine reactions is to use reversible inhibitors of MAO-A (RIMAs). Irreversible inhibition of MAO-A, as with the older MAOIs (Figure 7-54), prevents MAO-A from ever functioning again; enzyme activity returns only after new enzyme is synthesized. RIMAs, on the other hand, can be removed from the enzyme by competitive inhibition by MAO-A substrates (Figure 7-57). Thus, when tyramine releases norepinephrine, there is competition for MAO-A binding, and if norepinephrine levels are high enough, they can displace the RIMA from MAO-A and the enzyme activity is restored, allowing for the normal destruction of the extra norepinephrine and thereby reducing the risk of a tyramine reaction (Figure 7-57). However, the RIMA moclobemide still carries the dietary restriction warnings of irreversible MAOIs. A new

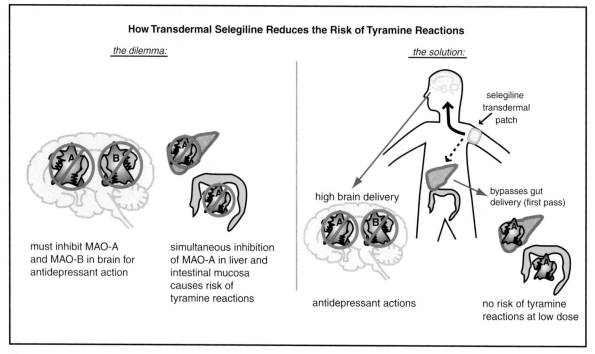

How Transdermal Selegiline Reduces the Risk of Tyramine Reactions

the dilemma:

the solution:

selegiline transdermal patch

high brain delivery

bypasses gut delivery (first pass)

must inhibit MAO-A and MAO-B in brain for antidepressant action

simultaneous inhibition of MAO-A in liver and intestinal mucosa causes risk of tyramine reactions

antidepressant actions

no risk of tyramine reactions at low dose

Figure 7-56. Transdermal selegiline. The selective monoamine oxidase B (MAO-B) inhibitor selegiline has antidepressant efficacy only when given at doses high enough also to inhibit monoamine oxidase A (MAO-A); yet when it is administered orally at these doses, it can also cause a tyramine reaction. How can selegiline inhibit both MAO-A and MAO-B in the brain, to have antidepressant effects, while inhibiting only MAO-B in the gut, so as to avoid a tyramine reaction? Transdermal administration of selegiline delivers the drug directly into the systemic circulation, hitting the brain in high doses and thus having antidepressant effects but avoiding a first pass through the liver and thus reducing risk of a tyramine reaction.

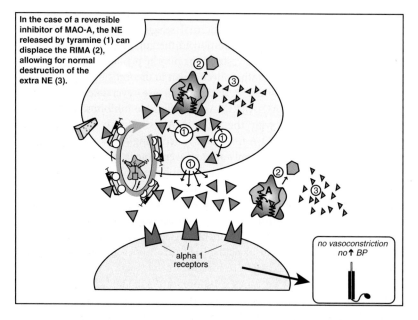

In the case of a reversible inhibitor of MAO-A, the NE released by tyramine (1) can displace the RIMA (2), allowing for normal destruction of the extra NE (3).

alpha 1 receptors

no vasoconstriction no↑ BP

Figure 7-57. Reversible inhibition of monoamine oxidase A (MAO-A). Shown in this figure is the combination of an MAO-A inhibitor and tyramine. However, in this case the MAO-A inhibitor is of the reversible type (reversible inhibitor of MAO-A, or RIMA). The accumulation of norepinephrine (NE) released by tyramine (1) can displace the RIMA (2), allowing for normal destruction of the extra NE (3).

RIMA in late-stage clinical testing is TriRima (CX157) which will hopefully not require dietary restrictions.

Drug–drug interactions for MAOIs

While MAOIs are famous for their tyramine reactions, drug–drug interactions are potentially more important clinically. MAOI drug–drug interactions may not only be more common, but also some interactions can be dangerous or even lethal. Drug interactions with MAOIs are poorly understood by many practitioners. Since most candidates for MAOI treatment will require treatment with many concomitant drugs over time, including treatment for coughs and colds, and for pain, this can prevent psychopharmacologists from prescribing an MAOI if they do not know which drugs are safe to give and which ones must be avoided.

There are two general types of potentially dangerous drug interactions with MAOIs for a practitioner to understand and avoid: those that can raise blood pressure by sympathomimetic actions, and those that can cause a potentially fatal serotonin syndrome by serotonin reuptake inhibition.

MAOIs and sympathomimetics to avoid or administer with caution

When drugs that boost adrenergic stimulation by a mechanism other than MAO inhibition are added to an MAOI, potentially dangerous hypertensive reactions can occur. For example, decongestants stimulate postsynaptic α_1 receptors directly or indirectly (Figure 7-58A); this constricts nasal blood vessels, but does not typically elevate blood pressure at therapeutic doses when the decongestants are given by themselves. MAOIs elevate norepinephrine, but this alone does not typically elevate blood pressure either (Figure 7-58B). However, the direct α_1 stimulation of a decongestant combined with the elevation of norepinephrine that occurs when taking an MAOI may be sufficient to cause hypertension or even hypertensive crisis (Figure 7-58C). This is less likely with topical/intranasal administration and less likely in those not vulnerable to hypertension, but must be monitored in any patient taking a decongestant with an MAOI. Other agents that can increase noradrenergic activity include stimulants, some antidepressants, and others listed in Table 7-4. For patients with colds/upper respiratory infections, who are on MAOIs, it is probably best to use

antihistamines, which are safe with the exception of those that are also serotonin reuptake inhibitors (e.g., brompheniramine and chlorpheniramine) (Table 7-4). Cough medicines with expectorants or codeine are safe, but avoid dextromethorphan, a weak serotonin reuptake inhibitor.

MAOI interactions with anesthetics

Both general anesthesia and local anesthetics that contain epinephrine can cause changes in blood pressure (Table 7-4). Thus, for a patient taking an MAO inhibitor who needs to have a local anesthetic, one should choose an agent that does not contain vasoconstrictors (Table 7-5). For elective surgery, one should wash out the MAO inhibitor 10 days prior to the surgery (Table 7-5). For urgent surgery or elective surgery when the patient is still taking an MAO inhibitor, one can cautiously use a benzodiazepine, mivacurium, rapacuronium, morphine, or codeine (Table 7-5).

Avoid MAOIs with serotonergic agents

A potentially much more dangerous combination than that of adrenergic stimulants and MAOIs is the combination of agents that inhibit serotonin reuptake with those that inhibit MAO. Inhibition of the serotonin transporter (SERT) leads to therapeutic levels of increased synaptic availability of serotonin (Figure 7-59A), as does inhibition of MAO-A (Figure 7-59B). However, in combination, these two mechanisms can cause excessive stimulation of postsynaptic serotonin receptors, which has the potential to cause a fatal *serotonin syndrome* or *serotonin toxicity* (Figure 7-59C). The general clinical features of serotonin toxicity can range from migraines, myoclonus, agitation, and confusion on the mild end of the spectrum, to hyperthermia, seizures, coma, cardiovascular collapse, permanent hyperthermic brain damage, and even death at the severe end of the spectrum. Early diagnostic criteria for serotonin toxicity (syndrome) were developed by Sternbach based on examination of published case reports (Table 7-6). However, these criteria can lack both sensitivity and specificity. The apparent limitations of the Sternbach criteria for serotonin toxicity prompted Gilman's group in Australia to develop a set of diagnostic criteria called the Hunter Serotonin Toxicity Criteria based on retrospective analysis of more than 2200 patients who experienced overdose from a serotonergic drug (Table 7-7). Only five of the clinical features associated

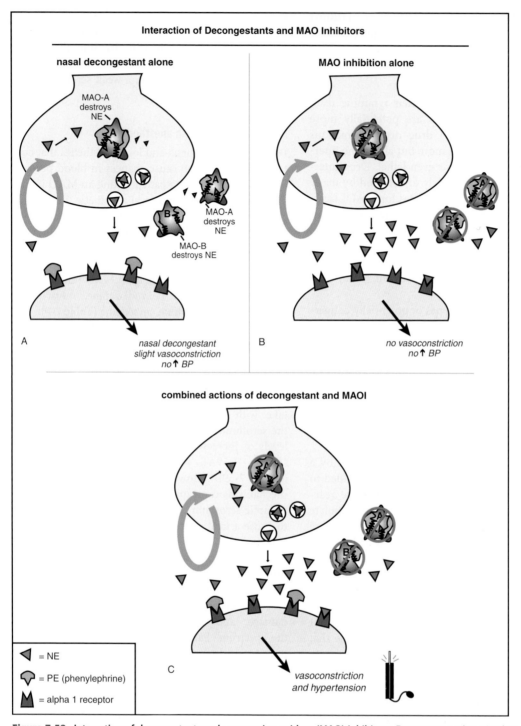

Figure 7-58. Interaction of decongestants and monoamine oxidase (MAO) inhibitors. Decongestants that stimulate postsynaptic α_1 receptors, such as phenylephrine, may interact with MAO inhibitors to increase risk of a tyramine reaction. Decongestants work by constricting nasal blood vessels, but they do not typically elevate blood pressure at the doses used (A). An MAO inhibitor given alone (and without the ingestion of tyramine) increases norepinephrine but does not usually cause vasoconstriction or hypertension (B). However, the noradrenergic actions of an MAO inhibitor combined with the direct α_1 stimulation of a decongestant may be sufficient to cause hypertension or even hypertensive crisis (C).

Table 7-4 Drugs that boost norepinephrine and thus should be used with caution with MAO inhibitors

The myth

If you're taking an MAOI, you can't take anything with norepinephrine reuptake inhibition, which means:

(1) You cannot have a local or a general anesthetic, so patients who need dental work, sutures, or surgery cannot take an MAOI.
(2) You can't take cold medications, such as decongestants, antihistamines, or cough medicines, so patients who get colds cannot take MAOIs.
(3) You can't take stimulants, so patients who need stimulants cannot take MAOIs.

The truth

Be careful using local anesthetics that contain epinephrine, and using general anesthesia, as these can cause blood pressure changes.

Sympathomimetic decongestants and stimulants should be used with caution while monitoring blood pressure in patients for whom the benefits are greater than the risks, and should be avoided only in high-risk/low-benefit populations.

The Owner's Manual: use with caution*

Decongestants	Stimulants	Antidepressants with norepineprhine reuptake inhibition	Other
Phenylephrine	Amphetamine	Most tricyclics	Phentermine
Pseudoephedrine	Methylphenidate	NRIs	Local anesthetics containing vasoconstrictors
	Modafinil	SNRIs	Tramadol, tapentadol
	Armodafinil	NDRIs	Cocaine, methamphetamine

* Some of these drugs may also have serotonergic properties that require contraindication with MAOIs.
NDRI, norepinephrine–dopamine reuptake inhibitor; NRI, norepinephrine reuptake inhibitor; SNRI, serotonin–norepinephrine reuptake inhibitor.

Table 7-5 The Owner's Manual: use of anesthetics

Local anesthetic	Elective surgery	Urgent or elective surgery when patient is still taking an MAO inhibitor
Choose an agent that does not contain vasoconstrictors	Wash out the MAO inhibitor 10 days prior to surgery	Cautiously use a benzodiazepine, mivacurium, rapacuronium, morphine, or codeine

Table 7-6 Serotonin toxicity: Sternbach criteria

Recent addition of or increase in a known serotonergic agent

Absence of other possible etiologies (infection, substance abuse, withdrawal, etc.)

No recent addition or increase of a neuroleptic agent

At least three of the following:

- Agitation
- Myoclonus
- Hyperreflexia
- Diaphoresis
- Shivering
- Tremor
- Diarrhea
- Ataxia/incoordination
- Fever

with serotonin toxicity were needed to make an accurate diagnosis: clonus, agitation, diaphoresis, tremor, and hyperreflexia. In addition, hypertonicity and hyperpyrexia were present in all life-threatening cases of serotonin toxicity. They also developed decision rules for diagnosis, based on the presence or absence of the seven clinical features (Table 7-7).

Drugs to avoid in combination with MAOIs in order to prevent serotonin toxicity are listed in Table 7-8. One can essentially never combine agents that have potent serotonin reuptake inhibition with

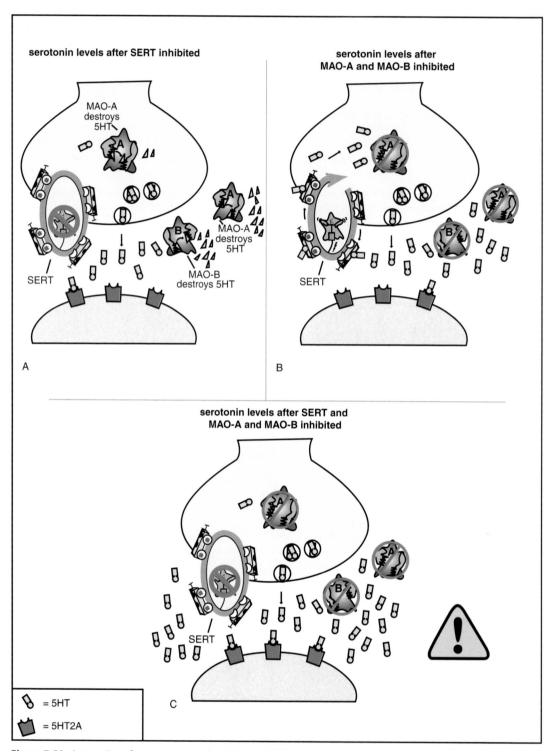

Figure 7-59. Interaction of serotonin reuptake inhibitors (SRIs) and monoamine oxidase (MAO) inhibitors. Inhibition of the serotonin transporter (SERT) leads to increased synaptic availability of serotonin (A). Similarly, inhibition of MAO leads to increased serotonin levels (B). These two mechanisms in combination can cause excessive stimulation of postsynaptic serotonin receptors, which may lead to hyperthermia, seizures, coma, cardiovascular collapse, or even death (C).

Table 7-7 Serotonin toxicity: Hunter criteria

Clinical features	Decision rules: in the presence of a serotonergic agent
Clonus	IF (spontaneous clonus = yes) THEN serotonin toxicity = YES
Agitation	OR ELSE IF (inducible clonus = yes) AND (agitation = yes) OR (diaphoresis = yes) THEN serotonin toxicity = YES
Diaphoresis	OR ELSE IF (ocular clonus = yes) AND (agitation = yes) OR (diaphoresis = yes) THEN serotonin toxicity = YES
Tremor	OR ELSE IF (tremor = yes) AND (hyperreflexia = yes) THEN serotonin toxicity = YES
Hyperreflexia	OR ELSE IF (hypertonic = yes) AND (temperature >38 °C) AND (ocular clonus = yes) OR (inducible clonus = yes) THEN serotonin toxicity = YES
Hypertonicity	OR ELSE serotonin toxicity = NO
Hyperpyrexia	

agents given in doses that cause substantial MAO inhibition. This includes any selective serotonin reuptake inhibitor (SSRI), any serotonin–norepinephrine reuptake inhibitor (SNRI), and the tricyclic antidepressant clomipramine. Opioids that block serotonin reuptake, especially meperidine but also tramadol, and dextromethorphan, must also be avoided when an MAO inhibitor is given (Table 7-8). Several drugs of abuse also block serotonin reuptake: thus, diligent questioning about drug use/abuse is necessary when considering prescribing an MAO inhibitor (Table 7-8). Although it is commonly believed that serotonin 1A partial agonism or the proserotonergic actions of lithium could also contribute to serotonin syndrome in combination with an MAOI, these mechanisms are not actually contraindications, and such medications can be administered with caution by experts in combination with an MAOI.

MAOI interactions with TCAs

MAOIs are formally contraindicated in the prescribing information for patients taking antidepressants that are norepinephrine reuptake inhibitors, such as most tricyclic antidepressants. This is because the sudden addition of noradrenergic reuptake blockade

Table 7-8 Drugs to avoid in combination with an MAO inhibitor due to the risk of serotonin syndrome/toxicity

The myth

You can't take any medications that block serotonin reuptake, which means you can't take any psychotropic medications. Since all patients who are candidates for an MAOI need concomitant medications, no one can take an MAOI.

Besides, you cannot get there from here because in order to start an MAOI, you have to disrupt everything, stopping all other meds for 2 weeks after taper. And, if you have to stop an MAOI to go back to a psychotropic medication, you have to go without all meds for another 2 weeks. This is an unacceptable risk and a hassle.

The truth

You must avoid only agents that block serotonin reuptake. There are many options for not only bridging between serotonin reuptake inhibitors and MAOIs, but also augmenting MAOIs.

The Owner's Manual: do not use

Antidepressants	Drugs of abuse	Opioids	Other
SSRIs	MDMA (ecstasy)	Meperidine	Non-subcutaneous sumatriptan
SNRIs	Cocaine	Tramadol	Chlorpheniramine
Clomipramine	Methamphetamine	Methadone	Brompheniramine
St. John's wort	High-dose or injected amphetamine	Fentanyl	Procarbazine?
			Dextromethorphan

MDMA, 3,4-methylenedioxymethamphetamine; SNRI, serotonin–norepinephrine reuptake inhibitor; SSRI, selective serotonin reuptake inhibitor.

in someone on an MAOI may result in a hypertensive reaction. However, with the exception of clomipramine, a potent serotonin reuptake inhibitor, other tricyclic antidepressants can be combined with MAOIs with caution for severely treatment-resistant patients by experts doing careful monitoring (Table 7-9). If this option is selected, one should start the MAO inhibitor at the same time as the tricyclic antidepressant (both at low doses) after an appropriate drug washout; then, one should alternately increase the doses of these agents every few days to a week as tolerated. The MAOI should not be started first.

Cyclobenzaprine, carbamazepine, and oxcarbazepine are structurally related to tricyclic antidepressants, and therefore some individuals believe they cannot be used with MAOIs; however, these agents do not block serotonin or norepinephrine reuptake and thus can be used with caution (Table 7-9).

MAOI interactions with opioids

Contrary to popular opinion, there is no dangerous pharmacological interaction between MAOIs and opioid mechanisms; instead, the reason why some opioids must be avoided is that certain agents (especially meperidine; possibly methadone and tramadol) have concomitant serotonin reuptake inhibition, while another (tapentadol) has norepinephrine reuptake inhibition (Table 7-10). Analgesics, including opioids, which are safe to administer with an MAOI are those lacking serotonin reuptake inhibiting properties, such as aspirin, acetaminophen, nonsteroidal anti-inflammatory drugs (NSAIDs), codeine, hydrocodone, and some others (Table 7-10).

Switching to and from MAOIs, and bridging medications to use during the switches

Because of the risk of serotonin toxicity, complete washout of a serotonergic drug is necessary before starting an MAO inhibitor (Figure 7-60). One must wait at least 5 half-lives after discontinuing the serotonergic drug before starting the MAO inhibitor. For most drugs, this means waiting 5–7 days; a notable exception is fluoxetine, for which one must wait 5 weeks because of

Table 7-9 The Owner's Manual: using tricyclic antidepressants with MAO inhibitors

Contraindicated	Use with caution
Clomipramine	Other tricyclic antidepressants
	Cyclobenzaprine
	Carbamazepine
	Oxcarbazepine

Table 7-10 Combining MAO inhibitors and pain medications

The myth
If you're taking an MAOI, you can't take painkillers because they will kill you, so patients who have sprained ankles, sore muscles, dental extractions, or surgeries cannot take MAOIs, as they must avoid all opioid and non-opioid painkillers.

The truth
There are a few things to avoid (which are easy to remember), and in practice, this is not really a problem.

The Owner's Manual				
Use with MAOIs				
Should be fine	Should be cautious	May sometimes be done by experts	Is not recommended	Is strictly prohibited
Acetaminophen	Buprenorphine	Hydromorphone	Fentanyl	Meperidine
Aspirin	Butophanol	Morphine	Methadone	
NSAIDs	Codeine	Oxycodone	Tapentadol	
	Hydrocodone	Oxymorphone	Tramadol	
	Nalbuphine			
	Pentazocine			

its long half-life and the long half-life of its active metabolite norfluoxetine.

When switching in the other direction, namely from an MAOI to a serotonin reuptake inhibitor, one must wait at least 14 days following the discontinuation of the MAO inhibitor before starting the serotonergic drug, to allow regeneration of sufficient MAO enzyme (Figure 7-61).

Because there is a required gap in antidepressant treatment when switching to or from an MAO inhibitor, clinicians may be concerned about managing symptoms during that time period. There are many medication options, depending on the individual patient's situation. These include benzodiazepines, Z-drug sedative hypnotics (e.g., zolpidem, eszopiclone, zaleplon), trazodone, lamotrigine, valproate, several other anticonvulsants, stimulants, and atypical antipsychotics (Table 7-11). Specifically, although trazodone does have serotonin reuptake inhibition at

Table 7-11 The Owner's Manual: how to bridge

Use these drugs with caution and careful monitoring while waiting to start an MAOI or when discontinuing an MAOI
Benzodiazepines
Z-drug hypnotics
Trazodone
Lamotrigine
Valproate
Gabapentin, pregabalin, topiramate, carbamazepine, oxcarbazepine
Stimulants
Atypical antipsychotics

Switching From a Serotonergic Drug to an MAOI

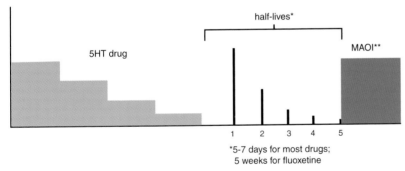

*5-7 days for most drugs; 5 weeks for fluoxetine

**titration schedule for MAOI may differ depending on the individual agent

Figure 7-60. Switching from a serotonergic drug to an MAOI. Because of the risk of serotonin toxicity, complete washout of a serotonergic drug is necessary before starting an MAOI. One must wait at least 5 half-lives after discontinuing the serotonergic drug before starting the MAOI. For most drugs, this means waiting 5–7 days; a notable exception is fluoxetine, for which one must wait 5 weeks due to its long half-life.

Switching From an MAOI to a Serotonergic Drug

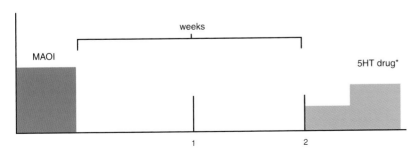

*titration schedule for 5HT drug may differ depending on the individual agent

Figure 7-61. Switching from an MAOI to a serotonergic drug. If one is switching from an MAOI to a serotonin reuptake inhibitor, one must wait at least 14 days following the discontinuation of the MAOI before starting the serotonergic drug.

341

antidepressant doses (i.e., 150 mg or higher), this property is not clinically relevant at the low doses used for insomnia while bridging an MAO inhibitor. The atypical antipsychotic ziprasidone also has serotonin reuptake inhibition, and is probably best avoided.

The bottom line for MAOIs

MAOIs should not be discounted as valuable treatment options for treatment-resistant depression and some treatment-resistant anxiety disorders such as panic disorder and social anxiety disorder. Although use of an MAOI does require a watchful eye over dietary intake, the restrictions are not as widespread as many believe. Likewise, although drug interactions can be serious and concomitant medication use must be stringently overseen, there are some mistaken beliefs regarding the extent of the medication mechanisms that must be avoided. Armed with knowledge of MAOI therapeutic, dietary, and drug-interaction mechanisms, clinicians may be able to revive these agents as therapeutic tools in the fight against treatment-resistant depression and anxiety.

Classic antidepressants: tricyclic antidepressants

The tricyclic antidepressants (TCAs) (Table 7-12; Figure 7-62) were so named because their chemical structure contains three rings. The TCAs were

Table 7-12 Some tricyclic antidepressants still in use

Generic name	Trade name
Clomipramine	Anafranil
Imipramine	Tofranil
Amitriptyline	Elavil; Endep; Tryprizol; Loroxyl
Nortriptyline	Pamelor; Endep; Aventyl
Protriptyline	Vivactil
Maprotiline	Ludiomil
Amoxapine	Asendin
Doxepin	Sinequan; Adapin
Desipramine	Norpramin; Pertofran
Trimipramine	Surmontil
Dothiepin	Prothiaden
Lofepramine	Deprimyl; Gamanil
Tianeptine	Coaxil; Stablon

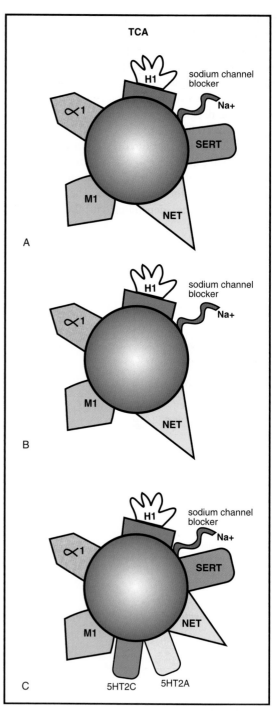

Figure 7-62. Icons of tricyclic antidepressants. All tricyclic antidepressants block reuptake of norepinephrine and are antagonists at H_1-histaminic, α_1-adrenergic, and muscarinic cholinergic receptors; they also block voltage-sensitive sodium channels (A, B, and C). Some tricyclic antidepressants are also potent inhibitors of the serotonin reuptake pump (A), and some may additionally be antagonists at serotonin 2A and 2C receptors (C).

synthesized about the same time as other three-ringed molecules which were shown to be effective tranquilizers for schizophrenia (i.e., the early antipsychotic neuroleptic drugs such as chlorpromazine) but were a disappointment when tested as antipsychotics. However, during testing for schizophrenia, they were discovered to be antidepressants. Long after their antidepressant properties were observed, the tricyclic antidepressants were discovered to block the reuptake pumps for norepinephrine (i.e., NET), or for both norepinephrine and serotonin (i.e., SERT) (Figures 7-62, 7-63, 7-64). Some tricyclics have equal or greater potency for SERT inhibition

(e.g., clomipramine: Figure 7-62A); others are more selective for NET inhibition (e.g., desipramine, maprotiline, nortriptyline, protriptyline: Figure 7-62B). Most, however, block both serotonin and norepinephrine reuptake to some extent. In addition, some tricyclic antidepressants have antagonist actions at $5HT_{2A}$ and $5HT_{2C}$ receptors which could contribute to their therapeutic profile (Figures 7-62C, 7-65, 7-66).

The major limitation to the tricyclic antidepressants has never been their efficacy: these are quite effective agents. The problem with drugs in this class is the fact that all of them share at least four other

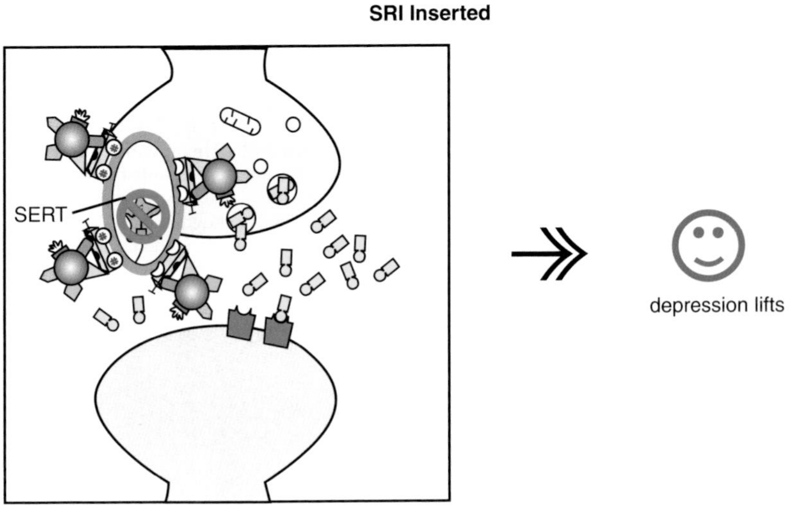

SRI Inserted

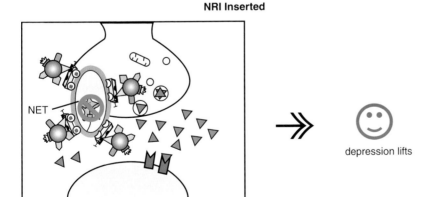

depression lifts

Figure 7-63. Therapeutic actions of tricyclic antidepressants (TCAs), part 1. In this figure, the TCA is shown with its serotonin reuptake inhibitor (SRI) portion inserted into the serotonin transporter (SERT), blocking it and causing an antidepressant effect.

NRI Inserted

depression lifts

Figure 7-64. Therapeutic actions of tricyclic antidepressants (TCAs), part 2. In this figure, the TCA is shown with its norepinephrine reuptake inhibitor (NRI) portion inserted into the norepinephrine transporter (NET), blocking it and causing an antidepressant effect. Thus both the serotonin reuptake portion (Figure 7-63) and the norepinephrine reuptake portion of the TCA act pharmacologically to cause an antidepressant effect.

5HT2A Inserted

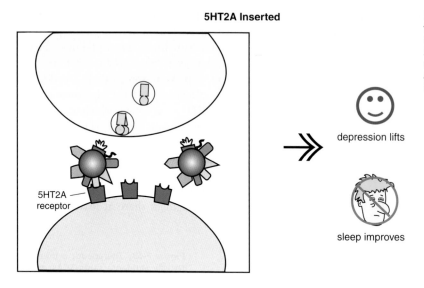

Figure 7-65. Therapeutic actions of tricyclic antidepressants (TCAs), part 3. In this figure, the TCA is shown with its $5HT_{2A}$ portion inserted into the $5HT_{2A}$ receptor, blocking it and causing an antidepressant effect as well as potentially improving sleep.

depression lifts

sleep improves

5HT2C Inserted

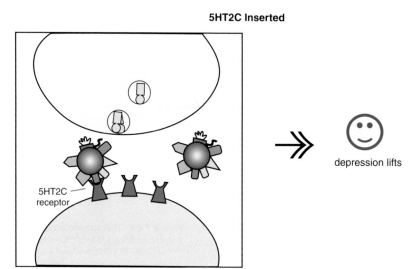

Figure 7-66. Therapeutic actions of tricyclic antidepressants (TCAs), part 4. In this figure, the TCA is shown with its $5HT_{2C}$ portion inserted into the $5HT_{2C}$ receptor, blocking it and causing an antidepressant effect.

depression lifts

unwanted pharmacologic actions, shown in Figure 7-62: namely, blockade of muscarinic cholinergic receptors, H_1-histaminic receptors, α_1-adrenergic receptors, and voltage-sensitive sodium channels (Figures 7-67 through 7-70).

Blockade of H_1-histaminic receptors, also called antihistaminic action, causes sedation and may cause weight gain (Figure 7-67). Blockade of M_1-muscarinic cholinergic receptors, also known as anticholinergic actions, causes dry mouth, blurred vision, urinary retention, and constipation (Figure 7-68). Blockade of α_1-adrenergic receptors causes orthostatic hypotension and dizziness (Figure 7-69). Tricyclic antidepressants also weakly block voltage-sensitive sodium channels (VSSCs) in heart and brain, and in overdose this action is thought to be the cause of coma and seizures due to central nervous system actions, and cardiac arrhythmias and cardiac arrest and death due to peripheral cardiac actions (Figure 7-70).

Tricyclic antidepressants are not merely antidepressants, since one of them (clomipramine)

H1 Inserted

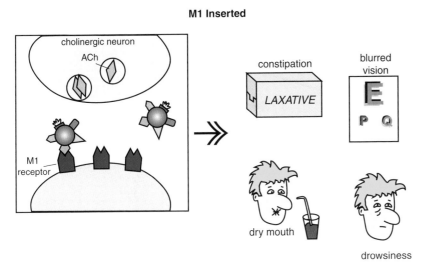

Figure 7-67. Side effects of tricyclic antidepressants (TCAs), part 1. In this figure, the TCA is shown with its antihistamine (H₁) portion inserted into histamine receptors, causing the side effects of weight gain and drowsiness.

M1 Inserted

Figure 7-68. Side effects of tricyclic antidepressants (TCAs), part 2. In this figure, the TCA is shown with its anticholinergic/antimuscarinic (M₁) portion inserted into acetylcholine receptors, causing the side effects of constipation, blurred vision, dry mouth, and drowsiness.

∝ 1 Inserted

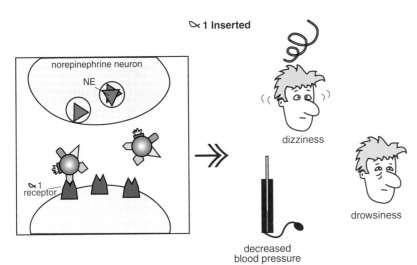

Figure 7-69. Side effects of tricyclic antidepressants (TCAs), part 3. In this figure, the TCA is shown with its α-adrenergic antagonist portion inserted into α₁-adrenergic receptors, causing the side effects of dizziness, drowsiness, and decreased blood pressure.

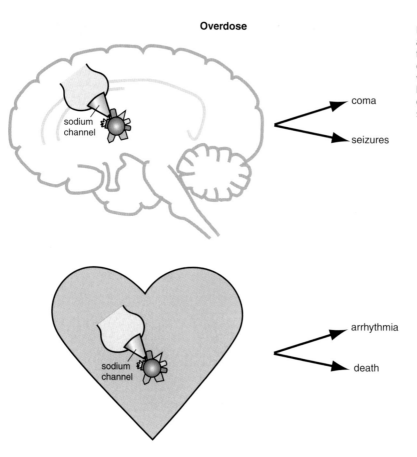

Overdose

coma

seizures

arrhythmia

death

Figure 7-70. Side effects of tricyclic antidepressants (TCAs), part 4. In this figure, the TCA is shown with its sodium channel blocker portion blocking voltage-sensitive sodium channels in the brain (top) and heart (bottom). In overdose, this action can lead to coma, seizures, arrhythmia, and even death.

has anti-obsessive–compulsive disorder effects and many of them have anti-panic effects at antidepressant doses and efficacy for neuropathic and low back pain at low doses. Because of their side effects and potential for death in overdose, tricyclic antidepressants have fallen into second-line use for depression.

Augmenting antidepressants

An increasing number of agents, devices, and procedures are now utilized alone or in combination with standard antidepressants to augment antidepressant efficacy in patients who do not attain full remission. The use of atypical antipsychotics as augmenting agents to antidepressants, and the hypothetical mechanism of their action in depression, is discussed extensively in Chapter 5. Above we have mentioned the combination of the 5HT$_{1A}$ partial agonist buspirone with SSRIs in the section covering vilazodone.

Lithium is discussed in Chapter 8 on mood stabilizers. Here, we mention various natural products, hormones, neurostimulation therapies, and psychotherapies as alternatives or as augmentation to antidepressants.

L-5-Methyltetrahydrofolate (L-methylfolate): monoamine modulator

L-Methylfolate, synthesized in the body from folate or dihydrofolate in the diet (Figure 7-71) or available as a medical food by prescription and called Deplin in the US, is an important regulator of a critical cofactor for monoamine neurotransmitter synthesis, namely tetrahydrobiopterin or BH4 (Figure 7-72). The monoamine synthetic enzymes that require BH4 as a cofactor are both tryptophan hydroxylase, the rate-limiting enzyme for serotonin synthesis, and tyrosine hydroxylase, the rate-limiting enzyme not only for dopamine synthesis but also for norepinephrine

Formation of L-methylfolate from Folic Acid (F)

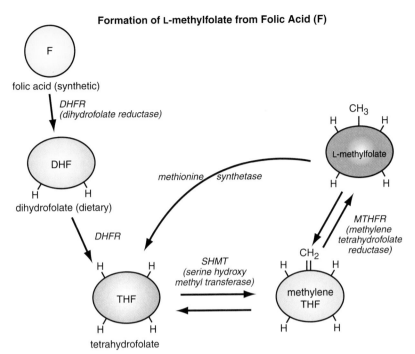

Figure 7-71. Formation of L-methylfolate from folic acid (F). L-Methylfolate is a monoamine modulator naturally synthesized from the vitamin folate for use within the central nervous system. Folic acid (synthetic) is converted to dihydrofolate (DHF) by the enzyme dihydrofolate reductase (DHFR), and DHF, in turn, is converted to tetrahydrofolate (THF), again by DHFR. Serine hydroxymethyl-transferase (SHMT) then converts THF to methylene THF. Finally, methylene THF is converted by methylene tetrahydrofolate reductase (MTHFR) to L-methylfolate.

BH4 Cofactor for Monoamine Neurotransmitter Synthesis

tyrosine hydroxlase

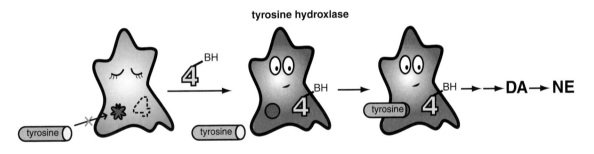

tryptophan hydroxlase

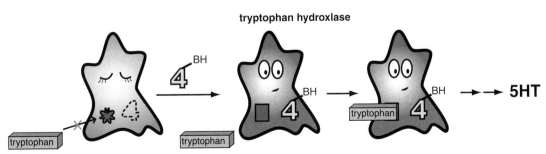

Figure 7-72. Tetrahydrobiopterin (BH4) cofactor for monoamine neurotransmitter synthesis. BH4 is a critical enzyme cofactor for tyrosine hydroxylase, the rate-limiting enzyme for dopamine and norepinephrine synthesis, and tryptophan hydroxylase, the rate-limiting enzyme for serotonin. Because L-methylfolate regulates BH4 production, it therefore plays an indirect role in regulating monoamine synthesis and concentrations.

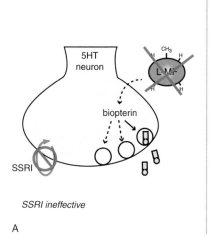

SSRI ineffective

A

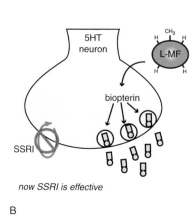

now SSRI is effective

B

Figure 7-73. Folate deficiency and monoamines. (A) Because L-methylfolate (L-MF) indirectly regulates monoamine neurotransmitter synthesis, deficiency of folate, from which it is derived, can lead to reduced monoamine levels and thus to symptoms of depression. Reduced synthesis of monoamines may mean that, even in the presence of a selective serotonin reuptake inhibitor (SSRI), serotonin levels may remain low. In fact, studies show that low levels of folate or L-MF may be linked to depression in some patients. (B) Administration of L-MF, folate, or folinic acid in conjunction with an antidepressant may boost the therapeutic effects of antidepressant monotherapy. High doses of oral L-MF may be the most efficient of these for boosting BH4 production in the central nervous system and thus enhancing brain monoamine neurotransmitter levels.

synthesis (Figure 7-72). Low amounts of L-methylfolate from genetic and/or environmental/dietary causes could theoretically lead to low synthesis of monoamines (Figures 7-73 and 7-74) and contribute to depression or to the resistance of some patients to treatment with antidepressants. That is, antidepressants such as SSRIs/SNRIs and others rely upon the continued synthesis of monoamines in order to work (Figure 7-73A). If there are no monoamines released, reuptake blockade is ineffective (Figure 7-73A). However, repletion of monoamine synthesis by L-methylfolate would theoretically make such patients responsive to antidepressants (Figure 7-73B).

A second mechanism involving L-methylfolate theoretically influences monoamine levels. That is, methylation of genes silences them, as discussed in Chapter 1 and illustrated in Figure 1-30. L-Methylfolate provides the methyl group for this silencing, so if L-methylfolate is low, potentially silencing of various genes could also be low. Specifically, if the silencing of the gene for the enzyme COMT (catechol-O-methyl-transferase) is low, more copies of this enzyme are made and enzyme activity goes up, causing dopamine levels to go down particularly in prefrontal cortex, potentially compromising information processing and causing symptoms such as cognitive dysfunction (Figure 7-74A). Hypothetically, silencing of COMT synthesis by L-methylfolate could result in higher dopamine levels in prefrontal cortex and improve symptoms linked to dopamine deficiency, such as cognitive deficits (Figure 7-74B).

What could cause problems in L-methylfolate availability that might lead to inefficient functioning of monoamine neurotransmitters? Some patients have dietary deficiencies severe enough to result in low levels of folate (or reciprocally high levels of homocysteine). In others, the deficiency in L-methylfolate may be more functional than manifest as low blood levels, and linked instead to genetic variants in folate metabolism. Several genetic variants exist in enzymes that regulate L-methylfolate levels:

- Methylene tetrahydrofolate reductase: MTHFR C677T; MTHFR A1298C
- Methionine synthase: MTR A2756G
- Methionine synthase reductase: MTRR A66G

Inheriting variants of these enzymes that lead to less availability of L-methylfolate could potentially compromise monoamine levels by impacting their synthesis and metabolism (Figures 7-73 and 7-74). This in turn could hypothetically contribute either to the cause of depression or some symptoms of depression, or be linked to treatment resistance. Evidence for this is only beginning to accumulate, including who might be the best candidates with depression for treatment with L-methylfolate (in contrast to folate) that would bypass these genetic variants. One hint comes from studies of MTHFR and COMT in schizophrenia (discussed in Chapter 4) and suggests that effects of some gene variants on the efficiency of information processing might be greater if variants in two or more particular genes are inherited together (see Figure 4-44).

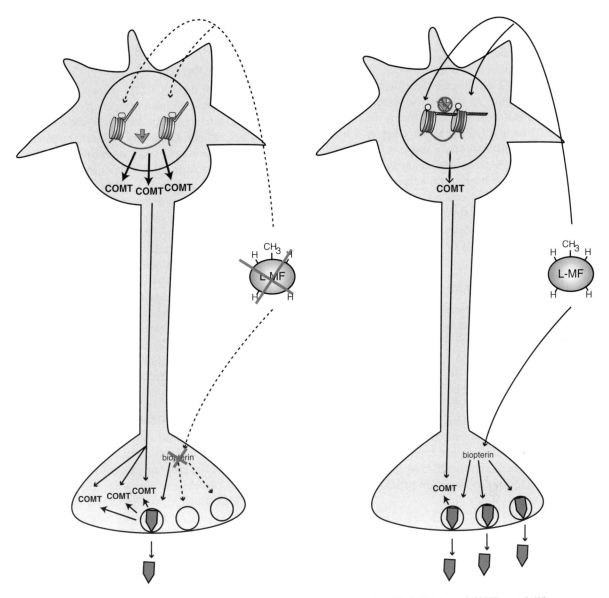

Figure 7-74A. L-Methylfolate and COMT, part 1. L-Methylfolate (L-MF) assists in the formation of tetrahydrobiopterin (biopterin), which is a critical cofactor for the synthesis of monoamines including dopamine. In addition, L-methylfolate could hypothetically lead to methylation of the promoter for the gene of the enzyme COMT (catechol-O-methyl-transferase), which inactivates dopamine and norepinephrine. This methylation silences the gene and decreases the synthesis of COMT enzyme, which reduces the metabolism of dopamine and norepinephrine. When L-methylfolate is deficient, biopterin formation is reduced and thus it is not sufficiently present to activate the enzyme that synthesizes dopamine, and dopamine levels are reduced. Furthermore, in the absence of L-methylfolate, methylation of the gene for COMT is reduced, leading to activation of this gene and thus increasing COMT synthesis. This in turn increases dopamine metabolism, further reducing dopamine levels.

Figure 7-74B. L-Methylfolate and COMT, part 2. When L-methylfolate (L-MF) is present, it can assist in the formation of tetrahydrobiopterin (biopterin), which is a critical cofactor for the synthesis of dopamine: thus dopamine levels will increase. In addition, L-methylfolate can hypothetically increase methylation of the promoter for the gene of the enzyme COMT (catechol-O-methyl-transferase), which inactivates dopamine. This methylation silences the COMT gene and thus decreases the synthesis of COMT, which reduces the metabolism of dopamine, increasing its levels.

The effects of two or more risk genes working together to increase the risk of an illness such as depression is called *epistasis*. There is some evidence that the T variant of MTHFR "conspires" with the Val variant of COMT to decrease the efficiency of information processing in the dorsolateral prefrontal cortex (DLPFC) during a cognitive load in schizophrenia ("having T with Val" in Chapter 4 and in Figure 4-44). This observation suggests the possibility that the same genetic interaction may be at play in some patients with depression, or treatment-resistant depression, or even depression with cognitive symptoms, and it is being explored as a potential genetic marker for who might be the best candidates for L-methylfolate treatment in depression.

S-adenosyl-methionine (SAMe)

L-Methylfolate is converted into methionine and finally into SAMe, which is the direct methyl donor for methylation reactions. If L-methylfolate is deficient, so might be SAMe, and it may be possible to administer methionine or SAMe to such patients as well as L-methylfolate. However, administering methionine or SAMe can cause build-up of the unwanted metabolite homocysteine that could theoretically interfere with epigenetic mechanisms, and can also eventually deplete precursors to SAMe. Nevertheless, high doses of SAMe may be effective in augmenting antidepressants in patients with major depression.

Thyroid

Thyroid hormones act by binding to nuclear ligand receptors to form a nuclear ligand-activated transcription factor. Abnormalities in thyroid hormone levels have long been associated with depression, and various forms and doses of thyroid hormones have long been utilized as augmenting agents to antidepressants, either to boost their efficacy in patients with inadequate response or to speed up their onset of action. Thyroid hormones have many complex cellular actions, including actions that may boost monoamine neurotransmitters as downstream consequences of thyroid's known abilities to regulate neuronal organization, arborization, and synapse formation, and this may account for how thyroid hormones enhance antidepressant action in some patients.

Brain stimulation: creating a perfect storm in brain circuits of depressed patients

Electroconvulsive therapy

Electroconvulsive therapy (ECT) is the classical therapeutic form of brain stimulation for depression. ECT is a highly effective treatment for depression whose mechanism of action remains a quandary. Failure to respond to a variety of antidepressants, singly or in combination, is a key factor for considering ECT, although it may also be utilized in urgent and severely disabling high-risk circumstances such as psychotic, suicidal, or postpartum depressions. ECT is the only therapeutic agent for the treatment of depression, with the possible exception of the experimental agents ketamine, scopolamine, and sleep deprivation, that is rapid in antidepressant onset, with therapeutic actions that can start after even a single treatment, and typically within a few days. The mechanism is unknown, but thought to be related to the probable mobilization of neurotransmitters caused by the seizure. Memory loss and social stigma are the primary problems associated with ECT and limit its use. There are striking regional and national differences across the world in the frequency of ECT use and in ECT techniques.

Transcranial magnetic stimulation

Transcranial magnetic stimulation (TMS) is another brain stimulation treatment approved for depression. It uses a rapidly alternating current passing through a small coil placed over the scalp that generates a magnetic field which in turn induces an electric current in the underlying areas of the brain. This electrical current depolarizes the affected cortical neurons, thereby causing nerve impulse flow out of the underlying brain areas (Figure 7-75). During the treatment the patient is awake and reclines comfortably in a chair while the magnetic coil is placed snugly against the scalp. There are few if any side effects except headache.

The TMS apparatus is localized in order to create an electrical impulse over the dorsolateral prefrontal cortex (DLPFC). Presumably, daily stimulation of this brain area for up to an hour over several weeks causes activation of various brain circuits that leads to an antidepressant effect (Figure 7-75). If this activates a brain circuit beginning in DLPFC, and connecting to other brain areas such as ventromedial prefrontal cortex (VMPFC) and amygdala, with connections to the brainstem centers of the monoamine neurotransmitter system, the net result would be monoamine

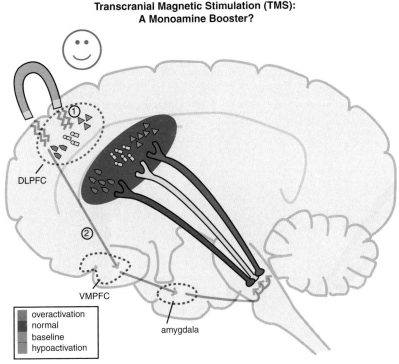

Transcranial Magnetic Stimulation (TMS): A Monoamine Booster?

DLPFC

VMPFC

amygdala

overactivation
normal
baseline
hypoactivation

Figure 7-75. Transcranial magnetic stimulation. Transcranial magnetic stimulation is a treatment in which a rapidly alternating current passes through a small coil placed over the scalp. This generates a magnetic field that induces an electrical current in the underlying areas of the brain (dorsolateral prefrontal cortex, DLPFC). The affected neurons then signal other areas of the brain. Presumably, stimulation of brain regions in which there is monoamine deficiency would lead to a boost in monoamine activity and thus alleviation of depressive symptoms.

modulation, especially for patients inadequately responsive to treatment with antidepressants (Figure 7-75, arrow 2). In this way, TMS would act through a mechanism unlike the known chemical antidepressants. However, TMS also releases neurotransmitters locally, in the area of the magnet, depolarizing them and releasing neurotransmitters from their axon terminals in the DLPFC (Figure 7-75, arrow 1). This is a second mechanism unlike chemical antidepressants, and may explain why TMS can be effective in patients who do not respond to chemical antidepressants. Finally, since all the effects of TMS are in the brain, there are no peripheral side effects such as nausea, weight gain, blood pressure changes, or sexual dysfunction. Lack of peripheral side effects plus the ability to help patients who do not respond to chemical antidepressants seem to be the particular advantages of TMS treatment of depression.

Deep brain stimulation

Deep brain stimulation (DBS) is an experimental treatment for the most severe forms of depression (Figure 7-76). Deep brain stimulation of neurons in some brain areas has proven effective for treatment of motor complications in Parkinson's disease and is now under study for treatment-resistant depression. The stimulation device is a battery-powered pulse generator implanted in the chest wall like a pacemaker. One or two leads are tunneled under the scalp and then into the brain, guided by neuroimaging and brain stimulation recording during the implantation procedure to facilitate the exact placement of the lead in the targeted brain area. The tip of each lead is composed of several contact areas that usually spread sequentially to cover additional parts of the intended anatomic target. The pulse generator delivers brief repeated pulses of current, which is adjusted based on individual tissue impedance.

The most common side effects are from the procedure itself. There is ongoing debate on where to place the stimulating electrodes for the treatment of depression, and how such stimulation might work to treat depression in patients inadequately responsive to antidepressants. Currently, one proposed location for electrodes in the treatment of depression with deep

Deep Brain Stimulation (DBS): A Monoamine Booster?

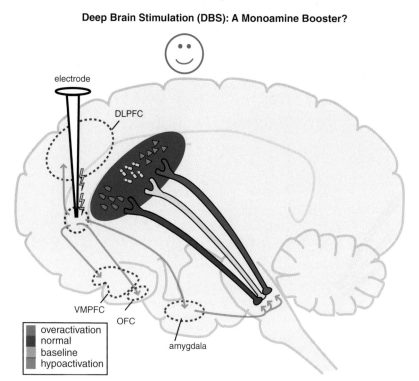

Figure 7-76. Deep brain stimulation. Deep brain stimulation involves a battery-powered pulse generator implanted in the chest wall. One or two leads are tunneled directly into the brain. The device then sends brief repeated pulses to the brain, which may have the result of boosting monoamine activity and thus alleviating depressive symptoms.

brain stimulation is in the subgenual area of the anterior cingulate cortex, part of the ventromedial prefrontal cortex (VMPFC: Figure 7-76). This brain area has important connections to other areas of prefrontal cortex, including other areas of ventromedial prefrontal cortex, orbitofrontal cortex (OFC), and dorsolateral prefrontal cortex, as well as amygdala (Figure 7-76). It is feasible that electrical stimulation of this brain area results in activation of circuits that lead back to brainstem monoamine centers, to act as a monoamine modulator in such patients. Reports of this treatment approach are encouraging.

Psychotherapy as an epigenetic "drug"

Psychotherapy has traditionally competed with psychopharmacology. As drugs have become the more dominant treatment, the pharmacological approach has been increasingly criticized as limited in scope, lacking in robust outcomes, and too heavily influenced by the pharmaceutical industry. However, drugs and psychotherapy may have a common neurobiological link since both can change brain circuits. It is not surprising, therefore, that both psychotherapy and psychopharmacology can be clinically effective for treating psychiatric disorders, or indeed that combining them can be therapeutically synergistic. Psychotherapy, like many other forms of learning, can hypothetically induce epigenetic changes in brain circuits that can enhance the efficiency of information processing in malfunctioning neurons to improve symptoms in psychiatric disorders, just like drugs.

Psychotherapies can thus be conceptualized as epigenetic "drugs," or at least as therapeutic agents that act epigenetically in a manner similar or complementary to drugs. Inefficient information processing in specific circuits correlates with specific psychiatric symptoms. Not only can genes and psychotropic drugs modify various neurotransmitter systems to alter the activity of these circuits and thus create or alleviate psychiatric symptoms by changing the efficiency of information processing in these circuits, but so can environmental experiences such as stress (see Figures 6-40 through 6-43), learning, and possibly even psychotherapy. Drugs can change gene expression in brain circuits as a downstream consequence of their immediate molecular properties, but so can the environment, hypothetically including psychotherapy. That is, both good and bad experiences can drive the production of epigenetic changes in gene expression, and indeed epigenetic changes in gene transcription seem to underlie long-term memories, good and bad. Bad memories of childhood trauma may trigger psychiatric disorders by causing unfavorable changes in brain circuits; good memories formed during psychotherapy may favorably alter the same brain circuits targeted by drugs, and similarly enhance the efficiency of information processing and thereby relieve symptoms (Figures 6-40 through 6-43).

Experimental animals have epigenetic mechanisms linked not only to spatial memory formation but also to fear conditioning and reward conditioning, models for mood, anxiety, and substance-abuse disorders. Both drugs and psychotherapy can facilitate the formation of new synapses that block memories of fear or reward and provide a potential explanation not only of how psychotherapy can hypothetically change symptoms by altering neuronal circuits, but how combining drugs that facilitate neurotransmission could potentially enhance the efficacy of psychotherapy in changing neuronal circuits, and thus reduce symptoms.

If both psychotropic drugs and psychotherapy converge upon brain circuits, maybe their combination can be harnessed for enhanced efficacy and better outcomes for patients with psychiatric disorders. The question is how to harness the potential of this approach and direct it most effectively to the relief of psychiatric symptoms. What are the techniques, what is the role of the therapist, what training is needed, how can this be standardized and made the most efficient over time with the fastest onset of action, how to measure the neurobiological and symptomatic results of this approach, how to assure that any progress is preserved? We still do not know when to expect greater benefits of psychotherapy alone, medications alone, or their combination, but at least now we have a conceptual basis for using both of them and even for combining them, since the two approaches converge neurobiologically. These and many more questions will form the research agenda for moving this approach forward as a central aspect of clinical therapeutics in psychiatry.

The best psychotherapy candidates to combine with drugs, particularly for the treatment of depression, are cognitive behavioral therapy and interpersonal therapy, which are often conducted by therapists who have read a training manual, been supervised administering it to patients, and who use a 12- to 24-week approach that follows a progression with a beginning, a middle, and an end. The new "trial-based therapy" described by de Oliveira is a version of cognitive psychotherapy that is intuitive, readily adapted by psychiatrists who are not necessarily sophisticated cognitive behavioral therapists, and can even be fun. In trial-based therapy the patient literally puts his psychiatric symptoms and core beliefs on trial. This idea is based on the universal principle portrayed in Franz Kafka's *The Trial* that human beings by their very nature are self-accusatory and this can lead to confusion, anxiety, and existential suffering. In fact, the central character of this novel, Joseph K, was arrested, put on trial, and convicted without ever knowing the crime of which he was accused. De Oliveira's technique is to take this universal truth and fit it into a modern courtroom paradigm. Here, during outpatient psychotherapy, a patient's self-accusations are put on trial as distorted schemas and core beliefs that have been developed about the self by the patient's "inner prosecutor," who convinces the patient that these beliefs are true, and because of this the patient suffers. Trial-based therapy seeks to point out to the patient that his symptoms and suffering are due to core beliefs that can be countered by activating his/her "inner defense attorney" to see things in a more balanced and realistic way and thereby relieve symptoms. One could hypothesize that, when successful, this approach is forming a synapse of the new perspective of the "inner defense attorney" to counter and inhibit the circuit mediating the activation of the first learning, namely the distorted core belief of the "inner prosecutor." Trial-based therapy is only one of the potential psychotherapies to combine with antidepressants for the treatment of major depression and to take us beyond the current plateau of pharmacotherapy. Combining psychotherapy with antidepressants has the potential of making the entire outcome greater than the sum of the parts, or $1 + 1 = 3$, the delightful "bad math" of therapeutic synergy.

How to choose an antidepressant
Evidence-based antidepressant selections

In theory, the best way to select a treatment for depression would be to follow the evidence. Unfortunately, there is little evidence for superiority of one option over another and a good deal of controversy about meta-analyses that compare antidepressants to each other. One general principle upon which most patients and prescribers agree, however, is when to switch versus when to augment. Thus, there is a preference for switching when the first treatment has intolerable side effects or when there is no response whatsoever, but to augment the first treatment with a second treatment when there is a partial response to the first treatment. Other than this guideline, there is little consistent evidence that one treatment option is better than another. All treatments subsequent to the first one seem to have diminishing returns in terms of chances to reach remission (Figure 7-4) or chances to remain in remission (Figure 7-6). Thus, evidence-based algorithms are not able to provide clear guidelines on how to choose an antidepressant, and what to do if an antidepressant does not work.

Symptom-based antidepressant selections

The neurobiologically informed psychopharmacologist may opt for adapting a symptom-based approach to selecting or combining a series of antidepressants (Figures 7-77 through 7-82). This strategy leads to the construction of a portfolio of multiple agents to treat all residual symptoms of unipolar depression until the patient achieves sustained remission.

First, symptoms are constructed into a diagnosis and then deconstructed into a list of specific symptoms that the individual patient is experiencing (Figure 7-77). Next, these symptoms are matched with the brain circuits that hypothetically mediate them (Figure 7-78) and then with the known neuropharmacological regulation of these circuits by neurotransmitters (Figure 7-79). Finally, available treatment options that target these neuropharmacological mechanisms are chosen to eliminate symptoms one by one (Figure 7-79). When symptoms persist, a treatment with a different mechanism is added or switched. No evidence proves that this is a superior approach, but it appeals not only to clinical intuition but also to neurobiological reasoning.

For example, in a patient with the symptoms of "problems concentrating" and "decreased interest" as well as "fatigue," this approach suggests targeting both NE and DA with first-line antidepressants plus augmenting agents that act on these neurotransmitters (Figure 7-79). This can also call for stopping the SSRI if this is partially the cause of these symptoms. On the other hand, for "insomnia," this symptom is hypothetically associated with an entirely different malfunctioning circuit regulated by different neurotransmitters (Figure 7-78); therefore, the treatment for this symptom calls for a different approach, namely the use of hypnotics that act on the GABA system or sedating antidepressants that work to block rather than boost the serotonin or histamine system (Figure 7-79). It is possible that any of these symptoms shown in Figure 7-79 would respond to whatever drug is administered, but this symptom-based approach can tailor the treatment portfolio to each individual patient, possibly finding a faster way of reducing specific symptoms with more tolerable treatment selections for that patient than a purely random approach.

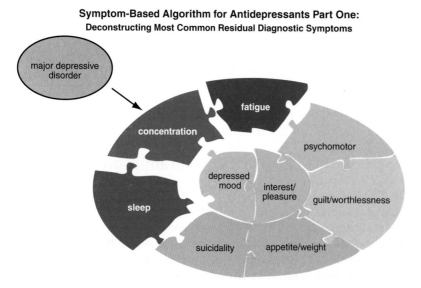

Symptom-Based Algorithm for Antidepressants Part One:
Deconstructing Most Common Residual Diagnostic Symptoms

Figure 7-77. Symptom-based algorithm for antidepressants, part 1. Shown here is the diagnosis of major depressive disorder deconstructed into its symptoms (as defined by formal diagnostic criteria). Of these, sleep disturbances, problems concentrating, and fatigue are the most common residual symptoms.

Symptom-Based Algorithm for Antidepressants Part Two:

Match Most Common Residual Symptoms to Hypothetically Malfunctioning Brain Circuits

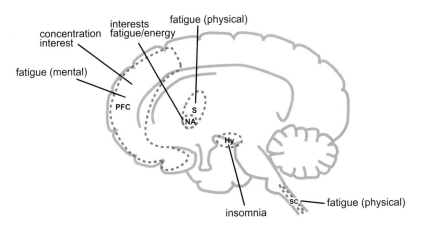

Figure 7-78. Symptom-based algorithm for antidepressants, part 2. In this figure the most common residual symptoms of major depression are linked to hypothetically malfunctioning brain circuits. Insomnia may be linked to the hypothalamus, problems concentrating to the dorsolateral prefrontal cortex (PFC), reduced interest to the PFC and nucleus accumbens (NA), and fatigue to the PFC, striatum (S), NA, and spinal cord (SC).

Symptom-Based Algorithm for Antidepressants Part Three:

Target Regulatory Neurotransmitters With Selected Pharmacological Mechanisms

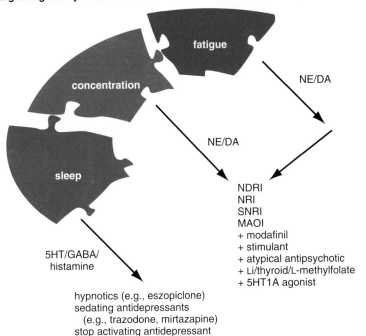

Figure 7-79. Symptom-based algorithm for antidepressants, part 3. Residual symptoms of depression can be linked to the neurotransmitters that regulate them and then, in turn, to pharmacological mechanisms. Fatigue and concentration are regulated in large part by norepinephrine (NE) and dopamine (DA), which are affected by many antidepressants, including norepinephrine–dopamine reuptake inhibitors (NDRIs), selective norepinephrine reuptake inhibitors (NRIs), serotonin–norepinephrine reuptake inhibitors (SNRIs), and monoamine oxidase inhibitors (MAOIs). Augmenting agents that affect NE and/or DA include modafinil, stimulants, atypical antipsychotics, lithium, thyroid hormone, L-methylfolate, and serotonin (5HT) 1A agonists. Sleep disturbance is regulated by 5HT, γ-aminobutyric acid (GABA), and histamine and can be treated with sedative hypnotics, with sedating antidepressants such as trazodone or mirtazapine, or by discontinuing an activating antidepressant.

The symptom-based approach for selecting antidepressants can also be applied to treating common associated symptoms of depression that are not components of the formal diagnostic criteria for depression (Figure 7-80). Five such symptoms are anxiety, pain, excessive daytime sleepiness/hypersomnia/problems with arousal and alertness, sexual dysfunction, and vasomotor symptoms (in women) (Figures 7-80 through 7-82).

The hypothetical pathways for the five additional associated symptoms of depression are shown in Figure 7-81. Sometimes it is said that for a good

Symptom-Based Algorithm for Antidepressants Part Four:
Deconstruct Into Common Non-DSM-IV Residual Symptoms

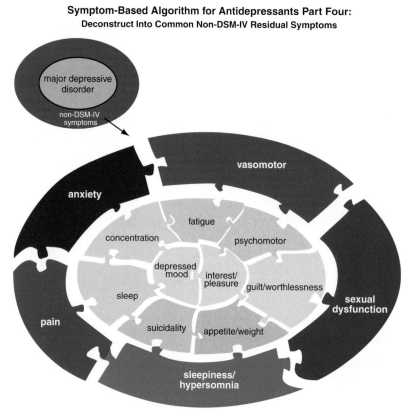

Figure 7-80. Symptom-based algorithm for antidepressants, part 4. There are several common symptoms of depression that are nonetheless not part of the formal diagnostic criteria for major depressive disorder. These include painful physical symptoms, excessive daytime sleepiness/hypersomnia with problems of arousal and alertness, anxiety, vasomotor symptoms, and sexual dysfunction.

clinician to get patients with major depression into remission, it requires targeting at least 14 of the 9 symptoms of depression!

Fortunately, psychiatric drug treatments do not respect the formal diagnostic criteria for psychiatric disorders. Treatments that target pharmacological mechanisms in specific brain circuits do so no matter what psychiatric disorder is associated with the symptom linked to that circuit. Thus, symptoms of one psychiatric disorder may be treatable with a proven agent that is known to treat the same symptom in another psychiatric disorder. For example, *anxiety* can be reduced in patients with major depression who do not have a full criterion anxiety disorder with the same serotonin and GABA mechanisms proven to work in anxiety disorders (Figure 7-82). *Sleepiness/hypersomnia* is a common associated symptom of depression, but frequently not detected because patients who have this problem surprisingly do not often complain about it, while patients with insomnia will much more commonly complain of that if they have that symptom. Problems with the arousal

mechanism in some patients with sleepiness/hypersomnia can also alter alertness and cognitive function, and such patients may respond to the same agents that are effective in sleep disorders, such as agents that can boost DA, NE, and/or histamine (Figure 7-82). We have already discussed *painful physical symptoms* and *vasomotor symptoms* in the section on SNRIs above, neither of which is included in the diagnostic criteria for major depression, both of which are nevertheless commonly associated with depression, and can be treated with SNRIs and other approaches (Figure 7-82). Finally, *sexual dysfunction* can be a complicated problem of many causes, and can range from lack of libido, to problems with arousal of peripheral genitalia, to lack of orgasm/ejaculation. Increasing DA or decreasing 5HT are the usual approaches to this set of problems whether the patient has major depression or not (Figure 7-82).

In summary, the symptom-based algorithm for selecting and combining antidepressants, and for building a portfolio of mechanisms until each diagnostic and associated symptom of depression is abolished, is

Symptom-Based Algorithm for Antidepressants Part Five:
Match Common Non-DSM-IV Residual Symptoms to
Hypothetically Malfunctioning Brain Circuits

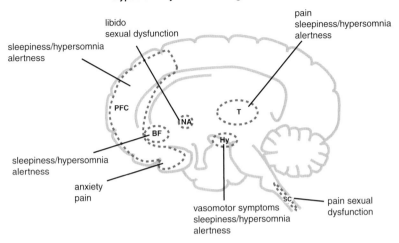

Figure 7-81. Symptom-based algorithm for antidepressants, part 5. In this figure common residual symptoms of major depression that are not part of formal diagnostic criteria are linked to hypothetically malfunctioning brain circuits. Painful physical symptoms are linked to the spinal cord (SC), thalamus (T), and ventral portions of the prefrontal cortex (PFC), while anxiety is associated with the ventral PFC. Vasomotor symptoms are mediated by the hypothalamus (Hy) and sexual dysfunction by the SC and nucleus accumbens (NA). Sleep symptoms that are part of the diagnostic criteria of depression involve mostly insomnia, linked to the hypothalamus; however, shown here are problems with hypersomnia and excessive daytime sleepiness, which may be beyond those symptoms included in the diagnostic criteria and be linked to problems with arousal and alertness and to arousal pathways not only in the hypothalamus but also the thalamus (T), basal forebrain (BF), and prefrontal cortex (PFC).

the modern psychopharmacologist's approach to major depression. This approach follows contemporary notions of neurobiological disease and drug mechanisms, with the goal of treatment being sustained remission.

Choosing an antidepressant for women based on their life cycle

Estrogen levels shift rather dramatically across the female life cycle in relation to various types of reproductive events (Figure 7-83). Such shifts are also linked to the onset or recurrence of major depressive episodes (Figures 7-83). In men, the incidence of depression rises in puberty, and then is essentially constant throughout life, despite a slowly declining testosterone level from age 25 onward (Figure 7-84). By contrast, in women, the incidence of depression in many ways mirrors their changes in estrogen across the life cycle (Figure 7-85). That is, as estrogen levels rise during puberty, the incidence of depression skyrockets in women, falling again after menopause (Figure 7-85). Thus, women have the same frequency of depression as men before puberty and after

menopause. However, during their childbearing years when estrogen is high and cycling, the incidence of depression in women is 2–3 times higher than in men (compare Figures 7-84 and 7-85). Choosing an antidepressant for women in the perimenopause or after the menopause is discussed above in the section on SNRIs.

Depression and its treatment during childbearing years and pregnancy

One of the most controversial and unsettled areas of modern psychopharmacology is the selection of therapeutic interventions for major depressive disorder and prevention of recurrence of depression in women during their childbearing years when they may be pregnant or may become pregnant. What about risks of treatment to the baby? Some antidepressants may pose risks to the fetus, including increased risk for serious congenital malformations if administered during the first trimester and increased risk for other fetal abnormalities and for fetal withdrawal symptoms after birth if administered during the third trimester, and increased risks of

Symptom-Based Algorithm for Antidepressants Part Six:
Target Regulatory Neurotransmitters With Selected Pharmacological Mechanisms

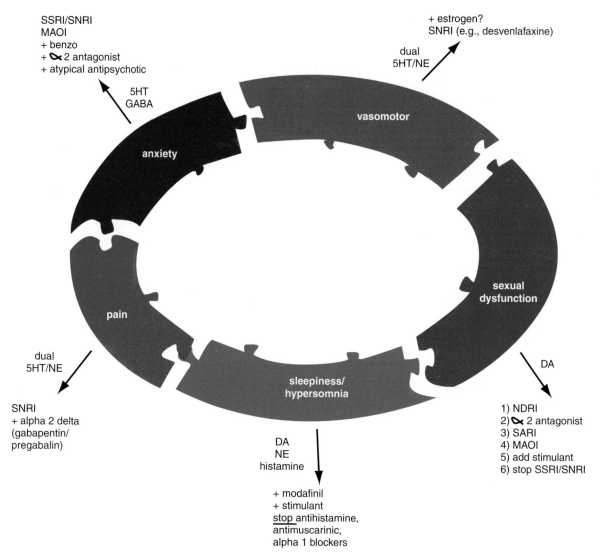

Figure 7-82. Symptom-based algorithm for antidepressants, part 6. Residual symptoms of depression can be linked to the neurotransmitters that regulate them and then, in turn, to pharmacological mechanisms. Painful physical symptoms are mediated by norepinephrine (NE) and to a lesser extent serotonin (5HT) and may be treated with serotonin–norepinephrine reuptake inhibitors (SNRIs) or $\alpha_2\delta$ ligands (pregabalin, gabapentin). Anxiety is related to 5HT and γ-aminobutyric acid (GABA); it can be treated with selective serotonin reuptake inhibitors (SSRIs), SNRIs, or monoamine oxidase inhibitors (MAOIs) as monotherapies, as well as by augmentation with benzodiazepines, α_2 antagonists, or atypical antipsychotics. Vasomotor symptoms may be modulated by NE and 5HT and treated with SNRIs; augmentation with estrogen therapy is also an option. Sexual dysfunction is regulated primarily by dopamine (DA) and may be treated with norepinephrine–dopamine reuptake inhibitors (NDRIs), α_2 antagonists, serotonin 2A antagonist/reuptake inhibitors (SARIs), MAOIs, addition of a stimulant, or by stopping an SSRI or SNRI. Hypersomnia and problems with arousal and alertness are regulated by DA, NE, and histamine and can be treated with activating agents such as modafinil or stimulants, or by stopping sedating agents with antihistamine, antimuscarinic, and/or α_1 blocking properties.

Risk of Depression Across Female Life Cycle

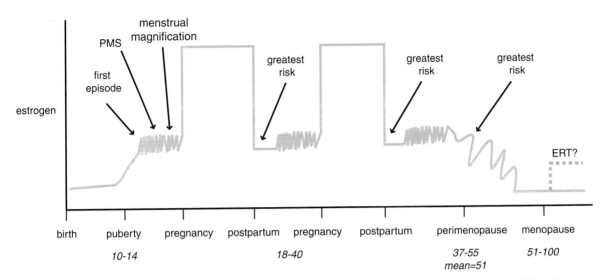

Figure 7-83. Risk of depression across the female life cycle. Several issues of importance in assessing women's vulnerability to the onset and recurrence of depression are illustrated here. These include first onset in puberty and young adulthood, premenstrual syndrome (PMS), and menstrual magnification as harbingers of future episodes or incomplete recovery states from prior episodes of depression. There are two periods of especially high vulnerability for first episodes of depression or for recurrence if a woman has already experienced an episode: namely, the postpartum period and the perimenopausal period. ERT, estrogen replacement therapy.

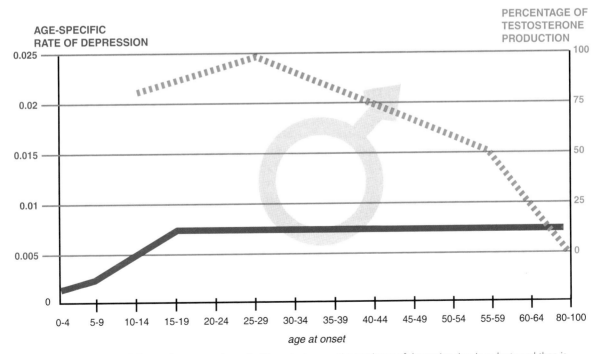

Figure 7-84. Incidence of depression across the male life cycle. In men, the incidence of depression rises in puberty and then is essentially constant throughout life, despite a slowly declining testosterone level from age 25 onward.

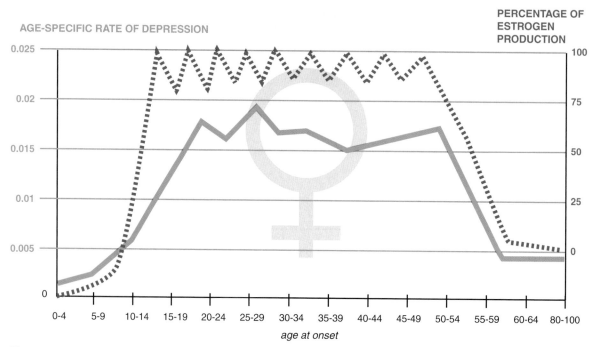

AGE-SPECIFIC RATE OF DEPRESSION

PERCENTAGE OF ESTROGEN PRODUCTION

Figure 7-85. Incidence of depression across the female life cycle. The incidence of depression in women mirrors their changes in estrogen across the life cycle. As estrogen levels rise during puberty, the incidence of depression also rises; it falls again during menopause, when estrogen levels fall. Thus before puberty and after menopause, women have the same frequency of depression as men (Figure 7-84). During their childbearing years, however, when estrogen is high and cycling, the incidence of depression in women is 2–3 times as high as it is in men (Figure 7-84).

prematurity, low birth weight, and possible long-term neurodevelopmental abnormalities if given any time during pregnancy (Table 7-13). At the same time, lack of treatment during pregnancy is not without risks to mother or baby (Table 7-13). For the mother with untreated depression, the risks include relapse or worsening of depression, poor self-care and possible self-harm including resorting to drug abuse of substances even more dangerous than antidepressants (Table 7-13). Not only is there risk of increased suicidality when young mothers are treated with antidepressants, there is also the risk of suicide when seriously depressed mothers of any age are not treated with antidepressants (Table 7-13). There are also numerous risks to the baby if the mother is not treated with antidepressants, including risk of poor prenatal care due to low motivation in the mother, risk of low birth weight and early developmental delay and disruption of maternal–infant bonding in children of women with untreated depression, and even risk of harm to the infant by

seriously depressed mothers in the postpartum period (Table 7-13).

Thus, in terms of treating pregnant patients with antidepressants, it seems that the psychopharmacologist is "damned if you do" and also "damned if you don't" (Table 7-13). Without clear guidelines, clinicians are best advised to assess risks and benefits for both child and mother on a case-by-case basis. For mild cases of depression, psychotherapy and psychosocial support may be sufficient. However, in many cases, the benefits of continuing antidepressant treatment during pregnancy outweigh the risks. L-Methylfolate and folate are actually administered as prenatal vitamins to many women and are deemed safe by most experts. Since patients with unipolar or bipolar depression may be prone to impulsive behavior (especially children and adolescents), it is a good idea for girls and women of childbearing potential who take antidepressants to receive counseling and possibly contraceptives to reduce the risk of unplanned pregnancies and first-trimester exposure of fetuses to antidepressants.

Table 7-13 Risks of antidepressant use or avoidance during pregnancy

Damned if you do

- Congenital cardiac malformations (especially first-trimester paroxetine)
- Newborn persistent pulmonary hypertension (third-trimester SSRIs)
- Neonatal withdrawal syndrome (third-trimester SSRIs)
- Prematurity, low birth weight
- Long-term neurodevelopmental abnormalities
- Increased suicidality of antidepressant use up to age 25
- Medical-legal risks of using antidepressants

Damned if you don't

- Relapse of major depression
- Increased suicidality of antidepressant non-use
- Poor self-care
- Poor motivation for prenatal care
- Disruption of maternal–infant bonding
- Low birth weight, developmental delay in children of women with untreated depression
- Self-harm
- Harm to infant
- Medical-legal risks of not using antidepressants

Depression and its treatment during the postpartum period and while breastfeeding

What about taking antidepressants during the postpartum period, when mothers are lactating and may be nursing? This is a very high-risk period for the onset or recurrence of a major depressive episode in women (Figure 7-83). Should a mother with depression avoid antidepressants in order to prevent risk of exposure of the baby to antidepressants in breast milk? How about a mother with past depression now in remission who is weighing the risk of her own relapse against the risk of exposing the baby to antidepressants in breast milk? In these circumstances there are no firm guidelines that fit all cases, and a risk–benefit ratio must be calculated for each situation, taking into consideration the risk of recurrence to the mother if she does not take antidepressants (given her own personal and family history of mood disorder), and the risk to her bonding to her baby if she does not breastfeed or to her baby if there is exposure to trace amounts of antidepressants in breast milk. Although estrogen replacement therapy (ERT) has been reported to be effective in some

patients with postpartum depression or postpartum psychosis, this is still considered experimental and should be reserved for use if at all only in patients resistant to antidepressants.

Whereas the risk to the infant of exposure to small amounts of antidepressants in breast milk is only now being clarified, it is quite clear that a mother with a prior postpartum depression who neglects to take antidepressants after a subsequent pregnancy has a 67% risk of recurrence if she does not take antidepressants and only one-tenth of that risk of recurrence if she does take antidepressants postpartum. Also, up to 90% of all postpartum psychosis and bipolar episodes occur within the first 4 weeks after delivery. Such high-risk patients will require appropriate treatment of their mood disorder, so the decision here is whether to breastfeed, not whether the mother should be treated.

Choosing an antidepressant on the basis of genetic testing

Genetic testing has the potential of assisting both in diagnosing psychiatric illnesses and in selecting psychotropic drugs. Genotyping is already entering other specialties in medicine, and is currently on the threshold of being introduced into routine mental health practice. In the not-too-distant future, experts foresee that most patients will have their entire genomes entered as part of their permanent electronic medical records. In the meantime, it is already possible to obtain from various laboratories genotyping of numerous genes that may be linked to psychiatric diagnoses and drug responses.

For example, several genetic forms of the cytochrome P450 (CYP) enzyme system can be obtained to predict high or low drug levels of substrate drugs (especially CYP 2D6, 2C19, and 3A4). Combined with therapeutic drug monitoring of actual drug levels, these CYP genotypes can potentially explain side effects and lack of therapeutic effects in some patients.

Treatment responses are not "all or none" phenomena, and genetic markers in psychopharmacology will potentially explain greater or lesser likelihood of response, nonresponse, or side effects, but not tell a clinician what drug to prescribe for a specific individual. More likely, the information will tell whether the patient is "biased" towards responding or not, tolerating or not, and along with past treatment response will help the clinician make a future treatment

Table 7-14 Genetic testing: genes that may help in therapeutic decision making

Gene	Protein	Biological function	Potential therapeutic implications
SLC 6A4 variation	SERT	Serotonin reuptake	Poor response, slow response, poor tolerability to SSRIs/SNRIs
$5HT_{2c}$ variation	$5HT_{2c}$ receptor	Regulates DA & NE release	Poor response, poor tolerability to atypical antipsychotics
DRD_2 variation	D_2 receptor	Mediates positive symptoms of psychosis, movements in Parkinsonism	Poor response, poor tolerability to atypical antipsychotics
COMT Val variation	COMT enzyme	Regulates DA levels in PFC; metabolizes DA and NE	Reduced executive functioning
MTHFR T variation	MTHFR enzyme	Regulates L-methylfolate levels and methylation	Reduced executive functioning, especially with Val COMT (T with Val)

recommendation that has a higher chance of success but is not guaranteed to be effective and tolerated. Some call this process the "weight of the evidence" and others "equipoise," where the genetic information will enrich the prescribing decision, but not necessarily dictate a single compelling choice.

Examples of this are shown in Table 7-14 for several candidate genes that are potentially helpful in weighing various treatment possibilities for patients with treatment-resistant depression. This is a rapidly expanding area of psychopharmacology and will likely impact drug selection dramatically in the next few years.

Should antidepressant combinations be the standard for treating unipolar major depressive disorder?

Given the disappointing number of patients who attain remission from a major depressive episode even after four consecutive treatments (Figure 7-4) and who can maintain that remission over the long run (Figure 7-6), the paradigm of prescribing a sequence of monotherapies each with a single mechanism of therapeutic action for major depression is rapidly changing to one of administering multiple simultaneous pharmacologic mechanisms, often with two or more therapeutic agents. In this respect, the pattern is following that of the treatment of bipolar disorder, which usually requires administration of more than one agent, and of illnesses such as HIV (human immunodeficiency virus) infection as well as tuberculosis. The question in the treatment of depression is not so much whether multiple pharmacologic

mechanisms should be simultaneously administered for patients with treatment-resistant depression, but rather whether multiple mechanisms and/or drugs should be given much earlier in the treatment sequence, or even from the time of initial treatment. Several specific suggestions of antidepressant combinations are shown in Figures 7-86 through 7-88. Many others can be constructed, but these particular combinations or "combos" have enjoyed widespread use even though there is little actual evidence-based data from clinical trials that their combination results in superior efficacy. Nevertheless, these suggestions may be useful for practicing clinicians to use in some patients.

Single-action and multiple-action monotherapies have already been extensively discussed in this chapter, and several combinations of SSRIs/SNRIs with other agents have been mentioned, from atypical antipsychotics (also discussed extensively in Chapter 5), to lithium, buspirone, trazodone, hypnotics, thyroid hormone, L-methylfolate, SAMe, neurostimulation, and psychotherapy. Several additional combos – called "heroic combos" because they have strong anecdotal experience of efficacy in some difficult cases of treatment-resistant depression – are shown in Figures 7-86 through 7-88, including several in which two antidepressants are added together.

Triple-action combo: SSRI/SNRI ± NDRI

If boosting one neurotransmitter is good, and two is better, maybe three boosted neurotransmitters is best (Figure 7-86). Triple-action antidepressant therapy with

Triple-Action Combos

SSRI + NDRI

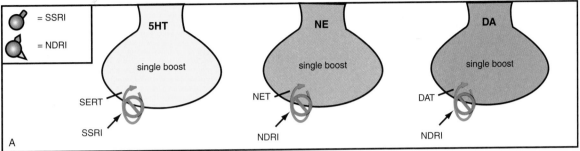

SNRI + NDRI

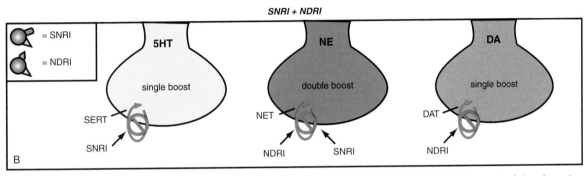

Figure 7-86. Heroic combos, part 1: SSRI/SNRI plus NDRI. A selective serotonin reuptake inhibitor (SSRI) plus a norepinephrine–dopamine reuptake inhibitor (NDRI) leads to a single boost for serotonin (5HT), norepinephrine (NE), and dopamine (DA). A serotonin–norepinephrine reuptake inhibitor (SNRI) plus a norepinephrine–dopamine reuptake inhibitor (NDRI) leads to a single boost for serotonin (5HT), a double boost for norepinephrine (NE), and a single boost for dopamine (DA).

modulation of all three monoamines (5HT, DA, and NE) would be predicted to occur by combining either an SSRI with an NDRI, perhaps the most popular combination in US antidepressant psychopharmacology, or by combining an SNRI with an NDRI, providing even more noradrenergic and dopaminergic action.

California rocket fuel: SNRI plus mirtazapine

This potentially powerful combination utilizes the pharmacologic synergy obtained by adding the enhanced serotonin and norepinephrine release from inhibition of both dual serotonin and norepinephrine reuptake by an SNRI to the disinhibition of both serotonin and norepinephrine release by the α_2 antagonist actions of mirtazapine (Figure 7-87). It is even possible that additional pro-dopaminergic actions result from the combination of norepinephrine reuptake blockade in prefrontal cortex due to SNRI actions with $5HT_{2C}$ actions of mirtazapine

disinhibiting dopamine release. This combination can provide very powerful antidepressant action for some patients with unipolar major depressive episodes. Mirtazapine combinations with various SSRIs and SNRIs have also been studied as potential treatments from the initiation of therapy in major depression.

Arousal combos

The frequent complaints of residual fatigue, loss of energy, motivation, sex drive, and problems concentrating/problems with alertness may be approached by combining either a stimulant or modafinil with an SNRI to recruit triple monoamine action and especially enhancement of dopamine (Figure 7-88). The stimulant lisdexamfetamine, which links the amino acid lysine to the stimulant *d*-amphetamine, and which slows the delivery and potentially reduces the abuse liability of *d*-amphetamine after oral

California Rocket Fuel

SNRI + mirtazapine

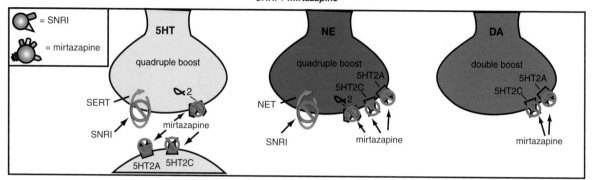

Figure 7-87. Heroic combos, part 2: California rocket fuel. A serotonin–norepinephrine reuptake inhibitor (SNRI) plus mirtazapine is a combination that has a great degree of theoretical synergy: norepinephrine reuptake blockade plus α_2 blockade, serotonin (5HT) reuptake plus $5HT_{2A}$ and $5HT_{2C}$ antagonism, and thus many 5HT actions plus norepinephrine (NE) actions. Specifically, 5HT is quadruple-boosted (with reuptake blockade, α_2 antagonism, $5HT_{2A}$ antagonism, and $5HT_{2C}$ antagonism), NE is quadruple-boosted (with reuptake blockade, α_2 antagonism, $5HT_{2A}$ antagonism, and $5HT_{2C}$ antagonism), and there may even be a double boost of dopamine (with $5HT_{2A}$ and $5HT_{2C}$ antagonism).

Arousal Combos

SNRI + stimulant

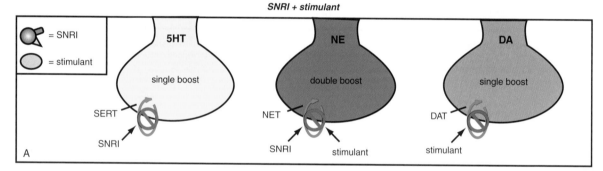

SNRI + modafinil

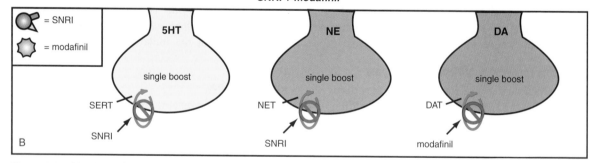

Figure 7-88. Heroic combos, part 3: SNRI plus stimulant or modafinil. A serotonin–norepinephrine reuptake inhibitor (SNRI) plus a stimulant means that serotonin (5HT) and dopamine (DA) are single-boosted and norepinephrine (NE) is double-boosted. With an SNRI in combination with modafinil, serotonin (5HT) and norepinephrine (NE) are single-boosted by the SNRI while dopamine (DA) is single-boosted by modafinil.

administration, is in late-stage clinical testing as an augmenting agent to SSRIs/SNRIs in treatment-resistant depression.

Future treatments for mood disorders

As mentioned in Chapter 6 and illustrated in Figure 6-39B, a number of agents that target stress and the HPA axis are in clinical testing, including *glucocorticoid antagonists, CRF-1 (corticotropin-releasing factor) antagonists* and *vasopressin-1B antagonists*.

Triple reuptake inhibitors (TRIs) or *serotonin–norepinephrine–dopamine reuptake inhibitors* (SNDRIs) are in clinical testing to confirm that if one mechanism is good (i.e., SSRI) and two mechanisms are better (i.e., SNRI), then maybe targeting all three mechanisms of the trimonoamine neurotransmitter system would be the best in terms of efficacy. Several different triple reuptake inhibitors (e.g., amitifidine, GSK-372475, BMS-820836, tasofensine, PRC200-SS, SEP-225289, and others) are in clinical development, some with additional pharmacologic properties (such as LuAA24530 with $5HT_{2C}$, $5HT_3$, $5HT_{2A}$, and α_{1A} antagonist properties), all differing in the amount of blockade of each of the three monoamine transporters SERT, NET, and DAT. It appears that too much dopamine activity can lead to a drug of abuse, and not enough DAT blockade means that the agent is essentially an SNRI. Perhaps the desirable profile is robust inhibition of the serotonin transporter and substantial inhibition of the norepinephrine transporter, like the known SNRIs, plus a little frosting on the cake of 10–25% inhibition of DAT. Further clinical trials will be necessary to clarify whether any of the "triples" will represent an advance over SSRIs or SNRIs in the treatment of depression.

Multimodal agents

It appears that combining multiple modes of monoaminergic action may enhance efficacy for some patients with depression. This can include reuptake blockade (at SERT, DAT, NET) with actions at G-protein receptors (e.g., $5HT_{1A}$, $5HT_{2C}$, $5HT_7$, α_2 receptors) with actions at ion-channel receptors ($5HT_3$ receptors and possibly NMDA receptors). One such agent already discussed is vilazodone (combination of SERT plus $5HT_{1A}$ partial agonist actions) (Figure 7-24). Another multimodal agent

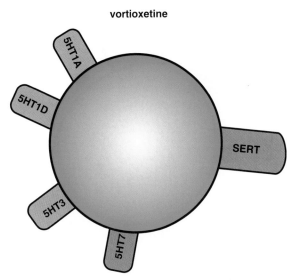

Figure 7-89. Vortioxetine. Vortioxetine is an antidepressant currently in development. It is a serotonin reuptake inhibitor and also has actions at several serotonin receptors, including $5HT_{1A}$ (partial agonist), $5HT_{1B/D}$ (partial agonist), $5HT_3$ (antagonist), and $5HT_7$ (antagonist).

in late-stage clinical development is vortioxetine (LuAA21004) (Figure 7-89). Vortioxetine acts via all three modes with a combination of five pharmacologic actions: reuptake blocking mode (SERT), G-protein receptor mode ($5HT_{1A}$ and $5HT_{1B/D}$ partial agonist, $5HT_7$ antagonist), and ion-channel mode ($5HT_3$ antagonist). In animal models vortioxetine increases the release of five different neurotransmitters: not only triple monoamine action on 5HT, NE, and DA release, but also increases in the release of acetylcholine and histamine. The clinical properties of vortioxetine suggest antidepressant efficacy without sexual dysfunction, and the pharmacologic properties suggest the potential for either pro-cognitive effects, or enhanced antidepressant efficacy compared to agents with fewer modes of action and effects on fewer neurotransmitters. Continued clinical testing will be necessary to see if vortioxetine fulfills its theoretical promise as an antidepressant.

NMDA blockade

One of the most interesting developments in recent years has been the observation that infusions of subanesthetic doses of ketamine can exert an immediate

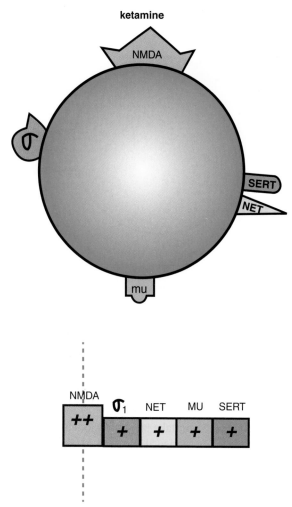

Figure 7-90. Ketamine. Ketamine is being studied for its potential therapeutic utility in depression. Ketamine is an NMDA (*N*-methyl-D-aspartate) receptor antagonist, with additional weak actions at σ_1 receptors, the norepinephrine transporter (NET), μ-opioid receptors, and the serotonin transporter (SERT).

antidepressant effect in patients with treatment-resistant unipolar or bipolar depression, and can immediately reduce suicidal thoughts. Unfortunately, the effects are not sustained for more than a few days, but this has led investigators to search for an oral ketamine-like agent that could have rapid onset and sustained efficacy in treatment-resistant patients.

Ketamine (Figure 7-90) acts as an open channel inhibitor at NMDA glutamate receptors (Figure 7-91), and causes downstream release of glutamate (Figure 7-92). Ketamine's actions at NMDA receptors are not unlike what is hypothesized to occur due to neurodevelopmental abnormalities that occur at NMDA synapses in schizophrenia (Figure 4-29B). This is not surprising, given that ketamine produces a schizophrenia-like syndrome in humans. When infused at subanesthetic doses in the study of depressed patients, ketamine does not induce psychosis, but is thought to produce downstream release in glutamate (Figure 7-92), which stimulates AMPA and mGluR subtypes of glutamate receptors while the NDMA receptors are being blocked by ketamine actions. One hypothesis for why ketamine has antidepressant actions proposes that the stimulation of AMPA receptors first activates the ERK/AKT signal transduction cascade (Figure 7-93A). This next triggers the mTOR (mammalian target of rapamycin) pathway (Figure 7-93A) and that causes the expression of synaptic proteins leading to an increased density of dendritic spines (Figure 7-93B), which can be seen soon after ketamine is administered in animals. Hypothetically, it is this increase in dendritic spines that causes the rapid-onset antidepressant effect.

Thus, investigators are looking for other agents that can trigger the pharmacologic changes that ketamine induces, from blocking NMDA receptors, to stimulating AMPA and various mGlu receptors, to inducing the mTOR pathway and an increase in dendritic spines. One candidate for an "oral ketamine" that acts on NMDA receptors is the cough medicine dextromethorphan (Figure 7-94). Both ketamine and dextromethorphan share actions not only at NMDA receptors, but also at σ receptors, μ-opioid receptors, SERT, and NET, but with different affinities (compare Figures 7-90 and 7-94). Dextromethorphan combined with quinidine (to prevent its metabolism to dextrorphan, which does not penetrate the brain effectively) is available in the US to treat unstable affect known as pseudo-bulbar affect, and could theoretically act in other disorders of mood and affect – but much more clinical testing is necessary. Many other agents that act on NMDA receptors as potential rapid-acting ketamine-like antidepressants are in early-stage clinical trials.

Site of Action of Ketamine: Binds to Open Channel at PCP Site to Block NMDA Receptor

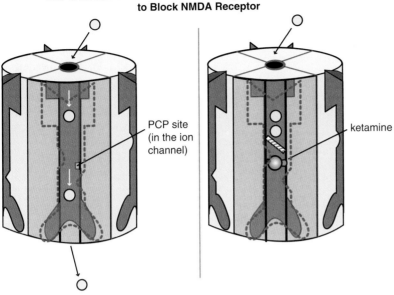

PCP site (in the ion channel)

ketamine

Figure 7-91. Site of action of ketamine. Ketamine binds to the open channel conformation of the *N*-methyl-D-aspartate (NMDA) receptor. Specifically, it binds to a site within the calcium channel of this receptor, which is often termed the PCP site because it is also where phencyclidine (PCP) binds. Blockade of NMDA receptors may prevent the excitatory actions of glutamate, which is postulated to be a therapeutic mechanism for treating depression. In fact, ketamine has demonstrated rapid, short-term antidepressant effects in both animal models and in humans.

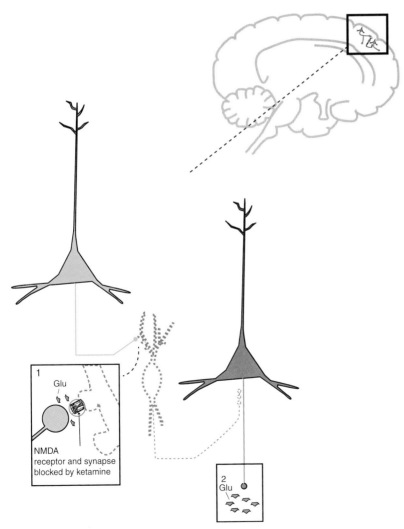

1
Glu

NMDA receptor and synapse blocked by ketamine

2
Glu

Figure 7-92. Mechanism of action of ketamine. Shown here are two cortical glutamatergic pyramidal neurons and a GABAergic interneuron. (1) If an *N*-methyl-D-aspartate (NMDA) receptor on a GABAergic interneuron is blocked by ketamine, this prevents the excitatory actions of glutamate (Glu) there. Thus, the GABA neuron is inactivated and does not release GABA (indicated by the dotted outline of the neuron). (2) GABA binding at the second cortical glutamatergic pyramidal neuron normally inhibits glutamate release: thus, the absence of GABA there means that the neuron is disinhibited and glutamate release is increased.

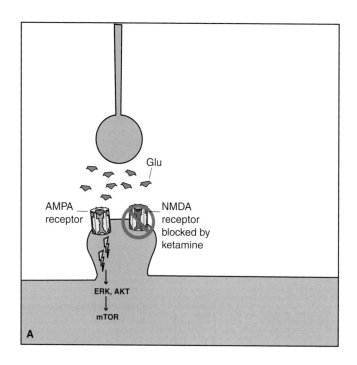

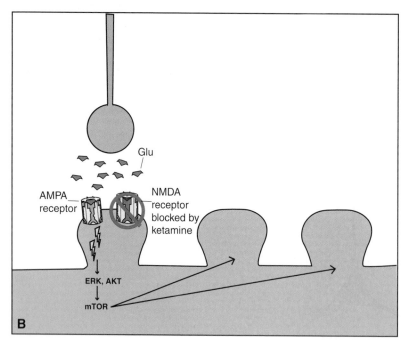

Figure 7-93. Ketamine, AMPA receptors, and mTOR. Glutamate activity heavily modulates synaptic potentiation; this is specifically modulated through NMDA (N-methyl-D-aspartate) and AMPA (α-amino-3-hydroxy-5-methyl-4-isoxazole-propionic acid) receptors. Ketamine is an NMDA receptor antagonist; however, its rapid antidepressant effects may also be related to indirect effects on AMPA receptor signaling and the mammalian target of rapamycin (mTOR) pathway. (A) It may be that blockade of the NMDA receptor leads to rapid activation of AMPA and mTOR signaling pathways. (B) This in turn would lead to rapid AMPA-mediated synaptic potentiation. Traditional antidepressants also cause synaptic potentiation; however, they do so via downstream changes in intracellular signaling. This may therefore explain the difference in onset of antidepressant action between ketamine and traditional antidepressants.

dextromethorphan

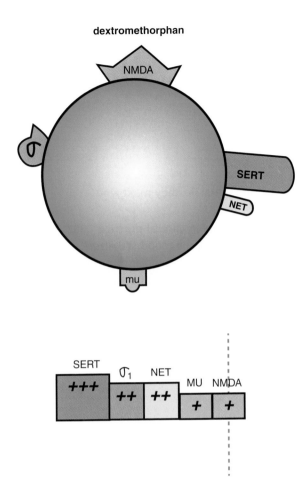

Figure 7-94. Dextromethorphan. Dextromethorphan is a weak *N*-methyl-ᴅ-aspartate (NMDA) receptor antagonist, with stronger binding affinity for the serotonin transporter (SERT), σ₁ receptors, and the norepinephrine transporter (NET). It also has some affinity for μ-opioid receptors. Dextromethorphan is approved to treat pseudobulbar affect (in combination with quinidine, which increases its bioavailability) and may have therapeutic utility in depression as well.

Summary

In this chapter, we began with an overview of antidepressant response, remission, relapse, and residual symptoms after treatment with antidepressants. The leading hypothesis for major depression for the past 40 years, namely the monoamine hypothesis, is discussed and critiqued. We have discussed the mechanisms of action of the major antidepressant drugs, including dozens of individual agents working by many unique mechanisms. The acute pharmacological actions of these agents on receptors and enzymes have been described, as well as the major hypothesis – modulation of serotonin, dopamine, and norepinephrine – which attempts to explain how all current antidepressants ultimately work.

Specific antidepressant agents which the reader should now understand include the selective serotonin reuptake inhibitors (SSRIs), serotonin partial agonist/reuptake inhibitors (SPARIs), serotonin–norepinephrine reuptake inhibitors (SNRIs), norepinephrine–dopamine reuptake inhibitors (NDRIs), selective norepinephrine reuptake inhibitors (selective NRIs), α_2 antagonists, serotonin antagonist/reuptake inhibitors (SARIs), MAOIs, tricyclic antidepressants, and melatonergic/monoaminergic antidepressants. We have also covered numerous antidepressant augmenting therapies: atypical antipsychotics, ʟ-methylfolate, SAMe, thyroid, lithium, $5HT_{1A}$ partial agonists, neurostimulation, psychotherapy, stimulants, and the combination of two antidepressants. We have provided some guidance for how to select and combine antidepressants by following a symptom-based algorithm for patients who do not remit on their first antidepressant. We have illustrated some options for combining drugs to treat such patients, and have provided a glimpse into the future by mentioning numerous novel antidepressants on the horizon.

Mood stabilizers

In this chapter, we will define mood stabilizers and will review the various pharmacological mechanisms of action proposed for mood stabilizers. We will also discuss concepts about how to use these drugs in clinical practice, including strategies for what to do if initial treatments fail and how to rationally combine mood stabilizers with another drug. Our treatment of mood stabilizers in this chapter is at the conceptual level, not at the pragmatic level. The reader should consult standard drug handbooks (such as the companion *Stahl's Essential Psychopharmacology: the Prescriber's Guide*) for details of doses, side effects, drug interactions, and other issues relevant to the prescribing of these drugs in clinical practice.

Definition of a mood stabilizer: a labile label

"There is no such thing as a mood stabilizer" – FDA
"Long live the mood stabilizers" – prescribers

What is a mood stabilizer? Originally, a mood stabilizer was a drug that treated mania and prevented recurrence of mania, thus "stabilizing" the manic pole of bipolar disorder. More recently, the concept of mood stabilizer has been defined in a wide-ranging manner, from "something that acts like lithium," to "an anticonvulsant used to treat bipolar disorder," to "an atypical antipsychotic used to treat bipolar disorder," with antidepressants considered as "mood de-stabilizers." With all this competing terminology, and with the number of drugs for the treatment of bipolar disorder exploding, the term *mood stabilizer* has become so confusing that regulatory authorities and some experts now suggest that it is best to use other terms for agents that treat bipolar disorder.

Rather than the term *mood stabilizers*, some would argue that there are drugs that can treat any or all of four distinct phases of the illness (Figures 8-1 and 8-2). Thus, a drug can be "mania-minded" and "treat from above" to reduce symptoms of mania, and/or "stabilize from above" to prevent relapse and recurrence of mania (Figure 8-1). Furthermore, drugs can be "depression-minded" and "treat from

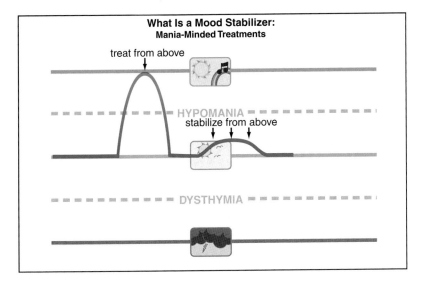

Figure 8-1. Mania-minded treatments. Although the ideal "mood stabilizer" would treat both mania and bipolar depression while also preventing episodes of either pole, in reality there is as yet no evidence to suggest that any single agent can achieve this consistently. Rather, different agents may be efficacious for different phases of bipolar disorder. As shown here, some agents seem to be "mania-minded" and thus able to "treat from above" and/or "stabilize from above" – in other words, to reduce and/or prevent symptoms of mania.

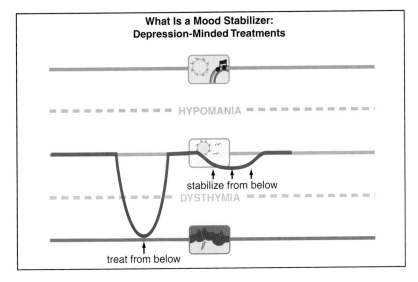

Figure 8-2. Depression-minded treatments. Although the ideal "mood stabilizer" would treat both mania and bipolar depression while also preventing episodes of either pole, as mentioned for Figure 8-1, in reality there is as yet no evidence to suggest that any single agent can achieve this consistently. Rather, different agents may be efficacious for different phases of bipolar disorder. As shown here, some agents seem to be "depression-minded" and thus able to "treat from below" and/or "stabilize from below" – in other words, to reduce and/or prevent symptoms of bipolar depression.

below" to reduce symptoms of bipolar depression, and/or "stabilize from below" to prevent relapse and recurrence of depression (Figure 8-2). Not all drugs proven to work in bipolar disorder have all four therapeutic actions. In this chapter, we will discuss agents that have one or more of these actions in bipolar disorder, and for historical purposes and simplification, refer to any of these agents as "mood stabilizers."

Lithium, the classic mood stabilizer

Bipolar disorder has classically been treated with lithium for more than 50 years. Lithium is an ion whose mechanism of action is not certain. Candidates for its mechanism of action are various signal transduction sites beyond neurotransmitter receptors (Figure 8-3). This includes second messengers, such as the phosphatidyl inositol system, where lithium inhibits the

Possible Mechanism of Lithium Action on Downstream Signal Transduction Cascades

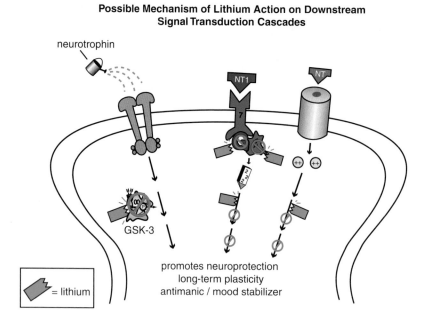

Figure 8-3. Lithium's mechanism of action. Although lithium is the oldest treatment for bipolar disorder, its mechanism of action is still not well understood. Several possible mechanisms exist and are shown here. Lithium may work by affecting signal transduction, perhaps through its inhibition of second-messenger enzymes such as inositol monophosphatase (right), by modulation of G proteins (middle), or by interaction at various sites within downstream signal transduction cascades (left).

enzyme inositol monophosphatase; modulation of G proteins; and most recently, regulation of gene expression for growth factors and neuronal plasticity by interaction with downstream signal transduction cascades, including inhibition of GSK-3 (glycogen synthase kinase 3) and protein kinase C (Figure 8-3).

However lithium works, it is proven effective in manic episodes and in maintenance of recurrence, especially for manic episodes and perhaps to a lesser extent for depressive episodes. Lithium is well established to help prevent suicide in patients with mood disorders. It is also used to treat depressive episodes in bipolar disorder as an augmenting agent to antidepressants for unipolar depression, as mentioned in Chapter 7, but is not formally approved for these uses. A number of factors have led to an unfortunate decline in the use of lithium in recent years, including the entry of multiple new treatment options into the therapeutic armamentarium for bipolar disorder, the side effects of lithium, and the monitoring burden that is part of prescribing lithium. The modern use of lithium by experts departs from its classic use as a high-dose monotherapy for euphoric mania, with lithium utilized now as one member of a portfolio of treatments, often allowing once-a-day administration and lower doses when combined with other mood stabilizers. Lithium has equal or better efficacy in bipolar disorder compared to valproate for manic, depressive, or mixed episodes, although valproate is often more frequently prescribed. Anticonvulsants including valproate have been controversially and not completely convincingly linked to causing suicidality, whereas lithium actually reduces suicide in patients with bipolar disorder. In fact, some provocative studies from Austria to Texas to Japan suggest that the more lithium mobilized by rain from rocks and soil and then dissolved in drinking water, the lower the suicide rate in the general population as well! Another potential use of lithium arises from the notion that inhibition of GSK-3 by lithium could theoretically inhibit the phosphorylation of tau (τ) proteins and thus slow the formation of plaques and tangles in Alzheimer's disease. A few studies have suggested that lithium can prevent progression from mild cognitive impairment to Alzheimer's disease and reduce phosphorylated τ levels, especially if given for a long period of time (> 1 year), and even at low doses. This remains controversial and needs replication in larger studies, but is certainly an interesting development to monitor.

Well-known side effects of lithium include gastrointestinal symptoms such as dyspepsia, nausea, vomiting, and diarrhea, as well as weight gain, hair loss, acne, tremor, sedation, decreased cognition, and incoordination. There are also long-term adverse effects upon the thyroid and kidney. Lithium has a narrow therapeutic window, requiring monitoring of plasma drug levels. Modern use of lithium often includes dosing at the lower end of the therapeutic window and combining lithium with other mood stabilizers.

Anticonvulsants as mood stabilizers

Based upon theories that mania may "kindle" further episodes of mania, a logical parallel with seizure disorders was drawn, since seizures can "kindle" more seizures. Thus, several anticonvulsants are used to treat bipolar disorder, some with better evidence of efficacy than others (Table 8-1). Since the first anticonvulsants tested, namely carbamazepine and valproate, proved effective in treating the manic phase of bipolar disorder, this has led to the idea than any anticonvulsant would be a mood stabilizer, especially for mania. However, this has not proven to be the case, as anticonvulsants do not all act by the same pharmacological mechanisms. Numerous anticonvulsants are discussed below, including not only those with proven efficacy in different phases of bipolar disorder but also those with dubious efficacy in bipolar disorder (Table 8-1).

Anticonvulsants with proven efficacy in bipolar disorder
Valproic acid

As for all anticonvulsants, the exact mechanism of action of valproic acid (also, valproate sodium, or valproate) is uncertain; however, even less may be known about the mechanism of valproate than for other anticonvulsants. Various hypotheses are discussed here, and summarized in Figures 8-4 though 8-7. At least three possibilities exist for how valproic acid works: inhibiting voltage-sensitive sodium channels (Figure 8-5), boosting the actions of the neurotransmitter GABA (γ-aminobutyric acid) (Figure 8-6), and regulating downstream signal transduction cascades (Figure 8-7). It is not known whether these actions explain the mood-stabilizing actions, the anticonvulsant actions, the anti-migraine actions, or the side effects of valproic acid. Obviously, this simple molecule has multiple and complex clinical effects, and research is trying to determine which of the various possibilities explain the mood-stabilizing effects of valproic acid so that new agents with more efficacy and fewer side effects can be developed by targeting the relevant pharmacological mechanism for bipolar disorder.

One hypothesis to explain mood-stabilizing antimanic actions is the possibility that valproate acts to

Table 8-1 Anticonvulsant mood stabilizers

Agent	Putative clinical actions				
	Epilepsy	Mania-minded		Depression-minded	
		Treat from above	Stabilize from above	Treat from below	Stabilize from below
Valproate	++++	++++	++	+	+/−
Carbamazepine	++++	++++	++	+	+/−
Lamotrigine	++++	+/−	++++	+++	++++
Oxcarbazepine/ licarbazepine	++++	++	+	+/−	+/−
Riluzole	+			+	+/−
Topiramate	++++	+/−	+/−		
Zonisamide	++++	+/−	+/−		
Gabapentin	++++	+/−	+/−		
Pregabalin	++++	+/−	+/−		
Levetiracetam	++++	+/−	+/−		

valproic acid

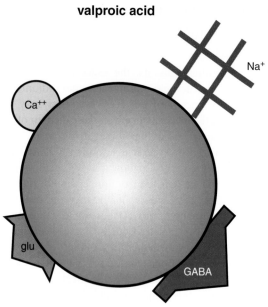

Figure 8-4. Valproic acid. Shown here is an icon of the pharmacological actions of valproic acid, an anticonvulsant used in the treatment of bipolar disorder. Valproic acid (also valproate) may work by interfering with voltage-sensitive sodium channels (VSSCs), enhancing the inhibitory actions of γ-aminobutyric acid (GABA), and regulating downstream signal transduction cascades, although which of these actions may be related to mood stabilization is not clear. Valproate may also interact with other ion channels, such as voltage-sensitive calcium channels (VSCCs), and also indirectly block glutamate actions.

diminish excessive neurotransmission by diminishing the flow of ions through voltage-sensitive sodium channels (VSSCs) (Figure 8-5). VSSCs are discussed in Chapter 3 and illustrated in Figures 3-19 through 3-21. No specific molecular site of action for valproate has been clarified, but it is possible that valproate may change the sensitivity of sodium channels by altering their phosphorylation, either by binding directly to the VSSC or its regulatory units or by inhibiting phosphorylating enzymes (Figure 8-5). If less sodium is able to pass into neurons, this may lead to diminished release of glutamate and therefore less excitatory neurotransmission, but this is only a theory. There may be additional effects of valproate on other voltage-sensitive ion channels, but these are poorly characterized and may relate to side effects as well as to therapeutic effects.

Another idea is that valproate enhances the actions of GABA, by increasing its release, decreasing its reuptake, or slowing its metabolic inactivation (Figure 8-6). The direct site of action of valproate that causes the enhancement of GABA remains unknown,

but there is good evidence that the downstream effects of valproate ultimately do result in more GABA activity, and thus more inhibitory neurotransmission, possibly explaining antimanic actions.

Finally, a number of downstream actions on complex signal transduction cascades have been described in recent years (Figure 8-7). Like lithium, valproate may inhibit GSK-3, but it may also target many other downstream sites, from blockade of phosphokinase C (PKC) and MARCKS (myristolated alanine-rich C kinase substrate), to activating various signals that promote neuroprotection and long-term plasticity such as ERK kinase (extracellular signal-regulated kinase), BCL2 (cytoprotective protein B-cell lymphoma/leukemia-2 gene), GAP43, and others (Figure 8-7). The effects of these signal transduction cascades are only now being clarified, and which of these possible effects of valproate might be relevant to mood-stabilizing actions is not yet understood.

Valproate is proven effective for the acute manic phase of bipolar disorder and is commonly used long term to prevent recurrence of mania, although its prophylactic effects have not been as well established as its acute effects in mania. Antidepressant actions of valproate have also not been well established, nor has it been shown to convincingly stabilize against recurrent depressive episodes, but there may be some efficacy for the depressed phase of bipolar disorder in some patients. Some experts believe valproic acid is more effective than lithium for rapid cycling and mixed episodes of mania. In reality, such episodes are very difficult to treat, and combinations of two or more mood stabilizers, including lithium plus valproate, are usually in order. As mentioned for lithium, valproate can also be utilized once a day in doses that are towards the bottom of the therapeutic range in combination with other mood stabilizers such as lithium to improve tolerability and compliance. For optimum efficacy, it may be ideal to push the dose of valproate, but no drug works if your patient refuses to take it, and valproic acid often has unacceptable side effects such as hair loss, weight gain, and sedation. Certain problems can be avoided by lowering the dose, but this will generally lower efficacy, and thus there may be the requirement to combine it with other mood stabilizers when valproate is given in lower doses. Some side effects may be related more to chronicity of exposure rather than to dose and thus may not be avoided by reducing the dose. This includes warnings for liver and pancreatic effects, fetal toxicities such as

Possible Sites of Action of Valproate on VSSCs

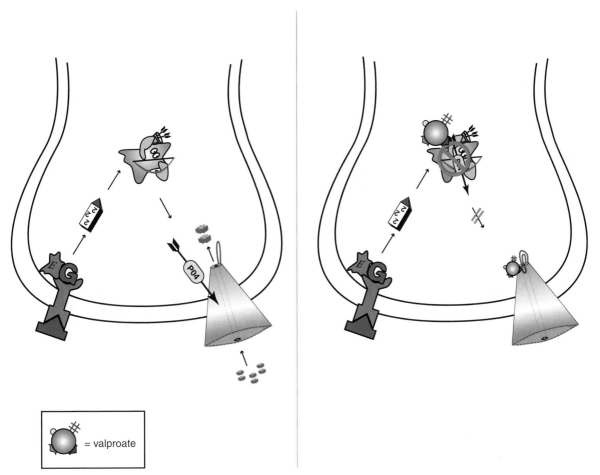

Figure 8-5. Possible sites of action of valproate on voltage-sensitive sodium channels (VSSCs). Valproate may exert antimanic effects by changing the sensitivity of VSSCs, perhaps by directly binding to channel subunits or inhibiting phosphorylating enzymes that regulate the sensitivity of these ion channels. Inhibition of VSSCs would lead to reduced sodium influx and, in turn, potentially to reduced glutamate excitatory neurotransmission, which is a possible mechanism for mania efficacy.

neural tube defects, concerns about weight gain and metabolic complications, and possible risk of amenorrhea and polycystic ovaries in women of childbearing potential. A syndrome of menstrual disturbances, polycystic ovaries, hyperandrogenism, obesity, and insulin resistance may be associated with valproic acid therapy in such women.

Carbamazepine

Carbamazepine (Figure 8-8) was actually the first anticonvulsant to be shown effective in the manic phase of bipolar disorder, but it did not receive formal FDA approval until recently as a once-daily

controlled-release formulation. Although carbamazepine and valproate both act effectively on the manic phase of bipolar disorder (Table 8-1), they appear to have different pharmacological mechanisms of action, including different side-effect profiles. Thus, carbamazepine is hypothesized to act by blocking voltage-sensitive sodium channels (VSSCs) (Figure 8-8), perhaps at a site within the channel itself, also known as the α subunit of VSSCs (Figure 8-9). As mentioned earlier, VSSCs are discussed in Chapter 3 and illustrated in Figures 3-19 through 3-21. The hypothesized action of carbamazepine upon the α subunit of VSSCs (Figure 8-9) is different from the

Possible Sites of Action of Valproate on GABA

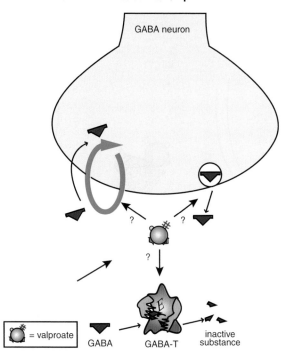

Figure 8-6. Possible sites of action of valproate on γ-aminobutyric acid (GABA). Valproate's antimanic effects may be due to enhancement of GABA neurotransmission, perhaps by inhibiting GABA reuptake, enhancing GABA release, or interfering with the metabolism of GABA by GABA transaminase (GABA-T).

hypothesized actions of valproate on these sodium channels (Figure 8-5), but may be similar to how the anticonvulsants oxcarbazepine and its active metabolite eslicarbazepine also act.

Although both carbamazepine and valproate are anticonvulsants and treat mania from above, there are many differences between these two anticonvulsants. For example, valproate is proven effective in migraine, but carbamazepine is proven effective in neuropathic pain. Furthermore, carbamazepine has a different side-effect profile than valproate, including suppressant effects upon the bone marrow, requiring initial monitoring of blood counts, and notable induction of the cytochrome P450 (CYP) enzyme 3A4. Carbamazepine is sedating and can cause fetal toxicity such as neural tube defects.

Lamotrigine

Lamotrigine (Figure 8-10) is approved as a mood stabilizer to prevent recurrence of both mania and depression. There are many curious things about

lamotrigine as a mood stabilizer. First, the FDA has not approved its use for bipolar depression, yet most experts believe that lamotrigine is effective for bipolar depression. In fact, given the growing concern about antidepressants inducing mania, causing mood instability, and increasing suicidality in bipolar disorder, lamotrigine has largely replaced antidepressants as a first-line recommendation in most treatment guidelines for bipolar depression. In that regard, lamotrigine has transformed the treatment of this difficult phase of bipolar disorder as one of the very few agents that seem to be effective for bipolar depression based upon results seen in clinical practice rather than from evidence derived from clinical trials.

A second interesting thing about lamotrigine is that even though it has some overlapping mechanistic actions with carbamazepine, namely binding to the open channel conformation of VSSCs (Figures 8-9 and 8-11), lamotrigine is not approved for bipolar mania. Perhaps its actions are not potent enough at sodium channels, or perhaps the long titration period required when starting this drug makes it difficult to show any useful effectiveness for mania, which generally requires treatment with drugs that can work quickly.

A third aspect of lamotrigine that is unusual for an antidepressant mood stabilizer is its tolerability profile. Lamotrigine is generally well tolerated for an anticonvulsant, except for its propensity to cause rashes, including (rarely) the life-threatening Stevens–Johnson syndrome (toxic epidermal necrolysis). Rashes caused by lamotrigine can be minimized by very slow up-titration of drug during initiation of therapy, avoiding or managing drug interactions such as those with valproate that raise lamotrigine levels, and by understanding how to identify and manage serious rashes, including being able to distinguish them from benign rashes (see discussion of lamotrigine in *Stahl's Essential Psychopharmacology: the Prescriber's Guide*).

Finally, lamotrigine seems to have some unique aspects to its mechanism of action (Figure 8-11), namely to reduce the release of the excitatory neurotransmitter glutamate. It is not clear whether this action is secondary to blocking the activation of VSSCs (Figure 8-11) or to some additional synaptic action. Reducing excitatory glutamatergic neurotransmission, especially if excessive during bipolar depression, may be a unique action of lamotrigine and

Possible Sites of Action of Valproate on Downstream Signal Transduction Cascades

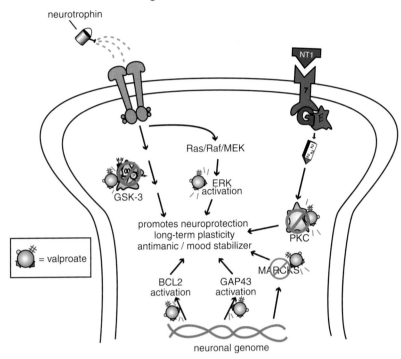

Figure 8-7. Possible sites of action of valproate on downstream signal transduction cascades. Valproate has been shown to have multiple downstream effects on signal transduction cascades, which may be involved in its antimanic effects. Valproate inhibits glycogen synthase kinase 3 (GSK-3), protein kinase C (PKC), and myristolated alanine-rich C kinase substrate (MARCKS). In addition, valproate activates signals that promote neuroprotection and long-term plasticity, such as extracellular signal-regulated kinase (ERK), cytoprotective protein B-cell lymphoma/leukemia-2 gene (BCL2), and GAP43.

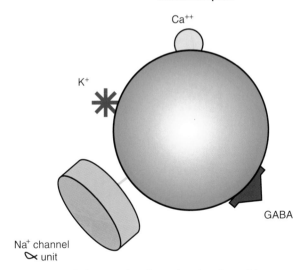

Figure 8-8. Carbamazepine. Shown here is an icon of the pharmacological actions of carbamazepine, an anticonvulsant used in the treatment of bipolar disorder. Carbamazepine may work by binding to the α subunit of voltage-sensitive sodium channels (VSSCs) and could perhaps have actions at other ion channels for calcium and potassium. By interfering with voltage-sensitive channels, carbamazepine may enhance the inhibitory actions of γ-aminobutyric acid (GABA).

explain why it has such a different clinical profile as a treatment from below and a stabilizer from below for bipolar depression.

Anticonvulsants with uncertain or doubtful efficacy in bipolar disorder

Oxcarbazepine/eslicarbazepine

Oxcarbazepine is structurally related to carbamazepine, but is not a metabolite of carbamazepine. Oxcarbazepine is actually not the active form of the drug, but a prodrug that is immediately converted into a 10-hydroxy derivative, also called the monohydroxy derivative, that most recently has been named licarbazepine. The active form of licarbazepine is the S enantiomer, known as eslicarbazepine. Thus, oxcarbazepine really works via conversion to eslicarbazepine.

Oxcarbazepine is well known as an anticonvulsant with a presumed mechanism of anticonvulsant action the same as that for carbamazepine, namely, binding to the open channel conformation of the VSSC at a

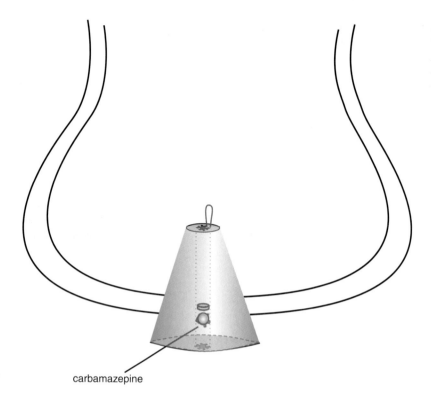

Figure 8-9. Binding site of carbamazepine. Carbamazepine is believed to bind to a site located within the open channel conformation of the voltage-sensitive sodium channel (VSSC) α subunit.

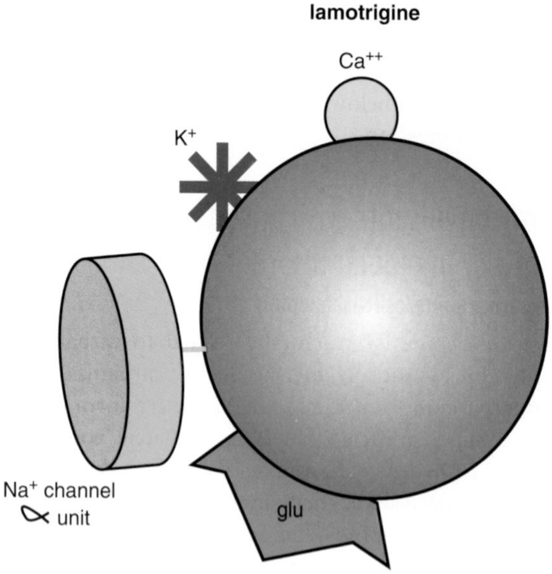

carbamazepine

lamotrigine

Ca++

K+

Na+ channel α unit

glu

Figure 8-10. Lamotrigine. Shown here is an icon of the pharmacological actions of lamotrigine, an anticonvulsant used in the treatment of bipolar disorder. Lamotrigine may work by blocking the α subunit of voltage-sensitive sodium channels (VSSCs) and could perhaps also have actions at other ion channels for calcium and potassium. Lamotrigine is also thought to reduce the release of the excitatory neurotransmitter glutamate.

Possible Sites of Action of Lamotrigine on Glutamate Release

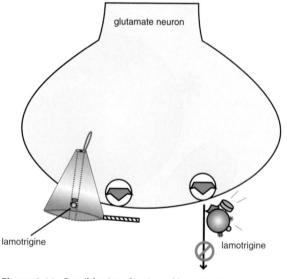

glutamate neuron

lamotrigine

lamotrigine

Figure 8-11. Possible site of action of lamotrigine on glutamate release. It is possible that lamotrigine reduces glutamate release through its blockade of voltage-sensitive sodium channels (VSSCs). Alternatively, lamotrigine may have this effect via an additional synaptic action that has not yet been identified.

site within the channel itself on the α subunit (as in Figure 8-9). However, oxcarbazepine seems to have some important differences from carbamazepine, including being less sedating, having less bone-marrow toxicity, and having fewer CYP 3A4 inter-actions, making it a more tolerable agent that is easier to dose. On the other hand, oxcarbazepine has never been proven to work as a mood stabilizer. Neverthe-less, because of a similar postulated mechanism of action but a better tolerability profile, oxcarbazepine has been utilized "off-label" by many clinicians, espe-cially for the manic phase of bipolar disorder. There is now active investigation of the active moiety eslicar-bazepine as a potential mood stabilizer.

Topiramate

Topiramate is another compound approved as an anticonvulsant and for migraine, and recently in com-bination with bupropion for weight loss in obesity. Topiramate has been tested in bipolar disorder, but with ambiguous results (Table 8-1). It does seem to be associated with weight loss and is sometimes given as an adjunct to mood stabilizers that cause weight gain, but can cause unacceptable sedation in some patients. Topiramate is also being tested in various substance-abuse disorders, including stimulant abuse and alco-holism. However, topiramate is not clearly effective as a mood stabilizer, neither from evidence-based ran-domized controlled trials (which are not consistently positive) nor from clinical practice.

The reason that topiramate may not have the robust efficacy of valproate or carbamazepine in the manic phase, nor of lamotrigine in the depressed and mainten-ance phases of bipolar disorder, is that it has a different mechanism of action from any of these agents. The exact binding site for topiramate is not known (see Figure 10-19), but it seems to enhance GABA function and reduce glutamate function by interfering with both sodium and calcium channels, but in a different way and at a different site than the previously discussed anticonvulsants. In addition, topiramate is a weak inhibitor of carbonic anhydrase. Topiramate is now considered an adjunctive treatment for bipolar disorder, perhaps helpful for weight gain, insomnia or anxiety, or possibly for comorbid substance abuse, but not neces-sarily as a mood stabilizer per se. It is also under investi-gation, in combination with phentermine, as a treatment for weight loss in obesity, which will be dis-cussed in Chapter 14.

Gabapentin and pregabalin

These anticonvulsants seem to have little or no action as mood stabilizers, yet are robust treatments for various pain conditions, from neuropathic pain to fibromyalgia, and for various anxiety disorders; they are discussed in more detail in Chapters 9 and 10, dealing with anxiety and pain. Gabapentin and pregabalin are now classified as α₂δ ligands, since they are known to bind selectively and with high affinity to the α₂δ site of voltage-sensitive calcium channels (VSCCs) (see discussion in Chapter 10, and Figures 10-14 through 10-18). It appears that blocking these VSCCs when they are open and in use causes improvement of seizures, pain, and anxiety but not stabilization of mood. That is, "use-dependent" blockade of VSCCs prevents the release of neurotrans-mitters such as glutamate in pain pathways and anxiety pathways and also prevents seizures, but does not appear to affect the mechanism involved in bipolar disorder, since clinical trials of these agents in bipolar disorder show unconvincing mood stabilization. How-ever, many bipolar patients do experience chronic pain, anxiety, and insomnia, and gabapentin and pregabalin may be useful adjunctive treatments to effective mood stabilizers, even though they do not appear to be robustly effective as mood stabilizers themselves. This is not surprising given the very different mechanism of action of these compounds as selective α₂δ ligands on calcium channels (Figures 10-14 through 10-18), com-pared to the mechanisms of proven mood stabilizers such as valproate, carbamazepine, and lamotrigine on sodium channels (discussed above).

Calcium channel blockers (L-type)

There are several types of calcium channels, not only the N or P/Q channels linked to secretion of neurotransmit-ters, targeted by α₂δ ligands, and discussed in Chapter 3 (see Figures 3-23 and 3-24) but also L channels localized on vascular smooth muscle that are targeted by various antihypertensive and antiarrhythmic drugs commonly called "calcium channel blockers." L-type channels are located on neurons where their function is still being debated, and some anecdotal evidence suggests that calcium channel blockers, especially dihydropyridine-type calcium channel blockers, may be useful for some patients with bipolar disorder.

Riluzole

This agent has anticonvulsant actions in preclinical models, but was developed to slow the progression of amyotrophic lateral sclerosis (ALS, or Lou Gehrig's disease). Theoretically, riluzole binds to VSSCs and prevents glutamate release in an action similar to that postulated for lamotrigine (Figure 8-11). The idea is that diminishing glutamate release in ALS would prevent the postulated excitotoxicity that may be causing death of motor neurons in ALS. Excessive glutamate activity may be occurring not only in ALS, but may also occur in bipolar depression, although not necessarily so severely as to cause widespread neuronal loss.

Due to riluzole's putative action on preventing glutamate release, it has been tested in case series in a number of treatment-resistant conditions hypothetically linked to excessive glutamate activity, including not only bipolar depression but also treatment-resistant unipolar depression and anxiety disorders, with some promising initial results. There is great need for another agent that has the same clinical effects as lamotrigine. The problem with riluzole is that it is quite expensive and has frequent liver-function abnormalities associated with its use.

Atypical antipsychotics as mood stabilizers: not just for psychotic mania

When atypical antipsychotics were approved for schizophrenia, it was not surprising that these agents would work for psychotic symptoms associated with mania, since the D_2 antagonist actions predict efficacy for psychosis in general (discussed in Chapter 5). However, it was somewhat surprising when these agents proved effective for the core nonpsychotic symptoms of mania and for maintenance treatment to prevent the recurrence of mania. These latter actions are similar to lithium and various anticonvulsants that act by very different mechanisms. More surprising yet is that some atypical antipsychotics are effective for bipolar depression. The question that arises is, how do atypical antipsychotics work as mood stabilizers? Also, do they act as mood stabilizers by the same pharmacologic mechanism as they do as antipsychotics? Finally, do they work for the symptoms of mania by the same pharmacologic mechanisms as they do for bipolar depression?

Putative pharmacologic mechanism of atypical antipsychotics in mania and bipolar depression

The answer to the question of how atypical antipsychotics work in mania is that we do not really know (Figure 5-36). In fact, theories about atypical

antipsychotic pharmacologic actions in bipolar disorder are less well developed than they are for schizophrenia, such as those discussed extensively in Chapter 5. Indeed, it is still a quandary how bipolar disorder itself can create seemingly opposite symptoms during various phases of the illness, as well as the combination of both manic and depressive symptoms simultaneously. Ideas about dysfunctional circuits in the depressed phase of bipolar disorder (discussed in Chapter 6 and illustrated in Figure 6-45) are contrasted with different dysfunctions in both overlapping and distinctive circuits during the manic phase of the illness (discussed in Chapter 6 and illustrated in Figure 6-48). Rather than being conceptualized as having activity that is simply "too low" in depression and "too high" in mania, the idea is that dysfunctional circuits in bipolar disorder are "out of tune" and chaotic. According to this notion, mood stabilizers have the ability to "tune" dysfunctional circuits, increasing the efficiency of information processing in symptomatic circuits, thus decreasing symptoms whether manic or depressed.

If so, the D_2 antagonist or partial agonist properties of atypical antipsychotics as well as conventional antipsychotics may account for reduction of psychotic symptoms in mania, but the $5HT_{2A}$ antagonist and $5HT_{1A}$ partial agonist properties of atypical antipsychotics may account for reduction of nonpsychotic manic and depressive symptoms by some (but not all) atypical antipsychotics. This could occur via reduction of glutamate hyperactivity from overly active pyramidal neurons by $5HT_{2A}$ antagonist actions (discussed in Chapter 5 and illustrated in Figure 5-15). This could reduce symptoms associated with glutamate hyperactivity, which could include both manic and depressive symptoms, depending upon the circuit involved. Anti-glutamate actions of atypical antipsychotics are consistent with the known pharmacologic mechanisms of several known anticonvulsants that are also mood stabilizers. Adding together different mechanisms that decrease excessive glutamate activity could explain the observed therapeutic benefits of combining atypical antipsychotics with proven anticonvulsant mood stabilizers.

Several other mechanisms are feasible explanations for how certain atypical antipsychotics work to improve symptoms in the depressed phase of bipolar disorder (discussed in Chapter 5 and illustrated in Figures 5-36, 5-37, 5-52, 5-60, 5-61). Thus, numerous mechanisms of different atypical antipsychotics can increase the availability of monoamine neurotransmitters serotonin, dopamine, and norepinephrine, known to be critical in the action of antidepressants in unipolar depression. There are very different pharmacologic properties of one atypical antipsychotic compared to another, and this could potentially explain not only why some atypical antipsychotics have different actions than others in bipolar disorder, but also why some bipolar patients respond to one atypical antipsychotic and not another. Thus, all atypical antipsychotics are approved for schizophrenia, and most are approved for mania, but only one for bipolar depression (quetiapine), with another one having multiple positive clinical trials in bipolar depression (lurasidone). Although these differences in mood-stabilizer approvals for individual atypical antipsychotics may be somewhat of an artifact of commercial considerations and lack of completion of clinical trials for some of the newer agents, it may also reflect differing portfolios of pharmacologic actions among those properties that might have antidepressant actions (Figure 5-36). Much further research must be completed before we will know the reason why atypical antipsychotics may work in mania or in bipolar depression. In the meantime, these agents as a class provide some of the broadest efficacy in bipolar disorder available, indeed broader than for most anticonvulsants and comparable or better than that for lithium. Increasingly, therefore, the treatment of bipolar disorder is not only with two or more agents, but with one of those agents being an atypical antipsychotic.

Other agents used in bipolar disorder

Benzodiazepines

Although benzodiazepines are not formally approved as mood stabilizers, they nevertheless provide valuable adjunctive treatment to proven mood stabilizers, especially in emergent situations. Intramuscular or oral administration of benzodiazepines can have a calming action immediately, and provide valuable time for mood stabilizers with a longer onset of action to begin working. Also, benzodiazepines are quite valuable for patients on an as-needed basis for intermittent agitation, insomnia and incipient manic symptoms. Skilled intermittent use can leverage the mood-stabilizing actions of concomitant mood stabilizers and prevent eruption of more severe symptoms and possibly avoid rehospitalization. Of course,

benzodiazepines should be administered with caution, especially acutely to patients with comorbid substance abuse, or chronically to any patient. The mechanism of action of benzodiazepines on $GABA_A$ receptors is discussed in further detail in Chapter 9.

Modafinil and armodafinil

The wake-promoting agents modafinil and the active enantiomer armodafinil have both been tested in bipolar depression with positive results. Large multicenter trials of armodafinil as adjunctive treatment to atypical antipsychotics in bipolar depression are promising. These agents, sometimes classified as stimulants but known to be blockers of the dopamine transporter (DAT), are discussed in greater detail in Chapter 11.

Hormones and natural products

The **omega-3 fatty acids** EPA (eicosapentanoic acid) and DHA (docosohexanoic acid) have been proposed as mood stabilizers, or as natural products that may boost the actions of proven mood stabilizers with few if any side effects. EPA is an essential fatty acid and can be metabolized to DHA, and is a normal component of a diet that contains fish. Both EPA and DHA are found in large quantity in the brain, especially in cell membranes. Recent investigations suggest that omega-3 fatty acids may inhibit PKC (protein kinase C), not unlike the actions described earlier for valproate and illustrated in Figure 8-7. Studies of omega-3 fatty acids are ongoing and suggestive, but they have not yet been proven effective in bipolar disorder.

Inositol is a natural product linked to second-messenger systems and signal transduction cascades, especially for the phosphatidyl inositol signals related to various neurotransmitter receptors such as the $5HT_{2A}$ receptor. Inositol has been studied in bipolar disorder and in treatment-resistant bipolar depression, where it may be as effective as an augmenting agent to antidepressants as approved mood stabilizers such as lamotrigine and risperidone. Further studies of inositol are necessary.

The centrally active form of the vitamin folate, L-**methylfolate**, is discussed extensively in Chapter 7 and illustrated in Figures 7-71 through 7-74. L-Methylfolate could theoretically boost monoamine neurotransmitter function in bipolar depression, but has not been widely studied in controlled trials. An additional rationale for utilizing L-methylfolate in bipolar disorder is because several anticonvulsants interfere with folate absorption or folate metabolism. Thus, bipolar patients who are partial responders to mood-stabilizing anticonvulsants (especially lamotrigine, valproate, and carbamazepine, but perhaps other anticonvulsants as well), or who lose their response, may be considered candidates for taking L-methylfolate.

Some investigators note that **thyroid hormone**, especially T_3, may stabilize mood in some patients with bipolar disorder. This is not well researched and is somewhat controversial, especially for long-term use.

Antidepressants: do they make you bipolar?

Increasingly, it seems that antidepressants either do not work, or may worsen the situation for some patients who have bipolar disorder, causing destabilization of mood with induction of mania or hypomania, rapid cycling or mixed states or even suicidality. There is even an ongoing debate about whether antidepressants can cause someone to develop bipolar disorder who does not have this condition prior to taking an antidepressant, proposing that bipolar disorder could even be a complication of antidepressant treatment. Although this possibility is still under investigation, there is now little debate about the possibility that antidepressants, perhaps especially tricyclic antidepressants, can activate bipolar disorder in patients known to have a bipolar spectrum disorder.

Based upon current evidence, it seems likely that someone who develops bipolar disorder after taking an antidepressant is an individual who already has bipolar disorder, but the condition may have been previously undiagnosed, wrongly diagnosed, or "unmasked," but not caused by antidepressant treatment. This is a particularly problematic issue for young patients, who may present with unipolar depressive symptoms before they express any manic or hypomanic symptoms, and who may be particularly vulnerable therefore both to misdiagnosis and to antidepressant-induced activation and suicidality.

So how do you know to whom you can give an antidepressant? Recommendations for use of antidepressants in patients with known bipolar disorder, who are at risk for bipolar disorder, or who have had activation of mania on antidepressants are still evolving. Currently, use of antidepressants for individuals in these situations must be considered on a case-by-case basis. Most experts agree that antidepressant monotherapy is generally to be avoided in such individuals, and that treatment of depression in bipolar disorder should start with other options such as lamotrigine, lithium, and/or atypical antipsychotics as monotherapies or in combination (Figure 8-12). Whether one can add an antidepressant to these agents in patients with bipolar depression who do not have robust treatment responses to these first-line agents is the subject of current debate. Many treatment guidelines do provide for use of antidepressants in combination with mood stabilizers, perhaps preferring bupropion the most and tricyclic antidepressants the least, but when to do this remains controversial, dependent somewhat on the results of ongoing studies, and upon where in the world you practice and were trained. Thus, common sense, integration of one's clinical experience, and keeping up with this evolving area of psychopharmacology is now considered the best practice.

Mood stabilizers in clinical practice
How do you choose a mood stabilizer?

Although many monotherapies are proven effective for one or more phases of bipolar disorder, few patients with a bipolar spectrum disorder can be maintained on monotherapy. Unfortunately for the practicing psychopharmacologist, almost all of the evidence for efficacy of mood stabilizers is based upon studies of monotherapies, whereas almost all patients with bipolar disorder are on combinations of therapeutic agents. In spite of having numerous evidence-based monotherapies, and learning all the lessons from empiric practice-based combinations of these treatments, bipolar disorder remains a highly recurrent, predominantly depressive illness with frequent comorbidities and residual symptoms. So, how does one get the best outcome for a bipolar patient? The answer proposed here is to learn the mechanisms of action of the known and putative mood stabilizers and their ancillary and adjunctive treatments, familiarize oneself with the evidence for their efficacy and safety in monotherapy trials, and then construct a unique portfolio of treatments one patient at a time. Evidence-based treatments for real-world management of bipolar disorder with combinations of mood stabilizers are relatively poorly researched. Many studies show that various atypical antipsychotics added to either lithium or valproate enhance antimanic efficacy. However, there are few studies of other combinations.

First-line treatments in bipolar disorder

Not all bipolar patients are complicated, especially at the onset of the illness, and when presenting in primary care in the depressed phase. So, before looking for complicated solutions, the best treatment choice for uncomplicated bipolar patients would first be to do no harm and thus to prescribe anything that avoids antidepressant monotherapy no matter what the current symptoms are. This begins with prudent determination of when depressive symptoms are due to bipolar versus unipolar depression, and if bipolar, may result in use of lamotrigine or an atypical antipsychotic or their combination while avoiding antidepressants.

Also, it should be appreciated that "mild mania" is not an oxymoron, and some bipolar patients present in this state, which suggests that treatment with either valproate, lithium, or an atypical antipsychotic monotherapy or their combination may reduce manic symptoms substantially. In primary care, there may be a wish to avoid valproate and lithium and even lamotrigine due to lack of familiarity with these agents, and to start with an atypical antipsychotic (while avoiding an antidepressant), with referral to a specialist if treatment results are not satisfactory.

That is the easy part. What about the majority of patients who present to psychopharmacologists with severe, recurrent, or mixed mania, rapid cycling symptoms, abundant comorbidity, and inadequate treatment responses with multiple residual symptoms after receiving all the treatments described above?

Combinations of mood stabilizers are the standard for treating bipolar disorder

Given the disappointing number of patients who attain remission from any phase of bipolar disorder after any given monotherapy or sequence of monotherapies, who can maintain that remission over the long run, and who can tolerate the treatment, it is not surprising that the majority of bipolar patients require treatment with several medications. Rather than have a simple regimen of one mood stabilizer at high doses and a patient with side effects but who is not in remission, it now seems highly preferable to have a patient in remission without symptoms no matter how many agents this takes. Furthermore, sometimes the doses of each agent can be lowered to

tolerable levels while the synergy among their therapeutic mechanisms provides more robust efficacy than single agents even in high doses.

Several specific suggestions of combinations, or "combos," have enjoyed widespread use, even though for many of them there is little actual evidence-based data from clinical trials that their combination results in superior efficacy (Figure 8-12). Because of the strong role of "eminence-based medicine" (with sometimes conflicting recommendations by different experts), rather than evidence-based medicine, for combination treatments, some of the options are discussed here with a bit of whimsy. Nevertheless, treatment of bipolar disorders with rational and empirically useful combinations is a serious business, and the reader may find that several of these suggestions are useful for practicing clinicians to use in the treatment of some patients.

The best evidence-based combinations consist of the addition of lithium or valproate to an atypical antipsychotic (Figure 8-12). Although lithium, lamotrigine, and valproate have all been available for a long time, there are remarkably few controlled studies of their use together. Nevertheless, they all have different mechanisms of action and different clinical profiles in the various phases of bipolar illness; they can therefore be usefully combined in clinical practice due to practice-based evidence as **li-vo** (lithium–valproate), **la-vo** (lamotrigine–valproate), **la-li** (lamotrigine–lithium), or even the triple combination **la-li-vo** (lamotrigine–lithium–valproate) (Figure 8-12). Combinations of lamotrigine and valproate need to be carefully monitored for the consequences of the drug interactions between the two, especially for elevations of lamotrigine levels and the possible increased risk of rashes, including serious rash, unless the lamotrigine dose is decreased by up to half. Carbamazepine, although sedating, has less weight gain than many other agents, and can be combined with lamotrigine despite the relative lack of controlled studies of combinations of carbamazepine with other agents. Attention to the fact that carbamazepine is an inducer of CYP 3A4 generally means not combining with drugs that are substrates of 3A4, such as certain atypical antipsychotics including lurasidone, clozapine, quetiapine, aripiprazole, and iloperidone (see Figures 2-20 and 2-21).

Lami-quel combines the two agents with arguably the best evidence as monotherapies. Lamotrigine by itself is a "stealth" approach to treating bipolar depression, given the long titration times (2 months or

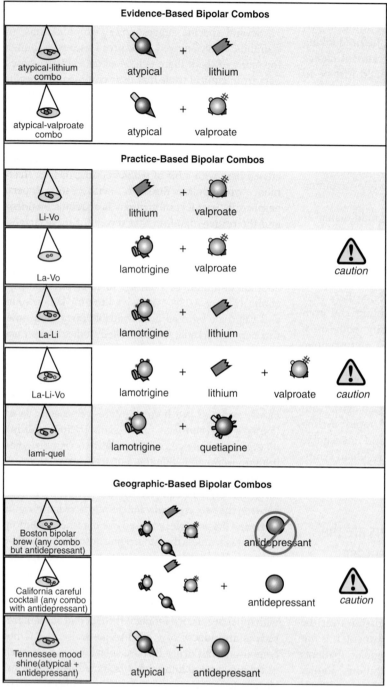

Combos for Bipolar Disorder

Figure 8-12. Bipolar disorder combinations. Most patients with bipolar disorder will require treatment with two or more agents. The combinations with the most evidence include addition of an atypical antipsychotic to either lithium (atypical–lithium combo) or valproate (atypical–valproate combo). Combinations that are not well studied in controlled trials but that have some practice-based evidence include lithium plus valproate (li-vo), cautious use of lamotrigine plus valproate (la-vo), lamotrigine plus lithium (la-li), cautious combination of lamotrigine, lithium, and valproate (la-li-vo), and combination of lithium plus quetiapine (lami-quel). Experts diverge in their opinions on how to treat bipolar depression, particularly when it comes to antidepressants. Some believe that even when combination treatment is required, it should never involve use of an antidepressant (Boston bipolar brew), while others recommend cautious addition of an antidepressant to one or more mood stabilizers (California careful cocktail). For patients who develop symptoms of activation during treatment with an antidepressant for unipolar depression, some experts suggest adding an atypical antipsychotic rather than discontinuing the antidepressant (Tennessee mood shine).

longer) and latency of onset of action once adequate dosing is reached (up to another 3 months). Thus, efficacy can appear to be clandestine and to sneak up on the patient over 3 or 4 months rather than dramatically boost mood soon after initiation of treatment. Rather than add an antidepressant to lamotrigine when there is inadequate response, or wait for many months for lamotrigine to work alone, an alternative approach would be to augment with quetiapine (the combination called "lami-quel" in Figure 8-12) or with any other atypical antipsychotic (for example, lurasidone for bipolar depression or depot long-acting risperidone injectable for rapid-cycling bipolar disorder). Other drugs may be useful adjuncts to help associated symptoms, but not to be mood stabilizing per se, including agents for substance abuse (naltrexone, acamprosate, varenicline), weight loss (zonisamide, topiramate), pain, anxiety, and sleep (gabapentin, pregabalin), agitation (benzodiazepines), and many others.

Armodafinil is emerging as another potential alternative to combine with atypical antipsychotics and/or lamotrigine in patients with bipolar depression insufficiently responsive to these other agents alone.

Some of the more innovative if "eminence-based" combinations from experts in various geographical regions are also frequently used (Figure 8-12). They include the **Boston bipolar brew** (Figure 8-12), so named because several experts, including many trained or working in Boston, are proponents of essentially *never* utilizing an antidepressant for bipolar patients. Thus, a "Boston bipolar brew" is any combination of mood stabilizers that does not include an antidepressant. By contrast, the **California careful cocktail** (Figure 8-12), arising from more laid-back experts in California, proposes the possibility of patients "earning" the right to add an antidepressant, but carefully, once exhausting other options for a bipolar depressed patient whose depression is not in remission. A "California careful cocktail" is the addition of an antidepressant to one or more mood stabilizers, particularly including one or more that has robust efficacy against mania and recurrence of mania. Finally, **Tennessee mood shine** (Figure 8-12) from experts there provides the option of treating bipolar depression that arises when giving an antidepressant and discovering that the patient either has activating side effects or treatment resistance, or that the diagnosis is changing from unipolar to bipolar depression as the condition is evolving. In this case, rather than stopping the antidepressant, an atypical antipsychotic is added.

Experimental and "off-label" combinations for bipolar depression with some evidence but not yet regulatory approval include combining lamotrigine with a dopamine agonist such as pramipexole or ropinirole. Finally, after trying all these options, continuing poor response in bipolar depression may reluctantly require augmentation of lamotrigine or a lamotrigine combination with an antidepressant. Given the promising data with lurasidone and armodafinil, these agents along with lamotrigine should probably be tried before using antidepressants.

Bipolar disorder and women

Although gender issues in bipolar disorder are less well investigated than they are in unipolar disorder, a brief discussion is in order for those special considerations known to be relevant to women with bipolar disorder. For example, in women, bipolar disorder is even more depressive in nature than it is in men, with more suicide attempts, mixed mania, and rapid cycling. Women have more thyroid dysfunction than men, and some experts believe that augmentation of bipolar patients with thyroid hormone (T_3), both in men but particularly in women, may enhance stability even in the absence of overt thyroid dysfunction. Women are more likely than men to report atypical or reverse vegetative symptoms during the depressed phase than men, especially increased appetite and weight gain. Comorbid anxiety and eating disorders are more frequent in bipolar women; comorbid substance-use disorders are more frequent in men.

There is some limited evidence that bipolar disorder may worsen during the premenstrual phase in some women, just as unipolar major depression may worsen premenstrually. Pregnancy is not protective against bipolar mood episodes, and the postpartum period is a very high-risk time for experiencing first onset and recurrence of depressive, manic, mixed, and psychotic episodes. There is little empirical study of bipolar disorder in perimenopausal or postmenopausal women, but there are suggestions that bipolar recurrence is more common during perimenopause and that estrogen may stabilize mood in perimenopausal women with bipolar disorder. No major gender differences have been consistently reported for mood stabilizers in terms of efficacy, but there are differences in side effects, including in women the possible risk from valproate of polycystic ovarian syndrome with amenorrhea, hyperandrogenism, weight gain, and insulin resistance.

During pregnancy, most anticonvulsant mood stabilizers and lithium are associated with risk for various fetal toxicities. Some may be mitigated by co-administration of folate. However, among the various options, it may be prudent to consider stabilizing bipolar women with atypical antipsychotics during pregnancy. If mood stabilizers are discontinued for pregnancy, this should not be done abruptly because it may increase the chance of recurrence. Of course, nontreatment of bipolar illness has its consequences, too, as discussed for nontreatment of unipolar depression during pregnancy in Chapter 7, with the problems outlined in Table 7-13. Many of the same considerations apply as well to the treatment of women with bipolar disorder during pregnancy, including the decision whether to continue or discontinue mood stabilizers during pregnancy, during postpartum periods, and during breastfeeding. Such decisions should be made on an individual basis after weighing the risks and benefits for a particular patient. Generally speaking, breastfeeding while taking lithium is not recommended, whereas breastfeeding while taking valproate, lamotrigine, carbamazepine, or atypical antipsychotics can be cautiously considered while carefully monitoring the infant and, if necessary, getting infant blood drug levels.

Children, bipolar disorder, and mood stabilizers

This is one of the great controversial areas of psychopharmacology today. As this textbook is not a child psychopharmacology textbook, only a few key issues will be mentioned here. Controversies in the treatment of unipolar depression in children and adolescents, such as increasing suicidality with antidepressants, are mentioned in Chapters 6 and 7. For bipolar disorder, there is debate about whether children even get this illness, and whether symptoms attributable to bipolar disorder should be treated at all with powerful psychotropic medications. In reality, it is increasingly clear that prepubertal and adolescent manias do exist and are more common than appreciated in the past, but that the symptoms are different from those of "classic" adult mania. That is, prepubertal mania is characterized by severe irritability, absence of discrete episodes, periodic "affective storms" with severe, persistent, and often violent outbursts, attacking behavior, and anger. Symptoms tend to be chronic and continuous rather than episodic and acute. Moods are only rarely euphoric, but there are high levels of hyperactivity and overactivity. It seems increasingly clear that pediatric mania may not be rare so much as difficult to diagnose and to distinguish from attention deficit hyperactivity disorder (ADHD), conduct disorder, and temper dysregulation, a newly proposed condition. Thus, an atypical picture of mania emerges for many children and adolescents with bipolar disorder, characterized by predominantly irritable mood, mania mixed with depression, and chronic course, which looks much different than the adult presentation of euphoric mania with a biphasic and episodic course.

Adolescent-onset mania may more frequently include euphoria, but otherwise has the symptom characteristics of childhood-onset rather than adult-onset mania. In fact, "mixed mania," affecting 20–30% of adults with bipolar mania, may often have its onset in childhood or adolescence with the additional characteristics of chronic course, high rate of suicide, poor response to treatment, and early history of cognitive symptoms highly suggestive of ADHD. Thus, pediatric mania may develop into adult mixed mania. In children, mania has considerable symptomatic overlap with ADHD, and it has been estimated that over half (and possibly up to 90%) of patients with pediatric mania also have ADHD. This is due not just to "distractibility, motor hyperactivity, and talkativeness," diagnostic symptoms that overlap with both mania and ADHD, but to true comorbidity. In such patients, it seems to be necessary to stabilize the mania before treating the ADHD to get best results, and also to combine mood stabilizers with ADHD treatments.

In children, conduct disorder is also strongly associated with mania. Most patients with mania qualify for the diagnosis of conduct disorder, making this association quite controversial if it leads to antipsychotic treatment of essentially all children with conduct disorder. However, there are differences in symptoms between the two groups, with physical restlessness and poor judgment more common in comorbid cases of conduct disorder and mania than in cases with mania alone. Finally, anxiety disorders, especially panic disorder and agoraphobia, are frequently comorbid with mania in children.

For treatment of bipolar disorder in children and adolescents, the best option is to use what has been proven in adults, but there is a striking paucity of evidence for how to treat bipolar disorder in children and adolescents. Much further study of mood stabilizers is required in children and adolescents.

Future mood stabilizers

As the pharmacologic targets for mood stabilizers are not well developed, new mood stabilizers tend to come from the same areas as current drugs: namely, new antipsychotics and new anticonvulsants. New research is also targeting novel ways to **block glutamate action** or to bind to the **sigma-1 (σ_1) site**. Both ketamine and dextromethorphan act at these sites and are discussed in Chapter 7 (see also Figures 7-90 through 7-94).

Summary

Mood stabilizers have evolved significantly in recent years. They include agents that are mania-minded and treat mania while preventing manic relapse, as well as agents that are depression-minded and treat bipolar depression while preventing depressive relapse. Numerous agents of diverse mechanisms of action are mood stabilizers, especially lithium, various anticonvulsants, and atypical antipsychotics. Because of limits to the efficacy and tolerability of current mood stabilizers, combination therapy is the rule and mood-stabilizer monotherapy the exception. Evidence is evolving for how to combine agents to relieve all symptoms of bipolar disorder and prevent relapse, but the treatment of bipolar disorder today remains as much a psychopharmacological art as a science.

Anxiety disorders and anxiolytics

This chapter will provide a brief overview of anxiety disorders and their treatments. Included here are descriptions of how the anxiety disorder subtypes overlap with each other and with major depressive disorder. Clinical descriptions and formal criteria for how to diagnose anxiety disorder subtypes are mentioned only in passing. The reader should consult standard reference sources for this material. The discussion here will emphasize how discoveries about the functioning of various brain circuits and neurotransmitters – especially those centered on the amygdala – impact our understanding of fear and worry, symptoms that cut across the entire spectrum of anxiety disorders.

The goal of this chapter is to acquaint the reader with ideas about the clinical and biological aspects of anxiety disorders in order to understand the mechanisms of action of the various treatments for these disorders discussed along the way. Many of these treatments are extensively discussed in other chapters. For details of mechanisms of anxiolytic agents used also for the treatment of depression (i.e., certain

antidepressants), the reader is referred to Chapter 7; for those anxiolytic agents used also for chronic pain (i.e., certain anticonvulsants), the reader is referred to Chapter 10. The discussion in this chapter is at the conceptual level, and not at the pragmatic level. The reader should consult standard drug handbooks (such as *Stahl's Essential Psychopharmacology: the Prescriber's Guide*) for details of doses, side effects, drug interactions, and other issues relevant to the prescribing of these drugs in clinical practice.

Symptom dimensions in anxiety disorders

When is anxiety an anxiety disorder?

Anxiety is a normal emotion under circumstances of threat and is thought to be part of the evolutionary "fight or flight" reaction of survival. Whereas it may be normal or even adaptive to be anxious when a saber-tooth tiger (or its modern-day equivalent) is attacking, there are many circumstances in which

Overlap of MDD and Anxiety Disorders

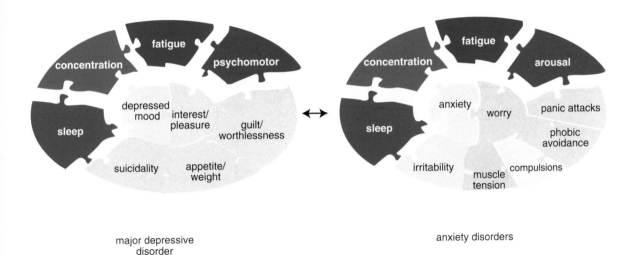

Figure 9-1. Overlap of major depressive disorder and anxiety disorders. Although the core symptoms of anxiety disorders (anxiety and worry) differ from the core symptoms of major depression (loss of interest and depressed mood), there is considerable overlap among the rest of the symptoms associated with these disorders (compare the "anxiety disorders" puzzle on the right to the "MDD" puzzle on the left). For example, fatigue, sleep difficulties, and problems concentrating are common to both types of disorders.

the presence of anxiety is maladaptive and constitutes a psychiatric disorder. The idea of anxiety as a psychiatric disorder is evolving rapidly, and is characterized by the concept of core symptoms of excessive fear and worry (symptoms at the center of anxiety disorders in Figure 9-1), compared to major depression, which is characterized by core symptoms of depressed mood or loss of interest (symptoms at the center of major depressive disorder in Figure 9-1).

Anxiety disorders have considerable symptom overlap with major depression (see those symptoms surrounding core features shown in Figure 9-1), particularly sleep disturbance, problems concentrating, fatigue, and psychomotor/arousal symptoms. Each anxiety disorder also has a great deal of symptom overlap with other anxiety disorders (Figures 9-2 through 9-5). Anxiety disorders are also extensively comorbid, not only with major depression, but also with each other, since many patients qualify over time for a second or even third concomitant anxiety disorder. Finally, anxiety disorders are frequently comorbid with many other conditions such as substance abuse, attention deficit hyperactivity disorder, bipolar disorder, pain disorders, sleep disorders, and more.

So, what is an anxiety disorder? These disorders all seem to maintain the core features of some form of anxiety or fear coupled with some form of worry, but

their natural history over time shows them to morph from one into another, to evolve into full syndrome expression of anxiety disorder symptoms (Figure 9-1) and then to recede into subsyndromal levels of symptoms only to reappear again as the original anxiety disorder, a different anxiety disorder (Figures 9-2 through 9-5), or major depression (Figure 9-1). If anxiety disorders all share core symptoms of fear and worry (Figures 9-1 and 9-6) and, as we shall see later in this chapter, are all basically treated with the same drugs, including many of the same drugs that treat major depression, the question now arises, what is the difference between one anxiety disorder and another? Also, one could ask, what is the difference between major depression and anxiety disorders? Are all these entities really different disorders, or are they instead different aspects of the same illness?

Overlapping symptoms of major depression and anxiety disorders

Although the core symptoms of major depression (depressed mood or loss of interest) differ from the core symptoms of anxiety disorders (fear and worry), there is a great deal of overlap with the other symptoms considered diagnostic both for a major depressive episode and for several different anxiety disorders

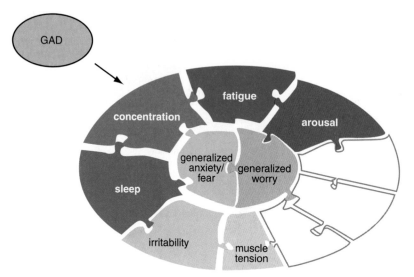

Figure 9-2. Generalized anxiety disorder (GAD). The symptoms typically associated with GAD are shown here. These include the core symptoms of generalized anxiety and worry as well as increased arousal, fatigue, difficulty concentrating, sleep problems, irritability, and muscle tension. Many of these symptoms, including the core symptoms, are present in other anxiety disorders as well.

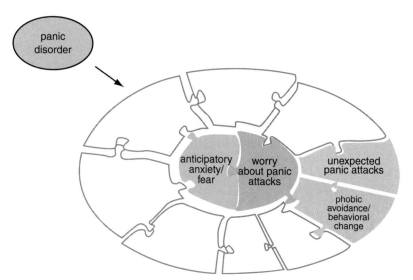

Figure 9-3. Panic disorder. The characteristic symptoms of panic disorder are shown here, with core symptoms of anticipatory anxiety as well as worry about panic attacks. Associated symptoms are the unexpected panic attacks themselves and phobic avoidance or other behavioral changes associated with concern over panic attacks.

(Figure 9-1). These overlapping symptoms include problems with sleep, concentration, and fatigue as well as psychomotor/arousal symptoms (Figure 9-1). It is thus easy to see how the gain or loss of just a few additional symptoms can morph a major depressive episode into an anxiety disorder (Figure 9-1) or one anxiety disorder into another (Figures 9-2 through 9-5).

From a therapeutic point of view, it may matter little what the specific diagnosis is across this spectrum of disorders (Figures 9-1 through 9-5). That is, first-line psychopharmacological treatments may not be much different for a patient who currently

qualifies for a major depressive episode plus the symptom of anxiety (but not an anxiety disorder) versus a patient who currently qualifies for a major depressive episode plus a comorbid anxiety disorder with full criteria anxiety symptoms. Although it can be useful to make specific diagnoses for following patients over time and for documenting the evolution of symptoms, the emphasis from a psychopharmacological point of view is increasingly to take a symptom-based therapeutic strategy to patients with any of these disorders because the brain is not organized according to the DSM, but according to brain

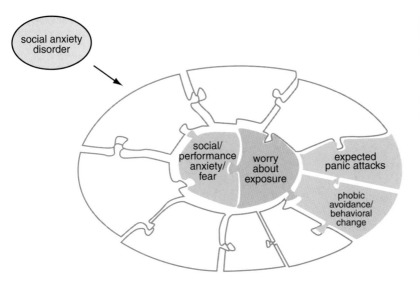

Figure 9-4. Social anxiety disorder. Symptoms of social anxiety disorder, shown here, include the core symptoms anxiety or fear over social performance plus worry about social exposure. Associated symptoms are panic attacks that are predictable and expected in certain social situations as well as phobic avoidance of those situations.

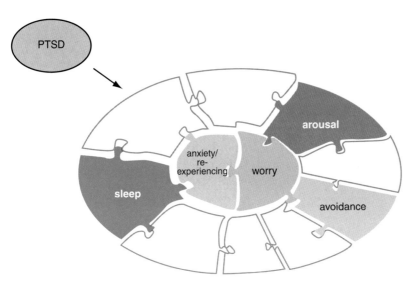

Figure 9-5. Posttraumatic stress disorder (PTSD). The characteristic symptoms of PTSD are shown here. These include the core symptoms of anxiety while the traumatic event is being re-experienced as well as worry about having the other symptoms of PTSD, such as increased arousal and startle responses, sleep difficulties including nightmares, and avoidance behaviors.

circuits with topographical localization of function. That is, specific treatments can be tailored to the individual patient by deconstructing whatever disorder the patient has into a list of the specific symptoms a given patient is experiencing (see Figures 9-2 through 9-5), and then matching these symptoms to hypothetically malfunctioning brain circuits regulated by specific neurotransmitters in order to rationally select and combine psychopharmacological treatments to eliminate all symptoms and get the patient to remission.

Overlapping symptoms of different anxiety disorders

Although there are different diagnostic criteria for different anxiety disorders (Figures 9-2 though 9-5), these are constantly changing, and many do not even consider obsessive–compulsive disorder to be an anxiety disorder any longer (OCD is discussed in Chapter 14 on impulsivity). All anxiety disorders have overlapping symptoms of anxiety/fear coupled with worry (Figure 9-6). Remarkable progress has been made in

Anxiety: The Phenotype

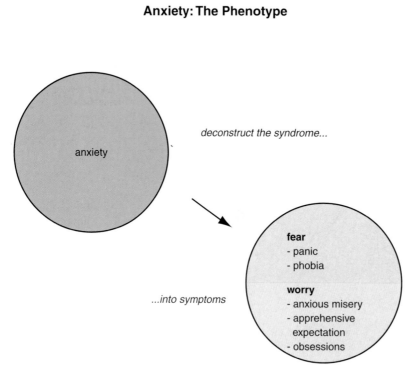

deconstruct the syndrome...

...into symptoms

Figure 9-6. Anxiety: the phenotype. Anxiety can be deconstructed, or broken down, into the two core symptoms of fear and worry. These symptoms are present in all anxiety disorders, although what triggers them may differ from one disorder to the next.

understanding the circuitry underlying the core symptom of anxiety/fear based upon an explosion of neurobiological research on the amygdala (Figures 9-7 through 9-14). The links between the amygdala, fear circuits, and treatments for the symptom of anxiety/ fear across the spectrum of anxiety disorders are discussed throughout the rest of this chapter.

Worry is the second core symptom shared across the spectrum of anxiety disorders (Figure 9-7). This symptom is hypothetically linked to the functioning of cortico-striato-thalamo-cortical (CSTC) loops. The links between the CSTC circuits, "worry loops," and treatments for the symptom of worry across the spectrum of anxiety disorders are discussed later in this chapter (see also Figures 9-15 through 9-17, 9-26, and 9-29). We shall see that what differentiates one anxiety disorder from another may not be the anatomical localization, or the neurotransmitters regulating fear and worry in each of these disorders (Figures 9-6 and 9-7), but the specific nature of malfunctioning within these same circuits in various anxiety disorders. That is, in generalized anxiety disorder (GAD), malfunctioning in the amygdala and CSTC worry loops may be hypothetically persistent, and unremitting, yet not severe (Figure 9-2), whereas malfunctioning may be theoretically intermittent but

catastrophic in an unexpected manner for panic disorder (Figure 9-3) or in an expected manner for social anxiety (Figure 9-4). Circuit malfunctioning may be traumatic in origin and conditioned in post-traumatic stress disorder (PTSD: Figure 9-5).

The amygdala and the neurobiology of fear

The amygdala, an almond-shaped brain center located near the hippocampus, has important anatomical connections that allow it to integrate sensory and cognitive information and then determine whether there will be a fear response. Specifically, the affect or feeling of fear may be regulated via reciprocal connections that the amygdala shares with key areas of prefrontal cortex that regulate emotions, namely the orbitofrontal cortex and the anterior cingulate cortex (Figure 9-8). However, fear is not just a feeling. The fear response can also include motor responses. Depending upon the circumstances and one's temperament, those motor responses could be fight, flight, or freezing in place. Motor responses of fear are regulated in part by connections between the amygdala and the periaqueductal gray area of the brainstem (Figure 9-9).

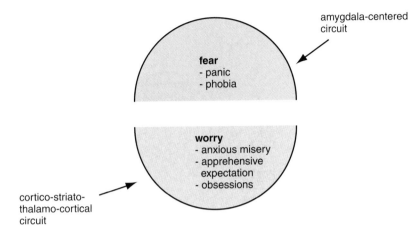

Associate Symptoms of Anxiety With Brain Regions and Circuits That Regulate Them

fear
- panic
- phobia

amygdala-centered circuit

worry
- anxious misery
- apprehensive expectation
- obsessions

cortico-striato-thalamo-cortical circuit

Figure 9-7. Linking anxiety symptoms to circuits. Anxiety and fear symptoms (e.g., panic, phobias) are regulated by an amygdala-centered circuit. Worry, on the other hand, is regulated by a cortico-striato-thalamo-cortical (CSTC) loop. These circuits may be involved in all anxiety disorders, with the different phenotypes reflecting not unique circuitry but rather divergent malfunctioning within those circuits.

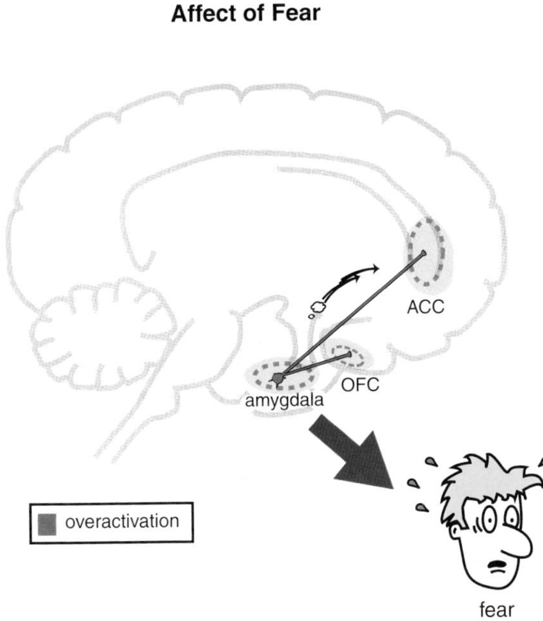

Affect of Fear

ACC

OFC

amygdala

■ overactivation

fear

Figure 9-8. Affect of fear. Feelings of fear are regulated by reciprocal connections between the amygdala and the anterior cingulate cortex (ACC) and the amygdala and the orbitofrontal cortex (OFC). Specifically, it may be that overactivation of these circuits produces feelings of fear.

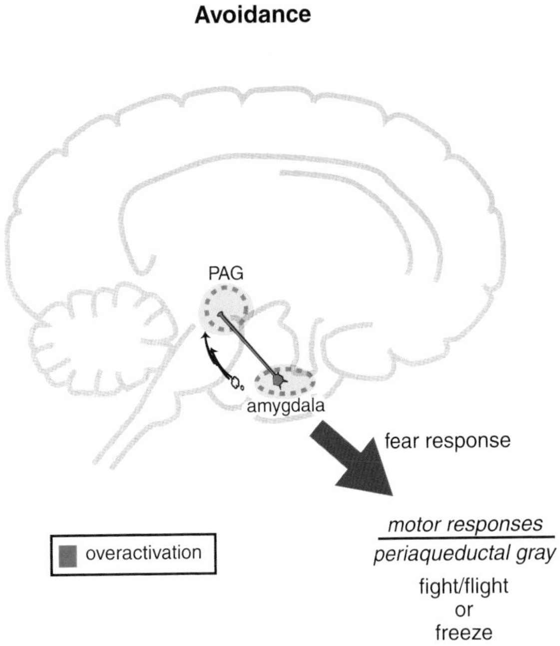

Avoidance

PAG

amygdala

fear response

■ overactivation

motor responses
periaqueductal gray
fight/flight
or
freeze

Figure 9-9. Avoidance. Feelings of fear may be expressed through behaviors such as avoidance, which is partly regulated by reciprocal connections between the amygdala and the periaqueductal gray (PAG). Avoidance in this sense is a motor response and may be analogous to freezing under threat. Other motor responses are to fight or to run away (flight) in order to survive threats from the environment.

393

Endocrine Output of Fear

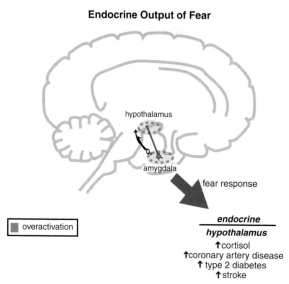

overactivation

fear response

endocrine
_____
hypothalamus
↑cortisol
↑coronary artery disease
↑ type 2 diabetes
↑ stroke

Figure 9-10. Endocrine output of fear. The fear response may be characterized in part by endocrine effects such as increases in cortisol, which occur because of amygdala activation of the hypothalamic–pituitary–adrenal (HPA) axis. Prolonged HPA activation and cortisol release can have significant health implications, such as increased risk of coronary artery disease, type 2 diabetes, and stroke.

Breathing Output

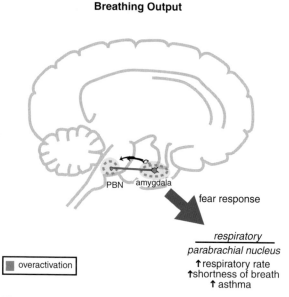

PBN   amygdala

fear response

overactivation

respiratory
_____
parabrachial nucleus
↑respiratory rate
↑shortness of breath
↑ asthma

Figure 9-11. Breathing output. Changes in respiration may occur during a fear response; these changes are regulated by activation of the parabrachial nucleus (PBN) via the amygdala. Inappropriate or excessive activation of the PBN can lead not only to increases in the rate of respiration but also to symptoms such as shortness of breath, exacerbation of asthma, or a sense of being smothered.

There are also endocrine reactions that accompany fear, in part due to connections between the amygdala and the hypothalamus, causing changes in the HPA (hypothalamic–pituitary–adrenal) axis, and thus of cortisol levels. A quick boost of cortisol may enhance survival when encountering a real but short-term threat. However, chronic and persistent activation of this aspect of the fear response can lead to increased medical comorbidity, including increased rates of coronary artery disease, type 2 diabetes, and stroke (Figure 9-10), and potentially to hippocampal atrophy as well (discussed in Chapter 6 and shown in Figure 6-39B). Breathing can also change during a fear response, regulated in part by the connections between amygdala and the parabrachial nucleus in the brainstem (Figure 9-11). An adaptive response to fear is to accelerate respiratory rate when having a fight/flight reaction to enhance survival, but in excess this can lead to unwanted symptoms of shortness of breath, exacerbation of asthma, or a false sense of being smothered (Figure 9-11), all symptoms common during anxiety, and especially during attacks of anxiety such as panic attacks.

The autonomic nervous system is attuned to fear, and is able to trigger responses from the cardiovascular system such as increased pulse and blood pressure for fight/flight reactions and survival during real threats. These autonomic and cardiovascular responses are mediated by connections between the amygdala and the locus coeruleus, home of the noradrenergic cell bodies (Figure 9-12; noradrenergic neurons are discussed in Chapter 6, and noradrenergic pathways and neurons are illustrated in Figures 6-25 through 6-30, and also Figure 6-32). When autonomic responses are repetitive and inappropriately or chronically triggered as part of an anxiety disorder, this can lead to increases in atherosclerosis, cardiac ischemia, hypertension, myocardial infarction, and even sudden death (Figure 9-12). "Scared to death" may not always be an exaggeration or a figure of speech! Finally, anxiety can be triggered internally from traumatic memories stored in the hippocampus and activated by connections with the amygdala (Figure 9-13), especially in conditions such as posttraumatic stress disorder.

The processing of the fear response is regulated by the numerous neuronal connections flowing into and out of the amygdala. Each connection utilizes specific neurotransmitters acting at specific receptors (Figure 9-14). What is known about these connections is that not only are several neurotransmitters involved in the production of symptoms of anxiety at the level of the amygdala, but numerous anxiolytic drugs have actions upon these specific neurotransmitter

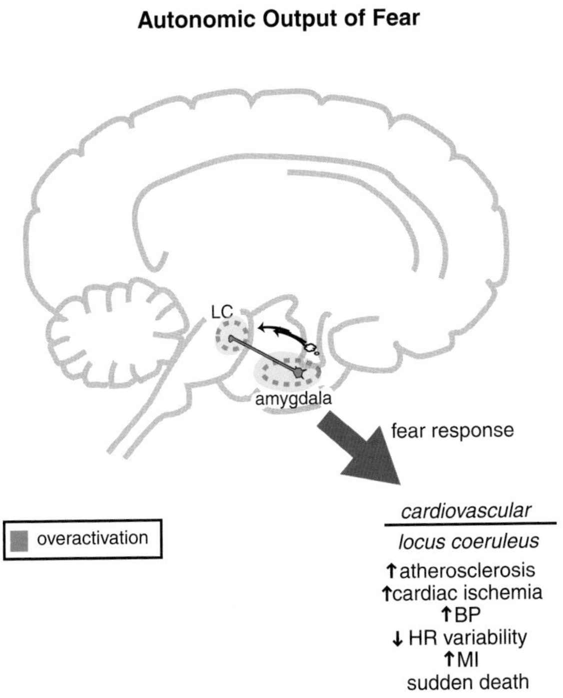

Autonomic Output of Fear

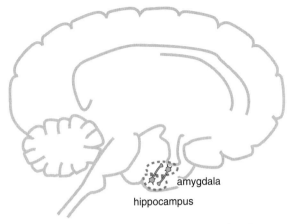

Figure 9-12. Autonomic output of fear. Autonomic responses are typically associated with feelings of fear. These include increases in heart rate (HR) and blood pressure (BP), which are regulated by reciprocal connections between the amygdala and the locus coeruleus (LC). Long-term activation of this circuit may lead to increased risk of atherosclerosis, cardiac ischemia, change in BP, decreased HR variability, myocardial infarction (MI), or even sudden death.

The Hippocampus: An Internal Fearmonger

Figure 9-13. The hippocampus and re-experiencing. Anxiety can be triggered not only by an external stimulus but also by an individual's memories. Traumatic memories stored in the hippocampus can activate the amygdala, causing the amygdala, in turn, to activate other brain regions and generate a fear response. This is termed re-experiencing, and it is a particular feature of posttraumatic stress disorder.

systems to relieve the symptoms of anxiety and fear (Figure 9-14). The neurobiological regulators of the amygdala, including the neurotransmitters GABA, 5HT, and NE, the voltage-gated calcium channels, and anxiolytics that act upon these neurotransmitters in order to mediate their therapeutic actions, are specifically discussed later in this chapter.

Cortico-striato-thalamo-cortical (CSTC) loops and the neurobiology of worry

Dopamine and born worried?

The second core symptom of anxiety disorders, worry, involves another unique circuit (Figure 9-15). Worry, which can include anxious misery, apprehensive expectations, catastrophic thinking, and obsessions, is linked to cortico-striato-thalamo-cortical (CSTC) feedback loops from the prefrontal cortex (Figures 9-15 and 9-16). Some experts theorize that similar CSTC feedback loops regulate the related symptoms of ruminations,

obsessions, and delusions, all of these symptoms being types of recurrent thoughts. Several neurotransmitters and regulators modulate these circuits, including serotonin, GABA, dopamine, norepinephrine, glutamate, and voltage-gated ion channels (Figure 9-15). These overlap greatly with many of the same neurotransmitters and regulators that modulate the amygdala (Figure 9-14). Since various genotypes for the enzyme COMT (catechol-O-methyl-transferase) regulate the availability of one of these neurotransmitters, namely dopamine, in the prefrontal cortex, differences in dopamine availability may impact the risk for worry and anxiety disorder and help to determine whether you are "born worried" and vulnerable to developing an anxiety disorder, particularly under stress (Figure 9-17).

Warriors versus worriers

In Chapter 4 the impact of genetic variants of COMT on cognitive functioning are mentioned in relation to schizophrenia. Specifically, normal controls with the Met variant of COMT have more efficient information processing in the dorsolateral prefrontal cortex (DLPFC) during a cognitive task such as the *n*-back test. These subjects have lower COMT activity, higher dopamine levels, and presumably better information processing during tasks of executive functioning that recruit circuits in the DLPFC. Because of

Associate Symptoms With Brain Regions, Circuits, and Neurotransmitters That Regulate Them

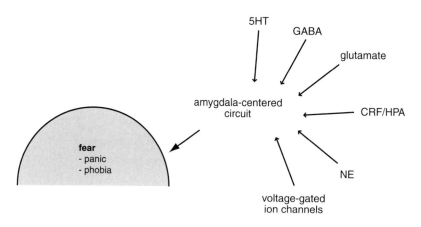

Figure 9-14. Linking anxiety symptoms to circuits to neurotransmitters. Symptoms of anxiety/fear are associated with malfunctioning of amygdala-centered circuits; the neurotransmitters that regulate these circuits include serotonin (5HT), γ-aminobutyric acid (GABA), glutamate, corticotropin-releasing factor (CRF), and norepinephrine (NE), among others. In addition, voltage-gated ion channels are involved in neurotransmission within these circuits.

Associate Symptoms With Brain Regions, Circuits, and Neurotransmitters That Regulate Them

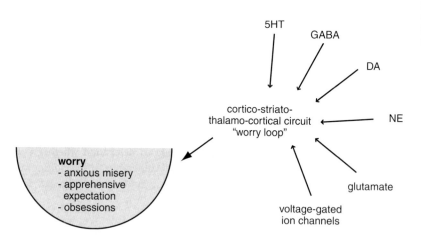

Figure 9-15. Linking worry symptoms to circuits to neurotransmitters. Symptoms of worry are associated with malfunctioning of cortico-striato-thalamo-cortical (CSTC) loops, which are regulated by serotonin (5HT), γ-aminobutyric acid (GABA), dopamine (DA), norepinephrine (NE), glutamate, and voltage-gated ion channels.

more efficient cognitive information processing, such subjects also have a lower risk for schizophrenia than subjects who are Val carriers of COMT (Figure 4-44).

At first glance, it would seem that all the biological advantages go to those with the Met variant of COMT. However, that is not necessarily true when it comes to processing stressors that cause dopamine release. With the Met genotype and its low COMT

activity and high dopamine levels, stressors can hypothetically produce too much dopamine activity, which actually decreases the efficiency of information processing under stress and creates the symptoms of anxiety and worry ("worriers"). Under stress, therefore, it appears that Val carriers of COMT with their higher enzyme activity and lower dopamine levels are hypothetically able to handle the increased dopamine

Worry/Obsessions

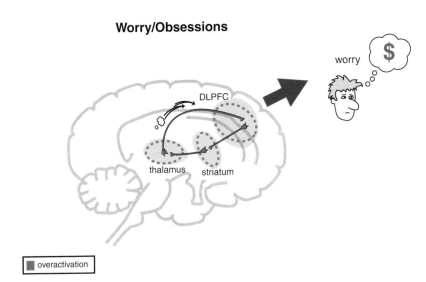

overactivation

Figure 9-16. Worry/obsessions circuit. Shown here is a cortico-striato-thalamo-cortical (CSTC) loop originating and ending in the dorsolateral prefrontal cortex (DLPFC). Overactivation of this circuit may lead to worry or obsessions.

release that comes with stress by optimizing their information processing; thus they are "warriors" who are not afraid or worried when stressed. Dopamine is just one of the potential regulators of worry circuits and CSTC loops.

GABA and benzodiazepines

GABA (γ-aminobutyric acid) is one of the key neurotransmitters involved in anxiety and in the anxiolytic action of many drugs used to treat the spectrum of anxiety disorders. GABA is the principal inhibitory neurotransmitter in the brain and normally plays an important regulatory role in reducing the activity of many neurons, including those in the amygdala and those in CSTC loops. Benzodiazepines, perhaps the best-known and most widely used anxiolytics, act by enhancing GABA actions at the level of the amygdala and at the level of the prefrontal cortex within CSTC loops to relieve anxiety. To understand how GABA regulates brain circuits in anxiety, and to understand how benzodiazepines exert their anxiolytic actions, it is important to understand the GABA neurotransmitter system, including how GABA is synthesized, how GABA action is terminated at the synapse, and the properties of GABA receptors (Figures 9-18 through 9-24).

Specifically, GABA is produced, or synthesized, from the amino acid glutamate (glutamic acid) via the actions of the enzyme glutamic acid decarboxylase, or GAD (Figure 9-18). Once formed in

presynaptic neurons, GABA is transported by vesicular inhibitory amino acid transporters (VIAATs) into synaptic vesicles, where GABA is stored until released into the synapse during inhibitory neurotransmission (Figure 9-18). GABA's synaptic actions are terminated by the presynaptic GABA transporter (GAT), also known as the GABA reuptake pump (Figure 9-19), analogous to similar transporters for other neurotransmitters discussed throughout this text. GABA action can also be terminated by the enzyme GABA transaminase (GABA-T), which converts GABA into an inactive substance (Figure 9-19).

There are three major types of GABA receptors and numerous subtypes. The major types are GABA$_A$, GABA$_B$, and GABA$_C$ receptors (Figure 9-20). GABA$_A$ and GABA$_C$ receptors are both ligand-gated ion channels and are part of a macromolecular complex that forms an inhibitory chloride channel (Figure 9-21). Various subtypes of GABA$_A$ receptors are targets of benzodiazepines, sedative hypnotics, barbiturates, and/or alcohol (Figure 9-21), and are involved with either tonic or phasic inhibitory neurotransmission at GABA synapses (Figure 9-22). The physiological role of GABA$_C$ receptors is not well clarified yet, but they do not appear to be targets of benzodiazepines. GABA$_B$ receptors, by contrast, are members of a different receptor class, namely, G-protein-linked receptors. GABA$_B$ receptors may be coupled to calcium and/or potassium channels, and may be involved in pain, memory, mood, and other CNS functions.

Born Worried? COMT Genetics and Life Stressors

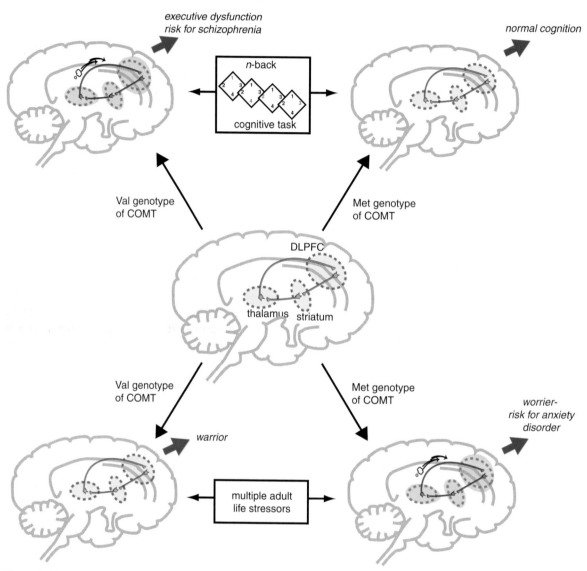

Figure 9-17. COMT genetics and life stressors. Activity in the cortico-striato-thalamo-cortical (CSTC) loop may vary during cognitive tasks depending on the variant of catechol-*O*-methyl-transferase (COMT) that an individual has (upper portion of figure). Thus, those with the Met genotype for COMT (i.e., those who have lower COMT activity and thus higher dopamine levels) may have "normal" activation and no problems with performance during a cognitive task, whereas those with the Val genotype may exhibit inefficiency of cognitive information processing, require overactivation of this circuit, and potentially make more errors during the same task. These latter individuals may also be at increased risk for schizophrenia. Similarly, the variant of COMT that an individual has may affect response to stress, since the CSTC loop also regulates worry. In this case, however, the beneficial genotype may be reversed. That is, because individuals with the Met genotype have lower COMT activity and thus higher dopamine levels, dopamine release in response to stress may be excessive and contribute to worry and risk for anxiety disorders. Those with the Val genotype, on the other hand, may be less reactive to stress because COMT can destroy the excess dopamine.

GABA is Produced

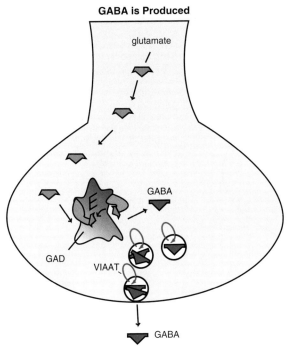

glutamate

GABA

GAD

VIAAT

GABA

GABA

Figure 9-18. Gamma-aminobutyric acid (GABA) is produced. The amino acid glutamate, a precursor to GABA, is converted to GABA by the enzyme glutamic acid decarboxylase (GAD). After synthesis, GABA is transported into synaptic vesicles via vesicular inhibitory amino acid transporters (VIAATs) and stored until its release into the synapse during neurotransmission.

GABA$_A$ receptor subtypes

GABA$_A$ receptors play a critical role in mediating inhibitory neurotransmission and as targets of the anxiolytic benzodiazepines. The molecular structure of GABA$_A$ receptors is shown in Figure 9-21. Each subunit of a GABA$_A$ receptor has four transmembrane regions (Figure 9-21A). When five subunits cluster together, they form an intact GABA$_A$ receptor with a chloride channel in the center (Figure 9-21B). There are many different subtypes of GABA$_A$ receptors, depending upon which subunits are present (Figure 9-21C). Subunits of GABA$_A$ receptors are sometimes also called isoforms, and include α (with six isoforms, α_1 to α_6), β (with three isoforms, β_1 to β_3), γ (with three isoforms, γ_1 to γ_3), δ, ϵ, π, θ, and ρ (with three isoforms, ρ_1 to ρ_3) (Figure 9-21C). What is important for this discussion is that, depending upon which subunits are present, the functions of a GABA$_A$ receptor can vary significantly.

Benzodiazepine-insensitive GABA$_A$ receptors

Benzodiazepine-insensitive GABA$_A$ receptors are those with α_4, α_6, γ_1, or δ subunits (Figure 9-21C). GABA$_A$ receptors with a δ subunit rather than a γ subunit, plus either α_4 or α_6 subunits, do not bind to

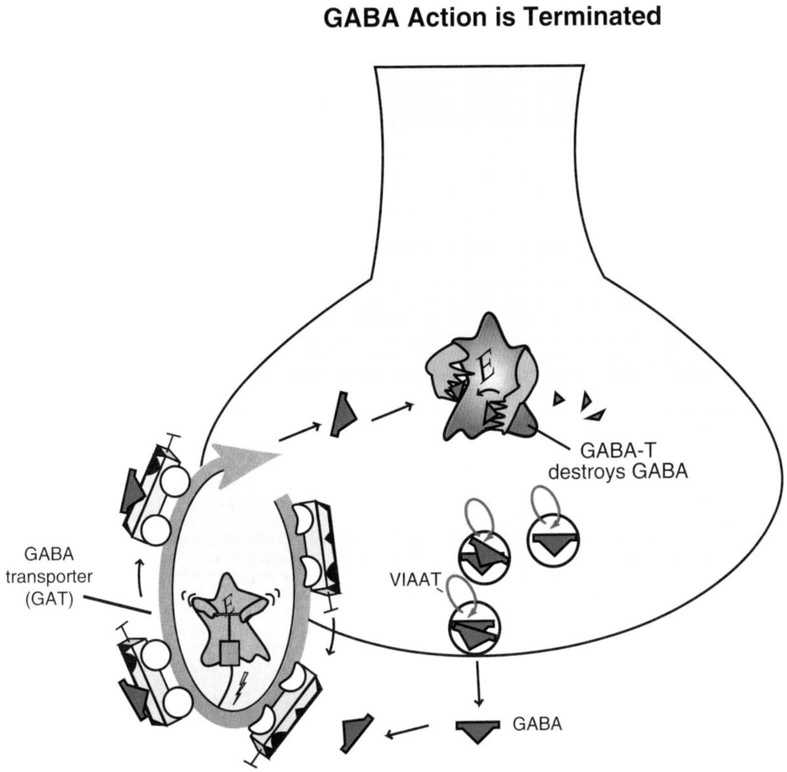

GABA Action is Terminated

GABA-T destroys GABA

GABA transporter (GAT)

VIAAT

GABA

GABA

Figure 9-19. Gamma-aminobutyric acid (GABA) action is terminated. GABA's action can be terminated through multiple mechanisms. GABA can be transported out of the synaptic cleft and back into the presynaptic neuron via the GABA transporter (GAT), where it may be repackaged for future use. Alternatively, once GABA has been transported back into the cell, it may be converted into an inactive substance via the enzyme GABA transaminase (GABA-T).

GABA Receptors

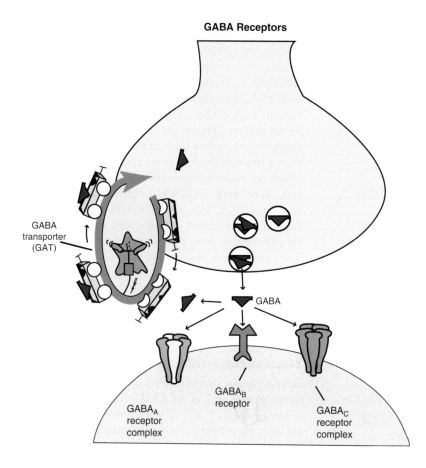

GABA transporter (GAT)

GABA

GABA$_A$ receptor complex

GABA$_B$ receptor

GABA$_C$ receptor complex

Figure 9-20. Gamma-aminobutyric acid (GABA) receptors. Shown here are receptors for GABA that regulate its neurotransmission. These include the GABA transporter (GAT) as well as three major types of postsynaptic GABA receptors: GABA$_A$, GABA$_B$, and GABA$_C$. GABA$_A$ and GABA$_C$ receptors are ligand-gated ion channels; they are part of a macromolecular complex that forms an inhibitory chloride channel. GABA$_B$ receptors are G-protein-linked receptors that may be coupled with calcium or potassium channels.

benzodiazepines. Such GABA$_A$ receptors do bind to other modulators, namely the naturally occurring neurosteroids, as well as to alcohol and to some general anesthetics (Figure 9-21C). The binding site for these non-benzodiazepine modulators is located between the α and the δ subunits, one site per receptor complex (Figure 9-21C). Two molecules of GABA bind per receptor complex, at sites located between the α and the β subunits, sometimes referred to as the GABA agonist site (Figure 9-21C). Since the site for the modulators is in a different location from the agonist sites for GABA, the modulatory site is often called *allosteric* (literally, "other site"), and the agents that bind there are called *allosteric modulators*.

Benzodiazepine-insensitive GABA$_A$ receptor subtypes (with δ subunits and α$_4$ or α$_6$ subunits) are located extrasynaptically, where they capture not only GABA that diffuses away from the synapse, but also neurosteroids synthesized and released by glia (Figure 9-22). Extrasynaptic, benzodiazepine-insensitive GABA$_A$ receptors are thought to mediate a type of inhibition at

the postsynaptic neuron that is *tonic*, in contrast to the *phasic* type of inhibition mediated by postsynaptic benzodiazepine-sensitive GABA$_A$ receptors (Figure 9-22). Thus, tonic inhibition may be regulated by the ambient levels of extracellular GABA molecules that have escaped presynaptic reuptake and enzymatic destruction. Tonic inhibition is thought to set the overall tone and excitability of the postsynaptic neuron, and to be important for certain regulatory events such as the frequency of neuronal discharge in response to excitatory inputs.

Since the GABA$_A$ receptors that modulate this action are not sensitive to benzodiazepines, they are not likely to be involved in the anxiolytic actions of benzodiazepines in various anxiety disorders. However, novel hypnotics as well as anesthetics have targeted these extrasynaptic benzodiazepine-insensitive GABA$_A$ receptors, and it is possible that novel synthetic neurosteroids that also target benzodiazepine-insensitive GABA$_A$ receptor subtypes could some day become novel anxiolytics. Indeed, anxiety itself may in part be dependent upon having the right amount of tonic

Structure of GABA_A Receptors

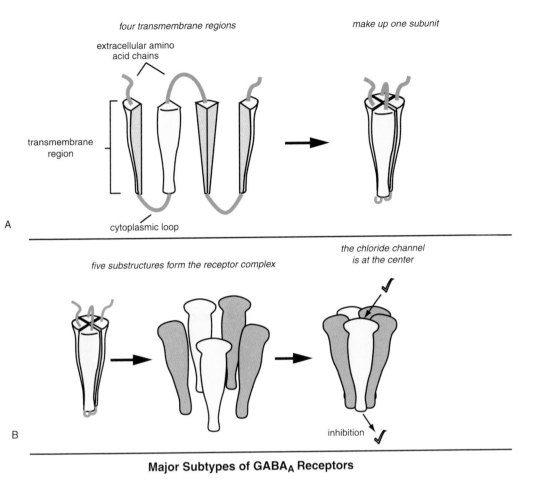

four transmembrane regions *make up one subunit*

extracellular amino acid chains

transmembrane region

cytoplasmic loop

A

five substructures form the receptor complex

the chloride channel is at the center

inhibition

B

Major Subtypes of GABA_A Receptors

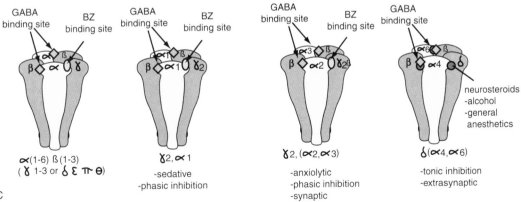

GABA binding site   BZ binding site

$\alpha(1\text{-}6)\ \beta(1\text{-}3)$
$(\gamma 1\text{-}3$ or $\delta\ \epsilon\ \pi\ \theta)$

GABA binding site   BZ binding site

$\gamma 2, \alpha 1$
-sedative
-phasic inhibition

GABA binding site   BZ binding site

$\gamma 2, (\alpha 2, \alpha 3)$
-anxiolytic
-phasic inhibition
-synaptic

GABA binding site

neurosteroids
-alcohol
-general anesthetics

$\delta(\alpha 4, \alpha 6)$
-tonic inhibition
-extrasynaptic

C

Figure 9-21. Gamma-aminobutyric acid-A (GABA_A) receptors. (A) Shown here are the four transmembrane regions that make up one subunit of a GABA_A receptor. (B) There are five copies of these subunits in a fully constituted GABA_A receptor, at the center of which is a chloride channel. (C) Different types of subunits (also called isoforms or subtypes) can combine to form a GABA_A receptor. These include six different alpha (α) isoforms, three different beta (β) isoforms, three different gamma (γ) isoforms, delta (δ), epsilon (ε), pi (π), theta (θ), and three different rho (ρ) isoforms. The ultimate type and function of each GABA_A receptor subtype will depend on which subunits it contains. Benzodiazepine-sensitive GABA_A receptors (middle two) contain γ and α_{1-3} subunits and mediate phasic inhibition triggered by peak concentrations of synaptically released GABA. Benzodiazepine-sensitive GABA_A receptors containing α_1 subunits are involved in sleep (second from left), while those that contain α_2 and/or α_3 subunits are involved in anxiety (second from right). GABA_A receptors containing α_4, α_6, γ_1, or δ subunits (far right) are benzodiazepine-insensitive, are located extrasynaptically, and regulate tonic inhibition.

Two Types of GABA$_A$ Mediated Inhibition

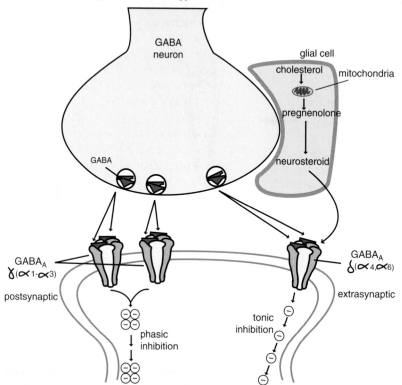

Figure 9-22. GABA$_A$ mediation of tonic and phasic inhibition. Benzodiazepine-sensitive GABA$_A$ receptors (those that contain γ and α$_{1-3}$ subunits) are postsynaptic receptors that mediate phasic inhibition, which occurs in bursts triggered by peak concentrations of synaptically released GABA. Benzodiazepine-insensitive GABA$_A$ receptors (those containing α$_4$, α$_6$, γ$_1$, or δ subunits) are extrasynaptic and capture GABA that diffuses away from the synapse as well as neurosteroids that are synthesized and released by glia. These receptors mediate inhibition that is tonic (i.e., mediated by ambient levels of extracellular GABA that has escaped from the synapse).

inhibition in key anatomic areas such as the amygdala and cortical areas of CSTC loops. Furthermore, naturally occurring neurosteroids may be important in setting that inhibitory tone in critical brain areas. If this tone becomes dysregulated, it is possible that abnormal neuronal excitability could become a factor in the development of various anxiety disorders.

Benzodiazepine-sensitive GABA$_A$ receptors

Benzodiazepine-sensitive GABA$_A$ receptors have several structural and functional features that make them distinct from benzodiazepine-insensitive GABA$_A$ receptors. In contrast to benzodiazepine-insensitive GABA$_A$ receptors, for a GABA$_A$ receptor to be sensitive to benzodiazepines, and thus to be a target for benzodiazepine anxiolytics, there must be two β units plus a γ unit of either the γ$_2$ or γ$_3$ subtype, plus two α units of the α$_1$, α$_2$, or α$_3$ subtype (Figure 9-21C). Benzodiazepines appear to bind to the region of the receptor between the γ$_{2/3}$ subunit and the α$_{1/2/3}$ subunit, one benzodiazepine molecule per receptor complex (Figure 9-21C). GABA itself binds with two molecules of GABA per receptor complex to the

GABA agonist sites in the regions of the receptor between the α and the β units (Figure 9-21C).

Benzodiazepine-sensitive GABA$_A$ receptor subtypes (with γ subunits and α$_{1-3}$ subunits) are thought to be postsynaptic in location and to mediate a type of inhibition at the postsynaptic neuron that is phasic, occurring in bursts of inhibition that are triggered by peak concentrations of synaptically released GABA (Figure 9-22). Theoretically, benzodiazepines acting at these receptors, particularly the α$_{2/3}$ subtypes clustered at postsynaptic GABA sites, should exert an anxiolytic effect due to enhancement of phasic postsynaptic inhibition. If this action occurs at overly active output neurons in the amygdala or in CSTC loops, it would theoretically cause anxiolytic actions with reduction of both fear and worry.

Not all benzodiazepine-sensitive GABA$_A$ receptors are the same. Notably, those benzodiazepine-sensitive GABA$_A$ receptors with α$_1$ subunits may be most important for regulating sleep and are the presumed targets of numerous sedative-hypnotic agents, including both benzodiazepine and non-benzodiazepine positive allosteric modulators of the GABA$_A$ receptor

(Figure 9-21C). The α_1 subtype of GABA$_A$ receptors and the drugs that bind to it are discussed further in Chapter 11 on sleep. Some of these agents are selective for only the α_1 subtype of GABA$_A$ receptor.

On the other hand, benzodiazepine-sensitive GABA$_A$ receptors with α_2 (and/or α_3) subunits may be most important for regulating anxiety and are the presumed targets of the anxiolytic benzodiazepines (Figure 9-21C). However, currently available benzodiazepines are nonselective for GABA$_A$ receptors with different α subunits. Thus, there is an ongoing search for selective $\alpha_{2/3}$ agents that could be utilized to treat anxiety disorders in humans. Such agents would theoretically be anxiolytic without being sedating. Partial agonists selective for $\alpha_{2/3}$ subunits of benzodiazepine-sensitive GABA$_A$ receptors hypothetically would cause less euphoria, be less reinforcing and thus less abusable, cause less dependence, and cause fewer problems in withdrawal. Such agents are being investigated but have not yet been introduced into clinical practice. Abnormally expressed γ_2, α_2, or δ subunits have all been associated with different types of epilepsy. Receptor subtype expression can change in response to chronic benzodiazepine administration and withdrawal, and could theoretically be altered in patients with various anxiety-disorder subtypes.

Benzodiazepines as positive allosteric modulators or PAMs

Since the benzodiazepine-sensitive GABA$_A$ receptor complex is regulated not only by GABA itself, but also by benzodiazepines at a highly specific allosteric modulatory binding site (Figure 9-23), this has led to the notion that there may be an "endogenous" or naturally occurring benzodiazepine synthesized in the brain (the brain's own Xanax!). However, the identity of any such substance remains elusive. Furthermore, it is now known that synthetic drugs that do not have a benzodiazepine structure also bind to the "benzodiazepine receptor." These developments have led to endless confusion with terminology, since non-benzodiazepines also bind to the "benzodiazepine receptor!" Thus, many experts now call the "benzodiazepine site" the GABA$_A$ *allosteric modulatory site* and anything that binds to this site, including benzodiazepines, *allosteric modulators*.

Acting alone, GABA can increase the frequency of opening of the chloride channel, but only to a limited extent (compare Figure 9-23A and B). The combination of GABA with benzodiazepines is thought to

increase the frequency of opening of inhibitory chloride channels but not to increase the conductance of chloride across individual chloride channels, nor to increase the duration of channel opening. The end result is more inhibition. More inhibition supposedly yields more anxiolytic action. How does this happen? The answer is that benzodiazepines act as agonists at the allosteric modulatory site of GABA binding. They are positive allosteric modulators, or PAMs, but have no activity on their own. Thus, when benzodiazepines bind to the allosteric modulatory site, they have no activity when GABA is not simultaneously binding to its agonist sites (compare Figure 9-23A and C).

So, how do benzodiazepines act as PAMs? This can occur only when GABA is binding to its agonist sites. The combination of benzodiazepines at the allosteric site plus GABA at its agonist sites increases the frequency of opening of the chloride channel to an extent not possible with GABA alone (compare Figure 9-23B and D).

The actions of benzodiazepines essentially as agonists at their positive allosteric sites can be reversed by the neutral antagonist flumazenil (Figure 9-24). Flumazenil is a short-acting intravenously administered antagonist to benzodiazepines that can reverse overdoses or anesthesia from benzodiazepines but can also induce seizures or withdrawal in patients dependent upon benzodiazepines.

Benzodiazepines as anxiolytics

A simplified notion of how benzodiazepine anxiolytics might modulate excessive output from the amygdala during fear responses in anxiety disorders is shown in Figure 9-25. Excessive amygdala activity (shown in Figures 9-8 through 9-12 and in Figure 9-25A) is theoretically reduced by enhancing the phasic inhibitory actions of benzodiazepine PAMs at postsynaptic GABA$_A$ receptors within the amygdala to blunt fear-associated outputs, hypothetically reducing the symptom of fear (Figure 9-25B). Benzodiazepines also theoretically modulate excessive output from worry loops (Figure 9-26A) by enhancing the actions of inhibitory interneurons in CSTC circuits (Figure 9-26B), hypothetically reducing the symptom of worry.

Alpha-2-delta ligands as anxiolytics

We have discussed voltage-sensitive calcium channels (VSCCs) in Chapter 3 and have illustrated presynaptic N and P/Q subtypes of VSCCs and

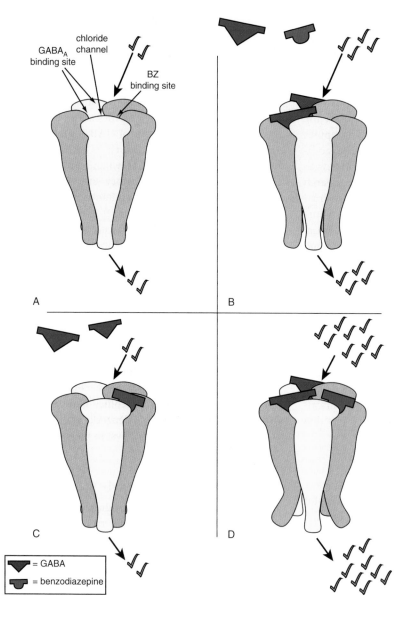

chloride
channel

GABA_A
binding site

BZ
binding site

A

B

C

D

= GABA

= benzodiazepine

Figure 9-23. Positive allosteric modulation of GABA_A receptors. (A) Benzodiazepine-sensitive GABA_A receptors, like the one shown here, consist of five subunits with a central chloride channel and have binding sites not only for GABA but also for positive allosteric modulators (e.g., benzodiazepines). (B) When GABA binds to its sites on the GABA_A receptor, it increases the frequency of opening of the chloride channel and thus allows more chloride to pass through. (C) When a positive allosteric modulator such as a benzodiazepine binds to the GABA_A receptor in the absence of GABA, it has no effect on the chloride channel. (D) When a positive allosteric modulator such as a benzodiazepine binds to the GABA_A receptor in the presence of GABA, it causes the channel to open even more frequently than when GABA alone is present.

their role in excitatory neurotransmitter release (see Figures 3-19 and 3-22 through 3-24). Gabapentin and pregabalin, also known as $\alpha_2\delta$ ligands, since they bind to the $\alpha_2\delta$ subunit of presynaptic N and P/Q VSCCs, block the release of excitatory neurotransmitters such as glutamate when neurotransmission is excessive, as postulated in the amygdala to cause fear (Figure 9-25A) and in CSTC circuits to cause worry (Figure 9-26A). Hypothetically, $\alpha_2\delta$ ligands bind to open, overly active VSCCs in the amygdala (Figure 9-25C) to reduce fear, and in CSTC circuits

(Figure 9-26C) to reduce worry. The $\alpha_2\delta$ ligands pregabalin and gabapentin have demonstrated anxiolytic actions in social anxiety disorder and panic disorder, and are also proven to be effective for the treatment of epilepsy and certain pain conditions, including neuropathic pain and fibromyalgia. The actions of $\alpha_2\delta$ ligands on VSCCs are discussed in Chapter 10 on pain and illustrated in Figures 10-17 through 10-19. $\alpha_2\delta$ ligands clearly have different mechanisms of action compared to serotonin reuptake inhibitors or benzodiazepines, and thus can be

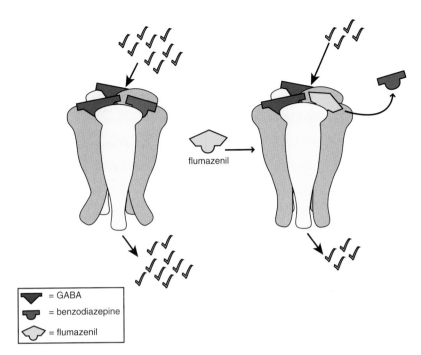

Figure 9-24. Flumazenil. The benzodiazepine receptor antagonist flumazenil is able to reverse a full agonist benzodiazepine acting at its site on the GABA$_A$ receptor. This may be helpful in reversing the sedative effects of full agonist benzodiazepines when administered for anesthetic purposes or when taken in overdose by a patient.

= GABA

= benzodiazepine

= flumazenil

useful for patients who do not do well on SSRIs/SNRIs or benzodiazepines. Also, $\alpha_2\delta$ ligands can be useful to combine with SSRIs/SNRIs or benzodiazepines in patients who are partial responders and are not in remission.

Serotonin and anxiety

Since the symptoms, circuits, and neurotransmitters linked to anxiety disorders overlap extensively with those for major depressive disorder (Figure 9-1), it is not surprising that drugs developed as antidepressants have proven to be effective treatments for anxiety disorders. Indeed, the leading treatments for anxiety disorders today are increasingly drugs originally developed as antidepressants. Serotonin is a key neurotransmitter that innervates the amygdala as well as all the elements of CSTC circuits, namely, prefrontal cortex, striatum, and thalamus, and thus is poised to regulate both fear and worry (serotonin pathways are discussed in Chapters 5 and 6 and illustrated in Figure 6-33). Antidepressants that can increase serotonin output by blocking the serotonin transporter (SERT) are also effective in reducing symptoms of anxiety and fear in every one of the anxiety disorders illustrated in Figures 9-2 through 9-5 – namely, GAD, panic disorder, social anxiety disorder, and PTSD. Such

agents include the well-known SSRIs (selective serotonin reuptake inhibitors; discussed in Chapter 7 and their mechanism of action illustrated in Figures 7-12 through 7-17), as well as the SNRIs (serotonin–norepinephrine reuptake inhibitors; also discussed in Chapter 7 and their mechanism of action illustrated in Figures 7-12 through 7-17 plus Figures 7-33 and 7-34).

A serotonin 1A (5HT$_{1A}$) partial agonist, buspirone, is recognized as a generalized anxiolytic, but not as a treatment for anxiety disorder subtypes. 5HT$_{1A}$ partial agonists as augmenting agents to antidepressants are discussed in Chapter 7, as are antidepressants combining 5HT$_{1A}$ partial agonism with serotonin reuptake inhibition (i.e., SPARIs and vilazodone: see Figures 7-25 through 7-29), which should theoretically be anxiolytic as well as antidepressant in action. The 5HT$_{1A}$ partial agonist properties of numerous atypical antipsychotics are discussed in Chapter 5 and illustrated in Figures 5-15, 5-16, 5-25, and 5-26.

The potential anxiolytic actions of buspirone could theoretically be due to 5HT$_{1A}$ partial agonist actions at both presynaptic and postsynaptic 5HT$_{1A}$ receptors (Figure 9-27 and Figures 5-15, 5-16, 5-25, 7-25 through 7-29), with actions at both sites resulting in enhanced serotonergic activity in projections to the amygdala (Figure 9-25D), prefrontal cortex, striatum, and thalamus (Figure 9-26D). SSRIs

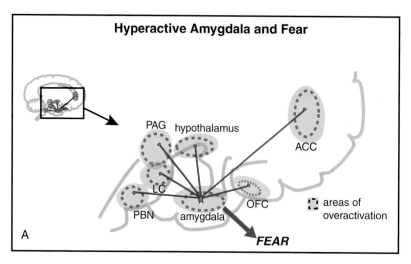

Hyperactive Amygdala and Fear

PAG hypothalamus

ACC

LC

PBN OFC

amygdala

□ areas of overactivation

FEAR

A

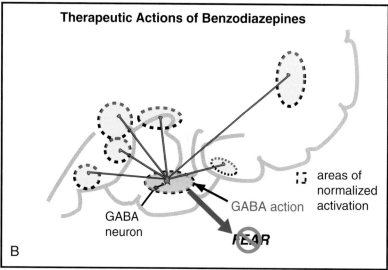

Therapeutic Actions of Benzodiazepines

□ areas of normalized activation

GABA action

GABA neuron

FEAR

B

Figure 9-25. Potential therapeutic actions of anxiolytics on anxiety/fear. (A) Pathological anxiety/fear may be caused by overactivation of amygdala circuits. (B) GABAergic agents such as benzodiazepines may alleviate anxiety/fear by enhancing phasic inhibitory actions at postsynaptic GABA_A receptors within the amygdala. (C) Agents that bind to the $\alpha_2\delta$ subunit of presynaptic N and P/Q voltage-sensitive calcium channels can block the excessive release of glutamate in the amygdala and thereby reduce the symptoms of anxiety. (D) The amygdala receives input from serotonergic neurons, which can have an inhibitory effect on some of its outputs. Thus, serotonergic agents may alleviate anxiety/fear by enhancing serotonin input to the amygdala.

and SNRIs theoretically do the same thing (Figures 9-25D and 9-26D). Since the onset of anxiolytic action for buspirone is delayed, just as it is for antidepressants, this has led to the belief that $5HT_{1A}$ agonists exert their therapeutic effects by virtue of adaptive neuronal events and receptor events (Figures 7-12 through 7-17 and 7-25 through 7-29), rather than simply by the acute occupancy of $5HT_{1A}$ receptors. In this way, the presumed mechanism of action of $5HT_{1A}$ partial agonists is analogous to the antidepressants – which are also presumed to act by adaptations in neurotransmitter receptors – and different from the benzodiazepine anxiolytics – which act relatively acutely by occupying benzodiazepine receptors.

Noradrenergic hyperactivity in anxiety

Norepinephrine is another neurotransmitter with important regulatory input to the amygdala (Figure 9-28) and to the prefrontal cortex and thalamus in CSTC circuits (Figure 9-29). Excessive noradrenergic output from the locus coeruleus can not only result in numerous peripheral manifestations of autonomic overdrive, as discussed above and illustrated in Figures 9-8 through 9-12, but can also trigger numerous central symptoms of anxiety and fear, such as nightmares, hyperarousal states, flashbacks, and panic attacks (Figure 9-28A). Excessive noradrenergic activity can also reduce the

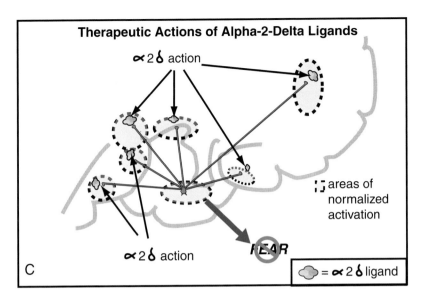

Therapeutic Actions of Alpha-2-Delta Ligands

∝2δ action

∝2δ action

FEAR

⊏⊐ areas of
normalized
activation

⊂⊃ = ∝2δ ligand

C

Figure 9-25. *(cont.)*

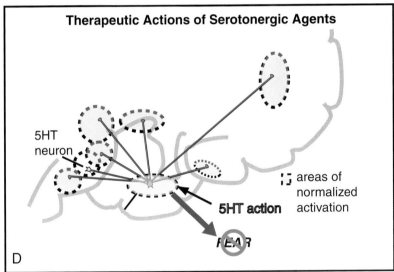

Therapeutic Actions of Serotonergic Agents

5HT
neuron

5HT action

FEAR

⊏⊐ areas of
normalized
activation

D

efficiency of information processing in the prefrontal cortex and thus in CSTC circuits and theoretically cause worry (Figure 9-29A). Hypothetically, these symptoms may be mediated in part by excessive noradrenergic input onto α_1- and β_1-adrenergic postsynaptic receptors in the amygdala (Figure 9-28A) or prefrontal cortex (Figure 9-29A). Symptoms of hyperarousal such as nightmares can be reduced in some patients with α_1-adrenergic blockers such as prazocin (Figure 9-28B); symptoms of fear (Figure 9-28C) and worry (Figure 9-29B) can be reduced by norepinephrine reuptake inhibitors (also called

NET or norepinephrine transporter inhibitors). The clinical effects of NET inhibitors can be confusing, because symptoms of anxiety can be made transiently worse immediately following initiation of an SNRI or selective NET inhibitor, when noradrenergic activity is initially increased but the postsynaptic receptors have not yet adapted. However, these same NET inhibitory actions, if sustained over time, will downregulate and desensitize postsynaptic NE receptors such as β_1 receptors, and actually reduce symptoms of fear and worry long term (Figure 9-29B).

Hyperactive CSTC Circuits and Worry

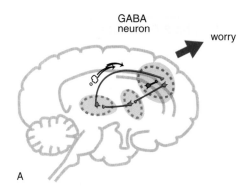

A

Therapeutic Actions of Benzodiazepines

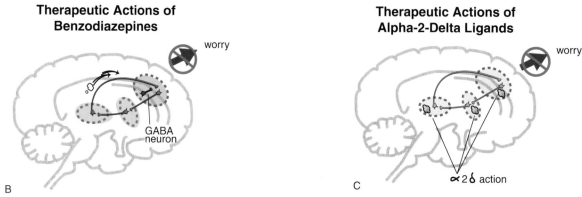

B

Therapeutic Actions of Alpha-2-Delta Ligands

C

Therapeutic Actions of Serotonergic Agents

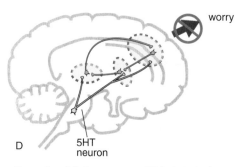

D

Figure 9-26. Potential therapeutic actions of anxiolytics on worry. (A) Pathological worry may be caused by overactivation of cortico-striato-thalamo-cortical (CSTC) circuits. (B) GABAergic agents such as benzodiazepines may alleviate worry by enhancing the actions of inhibitory GABA interneurons within the prefrontal cortex. (C) Agents that bind to the $\alpha_2\delta$ subunit of presynaptic N and P/Q voltage-sensitive calcium channels can block the excessive release of glutamate in CSTC circuits and thereby reduce the symptoms of worry. (D) The prefrontal cortex, striatum, and thalamus receive input from serotonergic neurons, which can have an inhibitory effect on output. Thus, serotonergic agents may alleviate worry by enhancing serotonin input within CSTC circuits.

Fear conditioning versus fear extinction
Fear conditioning

Fear conditioning is a concept as old as Pavlov's dogs. If an aversive stimulus such as footshock is coupled with a neutral stimulus such as a bell, the animal learns to associate the two and will develop fear when it hears a bell. In humans, fear is learned during stressful experiences associated with emotional trauma and is influenced by an individual's genetic predisposition as well as by an individual's prior exposure to environmental stressors that can cause

5HT1A Partial Agonist (SPA) Actions in Anxiety

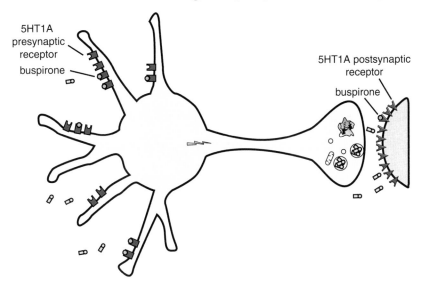

5HT1A
presynaptic
receptor

buspirone

5HT1A postsynaptic
receptor

buspirone

Figure 9-27. 5HT$_{1A}$ partial agonist actions in anxiety. 5HT$_{1A}$ partial agonists such as buspirone may reduce anxiety by actions both at presynaptic somatodendritic autoreceptors (left) and at postsynaptic receptors (right). The onset of action of buspirone, like that of antidepressants, is delayed, suggesting that the therapeutic effects are actually related to downstream adaptive changes rather than acute actions at these receptors.

stress sensitization of brain circuits (e.g., child abuse: see Chapter 6 and Figures 6-40 through 6-43). Often, fearful situations are managed successfully and then forgotten. Some fears are crucial for survival, such as appropriately fearing dangerous situations, and thus the mechanism of learned fear, called fear conditioning, has been extremely well conserved across species, including humans. However, other fears that are "learned" and not "forgotten" may hypothetically progress to anxiety disorders or a major depressive episode. This is a big problem, since almost 30% of the population will develop an anxiety disorder, due in large part to stressful environments, including exposure to fearful events during normal activities in twenty-first-century society, but in particular during war and natural disasters. Hearing an explosion, smelling burning rubber, seeing a picture of a wounded civilian, and seeing or hearing flood waters are all sensory experiences than can trigger traumatic re-experiencing and generalized hyperarousal and fear in PTSD. Panic associated with social situations will "teach" the patient to panic in social situations in social anxiety disorder. Panic randomly associated with an attack that happens to occur in a crowd, on a bridge, or in a shopping center will also trigger another panic attack when the same environment is encountered in panic disorder. These and other symptoms of anxiety disorders are all forms of learning known as fear conditioning (Figure 9-30).

The amygdala is involved in "remembering" the various stimuli associated with a given fearful situation. It does this by increasing the efficiency of neurotransmission at glutamatergic synapses in the lateral amygdala as sensory input about those stimuli comes in from the thalamus or sensory cortex (Figure 9-30). This input is then relayed to the central amygdala, where fear conditioning also improves the efficiency of neurotransmission at another glutamate synapse there (Figure 9-30). Both synapses are restructured and permanent learning is embedded into this circuit by NMDA receptors triggering long-term potentiation and synaptic plasticity, so that subsequent input from the sensory cortex and thalamus is very efficiently processed to trigger the fear response as output from the central amygdala every time there is sensory input associated with the original fearful event (Figure 9-30; see also Figures 9-8 through 9-13).

Input to the lateral amygdala is modulated by the prefrontal cortex, especially the ventromedial prefrontal cortex (VMPFC), and by the hippocampus. If the VMPFC is unable to suppress the fear response at the level of the amygdala, fear conditioning proceeds. The hippocampus remembers the context of the fear conditioning and makes sure fear is triggered when the fearful stimulus and all its associated stimuli are encountered. Most contemporary psychopharmacological treatments for anxiety and fear act by suppressing

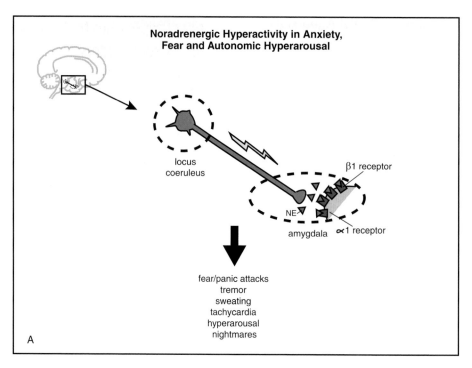

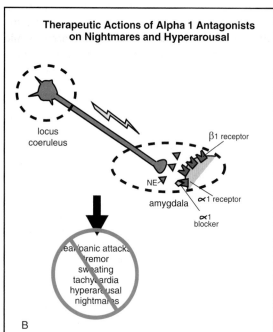

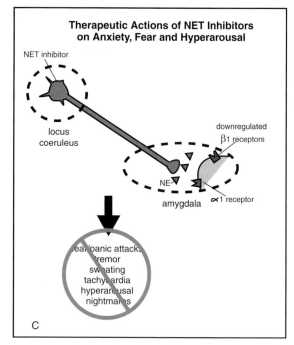

Figure 9-28. Noradrenergic hyperactivity in anxiety/fear. (A) Norepinephrine provides input not only to the amygdala but also to many regions to which the amygdala projects; thus it plays an important role in the fear response. Noradrenergic hyperactivation can lead to anxiety, panic attacks, tremors, sweating, tachycardia, hyperarousal, and nightmares. α_1- and β_1-adrenergic receptors may be specifically involved in these reactions. (B) Noradrenergic hyperactivity may be blocked by the administration of α_1-adrenergic blockers, which can lead to the alleviation of anxiety and other stress-related symptoms. (C) Noradrenergic hyperactivity may also be blocked by the administration of a norepinephrine transporter (NET) inhibitor, which can have the downstream effect of downregulating β_1-adrenergic receptors. Reduced stimulation via β_1-adrenergic receptors could therefore lead to the alleviation of anxiety and stress-related symptoms.

Hyperactive CSTC Circuits and Worry

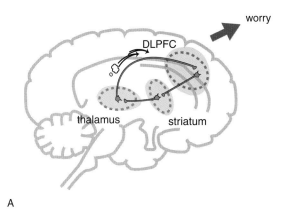

A

Delayed Therapeutic Actions of NET Inhibitors

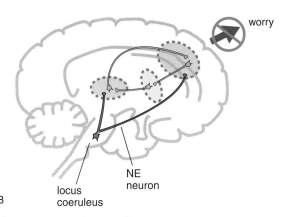

B

Figure 9-29. Noradrenergic hyperactivity in worry.
(A) Pathological worry may be caused by overactivation of cortico-striato-thalamo-cortical (CSTC) circuits. Specifically, excessive noradrenergic activity within these circuits can reduce the efficiency of information processing and theoretically cause worry.
(B) Noradrenergic hyperactivity in CSTC circuits may be blocked by the administration of a norepinephrine transporter (NET) inhibitor, which can have the downstream effect of downregulating β_1-adrenergic receptors. Reduced stimulation via β_1-adrenergic receptors could therefore lead to the alleviation of worry.

the fear output from the amygdala (Figures 9-25 and 9-28) and therefore are not cures, since the fundamental neuronal learning underlying fear conditioning in these patients remains in place.

Novel approaches to the treatment of anxiety disorders

Once fear conditioning is in place, it can be very difficult to reverse. Nevertheless, there may be two ways to neutralize fear conditioning: either by facilitating a process called *extinction* or by blocking a process called *reconsolidation*.

Fear extinction

Fear extinction is the progressive reduction of the response to a feared stimulus, and occurs when the stimulus is repeatedly presented without any adverse consequence. When fear extinction occurs, it appears that the original fear conditioning is not really "forgotten" even though the fear response can be profoundly reduced over time by the active process of fear extinction. Rather than reversing the synaptic changes described above for fear conditioning, it appears that a new form of learning with additional synaptic changes in the amygdala occurs during fear extinction. These changes can suppress symptoms of anxiety and fear by inhibiting the original learning but not by removing it (Figure 9-30). Specifically, activation of the amygdala by the VMPFC occurs while the hippocampus "remembers" the context in which the feared stimulus did not have any adverse consequences and fear is no longer activated (Figure 9-30). Fear extinction hypothetically occurs when inputs from the VMPFC and hippocampus activate glutamatergic neurons in the lateral amygdala that synapse upon an inhibitory GABAergic interneuron located within the intercalated cell mass of the amygdala (Figure 9-30). This sets up a gate within the central amygdala, with fear output occurring if the fear conditioning circuit predominates, and no fear output occurring if the fear extinction circuit predominates.

Fear extinction theoretically predominates over fear conditioning when synaptic strengthening and long-term potentiation in the new circuit are able to produce inhibitory GABAergic drive that can overcome the excitatory glutamatergic drive produced by the pre-existing fear conditioning circuitry (Figure 9-30). When fear extinction exists simultaneously with fear conditioning, memory for both are present, but the output depends upon which system is "stronger," better remembered," and has the most robust synaptic efficiency. These factors will determine which gate will open, the one with the fear response or the one that keeps the fear response in check. Unfortunately, over

Fear Conditioning vs. Fear Extinction

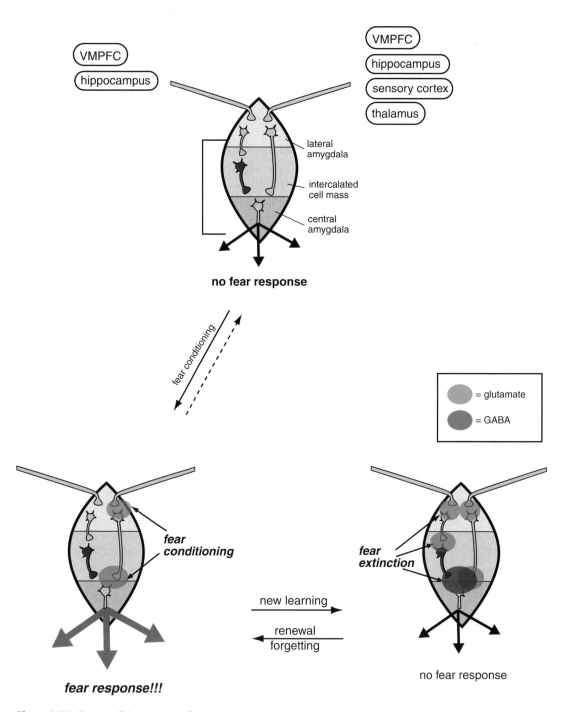

Figure 9-30. Fear conditioning versus fear extinction. When an individual encounters a stressful or fearful experience, the sensory input is relayed to the amygdala, where it is integrated with input from the ventromedial prefrontal cortex (VMPFC) and hippocampus, so that a fear response can be either generated or suppressed. The amygdala may "remember" stimuli associated with that experience by increasing the efficiency of glutamate neurotransmission, so that on future exposure to stimuli, a fear response is more efficiently triggered. If this is not countered by input from the VMPFC to suppress the fear response, fear conditioning proceeds. Fear conditioning is not readily reversed, but it can be inhibited through new learning. This new learning is termed fear extinction and is the progressive reduction of the response to a feared stimulus that is repeatedly presented without adverse consequences. Thus the VMPFC and hippocampus learn a new context for the feared stimulus and send input to the amygdala to suppress the fear response. The "memory" of the conditioned fear is still present, however.

time, fear conditioning may have the upper hand over fear extinction. Fear extinction appears to be more labile than fear conditioning, and tends to reverse over time. Also, fear conditioning can return if the old fear is presented in a context different than the one "learned" to suppress the fear during fear extinction, a process termed *renewal*.

Novel treatment approaches to anxiety disorders seek to facilitate fear extinction rather than just suppress the fear response triggered by fear conditioning, which is how current anxiolytic drugs work (Figures 9-25 through 9-30). Among currently effective treatments for anxiety, cognitive behavioral therapies that use exposure techniques and that require the patient to confront the fear-inducing stimuli in a safe environment may come closest to facilitating fear extinction, hypothetically because when these therapies are effective, they are able to trigger the learning of fear extinction in the amygdala (Figure 9-30). Unfortunately, because the hippocampus "remembers" the context of this extinction, such therapies are often context-specific and do not always generalize once the patient is outside the safe therapeutic environment; thus fear and worry may be "renewed" in the

real world. Current psychotherapy research is investigating how contextual cues can be used to strengthen extinction learning so that the therapeutic learning generalizes to other environments. Current psychopharmacology research is investigating how specific drugs might also strengthen extinction learning by pharmacologically strengthening the synapses on the fear-extinction side of the amygdala gate disproportionately to the synapses on the fear-conditioned side of the amygdala gate. How could this be done?

Based on successful animal experiments of extinction learning, one idea, shown in Figure 9-31, is to boost NMDA receptor activation at the very time when a patient receives systematic exposure to feared stimuli during cognitive behavioral therapy sessions. This can be done either with direct-acting agonists such as D-cycloserine or with indirect glycine-enhancing agents such as selective glycine reuptake inhibitors (SGRIs). This approach to boosting activity at NMDA synapses is discussed in Chapter 5 in relation to schizophrenia and is illustrated in Figure 5-90. As applied to novel anxiolytic therapy, the idea is that as therapy progresses, learning occurs, because glutamate release is provoked in the lateral

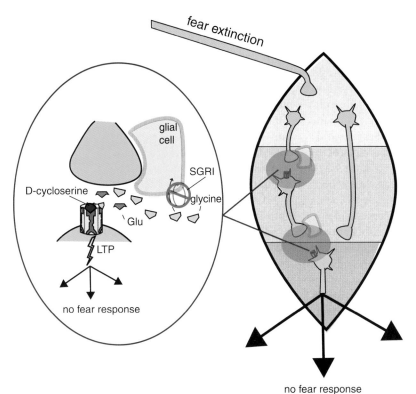

Figure 9-31. Facilitating fear extinction with NMDA receptor activation. Strengthening of synapses involved in fear extinction could help enhance the development of fear extinction learning in the amygdala and reduce symptoms of anxiety disorders. Administration of the N-methyl-D-aspartate (NMDA) coagonist D-cycloserine while an individual is receiving exposure therapy could increase the efficiency of glutamate neurotransmission at synapses involved in fear extinction. Likewise, administration of indirect glycine-enhancing agents such as selective glycine reuptake inhibitors (SGRIs) during exposure therapy could boost NMDA receptor activation. If this leads to long-term potentiation and synaptic plasticity while the synapses are activated by exposure therapy, it could result in structural changes in the amygdala associated with the fear extinction pathway and thus the predominance of the extinction pathway over the conditioned pathway.

amygdala and in the intercalated cell mass at inhibitory GABA neurons by the psychotherapy. If NMDA receptors at these two glutamate synapses could be pharmacologically boosted to trigger disproportionately robust long-term potentiation and synaptic plasticity, timed to occur at the exact time this learning and therapy is taking place and thus exactly when these synapses are selectively activated, it could theoretically result in the predominance of the extinction pathway over the conditioned pathway. Animal studies support this possibility, and early clinical studies are encouraging but not always robust or consistent to date. In the meantime, prudent psychopharmacologists are increasingly leveraging their current anxiolytic drug portfolio with concomitant psychotherapy, since many patients have already received enhanced therapeutic benefit from this combination.

Reconsolidation

Blocking reconsolidation of fear memories is a second mechanism that could theoretically be therapeutic for patients with anxiety disorders. Although classically, emotional memories that have been fear-conditioned were thought to last forever, recent animal experiments show that emotional memories can in fact be weakened or even erased at the time they are re-experienced. When fear is first conditioned, that memory is said to be "consolidated" via a molecular process that some have thought was essentially permanent. Hints at the mechanism of the initial consolidation of fear conditioning come from observations that both β blockers and opioids can potentially mitigate the conditioning of the original traumatic memory, even in humans, and some studies show that these agents can potentially reduce the chances of getting PTSD after a traumatic injury (Figure 9-32). Furthermore, once emotional memories have been consolidated as fear conditioning, animal experiments now show that they are not necessarily permanent, but can change when they are retrieved. Reconsolidation is the state in which reactivation of a consolidated fear memory makes it labile, and requires protein synthesis to keep the memory intact. Beta blockers disrupt reconsolidation of fear memories as well as formation of fear conditioning (Figure 9-32). Future research is trying to determine how to use psychotherapy to provoke emotional memories and reactivate them by producing a state where a pharmacologic agent could be administered to disrupt reconsolidation of these emotional memories and thereby relieve symptoms of anxiety. These are early days in terms of applying this concept in clinical settings, but this notion supports the growing idea that psychotherapy and psychopharmacology can be synergistic. Much more needs to be learned as to how to exploit this theoretical synergy.

Treatments for anxiety disorder subtypes

Generalized anxiety disorder

Treatments for generalized anxiety disorder (GAD) overlap greatly with those for other anxiety disorders and depression (Figure 9-33). First-line treatments include SSRIs and SNRIs, benzodiazepines, buspirone, and $\alpha_2\delta$ ligands such as pregabalin and gabapentin. Some prescribers are reluctant to give benzodiazepines for anxiety disorders in general and for GAD in particular, because of the long-term nature of GAD and the possibility of dependence, abuse, and withdrawal reactions with benzodiazepines.

While it is not a good idea to give benzodiazepines to a GAD patient who is abusing other substances, particularly alcohol, benzodiazepines can be useful when initiating an SSRI or SNRI, since these serotonergic agents are often activating, difficult to tolerate early in dosing, and have a delayed onset of action. $\alpha_2\delta$ ligands are a good alternative to benzodiazepines in some patients. Both benzodiazepines and $\alpha_2\delta$ ligands can have a role in some patients as augmenting agents, especially when initiating treatment with another agent that may be slower-acting or even activating. In other patients, benzodiazepines can be useful to "top up" an SSRI or SNRI for patients who have experienced only partial relief of symptoms. Benzodiazepines can also be useful for occasional intermittent use when symptoms surge and sudden relief is needed.

It should be noted that remission from all symptoms in patients with GAD who are taking an SSRI or SNRI may be slower in onset than it is in depression, and be delayed for 6 months or longer. If a GAD patient is not doing well after several weeks to months of treatment, switching to another SSRI/SNRI or buspirone or augmenting with a benzodiazepine or an $\alpha_2\delta$ ligand can be considered. Failure to respond to first-line treatments can lead to trials of sedating antidepressants such as mirtazapine, trazodone, or tricyclic antidepressants, or even sedating antihistamines such as hydroxyzine. Although not well studied, the SPARI vilazodone should theoretically have

Beta blockers prevent fear conditioning and reconsolidation of fear

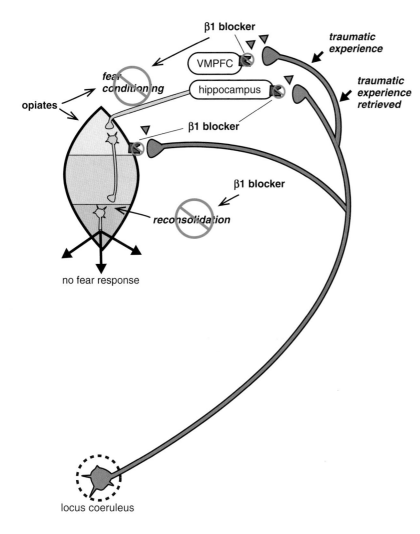

Figure 9-32. Blocking fear conditioning and reconsolidation. When fear is first conditioned, the memory is said to be "consolidated" via a molecular process that once was thought to be permanent. However, there is some research to suggest that administration of either β-adrenergic blockers or opioids can potentially mitigate the conditioning of the original traumatic memory. Furthermore, research also now shows that even when emotional memories have been consolidated as fear conditioning, they can change when they are retrieved. Reconsolidation is the state in which reactivation of a consolidated fear memory makes it labile. This requires protein synthesis to keep the memory intact and, like fear conditioning, may also be disrupted by β blockers.

efficacy for GAD and can be considered as a second-line agent as well. Adjunctive treatments that can be added to first- or second-line therapies for GAD include hypnotics for continuing insomnia, atypical antipsychotics for severe, refractory, and disabling symptoms unresponsive to aggressive treatment, and cognitive behavioral psychotherapy. Old-fashioned treatments for anxiety such as barbiturates and meprobamate are not considered appropriate today, given the other choices shown in Figure 9-33.

Panic disorder

Panic attacks occur in many conditions, not just panic disorder, and panic disorder is frequently comorbid with the other anxiety disorders and with major depression. It is thus not surprising that contemporary treatments for panic disorder overlap significantly with those for the other anxiety disorders and with those for major depression (Figure 9-34). First-line treatments include SSRIs and SNRIs, as well as benzodiazepines and α$_2$δ ligands, although benzodiazepines

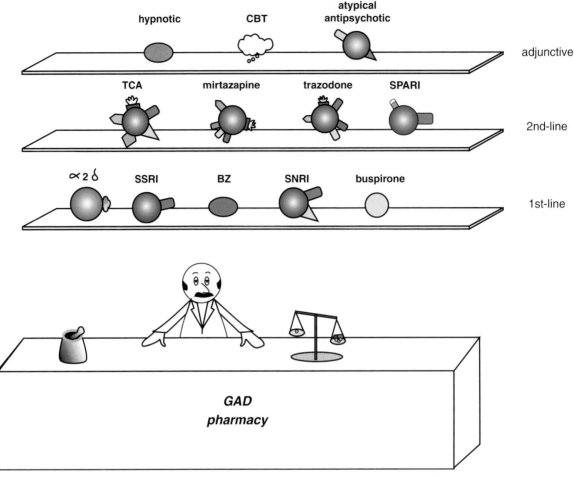

Figure 9-33. Generalized anxiety disorder (GAD) pharmacy. First-line treatments for GAD include $\alpha_2\delta$ ligands, selective serotonin reuptake inhibitors (SSRIs), benzodiazepines (BZs), serotonin–norepinephrine reuptake inhibitors (SNRIs), and buspirone. Second-line treatments include tricyclic antidepressants (TCAs), mirtazapine, trazodone, and serotonin partial agonist/reuptake inhibitors (SPARIs, e.g., vilazodone). Adjunctive medications that may be helpful include hypnotics or an atypical antipsychotic; cognitive behavioral therapy (CBT) is also an important component of anxiety treatment.

are often used second line, during treatment initiation with an SSRI/SNRI, for emergent use during a panic attack, or for incomplete response to an SSRI/SNRI. $\alpha_2\delta$ ligands are approved for the treatment of anxiety in Europe and other countries but not in the US.

Second-line treatments include older antidepressants such as tricyclic antidepressants. Mirtazapine and trazodone are sedating antidepressants that can be helpful in some cases, and are occasionally used as augmenting agents to SSRIs/SNRIs when these first-line agents have only a partial treatment response. The MAO inhibitors, discussed in Chapter 7, are much neglected in psychopharmacology in general and for the treatment of panic disorder in particular.

However, these agents can have powerful efficacy in panic disorder and should be considered when first-line agents and various augmenting strategies fail.

Cognitive behavioral psychotherapy can be an alternative or an augmentation to psychopharmacologic approaches, and can help modify cognitive distortions and, through exposure, diminish phobic avoidance behaviors.

Social anxiety disorder

The treatment options for this anxiety disorder (Figure 9-35) are very similar to those for panic disorder, with a few noteworthy differences. The

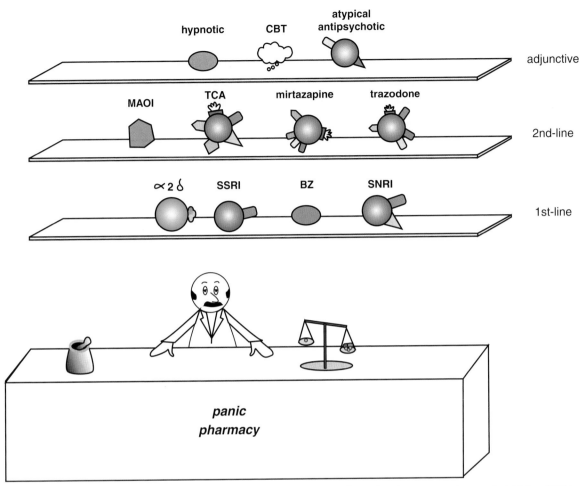

Figure 9-34. Panic pharmacy. First-line treatments for panic disorder include α₂δ ligands, selective serotonin reuptake inhibitors (SSRIs), benzodiazepines (BZs), and serotonin–norepinephrine reuptake inhibitors (SNRIs). Second-line treatments include monoamine oxidase inhibitors (MAOIs), tricyclic antidepressants (TCAs), mirtazapine, and trazodone. Cognitive behavioral therapy (CBT) may be beneficial for many patients. In addition, adjunctive medications for residual symptoms may include hypnotics or an atypical antipsychotic.

SSRIs and SNRIs and α₂δ ligands are certainly first-line therapies, but the utility of benzodiazepine monotherapy for first-line treatment is not generally as widely accepted as it might be for GAD and panic disorder. There is also less evidence for the utility of older antidepressants for social anxiety disorder, particularly the tricyclic antidepressants, but also other sedating antidepressants such as mirtazapine and trazodone. Beta blockers, sometimes with benzodiazepines, can be useful for some patients with very discrete types of social anxiety, such as performance anxiety. Listed as adjunctive treatments are agents for alcohol dependence/abuse, such as naltrexone and acamprosate, since many patients may discover the utility of alcohol in relieving their social anxiety symptoms and develop alcohol dependence/abuse. Cognitive behavioral psychotherapy can be a powerful intervention, sometimes better than drugs for certain patients, and often helpful in combination with drugs.

Posttraumatic stress disorder

Although many treatments are shown in Figure 9-36, psychopharmacologic treatments for PTSD in general may not be as effective as these same

417

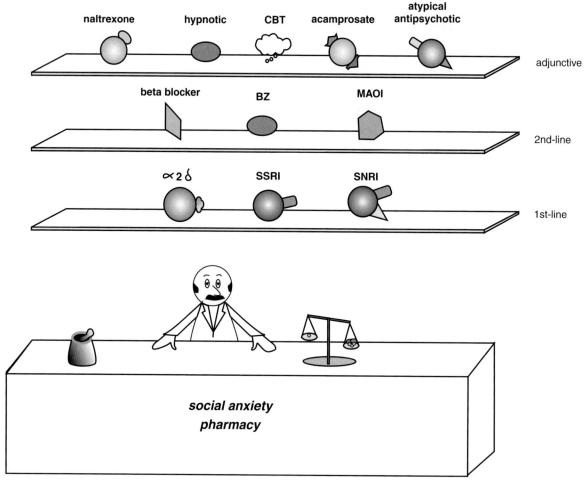

Figure 9-35. Social anxiety pharmacy. First-line treatments for social anxiety disorder include $\alpha_2\delta$ ligands, selective serotonin reuptake inhibitors (SSRIs), and serotonin–norepinephrine reuptake inhibitors (SNRIs). Monoamine oxidase inhibitors (MAOIs) have been shown to be beneficial and may be a second-line option; other second-line options include benzodiazepines (BZs) and β blockers. Several medications may be used as adjuncts for residual symptoms; cognitive behavioral therapy may (CBT) be useful as well.

treatments are in other anxiety disorders. Also, PTSD is so highly comorbid that many of the psychopharmacologic treatments are more effectively aimed at comorbidities such as depression, insomnia, substance abuse, and pain than at core symptoms of PTSD. SSRIs and SNRIs are proven effective and are considered first-line treatments, but often leave the patient with residual symptoms, including sleep problems. Thus, most patients with PTSD do not take monotherapy. Benzodiazepines are to be used with caution, not only because of limited evidence from clinical trials for efficacy in PTSD, but also because many PTSD patients abuse alcohol and other substances. A unique treatment

for PTSD is the administration of α_1 antagonists at night to prevent nightmares. Pre-emptive treatment with β blockers or opioids is discussed above, but is not a proven or practical treatment option at this point. Much more effective treatments for PTSD are greatly needed.

Much of the advance in treatment of PTSD has been in using drugs to treat comorbidities and psychotherapies to treat core symptoms. Exposure therapy is perhaps most effective among psychotherapies, but many forms of CBT are being investigated and used in clinical practice, depending upon the training of the therapist and the specific needs of the individual.

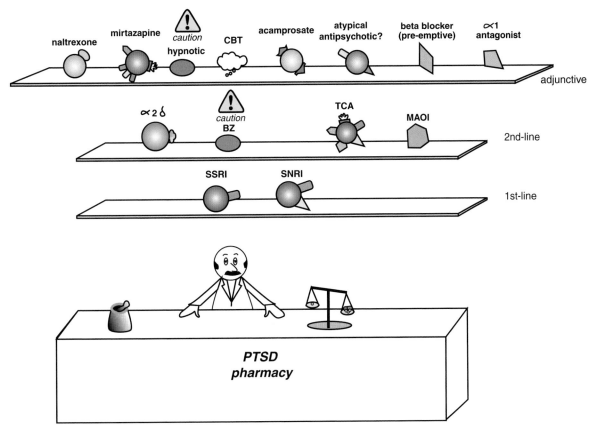

Figure 9-36. Posttraumatic stress disorder (PTSD) pharmacy. First-line pharmacological options for PTSD are selective serotonin reuptake inhibitors (SSRIs) and serotonin–norepinephrine reuptake inhibitors (SNRIs). In PTSD, unlike other anxiety disorders, benzodiazepines (BZs) have not been shown to be as helpful, although they may be considered with caution as a second-line option. Other second-line treatments include α₂δ ligands, tricyclic antidepressants (TCAs), and monoamine oxidase inhibitors (MAOIs). Several medications may be used as adjuncts for residual symptoms, and cognitive behavioral therapy (CBT) is typically recommended as well.

Summary

Anxiety disorders have core features of fear and worry that cut across the entire spectrum of anxiety disorder subtypes, from generalized anxiety disorder to panic disorder, social anxiety disorder, and posttraumatic stress disorder. The amygdala plays a central role in the fear response, and cortico-striato-thalamo-cortical (CSTC) circuits are thought to play a key role in mediating the symptom of worry. Numerous neurotransmitters are involved in regulating the circuits that underlie the anxiety disorders. GABA (γ-aminobutyric acid) is a key neurotransmitter in anxiety and the benzodiazepine anxiolytics act upon this neurotransmitter system. Serotonin, norepinephrine, $\alpha_2\delta$ ligands for voltage-gated calcium channels, and other regulators of anxiety circuits are also discussed as approaches to the treatment of anxiety disorders. The concept of opposing actions of fear conditioning versus fear extinction within amygdala circuits hypothetically is linked to the production and maintenance of symptoms in anxiety disorder and provides a substrate for potential novel therapeutics combining psychotherapy and drugs. Numerous treatments are available for anxiety disorders, most of which are similar for the entire anxiety disorder spectrum and are also used for the treatment of depression.

This chapter will provide a brief overview of chronic pain conditions associated with different psychiatric disorders and treated with psychotropic drugs. Included here are discussions of the symptomatic and pathophysiologic overlap between disorders with pain and many other disorders treated in psychopharmacology, especially depression and anxiety. Clinical descriptions and formal criteria for how to diagnose painful conditions are only mentioned here in passing. The reader should consult standard reference sources for this material. The discussion here will emphasize how discoveries about the functioning of various brain circuits and neurotransmitters – especially those acting upon the central processing of pain – have impacted our understanding of the pathophysiology and treatment of many painful conditions that may occur with or without various psychiatric disorders. The goal of this chapter is to acquaint the reader with ideas about the clinical and biological aspects of the symptom of pain, how it can be hypothetically caused by alterations of pain processing within the central nervous system (CNS), how it can be associated with many of the symptoms of depression and anxiety, and finally how it can be treated with several of the same agents that can treat

depression and anxiety. The discussion in this chapter is at the conceptual level, not at the pragmatic level. The reader should consult standard drug handbooks (such as *Stahl's Essential Psychopharmacology: the Prescriber's Guide*) for details of doses, side effects, drug interactions, and other issues relevant to the prescribing of these drugs in clinical practice.

What is pain?

No experience rivals pain for its ability to capture our attention, focus our actions, and cause suffering (see Table 10-1 for some useful definitions regarding pain). The powerful experience of pain, especially acute pain, can serve a vital function – to make us aware of damage to our bodies, and to rest the injured part until it has healed. When acute pain is *peripheral* in origin (i.e., originating outside of the CNS) but continues as chronic pain, it can cause changes in CNS pain mechanisms that enhance or perpetuate the original peripheral pain. For example, osteoarthritis, low back pain, and diabetic peripheral neuropathic pain begin as peripheral pain, but over time these conditions can trigger central pain mechanisms that amplify peripheral pain and generate additional pain centrally. This may

Table 10-1 Pain: some useful definitions

Pain	An unpleasant sensory and emotional experience associated with actual or potential tissue damage, or described in terms of such damage
Acute pain	Pain that is of short duration and resolves; usually directly related to the resolution or healing of tissue damage
Chronic pain	Pain that persists for longer than would be expected; an artificial threshold for chronicity (e.g., 1 month) is not appropriate
Neuropathic pain	Pain that arises from damage to, or dysfunction of, any part of the peripheral or central nervous system
Nociception	The process by which noxious stimuli produce activity in the sensory pathways that convey "painful" information
Allodynia	Pain caused by a stimulus that does not normally provoke pain
Hyperalgesia	An increased response to a stimulus that is normally painful
Analgesia	Any process that reduces the sensation of pain, while not affecting normal touch
Local anesthesia	Blockade of all sensation (innocuous and painful) from a local area
Noxious stimulus	Stimulus that inflicts damage, or would potentially inflict damage, on tissues of the body
Primary afferent neuron (PAN)	The first neuron in the somatosensory pathway; detects mechanical, thermal, or chemical stimuli at its peripheral terminals and transmits action potentials to its central terminals in the spinal cord; all PANs have a cell body in the dorsal root ganglion
Nociceptor	A primary afferent (sensory) neuron that is only activated by a noxious stimulus
Nociception	The process by which a nociceptor detects a noxious stimulus and generates a signal (action potentials) that is propagated towards higher centers in the nociceptive pathway
Dorsal root ganglion (DRG)	Contains the cell bodies of primary afferent neurons; proteins, including transmitters, receptors, and structural proteins, are synthesized here and transported to peripheral and central terminals
Interneuron	Neuron with its cell body, axon and dendrites within the spinal cord; can be excitatory (e.g., containing glutamate) or inhibitory (e.g., containing GABA)
Projection neurons	Neuron in the dorsal horn that receives input from PANs and/or interneurons, and projects up the spinal cord to higher processing centers
Spinothalamic tract	Tract of neurons that project from the spinal cord to the thalamus
Spinobulbar tracts	Several different tracts of neurons that project from the spinal cord to brainstem nuclei
Somatosensory cortex	Region of the cerebral cortex that receives input mainly from cutaneous sensory nerves; the cortex is topographically arranged, with adjacent areas receiving input from adjacent body areas; stimulation of the somatosensory cortex creates sensations from the body part that projects to it

explain why research has recently shown that chronic pain conditions of peripheral origin can be successfully targeted for relief by psychotropic drugs that work on central pain mechanisms.

Many other chronic pain conditions may start *centrally* and never have a peripheral causation to the pain, especially conditions associated with multiple unexplained painful physical symptoms such as depression, anxiety, and fibromyalgia. Because these centrally mediated pain conditions are associated with emotional symptoms, this type of pain has until recently often been considered not to be "real" but rather a nonspecific outcome of unresolved psychological conflicts that would improve when the associated psychiatric condition improved; therefore, there was not a perceived need to target this type of pain. Today, however, many painful conditions without identifiable peripheral lesions and that were once

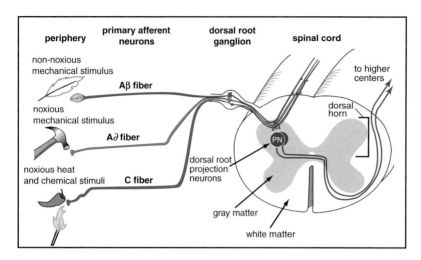

Figure 10-1. Activation of nociceptive nerve fibers. Detection of a noxious stimulus occurs at the peripheral terminals of primary afferent neurons and leads to generation of action potentials that propagate along the axon to the central terminals. Aβ fibers respond only to non-noxious stimuli, Aδ fibers respond to noxious mechanical stimuli and subnoxious thermal stimuli, and C fibers respond only to noxious mechanical, heat, and chemical stimuli. Primary afferent neurons have their cell bodies in the dorsal root ganglion and send terminals into that spinal cord segment as well as sending less dense collaterals up the spinal cord for a short distance. Primary afferent neurons synapse onto several different classes of dorsal horn projection neurons (PN), which project via different tracts to higher centers.

linked only to psychiatric disorders are now hypothesized to be forms of chronic neuropathic pain syndromes that can be successfully treated with the same agents that treat neuropathic pain syndromes not associated with psychiatric disorders. These treatments include the SNRIs (serotonin–norepinephrine reuptake inhibitors: discussed in Chapter 7 on antidepressants) and the $\alpha_2\delta$ ligands (anticonvulsants that block voltage-gated calcium channels or VSCCs: discussed in Chapter 8 on mood stabilizers and in Chapter 9 on anxiety disorders). Additional psychotropic agents acting centrally at various other sites are also used to treat a variety of chronic pain conditions and will be mentioned below. Many additional drugs are being tested as potential novel pain treatments as well.

Since pain is clearly associated with some psychiatric disorders, and psychotropic drugs that treat various psychiatric conditions are also effective for a wide variety of pain conditions, the detection, quantification, and treatment of pain are rapidly becoming standardized parts of a psychiatric evaluation. Modern psychopharmacologists increasingly consider pain to be a psychiatric "vital sign," thus requiring routine evaluation and symptomatic treatment. In fact, elimination of pain is increasingly recognized as necessary in order to have full symptomatic remission not only of chronic pain conditions, but also of many psychiatric disorders.

"Normal" pain and the activation of nociceptive nerve fibers

The nociceptive pain pathway is the series of neurons that begins with detection of a noxious stimulus and ends with the subjective perception of pain. This so-called *nociceptive pathway* starts from the periphery, enters the spinal cord, and projects to the brain (Figure 10-1). It is important to understand the processes by which incoming information can be modulated to increase or decrease the perception of pain associated with a given stimulus, because these processes can explain not only why maladaptive pain states arise but also why drugs that work in psychiatric conditions such as depression and anxiety can also be effective in reducing pain.

Nociceptive pathway to the spinal cord

Primary afferent neurons detect sensory inputs including pain (Figure 10-1). They have their cell bodies in the dorsal root ganglia located along the spinal column outside of the CNS and thus are considered peripheral and not central neurons (Figure 10-1). Nociception begins with transduction – the process by which specialized membrane proteins located on the peripheral projections of these neurons detect a stimulus and generate a voltage change at their peripheral neuronal membranes. A sufficiently strong stimulus will lower the voltage at the membrane (i.e., depolarize the membrane) enough to activate voltage-sensitive sodium channels (VSSCs) and trigger an action potential that will be propagated along the length of the axon to the central terminals of the neuron in the spinal cord (Figure 10-1). VSSCs are introduced in Chapter 3 and illustrated in Figures 3-19 and 3-20. Nociceptive impulse flow from primary afferent neurons into the CNS can be reduced or stopped when VSSCs are blocked by peripherally administered local anesthetics such as lidocaine.

The specific response characteristics of primary afferent neurons are determined by the specific receptors and channels expressed by that neuron in the periphery (Figure 10-1). For example, primary afferent neurons that express a stretch-activated ion channel are mechanosensitive; those that express the vanillinoid receptor 1 (VR1) ion channel are activated by capsaicin, the pungent ingredient in chili peppers, and also by noxious heat, leading to the burning sensation both these stimuli evoke. These functional response properties are used to classify primary afferent neurons into three types: Aβ, Aδ, and C-fiber neurons (Figure 10-1). Aβ fibers detect small movements, light touch, hair movement, and vibrations; C-fiber peripheral terminals are bare nerve endings that are only activated by noxious mechanical, thermal, or chemical stimuli; Aδ fibers fall somewhere in between, sensing noxious mechanical stimuli and subnoxious thermal stimuli (Figure 10-1). Nociceptive input and pain can thus be caused by activating primary afferent neurons peripherally, such as from a sprained ankle or a tooth extraction. NSAIDs (nonsteroidal anti-inflammatory drugs) can reduce painful input from these primary afferent neurons, presumably via their peripheral actions. Opioids can also reduce such pain, but from central actions, as explained below.

Nociceptive pathway from the spinal cord to the brain

The central terminals of peripheral nociceptive neurons synapse in the dorsal horn of the spinal cord onto the next cells in the pathway – dorsal horn neurons, which receive input from many primary afferent neurons and then project to higher centers (Figure 10-3). For this reason, they are sometimes also called dorsal horn projection neurons (PN in Figures 10-1, 10-2, and 10-3). Dorsal horn neurons are thus the first neurons of the nociceptive pathway that are located entirely within the CNS, and are therefore a key site for modulation of nociceptive neuronal activity as it comes into the CNS. A vast number of neurotransmitters have been identified in the dorsal horn, some of which are shown in Figure 10-2.

Neurotransmitters in the dorsal horn are synthesized not only by primary afferent neurons, but by the other neurons in the dorsal horn as well, including descending neurons and various interneurons (Figure 10-2). Some neurotransmitter systems in the dorsal horn are successfully targeted by known pain-relieving drugs, especially opioids, serotonin- and norepinephrine-boosting SNRIs (serotonin–norepinephrine reuptake inhibitors), and $\alpha_2\delta$ ligands acting at voltage-sensitive calcium channels (VSCCs). All of the neurotransmitter systems acting in the dorsal horn are potential targets for novel pain-relieving drugs (Figure 10-2), and a plethora of such novel agents is currently in clinical and preclinical development.

There are several classes of dorsal horn neurons: some receive input directly from primary sensory neurons, some are interneurons, and some project up the spinal cord to higher centers (Figure 10-3). There are several different tracts in which these projection neurons can ascend, which can be crudely divided into two functions: the sensory/discriminatory pathway and the emotional/motivational pathway (Figure 10-3).

In the sensory/discriminatory pathway, dorsal horn neurons ascend in the spinothalamic tract; then, thalamic neurons project to the primary somatosensory cortex (Figure 10-3). This particular pain pathway is thought to convey the precise location of the nociceptive stimulus and its intensity. In the emotional/motivational pathway, other dorsal horn neurons project to brainstem nuclei, and from there to limbic regions (Figure 10-3). This second pain pathway is thought to convey the affective component that nociceptive stimuli evoke. Only when these two aspects of sensory discrimination and emotions come together and the final, subjective perception of pain is created can we use the word *pain* to describe the modality ("ouch" in Figure 10-3). Before this point, we are simply discussing activity in neural pathways, which should be described as noxious-evoked or nociceptive neuronal activity but not necessarily as pain.

Neuropathic pain

The term *neuropathic pain* describes pain that arises from damage to, or dysfunction of, any part of the peripheral or central nervous system, whereas "normal" pain (so-called *nociceptive pain*, just discussed in the section above) is caused by activation of nociceptive nerve fibers.

Peripheral mechanisms in neuropathic pain

Normal transduction and conduction in peripheral afferent neurons can be hijacked in certain neuropathic pain states to maintain nociceptive signaling

Multiple Neurotransmitters Modulate Pain Processing
in the Spinal Cord

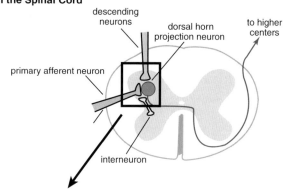

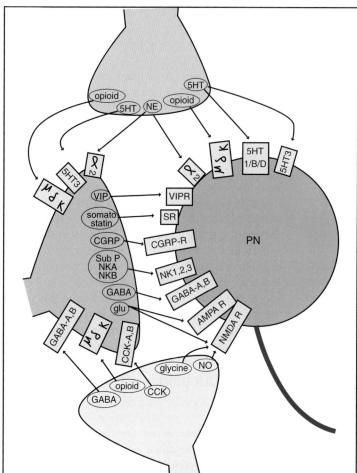

Figure 10-2. Multiple neurotransmitters modulate pain processing in the spinal cord. There are many neurotransmitters and their corresponding receptors in the dorsal horn. Neurotransmitters in the dorsal horn may be released by primary afferent neurons, by descending regulatory neurons, by dorsal horn projection neurons (PN) and by interneurons. Neurotransmitters present in the dorsal horn that have been best studied in terms of pain transmission include substance P (NK1, 2, and 3 receptors), endorphins (μ-opioid receptors), norepinephrine (α_2-adrenergic receptors), and serotonin ($5HT_{1B/D}$ and $5HT_3$ receptors). Several other neurotransmitters are also represented, including VIP (vasopressin inhibitory protein and its receptor VIPR); somatostatin and its receptor SR; calcitonin-gene-related peptide (CGRP and its receptor CGRP-R); GABA and its receptors $GABA_A$ and $GABA_B$; glutamate and its receptors AMPA-R (α-amino-3-hydroxy-5-methyl-4-isoxazole propionic acid receptor) and NMDA-R (N-methyl-D-aspartate receptor); nitric oxide (NO); cholecystokinin (CCK and its receptors CCK-A and CCK-B); and glycine and its receptor NMDA-R.

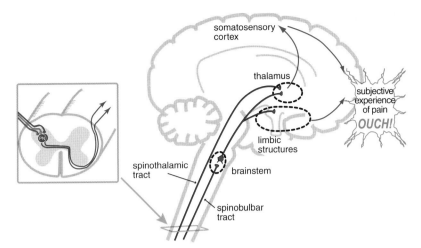

Figure 10-3. From nociception to pain. Dorsal horn neurons in the spinothalamic tract project to the thalamus and then to the primary somatosensory cortex. This pathway carries information about the intensity and location of the painful stimuli and is termed the discriminatory pathway. Neurons ascending in the spinobulbar tract project to brainstem nuclei and then to both the thalamus and limbic structures. These pathways convey the emotional and motivational aspects of the pain experience. Only when information from the discriminatory (thalamocortical) and emotional/motivational (limbic) pathways combine is the human subjective experience of pain formed ("ouch").

in the absence of a relevant noxious stimulus. Neuronal damage by disease or trauma can alter electrical activity of neurons, allow cross-talk between neurons, and initiate inflammatory processes to cause *peripheral sensitization*. In this chapter, we will not emphasize peripheral sensitization disorders and mechanisms, but rather central sensitization disorders and mechanisms.

Central mechanisms in neuropathic pain

At each major relay point in the pain pathway (Figure 10-3), the nociceptive pain signal is susceptible to modulation by endogenous processes to either dampen down the signal or amplify it. This happens not only peripherally at primary afferent neurons, as has just been discussed, but also at central neurons in the dorsal horn of the spinal cord as well as in numerous brain regions. The events in the dorsal horn of the spinal cord are better understood than those in brain regions of nociceptive pathways, but pain processing in the brain may be the key to understanding the generation and amplification of central pain in disorders of chronic peripheral pain such as osteoarthritis, low back pain, and diabetic peripheral neuropathic pain, as well as painful physical symptoms in affective and anxiety disorders and in fibromyalgia.

"Segmental" central sensitization is a process thought to be caused when plastic changes occur in the dorsal horn, classically in conditions such as phantom pain after limb amputation. Specifically, this type of neuronal plasticity in the dorsal horn is called activity-dependent or use-dependent, because it

requires constant firing of the pain pathway in the dorsal horn. The consequence of this constant input of pain is eventually to cause exaggerated (hyperalgesic) or prolonged responses to any noxious input – a phenomenon sometimes called "wind-up" – as well as painful responses to normally innocuous inputs (called allodynia). Phosphorylation of key membrane receptors and channels in the dorsal horn appears to increase synaptic efficiency and thus to trip a master switch, opening the gate to the pain pathway and turning on central sensitization that acts to amplify or create the perception of pain even if there is no pain input coming from the periphery. The gate can also close, as conceptualized in the classic "gate theory" of pain, in order to explain how innocuous stimulation (e.g., acupuncture, vibration, rubbing) away from the site of an injury can close the pain gate and reduce the perception of the injury pain.

In segmental central sensitization, a definite peripheral injury (Figure 10-4A) is combined with central sensitization at the spinal cord segment receiving nociceptive input from the damaged area of the body (Figure 10-4B). Segmental central sensitization syndromes are thus "mixed" states where the insult of central segmental changes (Figure 10-4B) is added to peripheral injuries such as low back pain, diabetic peripheral neuropathic pain, and painful cutaneous eruptions of herpes zoster (shingles) (Figure 10-4A).

"Suprasegmental" central sensitization is hypothesized to be linked to plastic changes that occur in brain sites within the nociceptive pathway, especially the thalamus and cortex, in the presence of known peripheral causes (Figure 10-5A) or even in the absence of identifiable triggering events (Figure 10-5B). In the

Onset of Acute Pain from Painful Peripheral Conditions

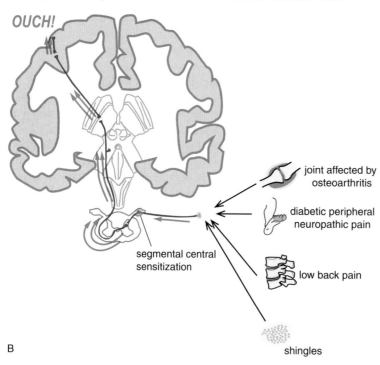

Figure 10-4. Acute pain and development of segmental central sensitization. (A) When peripheral injury occurs, nociceptive impulse flow from primary afferent neurons is transmitted via dorsal horn neurons to higher brain centers, where it can ultimately be interpreted as pain (represented by the "ouch"). (B) In some cases, injury or disease directly affecting the nervous system may result in plastic changes that lead to sensitization within the central nervous system, such that the experience of pain continues even after tissue damage is resolved. Impulses may be generated at abnormal locations either spontaneously or via mechanical forces. At the level of the spinal cord, this process is termed segmental central sensitization. This mechanism underlies conditions such as diabetic peripheral neuropathic pain and shingles.

Development of Segmental Central Sensitization and Increased Pain

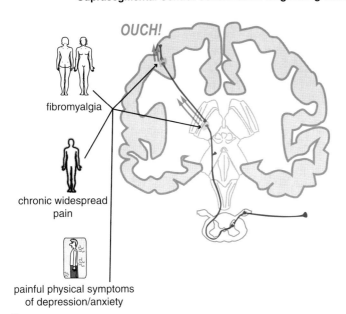

Chronic Pain with Suprasegmental Central Sensitization from Peripheral Injury

OUCH!

suprasegmental central sensitization

joint affected by osteoarthritis

diabetic peripheral neuropathic pain

low back pain

A

shingles

Suprasegmental Central Sensitization Originating in the Brain

OUCH!

fibromyalgia

chronic widespread pain

painful physical symptoms of depression/anxiety

B

Figure 10-5. Suprasegmental central sensitization. Plastic changes in brain sites within the nociceptive pathway can cause sensitization, for instance at the level of the thalamus or the sensory cortex. This process within the brain is termed suprasegmental central sensitization. This can occur following peripheral injury (A) or even in the absence of identifiable triggering events (B). This mechanism is believed to underlie conditions such as fibromyalgia, chronic widespread pain, and painful symptoms in depression and anxiety disorders.

The Spectrum from Mood and Anxiety Disorders to Painful Functional Somatic Symptoms

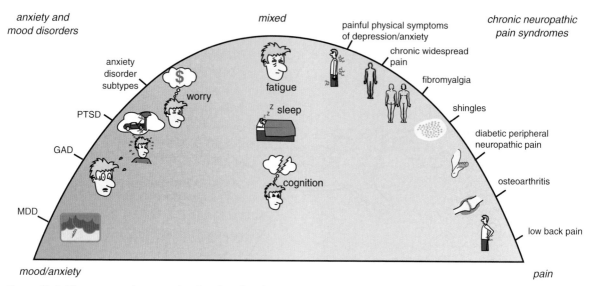

Figure 10-6. **The spectrum from mood and anxiety disorders to painful functional somatic syndromes.** Affective spectrum disorders include mood and anxiety disorders, while "functional somatic syndrome" is a term used to describe disorders such as fibromyalgia and chronic widespread pain. Pain, though not a formal diagnostic feature of depression or anxiety disorders, is nonetheless frequently present in patients with these disorders. Similarly, depressed mood, anxiety, and other symptoms identified as part of depression and anxiety disorders are now recognized as being common in functional somatic syndromes. Thus, rather than being discrete groups of illnesses, affective spectrum disorders and functional somatic syndromes may instead exist along the same spectrum.

case of peripherally activated suprasegmental central sensitization, it is as though the brain "learns" from its experience of pain, and decides not only to keep the process going, but also to enhance it and make it permanent. In the case of pain that originates centrally without peripheral input, it is as though the brain has figured out how to spontaneously activate its pain pathways. Interrupting this process of sensitized brain pathways for pain and getting the CNS to "forget" its molecular memories may be one of the greatest therapeutic opportunities in psychopharmacology today, not only because this may be a therapeutic strategy for various chronic neuropathic pain conditions, as discussed here, but also because it may be a viable approach to treating the hypothesized molecular changes that may underlie disease progression in a wide variety of disorders, from schizophrenia to stress-induced anxiety and affective disorders, to addictive disorders. Conditions hypothesized to be caused by suprasegmental central sensitization syndromes of pain originating in the brain without peripheral pain input include fibromyalgia, the syndrome of chronic widespread pain, and painful

physical symptoms of depression and anxiety disorders, especially PTSD (Figure 10-5B).

The spectrum of mood and anxiety disorders with pain disorders

A large group of overlapping disorders can have emotional symptoms, painful physical symptoms, or both (Figure 10-6). Although pain in the absence of emotional symptoms has long been seen as a neurological disorder, and pain in the presence of emotional symptoms as a psychiatric disorder, it is now clear that pain is a symptom that can be mapped onto inefficient information processing within the pain circuit, and is largely considered the same symptom with the same treatments whether occurring by itself or as part of any number of syndromes (Figure 10-6). Thus, pain (Figure 10-6, on the right) can occur not only by itself, but also concomitantly with the emotional symptoms of depressed mood and anxiety (Figure 10-6, on the left), and with the physical symptoms of fatigue, insomnia, and problems concentrating (Figure 10-6, in the middle). No matter whether pain occurs by itself or with additional concomitant emotional or physical symptoms, or in the presence of full syndromal psychiatric disorders such as major depressive disorder, generalized anxiety disorder, or PTSD (Figure 10-6, on the left), it must be treated – and the treatments are the same across the spectrum (Figure 10-6), namely SNRIs and $\alpha_2\delta$ ligands, as will be explained below.

Fibromyalgia

Fibromyalgia has emerged as a diagnosable (Table 10-2) and treatable pain syndrome with tenderness but no structural pathology in muscles, ligaments, or joints. Fibromyalgia is recognized as a chronic, widespread pain syndrome associated with fatigue, nonrestorative sleep and tenderness at 11 or more of 18 designated "trigger points" where ligaments, tendons, and muscle attach to bone (Figure 10-7). It is the second most common diagnosis in rheumatology clinics, and may affect 2–4% of the population. Although symptoms of fibromyalgia are chronic and debilitating, they are not necessarily progressive. There is no known cause and there is no known pathology identifiable in the muscles or joints. This syndrome can be deconstructed into its component symptoms (Figure 10-8), and then matched with hypothetically malfunctioning brain circuits (Figure 10-9). Some studies suggest that 75–90% of

identified patients are women, especially Caucasian women. A related syndrome, called chronic widespread pain, is essentially pain without the tenderness, sometimes called "male fibromyalgia" because many men often do

Table 10-2 American College of Rheumatology (ACR) 1990 criteria for fibromyalgia (Wolfe F, *et al. Arthritis Rheum* 1990; **33**: 160–72).

History of widespread pain
Considered widespread when present in all of the following:
Left side of the body
Right side of the body
Above the waist
Below the waist
Axial skeleton (cervical spine, anterior chest, thoracic spine, or low back)
Must be present for at least 3 months
Pain in 11 of 18 tender point sites on digital palpation
Digital palpation should be performed with an approximate force of 4 kg
For a tender point to be considered positive, the subject must state that the palpation was painful

Tender Points for the Diagnosis of Fibromyalgia

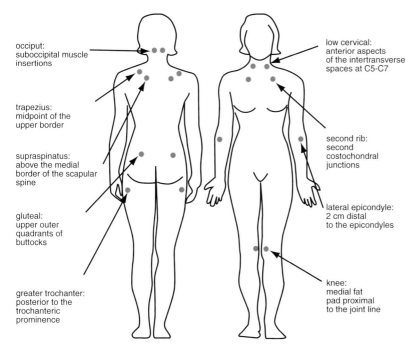

occiput:
suboccipital muscle
insertions

trapezius:
midpoint of the
upper border

supraspinatus:
above the medial
border of the scapular
spine

gluteal:
upper outer
quadrants of
buttocks

greater trochanter:
posterior to the
trochanteric
prominence

low cervical:
anterior aspects
of the intertransverse
spaces at C5-C7

second rib:
second
costochondral
junctions

lateral epicondyle:
2 cm distal
to the epicondyles

knee:
medial fat
pad proximal
to the joint line

Figure 10-7. Tender points for the diagnosis of fibromyalgia. Fibromyalgia is a chronic widespread pain syndrome formally diagnosed based on tenderness in at least 11 of 18 designated "trigger points" where ligaments, tendons, and muscle attach to bone. Other diagnostic features include fatigue and nonrestorative sleep.

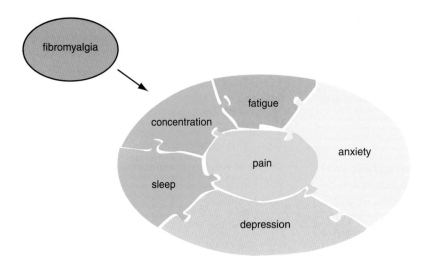

Figure 10-8. Symptoms of fibromyalgia. In addition to pain as a central feature of fibromyalgia, many patients experience fatigue, anxiety, depression, disturbed sleep, and problems concentrating.

Match Each Symptom of Fibromyalgia to Hypothetically Malfunctioning Brain Circuits

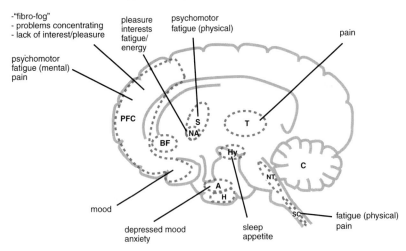

Figure 10-9. Symptom-based algorithm for fibromyalgia. A symptom-based approach to treatment selection for fibromyalgia follows the theory that each of a patient's symptoms can be matched with malfunctioning brain circuits and neurotransmitters that hypothetically mediate those symptoms; this information is then used to select a corresponding pharmacological mechanism for treatment. Pain is linked to transmission of information via the thalamus (T), while physical fatigue is linked to the striatum (S) and spinal cord (SC). Problems concentrating and lack of interest (termed "fibro-fog") as well as mental fatigue are linked to the prefrontal cortex (PFC), specifically the dorsolateral PFC. Fatigue, low energy, and lack of interest may all also be related to the nucleus accumbens (NA). Disturbances in sleep and appetite are associated with the hypothalamus (Hy), depressed mood with the amygdala (A) and orbitofrontal cortex, and anxiety with the amygdala.

not experience (or at least do not report) tenderness on examination of areas of pain.

Decreased gray matter in chronic pain syndromes?

Some very troubling preliminary reports suggest that chronic pain may even "shrink the brain" in the DLPFC (dorsolateral prefrontal cortex) (Figure 10-10)

and thereby contribute to cognitive dysfunction in certain pain states such as fibromyalgia (Figure 10-8) and low back pain. Brain atrophy is discussed in relation to stress and anxiety disorders in Chapter 6 and illustrated in Figure 6-39. It would not be surprising if stressful conditions that cause pain, as well as pain that causes distress, are all involved in causing brain atrophy and/or cognitive dysfunction in fibromyalgia and other chronic pain states.

Gray-matter loss in chronic pain

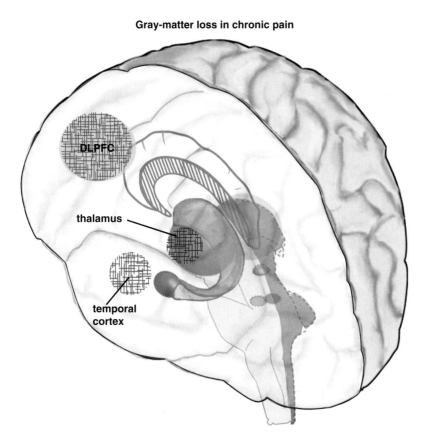

Figure 10-10. Gray-matter loss in chronic pain. Research suggests that chronic pain, like anxiety and stress-related disorders, may lead to brain atrophy. Specifically, there are data showing gray-matter loss in the dorsolateral prefrontal cortex (DLPFC), the thalamus, and the temporal cortex in patients with chronic pain conditions.

Chronic back pain, for example, has also been reported to be associated with decreased prefrontal and thalamic gray-matter density (Figure 10-10). Some experts have hypothesized that in fibromyalgia and other chronic neuropathic pain syndromes, the persistent perception of pain could lead to overuse of DLPFC neurons, excitotoxic cell death in this brain region, and reduction of the corticothalamic "brake" on nociceptive pathways. Such an outcome could cause not only increased pain perception, but diminished executive functioning, sometimes called "fibro-fog" in fibromyalgia. In Chapter 6 we discussed how stress-related HPA (hypothalamic–pituitary–adrenal) axis abnormalities in CRH-ACTH-cortisol regulation may be linked to hippocampal atrophy (see Figure 6-39), possibly linked to reduced availability of growth factors (Figures 6-37 and 6-38). Alterations in growth factors may be linked to the reports of reduction in gray-matter volume in chronic pain syndromes (fibromyalgia and low back pain), but in different brain regions (DLPFC, temporal cortex, and thalamus: Figure 10-10) than reported for

depression (Figure 6-39B). Gray matter may actually be increased in other brain regions in chronic pain.

Although still preliminary, these findings suggest a possibly structural consequence to suprasegmental central sensitization (Figure 10-10) not unlike that suspected for depression and stress (Figure 6-39). Abnormal pain processing, exaggerated pain responses, and perpetual pain could hypothetically be linked to deficiencies in the DLPFC circuit and its regulation by dopamine, and provide a potential explanation for the cognitive difficulties associated with chronic pain, especially so-called "fibro-fog" in fibromyalgia (Figure 10-8). Thalamic abnormalities could hypothetically be linked to problems sleeping and nonrestorative sleep seen in chronic pain syndromes as well (Figure 10-8). Thus, chronic pain syndromes not only cause pain, but also problems with fatigue, mental concentration, and sleep as well as depression and anxiety (Figure 10-8). Structural brain abnormalities associated with inefficient information processing in brain areas that mediate these symptoms (Figure 10-9) may explain why these various symptoms (Figure 10-8) are frequently associated with chronic pain syndromes.

Descending spinal synapses in the dorsal horn and the treatment of chronic pain

The periaqueductal gray (PAG) is the site of origin and regulation of much of the descending inhibition that projects down the spinal cord to the dorsal horn (Figure 10-2). The periaqueductal gray is discussed in relation to its connections with the amygdala and the motor component of the fear response in Chapter 9 and illustrated in Figure 9-9. The periaqueductal gray also integrates inputs from nociceptive pathways and limbic structures such as the amygdala and limbic cortex, and sends outputs to brainstem nuclei and the rostroventromedial medulla to drive descending inhibitory pathways. Some of these descending pathways release endorphins, which act via mostly presynaptic μ-opioid receptors to inhibit neurotransmission from nociceptive primary afferent neurons (Figure 10-2). Spinal μ-opioid receptors are one target of opioid analgesics; so are μ-opioid receptors in the periaqueductal gray itself (Figure 10-11). Interestingly, since Aβ fibers (Figure 10-1) do not express μ-opioid receptors, this may explain why opioid analgesics spare normal sensory input. Enkephalins, which also act via δ-opioid receptors, are also antinociceptive, whereas dynorphins, acting at κ-opioid receptors, can be either anti- or pronociceptive. Interesting also is that opioids in general are not only no more effective for chronic neuropathic pain states than SNRIs or $α_2δ$ ligands, but in many cases, such as in fibromyalgia, are not proven to be effective at all.

Two other important descending inhibitory pathways are also shown in Figure 10-2. One is the descending spinal norepinephrine (NE) pathway (Figure 10-12), which originates in the locus coeruleus (LC), and especially from noradrenergic cell bodies in the lower (caudal) parts of the brainstem neurotransmitter center (lateral tegmental norepinephrine cell system) (Figure 6-32). The other important descending pathway is the descending spinal serotonergic (5HT) pathway (Figure 10-13), which originates in the nucleus raphe magnus of the rostroventromedial medulla and especially the lower (caudal) serotonin nuclei (raphe magnus, raphe pallidus, and raphe obscuris) (Figure 6-33).

Descending noradrenergic neurons inhibit neurotransmitter release from primary afferents directly via inhibitory $α_2$-adrenergic receptors (Figure 10-2), explaining why direct-acting $α_2$ agonists such as clonidine can be useful in relieving pain in some patients. Serotonin inhibits primary afferent terminals via postsynaptic $5HT_{1B/D}$ receptors (Figure 10-2). These inhibitory receptors are G-protein-coupled, and indirectly influence ion channels to hyperpolarize the nerve terminal and inhibit nociceptive neurotransmitter release. However, serotonin is also a major transmitter in descending *facilitation* pathways to the spinal cord. Serotonin released onto some primary afferent neuron terminals in certain areas of the dorsal horn acts predominantly via excitatory $5HT_3$ receptors to enhance neurotransmitter release from these primary afferent neurons (Figure 10-2). The combination of both inhibitory and facilitatory actions of serotonin may explain why SSRIs, with actions that increase only serotonin levels, are not consistently useful in the treatment of pain, whereas SNRIs, with actions on both serotonin and norepinephrine, are now proven to be effective in various neuropathic pain states, including diabetic peripheral neuropathic pain and fibromyalgia.

Descending inhibition, mostly via serotonergic and noradrenergic pathways, is normally active at rest and is thought to act physiologically to mask perception of irrelevant nociceptive input (e.g., from digestion, joint movement, etc.: Figures 10-12A and 10-13A). One hypothesis for why patients with depression or fibromyalgia or related chronic pain disorders perceive pain when there is no obvious sign of peripheral trauma is that descending inhibition may not be acting adequately to mask irrelevant nociceptive input. This leads to the perception of pain from what is actually normal input that is ordinarily ignored (Figures 10-12B and 10-13B). If this descending monoaminergic inhibition is enhanced with an SNRI, irrelevant nociceptive inputs from joints, muscles, and the back in fibromyalgia and depression, and from digestion and the gastrointestinal tract in irritable bowel syndrome, are hypothetically once again ignored and thus are no longer perceived as painful (Figures 10-12C and 10-13C). SNRIs include duloxetine, milnacipran, venlafaxine, desvenlafaxine, and some tricyclic antidepressants (TCAs). SNRIs and TCAs are discussed extensively in Chapter 7.

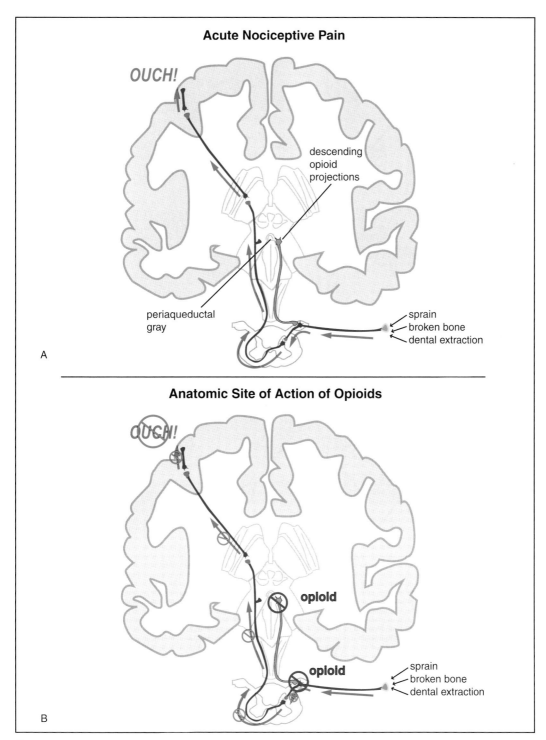

Figure 10-11. Acute nociceptive pain and opioids. Descending opioid projections are activated by severe injury or "danger" to inhibit nociceptive neurotransmission in the dorsal horn, which allows the individual to escape any immediate danger without being compromised. (A) Shown here is nociceptive input from a peripheral injury being transmitted to the brain and interpreted as pain. The descending opioid projection is not activated and thus is not inhibiting the nociceptive input. (B) Endogenous opioid release in the descending opioid projection, or exogenous administration of an opioid, can cause inhibition of nociceptive neurotransmission in the dorsal horn or in the periaqueductal gray and thus prevent or reduce the experience of pain.

Descending NE Inhibition of Pain

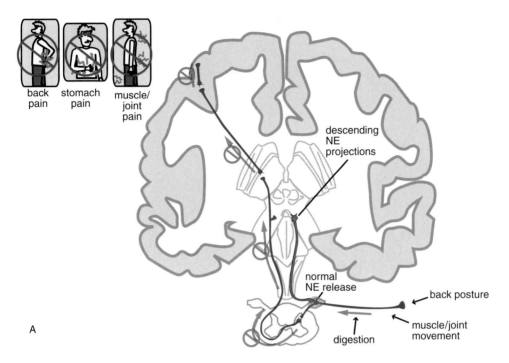

Deficient NE Inhibition Leads to Pain

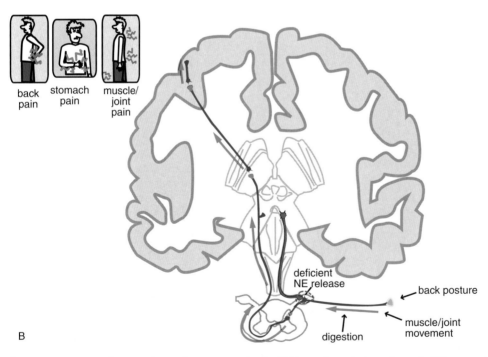

Figure 10-12. Descending noradrenergic neurons and pain. (A) Descending spinal noradrenergic (NE) neurons inhibit neurotransmitter release from primary afferent neurons via presynaptic α_2-adrenergic receptors, and inhibit activity of dorsal horn neurons via postsynaptic α_2-adrenergic receptors. This suppresses bodily input (e.g., regarding muscles/joints or digestion) from reaching the brain and thus prevents it from being interpreted as painful. (B) If descending NE inhibition is deficient, then it may not be sufficient to mask irrelevant nociceptive input, potentially leading to perception of pain from input that is normally ignored. This may be a contributing factor for painful somatic symptoms in fibromyalgia, depression, irritable bowel syndrome, and anxiety disorders.

SNRI Action Boosts NE Inhibition of Pain

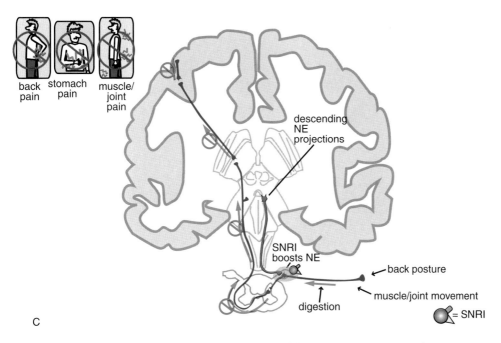

Figure 10-12. (*cont.*) (C) A serotonin–norepinephrine reuptake inhibitor (SNRI) can increase noradrenergic neurotransmission in the descending spinal pathway to the dorsal horn, and thus may enhance inhibition of bodily input so that it does not reach the brain and get interpreted as pain.

Descending inhibition is also activated during severe injury by incoming nociceptive input, and in dangerous "conflict" situations via limbic structures, causing the release of endogenous opioid peptides (Figure 10-11B), serotonin (Figure 10-13A), and nor-epinephrine (Figure 10-12A). When this happens, this reduces not only the release of nociceptive neurotransmitters in the dorsal horn (Figure 10-2) but also the transmission of nociceptive impulses up the spinal cord into the brain (Figure 10-3), thereby reducing the perception of pain, dulling it to allow escape from the situation without the injury com-promising physical performance in the short run (reduction of "ouch" in Figure 10-3). On return to safety, descending facilitation replaces the inhibition to redress the balance, increases awareness of the injury, and forces rest of the injured part (lots of "ouch" in Figure 10-3).

The power of this system can be seen in humans persevering through severe injury on the sports field and on the battlefield. The placebo effect may also involve endogenous opioid release from these des-cending inhibitory neurons (Figure 10-11B), since activation of a placebo response to pain is reversible by the μ-opioid antagonist naloxone. These are adap-tive changes within the pain pathways that facilitate survival and enhance function for the individual. However, maladaptive changes can also hijack these same mechanisms to inappropriately maintain pain without relevant tissue injury, as may occur in various forms of neuropathic pain ranging from diabetes to fibromyalgia and beyond.

Targeting sensitized circuits in chronic pain conditions

Chronic pain perpetuated as a marker of an irrevers-ible sensitization process within the central nervous system has already been discussed as a disorder trig-gered by progressive molecular changes due to abnor-mal neuronal activity within the pain pathway, sometimes called central sensitization. When this occurs at the spinal or segmental level, it is likely linked to the multiple different neurotransmitters released there, with each neurotransmitter's release

Descending 5HT Inhibition of Pain

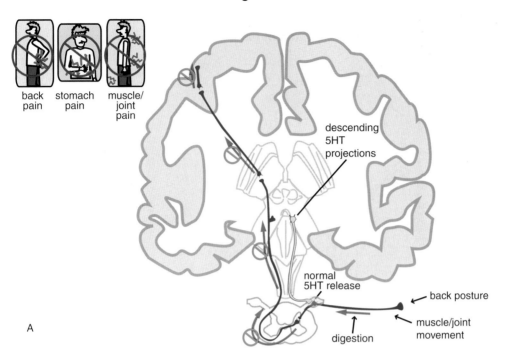

A

Deficient 5HT Inhibition Leads to Pain

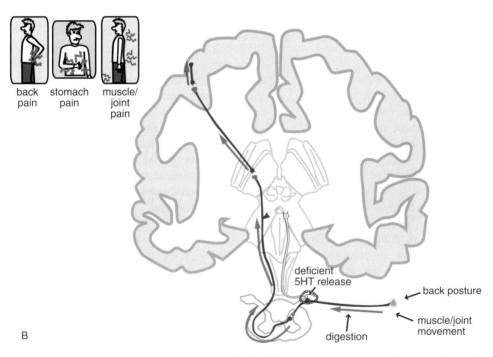

B

Figure 10-13. Descending serotonergic neurons and pain. (A) Descending serotonergic (5HT) neurons directly inhibit activity of dorsal horn neurons, predominantly via 5HT$_{1B/D}$ receptors. This suppresses bodily input (e.g., regarding muscles/joints or digestion) from reaching the brain and thus prevents it from being interpreted as painful. (B) If descending 5HT inhibition is deficient, it may not be sufficient to mask irrelevant nociceptive input, potentially leading to perception of pain from input that is normally ignored. This may be a contributing factor for painful somatic symptoms in fibromyalgia, depression, irritable bowel syndrome, and anxiety disorders. (C) A serotonin–norepinephrine reuptake inhibitor (SNRI) can increase serotonergic neurotransmission in the descending spinal pathway to the dorsal horn, and thus may enhance inhibition of bodily input so that it does not reach the brain and get interpreted as pain. However, the noradrenergic effects of SNRIs may be more relevant to suppression of nociceptive input.

SNRI Action Boosts 5HT Inhibition of Pain

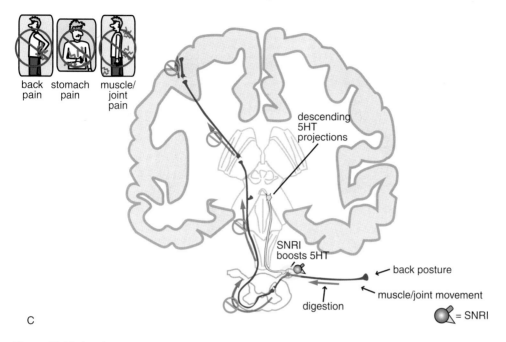

back pain   stomach pain   muscle/ joint pain

descending 5HT projections

SNRI boosts 5HT

back posture

muscle/joint movement

digestion

= SNRI

C

Figure 10-13. *(cont.)*

mechanism requiring presynaptic depolarization and activation of N-type and P/Q-type voltage-sensitive calcium channels (VSCCs: Figures 10-14 and 10-15), which is often coupled to the release of glutamate but also to aspartate, substance P (SP), calcitonin-gene-related peptide (CGRP), and other neurotransmitters (Figure 10-2). When this occurs at suprasegmental levels in the thalamus and cortex, it is likely linked to release mostly of glutamate via the same N-type and P/Q-type VSCCs (Figures 10-14 and 10-15). The idea is that low release of neurotransmitter creates no pain response because there is insufficient neurotransmitter release to stimulate the postsynaptic receptors (Figure 10-14A). However, normal amounts of neurotransmitter release cause a full nociceptive pain response and acute pain (Figure 10-14B). Hypothetically, in states of central sensitization there is excessive and unnecessary ongoing nociceptive activity causing neuropathic pain (Figure 10-15A). Blocking VSCCs with the $\alpha_2\delta$ ligands gabapentin or pregabalin (Figure 10-16) inhibits release of various neurotransmitters in the dorsal horn (Figures 10-2, 10-15B, 10-17A) or in the thalamus and cortex (Figures 10-15B and 10-17B) and has indeed proven to be an effective treatment for various disorders causing neuropathic pain (Figure 10-15B). Gabapentin

and pregabalin (Figure 10-16), may more selectively bind the "open channel" conformation of VSCCs (Figure 10-18), and thus be particularly effective in blocking those channels that are the most active, with a "use-dependent" form of inhibition (Figures 10-15B, 10-17, 10-18B). This molecular action predicts more affinity for centrally sensitized VSCCs that are actively conducting neuronal impulses within the pain pathway, and thus having a selective action on those VSCCs causing neuropathic pain, ignoring other VSCCs that are not open, and thus not interfering with normal neurotransmission in central neurons uninvolved in mediating the pathological pain state.

Treatment of pain, including neuropathic pain conditions, may be less costly when you "pay" for it in advance, or at least early in the game. The hope is that early treatment of pain could interfere with the development of chronic persistent painful conditions by blocking the ability of painful experiences to imprint themselves upon the central nervous system by not allowing triggering of central sensitization. Thus, the mechanisms whereby symptomatic suffering of chronic neuropathic pain is relieved – such as with SNRIs or $\alpha_2\delta$ ligands – may also be the same mechanisms that could prevent disease progression to chronic persistent pain states. This notion calls for aggressive

Subthreshold Pain Response

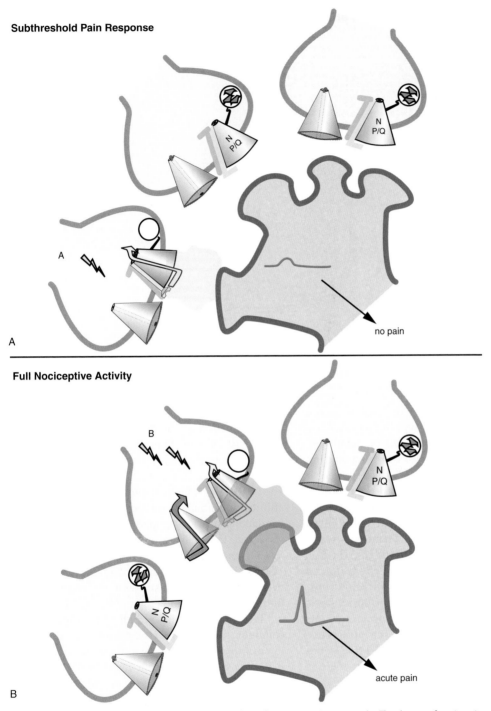

Full Nociceptive Activity

Figure 10-14. Activity-dependent nociception in pain pathways, part 1: acute pain. The degree of nociceptive neuronal activity in pain pathways determines whether one experiences acute pain. An action potential on a presynaptic neuron triggers sodium influx, which in turn leads to calcium influx and ultimately release of neurotransmitter. (A) In some cases, the action potential generated at the presynaptic neuron causes minimal neurotransmitter release; thus the postsynaptic neuron is not notably stimulated and the nociceptive input does not reach the brain (in other words, there is no pain). (B) In other cases, a stronger action potential at the presynaptic neuron may cause voltage-sensitive calcium channels to remain open longer, allowing more neurotransmitter release and more stimulation of the postsynaptic neuron. Thus, the nociceptive input is transmitted to the brain and acute pain occurs.

**Central Sensitization and
Excessive Nociceptive Activity**

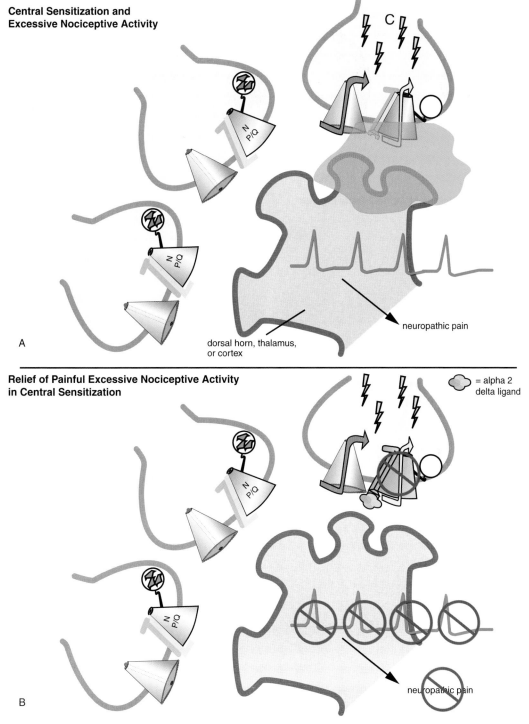

**Relief of Painful Excessive Nociceptive Activity
in Central Sensitization**

Figure 10-15. Activity-dependent nociception in pain pathways, part 2: neuropathic pain. (A) Strong or repetitive action potentials can cause prolonged opening of calcium channels, which may lead to excessive release of neurotransmitter into the synaptic cleft, and consequently to excessive stimulation of postsynaptic neurons. Ultimately this may induce molecular, synaptic, and structural changes, including sprouting, which are the theoretical substrates for central sensitization syndromes. In other words, this can lead to neuropathic pain. (B) $\alpha_2\delta$ ligands such as gabapentin or pregabalin bind to the $\alpha_2\delta$ subunit of voltage-sensitive calcium channels, changing their conformation to reduce calcium influx and therefore reduce excessive stimulation of postsynaptic receptors.

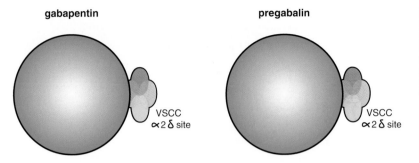

gabapentin

pregabalin

Figure 10-16. Gabapentin and pregabalin. Shown here are icons of the pharmacological actions of gabapentin and pregabalin, two anticonvulsants that also have efficacy in chronic pain. These agents bind to the $\alpha_2\delta$ subunit of voltage-sensitive calcium channels (VSCCs).

Anatomic Actions of Alpha-2-Delta Ligands

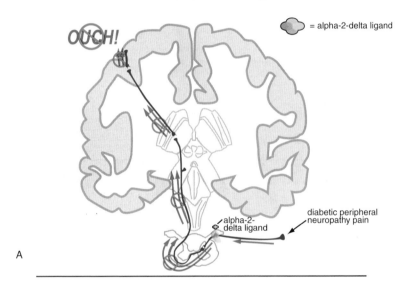

A

Figure 10-17. Anatomic actions of $\alpha_2\delta$ ligands. (A) $\alpha_2\delta$ ligands may alleviate chronic pain associated with sensitization at the level of the dorsal horn. As illustrated here, $\alpha_2\delta$ ligands may bind to voltage-sensitive calcium channels (VSCCs) in the dorsal horn to reduce excitatory neurotransmission and thus alleviate pain. (B) $\alpha_2\delta$ ligands may also alleviate chronic pain associated with sensitization at the level of the thalamus or cortex. As illustrated here, $\alpha_2\delta$ ligands may bind to VSCCs in the thalamus and cortex to reduce excitatory neurotransmission and thus alleviate pain.

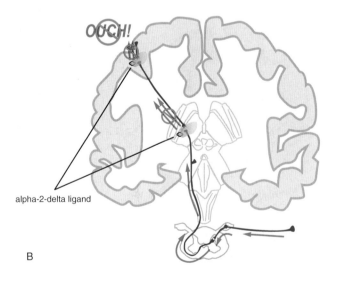

B

Molecular Action of Alpha-2-Delta Ligands

A. Open conformation of VSCC

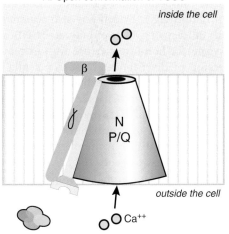

B. Alpha-2-delta ligand binding to open conformation and inhibiting VSCC

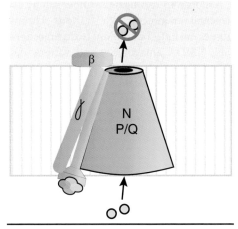

C. Closed conformation of VSCC

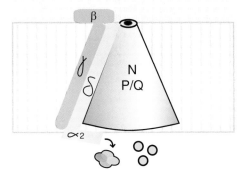

Figure 10-18. Binding of $\alpha_2\delta$ ligands. (A) Calcium influx occurs when voltage-sensitive calcium channels (VSCCs) are in the open-channel conformation. (B) $\alpha_2\delta$ ligands such as gabapentin and pregabalin have greatest affinity for the open-channel conformation and thus block those channels that are most active. (C) When VSCCs are in the closed conformation $\alpha_2\delta$ ligands do not bind and thus do not disrupt normal neurotransmission.

treatment of painful symptoms in these conditions that theoretically have their origin within the CNS, thus "intercepting" the central sensitization process before it is durably imprinted into angry circuits. Thus, major depression and anxiety disorders and fibromyalgia can all be treated with SNRIs and/or $\alpha_2\delta$ ligands to eliminate painful physical symptoms and thereby improve the chances of reaching full symptomatic remission. The opportunity to prevent permanent pain syndromes or progressive worsening of pain is one reason why pain is increasingly being considered a psychiatric "vital sign" that must be assessed routinely in the evaluation and treatment of psychiatric disorders by psychopharmacologists. Future testing of agents capable of reducing pain should be done to determine whether eliminating painful symptoms early in the course of psychiatric and functional somatic illnesses will improve outcomes, including preventing symptomatic relapses, the development of treatment resistance, or even brain atrophy from stress in pain states (Figure 10-10) and hippocampal atrophy from stress in anxiety and affective disorders (Figure 6-39). Pre-emptively treating pain before it occurs, or at least rescuing centrally mediated and sensitizing pain by intercepting such pain before it becomes permanent, may represent some of the most promising therapeutic applications of dual reuptake inhibitors and $\alpha_2\delta$ ligands, and it deserves careful clinical evaluation.

Targeting ancillary symptoms in fibromyalgia

We have repeatedly mentioned the proven usefulness of the $\alpha_2\delta$ ligands gabapentin and pregabalin and the SNRIs duloxetine, milnacipran, venlafaxine, and desvenlafaxine for treating the painful symptoms of fibromyalgia, yet these two classes have not been studied extensively in combination. Nevertheless, they are frequently used together in clinical practice on an empiric basic and anecdotally have been shown to give additive improvement in relieving pain. Each class of drug may also help different ancillary symptoms in fibromyalgia, so the combination of $\alpha_2\delta$ ligands with SNRIs may lead to broader symptom relief than using either alone, although both are effective for pain in fibromyalgia. That is, $\alpha_2\delta$ ligands may reduce symptoms of anxiety in fibromyalgia (see discussion of $\alpha_2\delta$ ligands in anxiety in Chapter 9, illustrated in Figures 9-25C and 9-26C) and for improving the slow-wave sleep disorder of fibromyalgia (sleep disorders and their treatment are discussed in further detail in Chapter 11). SNRIs can be useful in reducing symptoms of depression and anxiety in fibromyalgia (see Chapter 7 on antidepressants and Figures 7-30 through 7-34; see also Chapter 9 on anxiety and Figures 9-25D and 9-26D) and for treating fatigue as well as the cognitive symptoms associated with fibromyalgia, sometimes also called "fibro-fog."

Problems with executive functioning in a wide variety of clinical conditions are generally linked to inefficient information processing in the dorsolateral prefrontal cortex (DLPFC), where dopamine neurotransmission is important in regulating brain circuits (see Chapter 4 on schizophrenia and Figure 4-41; see Chapter 6 on depression and Figures 6-45, 6-48, and 6-49; see Chapter 9 on anxiety disorders and Figure 9-17). This concept of dopaminergic regulation of cognition in DLPFC and the role of boosting dopamine neurotransmission to improve executive dysfunction is also discussed in Chapter 12 on attention deficit hyperactivity disorder. Since SNRIs increase dopamine concentrations in DLPFC (see Figure 7-34C), they can also potentially improve symptoms of "fibro-fog" in fibromyalgia patients. This may be particularly so for the SNRI milnacipran, which has potent norepinephrine reuptake binding properties at all clinically effective doses (Figure 7-32), or for higher doses of the SNRIs duloxetine (Figure 7-31), venlafaxine, and desvenlafaxine (Figure 7-30), which have increased norepinephrine reuptake blocking properties and thus act to increase concentrations of dopamine in the DLPFC (Figure 7-34C). Other strategies for improving fibro-fog in fibromyalgia patients include the same ones used to treat cognitive dysfunction in depression, including modafinil, armodafinil, selective norepinephrine reuptake inhibitors (NRIs) such as atomoxetine, norepinephrine–dopamine reuptake inhibitors (NDRIs) such as bupropion, and, with caution, stimulants. SNRIs, sometimes augmented with modafinil, stimulants, or bupropion, can also be useful for symptoms of physical fatigue as well as mental fatigue in fibromyalgia patients.

Second-line treatments for pain in fibromyalgia can include mirtazapine and tricyclic antidepressants,

as well as the tricyclic muscle relaxant cyclobenzaprine. Sleep aids such as benzodiazepines, hypnotics, and trazodone can be helpful in relieving sleep disturbance in fibromyalgia. Evidence is also accumulating for the efficacy of γ-hydroxybutyrate (GHB or sodium oxybate) in fibromyalgia (use with extreme caution because of diversion and abuse potential). GHB is approved for narcolepsy, enhances slow-wave sleep, and is discussed in Chapter 11 on sleep. In heroic cases the use of GHB by experts for the treatment of severe and treatment-resistant cases of fibromyalgia may be justified. A number of anticonvulsants other than the $\alpha_2\delta$ ligands (Figure 10-19) are also used second line for chronic neuropathic pain states, including fibromyalgia. These agents are thought to target voltage-gated sodium channels rather than voltage-gated calcium channels (Figure 10-19) and thus seem to have a different mechanism of action than $\alpha_2\delta$ ligands and may be effective in patients with inadequate response to $\alpha_2\delta$ ligands. Other adjunctive or experimental treatments for various chronic pain syndromes include botulinum toxin injections, cannabinoids, NMDA antagonists, and various new anticonvulsants.

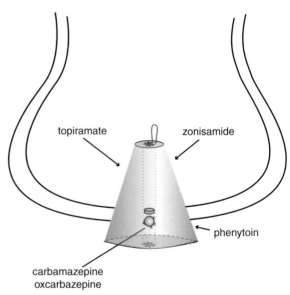

Figure 10-19. Anticonvulsants in chronic pain. A number of anticonvulsants other than the $\alpha_2\delta$ ligands are also used second line for chronic neuropathic pain states, including fibromyalgia. These agents are thought to target voltage-sensitive sodium channels (VSSCs) rather than voltage-sensitive calcium channels (VSCCs) and thus seem to have a different mechanism of action than $\alpha_2\delta$ ligands.

Summary

This chapter has defined pain, and has explained the processing of nociceptive neuronal activity into the perception of pain by pathways that lead to the spinal cord, and then up the spinal cord to the brain. Neuropathic pain is discussed extensively, including both peripheral and central mechanisms, and the concept of central sensitization. The key role of descending inhibitory pathways that reduce the activity of nociceptive pain neurons with the release of serotonin and norepinephrine is explained, and shown to be the basis for the actions of serotonin–norepinephrine reuptake inhibitors (SNRIs) as agents that reduce the perception of pain in conditions ranging from major depression to fibromyalgia to diabetic peripheral neuropathic pain, low back pain, osteoarthritis, and related conditions. The critical role of voltage-sensitive calcium channels (VSCCs) is also explained, providing the basis for the actions of $\alpha_2\delta$ ligands as agents that also reduce the perception of pain in diabetic peripheral neuropathic pain, fibromyalgia, painful physical symptoms of depression and anxiety disorders, shingles, and other neuropathic pain conditions. Finally, the spectrum of conditions from affective disorders to chronic neuropathic pain disorders is introduced, with emphasis on the condition of fibromyalgia and its newly evolving psychopharmacological treatments.

Disorders of sleep and wakefulness and their treatment

This chapter will provide a brief overview of the psychopharmacology of disorders of sleep and wakefulness. Included here are short discussions of the symptoms, diagnostic criteria, and treatments for disorders that cause insomnia, excessive daytime sleepiness, or both. Clinical descriptions and formal criteria for how to diagnose sleep disorders are mentioned here only in passing. The reader should consult standard reference sources for this material. The discussion here will emphasize the links between various brain circuits and their neurotransmitters and disorders that cause insomnia or sleepiness. The goal of this chapter is to acquaint the reader with ideas about the clinical and biological aspects of sleep and wakefulness, how various disorders can alter sleep and wakefulness, and how many new and evolving treatments can resolve the symptoms of insomnia and sleepiness.

The detection, assessment, and treatment of sleep/wake disorders are rapidly becoming standardized parts of a psychiatric evaluation. Modern psychopharmacologists increasingly consider sleep to be a psychiatric "vital sign," requiring routine evaluation and symptomatic treatment whenever sleep disorders are encountered. This is similar to the situation of pain (Chapter 10), which is also increasingly being considered as another psychiatric "vital sign." That is, disorders of sleep (and pain) are so important, so pervasive, and cut across so many psychiatric conditions that the elimination of these symptoms – no matter what psychiatric disorder may be present – is increasingly recognized as necessary in order to achieve full symptomatic remission for the patient.

Many of the treatments discussed in this chapter are covered in previous chapters. For details of mechanisms of insomnia treatments that are also used for the treatment of depression, the reader is referred to Chapter 7. For those insomnia treatments that are benzodiazepines and share the same mechanism of action with various benzodiazepine anxiolytics, the reader is referred to Chapter 9. For various hypersomnia treatments, especially stimulants, the reader is referred to Chapter 12 on ADHD and to Chapter 14 on drug abuse, which also discuss the use and abuse of stimulants. The discussion in this chapter is at the conceptual level, and not at the pragmatic level. The reader should consult standard drug handbooks (such as *Stahl's Essential Psychopharmacology: the Prescriber's Guide*) for details of doses, side effects, drug interactions, and other issues relevant to the prescribing of these drugs in clinical practice.

Neurobiology of sleep and wakefulness
The arousal spectrum

Although many experts approach insomnia and sleepiness by emphasizing the separate and distinct *disorders* that cause them, many pragmatic psychopharmacologists approach insomnia or excessive daytime sleepiness as important *symptoms* that cut across many conditions and that occur along a spectrum from deficient arousal to excessive arousal (Figure 11-1). In this conceptualization, an awake, alert, creative and problem-solving person has the right balance between too much and too little arousal (baseline brain functioning in gray at the middle of the spectrum in Figure 11-1). As arousal increases beyond normal, during the day there is hypervigilance (Figure 11-1); if this increased, arousal occurs at night and there is insomnia (Figure 11-1, and overactivation of the brain in red at the right-hand side of the spectrum in Figure 11-2). From a treatment perspective, insomnia can be conceptualized as a disorder of excessive nighttime arousal, with hypnotics moving the patient from too much arousal to sleep (Figure 11-2).

On the other hand, as arousal diminishes, symptoms crescendo from mere inattentiveness to more severe forms of cognitive disturbances until the patient has excessive daytime sleepiness with sleep attacks (Figure 11-1, and hypoactivation of the brain in blue at the left-hand side of the spectrum in Figure 11-3). From a treatment perspective, sleepiness can be conceptualized as a disorder of deficient daytime arousal, with wake-promoting agents moving the patient from too little arousal to awake with normal alertness (Figure 11-3).

Note in Figure 11-1 that cognitive disturbance is the product of both too little and too much arousal, consistent with the need of cortical pyramidal neurons to be optimally "tuned," with too much activity making them just as out of tune as too little. Note also in Figures 11-1 through 11-3 that the arousal spectrum is linked to the actions of five neurotransmitters shown in the brains represented in these figures (i.e., histamine, dopamine,

norepinephrine, serotonin, and acetylcholine). Sometimes these neurotransmitter circuits as a group are called the ascending reticular activating system, because they are known to work together to regulate arousal. This same ascending neurotransmitter system is blocked at several sites by many agents that cause sedation. Actions of sedating drugs on these neurotransmitters are discussed in Chapter 5 on antipsychotics and illustrated in Figure 5-38. Figure 11-1 also shows that excessive arousal can extend past insomnia to panic, hallucinations, and all the way to frank psychosis (far right-hand side of the spectrum).

The sleep/wake switch

We have discussed how the ascending neurotransmitter systems from the brainstem regulate a cortical arousal system on a smooth continuum like a rheostat on a lighting system or a volume button on a radio. There is another set of circuits in the hypothalamus that regulate sleep and wake discontinuously, like an on/off switch. Not surprisingly, this circuitry is called the *sleep/wake switch* (Figure 11-4). The "on" switch is known as the *wake promoter* and is localized within the tuberomammillary nucleus (TMN) of the hypothalamus (Figure 11-4A). The "off" switch is known as the *sleep promoter* and is localized within the ventrolateral preoptic (VLPO) nucleus of the hypothalamus (Figure 11-4B).

Two other sets of neurons are shown in Figure 11-4 as regulators of the sleep/wake switch: orexin-containing neurons of the lateral hypothalamus (LAT) and melatonin-sensitive neurons of the suprachiasmatic nucleus (SCN). The lateral hypothalamus serves to stabilize and promote wakefulness via a peptide neurotransmitter known by two different names: orexin and hypocretin. These lateral hypothalamic neurons and their orexin are lost in narcolepsy, especially narcolepsy with cataplexy. New hypnotics on the horizon (orexin antagonists) block the receptors for these neurotransmitters and are discussed later in this chapter. The SCN is the brain's internal clock, or pacemaker, and regulates circadian input to the sleep/wake switch in response to how it is programmed by hormones such as melatonin and by the light/dark cycle. Circadian rhythms and the SCN are discussed in Chapter 7 on antidepressants and illustrated in Figures 7-39 to 7-42.

Arousal Spectrum of Sleep and Wakefulness

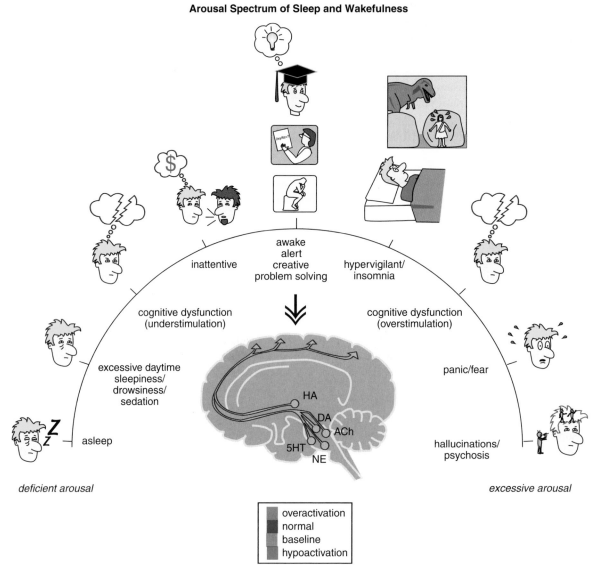

Figure 11-1. Arousal spectrum of sleep and wakefulness. One's state of arousal is more complicated than simply being "awake" or "asleep." Rather, arousal exists as if on a dimmer switch, with many phases along the spectrum. Where on the spectrum one lies is influenced in large part by five key neurotransmitters: histamine (HA), dopamine (DA), norepinephrine (NE), serotonin (5HT), and acetylcholine (ACh). When there is good balance between too much and too little arousal (depicted by the gray [baseline] color of the brain), one is awake, alert, and able to function well. As the dial shifts to the right there is too much arousal, which may cause hypervigilance and consequently insomnia at night. As arousal further increases this can cause cognitive dysfunction, panic, and in extreme cases perhaps even hallucinations. On the other hand, as arousal diminishes, individuals may experience inattentiveness, cognitive dysfunction, sleepiness, and ultimately sleep.

The circadian wake drive is shown in Figure 11-5 over two full 24-hour cycles. Also shown in Figure 11-5 is the ultradian sleep cycle (a cycle faster than a day, showing cycling in and out of REM and slow-wave sleep several times during the night). Homeostatic sleep drive, illustrated as well in Figure 11-5, increases the drive for sleep as the day goes on, presumably due to fatigue, and diminishes at night with rest. The novel neurotransmitter adenosine is linked to homeostatic drive, and appears to accumulate as this drive increases during the day, and to diminish at night. Caffeine is now known to be an antagonist of

Insomnia: Excessive Nighttime Arousal?

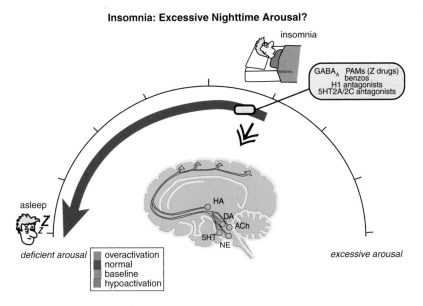

Figure 11-2. Insomnia: excessive nighttime arousal? Insomnia is conceptualized as being related to hyperarousal at night, depicted here as the brain being red (overactive). Agents that reduce brain activation, such as positive allosteric modulators of GABA$_A$ receptors (e.g., benzodiazepines, "Z drugs"), histamine 1 antagonists, and serotonin 2A/2C antagonists, can shift one's arousal state from hyperactive to sleep.

Excessive Daytime Sleepiness: Deficient Daytime Arousal?

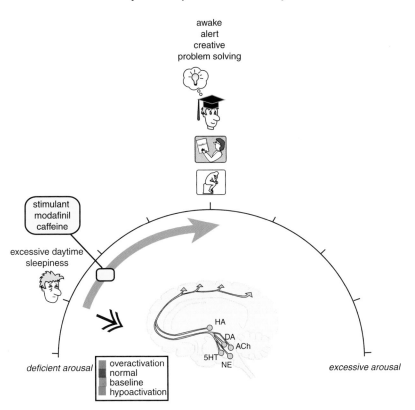

Figure 11-3. Excessive daytime sleepiness: deficient daytime arousal. Excessive sleepiness is conceptualized as being related to hypoarousal during the day, depicted here as the brain being blue (hypoactive). Agents that increase brain activation, such as the stimulants, modafinil, and caffeine, can shift one's arousal state from hypoactive to awake with normal alertness.

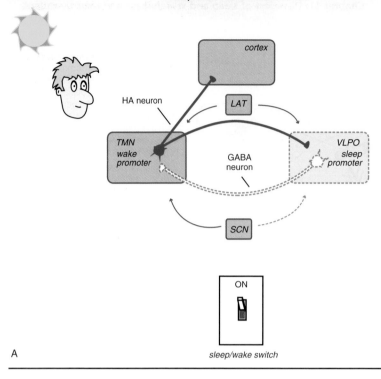

A   *sleep/wake switch*

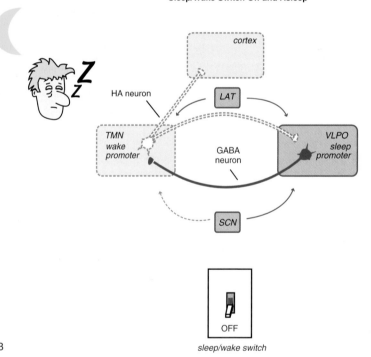

B   *sleep/wake switch*

Figure 11-4. Sleep/wake switch. The hypothalamus is a key control center for sleep and wake, and the specific circuitry that regulates sleep/wake (i.e., whether the dimmer switch is set all the way to the left for sleep or is somewhere else along the continuum for wake) is called the sleep/wake switch. The "off" setting, or sleep promoter, is localized within the ventrolateral preoptic nucleus (VLPO) of the hypothalamus, while "on" – the wake promoter – is localized within the tuberomammillary nucleus (TMN) of the hypothalamus. Two key neurotransmitters regulate the sleep/wake switch: histamine from the TMN and GABA from the VLPO. (A) When the TMN is active and histamine is released to the cortex and the VLPO, the wake promoter is on and the sleep promoter inhibited. (B) When the VLPO is active and GABA is released to the TMN, the sleep promoter is on and the wake promoter inhibited. The sleep/wake switch is also regulated by orexin/hypocretin neurons in the lateral hypothalamus (LAT), which stabilize wakefulness, and by the suprachiasmatic nucleus (SCN) of the hypothalamus, which is the body's internal clock and is activated by melatonin, light, and activity to promote either sleep or wake.

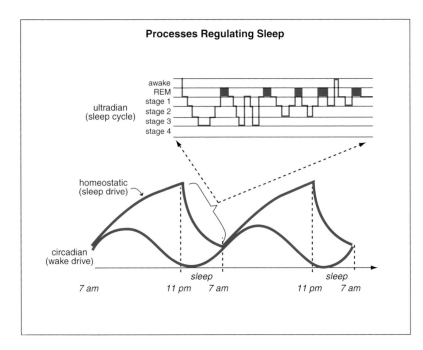

Processes Regulating Sleep

Figure 11-5. Processes regulating sleep. Several processes that regulate sleep/wake are shown here. The circadian wake drive is a result of input (light, melatonin, activity) to the suprachiasmatic nucleus. Homeostatic sleep drive increases the longer one is awake and decreases with sleep. As the day progresses, circadian wake drive diminishes and homeostatic sleep drive increases until a tipping point is reached and the ventrolateral preoptic sleep promoter (VLPO) is triggered to release GABA in the tuberomammillary nucleus (TMN) and inhibit wakefulness. Sleep itself consists of multiple phases that recur in a cyclical manner; this process is known as the ultradian cycle, and is depicted at the top of this figure.

adenosine, and this may explain in part its ability to promote wakefulness and diminish fatigue, namely by opposing endogenous adenosine's regulation of the homeostatic sleep drive.

Two key neurotransmitters regulate the sleep/wake switch: histamine from the TMN and GABA (γ-aminobutyric acid) from the VLPO. Thus, when the sleep/wake switch is on, the wake promoter TMS is active and histamine is released (Figure 11-4). This occurs both in the cortex to facilitate arousal, and in the VLPO to inhibit the sleep promoter. As the day progresses, circadian wake drive diminishes and homeostatic sleep drive increases (Figure 11-5); eventually a tipping point is reached, and the VLPO sleep promoter is triggered, the sleep/wake switch is turned off, and GABA is released in the TMN to inhibit wakefulness (Figure 11-4).

Disorders characterized by excessive daytime sleepiness can be conceptualized as the sleep/wake switch being off during the daytime. Wake-promoting treatments such as modafinil given during the day tip the balance back to wakefulness by promoting the release of histamine from TMN neurons. The exact mechanism of this enhancement of histamine release by modafinil or stimulants is not known, but is currently hypothesized to be related in part to a downstream consequence of the actions of wake-promoting drugs on dopamine

neurons, especially by blocking the dopamine transporter DAT.

On the other hand, disorders characterized by insomnia can be conceptualized as the sleep/wake switch being on at night. Insomnia can be treated either by agents that enhance GABA actions, and thus inhibit the wake promoter, or by agents that block the action of histamine released from the wake promoter and act at postsynaptic H_1 receptors.

Disorders characterized by a disturbance in circadian rhythm can be conceptualized as either "phase delayed," with the wake promoter and sleep/wake switch being turned on too late in a normal 24-hour cycle, or "phase advanced," with the wake promoter and sleep/wake switch being turned on too early in a normal 24-hour cycle. That is, individuals who are phase delayed, including many depressed patients and many normal adolescents, still have their sleep/wake switch off when it is time to get up (see discussion in Chapter 7 and Figure 7-39). Giving such individuals morning light and evening melatonin can reset the circadian clock in the SCN so that it wakes the person up earlier. Other individuals may be phase advanced, including many normal elderly people. Giving these individuals evening light and morning melatonin can reset their SCNs so that the sleep/wake switch stays off a bit longer, returning the patient to a normal rhythm.

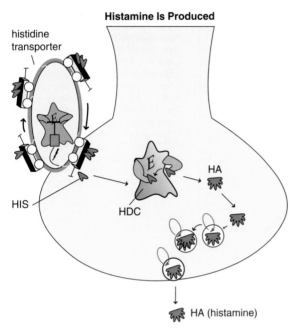

Figure 11-6. Histamine is produced. Histidine (HIS), a precursor to histamine, is taken up into histamine nerve terminals via a histidine transporter and converted into histamine by the enzyme histidine decarboxylase (HDC). After synthesis, histamine is packaged into synaptic vesicles and stored until its release into the synapse during neurotransmission.

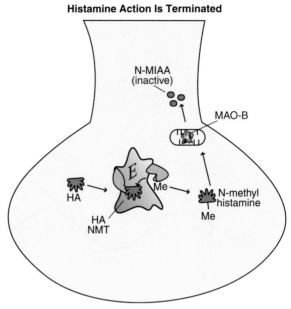

Figure 11-7. Histamine's action is terminated. Histamine can be broken down intracellularly by two enzymes. Histamine N-methyl-transferase (histamine NMT) converts histamine into N-methyl-histamine, which is then converted by monoamine oxidase B (MAO-B) into the inactive substance N-methyl-indole-acetic acid (N-MIAA).

Histamine

Histamine is one of the key neurotransmitters regulating wakefulness, and is the ultimate target of many wake-promoting drugs (via downstream histamine release) and sleep-promoting drugs (antihistamines). Histamine is produced from the amino acid histidine, which is taken up into histamine neurons and converted to histamine by the enzyme histidine decarboxylase (Figure 11-6). Histamine's action is terminated by two enzymes working in sequence: histamine N-methyl-transferase, which converts histamine to N-methyl-histamine, and MAO-B, which converts N-methyl-histamine into N-MIAA (N-methyl-indole-acetic acid), an inactive substance (Figure 11-7). Additional enzymes such as diamine oxidase can also terminate histamine action outside of the brain. Note that there is no apparent reuptake pump for histamine. Thus, histamine is likely to diffuse widely away from its synapse, just like dopamine does in prefrontal cortex.

There are a number of histamine receptors (Figures 11-8 through 11-11). The postsynaptic histamine 1 (H_1) receptor is best known (Figure 11-9A)

because it is the target of "antihistamines" (i.e., H_1 antagonists) (Figure 11-9B). When histamine itself acts at H_1 receptors, it activates a G-protein-linked second-messenger system that activates phosphatidyl inositol, and the transcription factor cFOS, and results in wakefulness, normal alertness, and pro-cognitive actions (Figure 11-9A). When these H_1 receptors are blocked in the brain, they interfere with the wake-promoting actions of histamine, and thus can cause sedation, drowsiness, or sleep (Figure 11-9B).

Histamine 2 (H_2) receptors, best known for their actions in gastric acid secretion and the target of a number of anti-ulcer drugs, also exist in the brain (Figure 11-10). These postsynaptic receptors also activate a G-protein second-messenger system with cAMP, phosphokinase A, and the gene product CREB. The function of H_2 receptors in brain is still being clarified, but apparently is not linked directly to wakefulness.

A third histamine receptor is present in brain, namely the H_3 receptor (Figures 11-8 and 11-11). Synaptic H_3 receptors are presynaptic (Figure 11-11A) and function as autoreceptors (Figure 11-11B). That is, when histamine binds to these receptors, it turns

Histamine Receptors

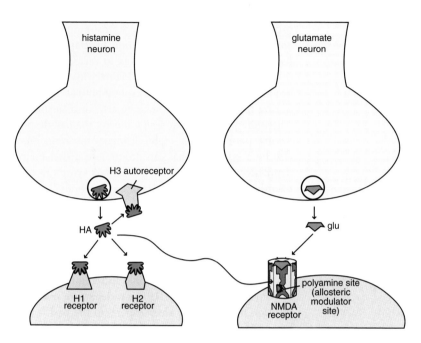

Figure 11-8. Histamine receptors. Shown here are receptors for histamine that regulate its neurotransmission. Histamine 1 and histamine 2 receptors are postsynaptic, while histamine 3 receptors are presynaptic autoreceptors. There is also a binding site for histamine on NMDA receptors – it can act at the polyamine site, which is an allosteric modulatory site.

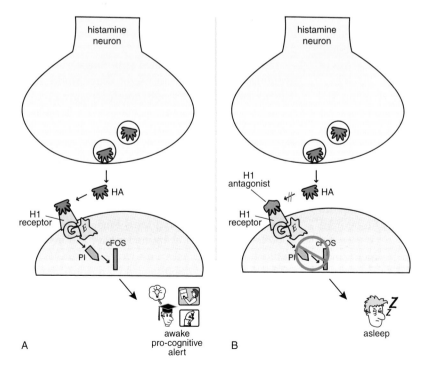

Figure 11-9. Histamine 1 receptors. (A) When histamine binds to postsynaptic histamine 1 receptors, it activates a G-protein-linked second-messenger system that activates phosphatidyl inositol and the transcription factor cFOS. This results in wakefulness and normal alertness. (B) Histamine 1 antagonists prevent activation of this second messenger and thus can cause sleepiness.

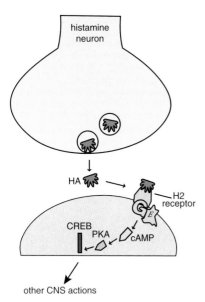

Figure 11-10. Histamine 2 receptors. Histamine 2 receptors are present both in the body and in the brain. When histamine binds to postsynaptic histamine 2 receptors it activates a G-protein-linked second-messenger system with cAMP, phosphokinase A, and the gene product CREB. The function of histamine 2 receptors in the brain is not yet elucidated but does not appear to be directly linked to wakefulness.

off further release of histamine (Figure 11-11B). One novel approach to new wake-promoting and pro-cognitive drugs is to block these receptors, thus facilitating the release of histamine, allowing histamine to act at H_1 receptors to produce the desired effects (Figure 11-11C). Several H_3 antagonists are in clinical development.

There is a fourth type of histamine receptor, H_4, but these are not known to occur in the brain. Finally, histamine acts also at NMDA (*N*-methyl-D-aspartate) receptors (Figure 11-8). Interestingly, when histamine diffuses away from its synapse to a glutamate synapse containing NMDA receptors, it can act at an allosteric modulatory site called the polyamine site, to alter the actions of glutamate at NMDA receptors (Figure 11-8). The role of histamine and function of this action are not well clarified.

Histamine neurons all arise from a single small area of the hypothalamus known as the tuberomammillary nucleus (TMN), which is part of the sleep/wake switch illustrated in Figure 11-4. Thus, histamine plays an important role in arousal, wakefulness, and sleep. The TMN is a small bilateral nucleus that provides histaminergic input to most brain regions and to the spinal cord (Figure 11-12).

Insomnia and hypnotics
What is insomnia?

Insomnia has many causes, including both sleep disorders and psychiatric disorders. Insomnia can also contribute to the onset, exacerbation, or relapse of many psychiatric disorders and is linked to various dysfunctions in many medical illnesses. Primary insomnia may be a condition with too much arousal both at night and during the day, and thus may be a form of insomnia where the patient is not sleepy during the day despite having poor sleep at night. Primary insomnia may also be a symptom that can progress to a first major depressive episode. Thus, is insomnia a symptom or a disorder? The answer appears to be "yes, both."

Chronic treatment for chronic insomnia?

A major reconceptualization of insomnia has recently occurred among experts, with a newly formed consensus that insomnia can be chronic and that it may need to be treated chronically. This is a departure from the position held by many sleep experts in the past – that insomnia was treated by attacking its underlying cause, and not by giving chronic "symptomatically masking" treatment with hypnotics. The old guidelines recommending short-term use of hypnotics for insomnia were the product of safety concerns for hypnotics identified first during the barbiturate era and then during the benzodiazepine era.

Other problems associated with long-term use of hypnotics have to do with use of drugs whose half-lives are not ideal for use as hypnotics (Figure 11-13A, B, and C). That is, many agents used as hypnotics, particularly in the past, have half-lives that are too long (Figure 11-13A and B). This can cause drug accumulation and hip fractures from falls, especially in the elderly, when such agents are used every night (Figure 11-13A). Long half-life can also cause next-day carryover effects and sedation and memory problems from residual daytime drug levels (Figure 11-13A and B). Other agents used as hypnotics have half-lives that are too short, and their effects can wear off before it is time to wake up, causing insufficient sleep maintenance and nocturnal awakenings, as well as restless and disturbed sleep in some patients (Figure 11-13C). More recently, however, the hypnotics given most frequently for chronic use are those that have optimized half-lives targeting rapid onset of action, and plasma drug levels above the minimally effective concentration, but only until it is time to

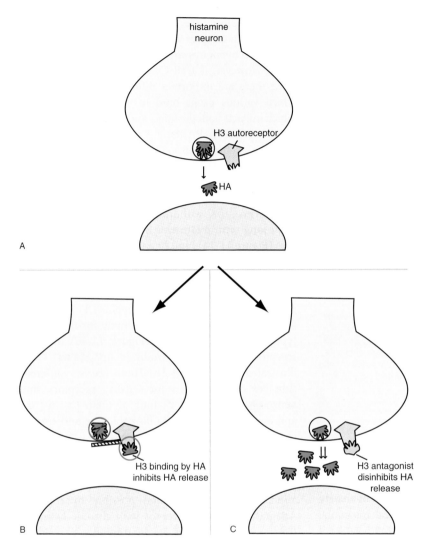

histamine
neuron

H3 autoreceptor

HA

A

H3 binding by HA
inhibits HA release

B

H3 antagonist
disinhibits HA
release

C

Figure 11-11. Histamine 3 receptors. Histamine 3 receptors are presynaptic autoreceptors (A), which means that when histamine binds to these receptors it turns off further histamine release (B). Antagonists of these receptors, which are in development, therefore disinhibit histamine release (C) and may hypothetically enhance alertness and cognition.

wake up (Figure 11-13D). Perhaps no therapeutic area of psychopharmacology is as critically dependent upon plasma drug levels, and thus the pharmacokinetics of the drug, as is the use of hypnotics. This fact may be related to the nature of the arousal system and of the sleep/wake switch, which requires pharmacologic action to a degree sufficient to reach the critical tipping point that trips the switch "off" to allow sleep, but only at night.

Other reasons for short-term restrictions on benzodiazepine hypnotics (Figure 11-14) in the past had to do with their long-term effects, including loss of efficacy over time (tolerance) and withdrawal effects, including rebound insomnia in some patients worse than their original insomnia (Figure 11-15A). Recent investigations have shown that some non-

benzodiazepine hypnotics may not have these problems (Figure 11-15B). These include the GABA$_A$ positive allosteric modulators (PAMs), sometimes also called "Z drugs" (because they all start with the letter Z: zaleplon, zolpidem, zopiclone) (Figure 11-16). Perhaps the best long-term studies have been done with eszopiclone, which shows little or no tolerance, dependence, or withdrawal with use for many months (Figure 11-15B). This is probably also the case for long-term use of zolpidem, zolpidem CR, and the melatonergic agent ramelteon, as well as for "off-label" use of the sedating antidepressant trazodone, none of which have restrictions against chronic use. For these reasons, it is now recognized that chronic insomnia may need chronic treatment with certain hypnotics.

Histaminergic Projections from the Hypothalamus

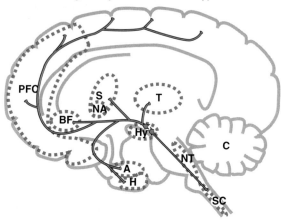

the histamine center is in the hypothalamus (TMN, tuberomammillary nucleus), which provides input to most brain regions and the spinal cord

Figure 11-12. Histaminergic projections from the hypothalamus. In the brain, histamine (HA) is produced solely by cells in the tuberomammillary nucleus (TMN) of the hypothalamus (Hy). From the TMN, histaminergic neurons project to various brain regions including the prefrontal cortex (PFC), the basal forebrain (BF), the striatum (S) and nucleus accumbens (NA), the amygdala (A) and hippocampus (H), brainstem neurotransmitter centers (NT), and spinal cord (SC).

Benzodiazepine hypnotics

There are at least five benzodiazepines approved specifically for insomnia in the US (Figure 11-14), although there are several others in different countries. Various benzodiazepines developed for the treatment of anxiety disorders are also frequently used to treat insomnia. Benzodiazepine anxiolytics are discussed in Chapter 9 and their mechanism of action is illustrated in Figure 9-23. Because benzodiazepines do not have ideal half-lives for many patients (Figure 11-13A, B, and C), and can cause long-term problems (Figure 11-15A), they are generally considered second-line agents for use as hypnotics. However, when first-line agents fail to work, benzodiazepines still have a place in the treatment of insomnia, particularly for insomnia associated with various psychiatric and medical illnesses.

GABA$_A$ positive allosteric modulators (PAMs) as hypnotics

These hypnotics act at GABA$_A$ receptors to enhance the action of GABA by binding to a site different from where GABA itself binds to this receptor.

Benzodiazepines are classified as GABA$_A$ PAMs (discussed in Chapter 9 and illustrated in Figure 9-23). Barbituate hypnotics are yet another type of GABA$_A$ PAM. However, not all GABA$_A$ PAMs are the same, since there are important differences in the ways in which various drugs bind to the GABA$_A$ receptor, which impacts both the safety and the efficacy of various classes of GABA$_A$ PAMs.

That is, the GABA$_A$ PAMs zaleplon, zolpidem, and zopiclone (Figure 11-16) appear to bind to the GABA$_A$ receptor in a way that does not cause a high degree of tolerance to their therapeutic actions, dependence, or withdrawal upon discontinuation from long-term treatment. By contrast, benzodiazepines (Figure 11-14) bind in a manner that changes the conformation of the GABA$_A$ receptor such that tolerance generally develops, as well as some degree of dependence and withdrawal, especially for some patients and for some benzodiazepines. Furthermore, for some Z drugs, there is specificity for the α_1 subtype of GABA$_A$ receptor (Figure 11-16). GABA$_A$ receptor subtypes are introduced in Chapter 9 and illustrated in Figure 9-21. There are six different subtypes of α subunits for GABA$_A$ receptors, and benzodiazepines bind to four of them (α_1, α_2, α_3, and α_5) (Figure 11-14), as do zopiclone and eszopiclone (Figure 11-16). The α_1 subtype is known to be critical for producing sedation and thus is targeted by every effective GABA$_A$ PAM hypnotic. The α_1 subtype is also linked to daytime sedation, anticonvulsant actions, and possibly to amnesia. Adaptations of this receptor with chronic hypnotic treatments that target it are thought to lead to tolerance and withdrawal. The α_2 and α_3 receptor subtypes are linked to anxiolytic, muscle relaxant, and alcohol-potentiating actions. Finally, the α_5 subtype, mostly in the hippocampus, may be linked to cognition and other functions. Zaleplon and zolpidem are α_1 selective (Figure 11-16). The functional significance of selectivity is not yet proven, but may contribute to the lower risk of tolerance and dependence of these agents.

Modifications of two of the Z drugs, zolpidem and zopiclone, are available for clinical use. For zolpidem, a controlled-release formulation known as zolpidem CR (Figure 11-16) extends the duration of action of zolpidem immediate-release from about 2–4 hours (Figure 11-13B) to a more optimized duration of 6–8 hours, improving sleep maintenance (Figure 11-13D). An alternative dosage formulation of zolpidem for

Ultralong Half-Life Hypnotics Cause Drug Accumulation (Toxicity)

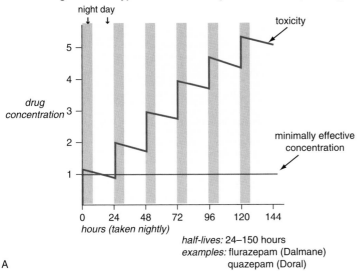

half-lives: 24–150 hours
examples: flurazepam (Dalmane)
quazepam (Doral)

A

**Moderately Long Half-Life Hypnotics Do Not Wear off Until
After Time to Awaken (Hangover)**

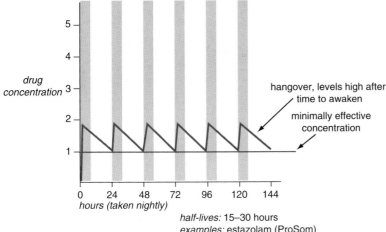

half-lives: 15–30 hours
examples: estazolam (ProSom)
temazepam (Restoril)
most TCAs
mirtazapine (Remeron)
olanzapine (Zyprexa)

B

Figure 11-13. Half-lives of hypnotics. The half-lives of hypnotics can have an important impact on their tolerability and efficacy profiles. (A) Hypnotics with ultra-long half-lives (greater than 24 hours: for example, flurazepam and quazepam) can cause drug accumulation with chronic use. This can cause impairment that has been associated with increased risk of falls, particularly in the elderly. (B) Hypnotics with moderate half-lives (15–30 hours: estazolam, temazepam, most tricyclic antidepressants, mirtazapine, olanzapine) may not wear off until after the individual needs to awaken and thus may have "hangover" effects (sedation, memory problems). (C) Hypnotics with ultra-short half-lives (1–3 hours: triazolam, zaleplon, zolpidem, melatonin, ramelteon) can wear off before the individual needs to awaken and thus cause loss of sleep maintenance. (D) Hypnotics with half-lives that are short but not ultra-short (approximately 6 hours: zolpidem CR and perhaps low doses of trazodone or doxepin) may provide rapid onset of action and plasma levels above the minimally effective concentration only for the duration of a normal night's sleep.

sublingual administration with faster onset and given at a fraction of the usual nighttime dose is also available for middle-of-the-night administration for patients who have middle insomnia. For zopiclone, a racemic mixture of both R and S zopiclone, there is the introduction of the S enantiomer, eszopiclone (Figure 11-16). Clinically meaningful differences between the active enantiomer and the racemic mixture are debated.

Psychiatric insomnia and the GABA$_A$ PAMs

In many ways, the introduction of the Z drugs has contributed to the reconceptualization of the treatment of chronic insomnia. That is, optimized pharmacokinetic durations of action (Figure 11-13D) coupled with studies establishing safety in long-term use without a high incidence of tolerance or dependence (Figure 11-15B) have opened the door to the treatment of chronic insomnia

455

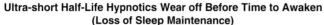

Figure 11-13. (*cont.*)

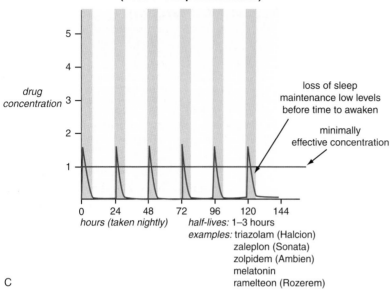

Ultra-short Half-Life Hypnotics Wear off Before Time to Awaken (Loss of Sleep Maintenance)

drug concentration

loss of sleep maintenance low levels before time to awaken

minimally effective concentration

hours (taken nightly)

half-lives: 1–3 hours

examples: triazolam (Halcion)
zaleplon (Sonata)
zolpidem (Ambien)
melatonin
ramelteon (Rozerem)

C

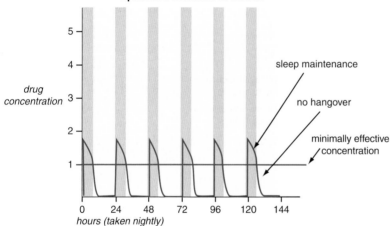

Optimized Duration of Action

drug concentration

sleep maintenance

no hangover

minimally effective concentration

hours (taken nightly)

half-lives/duration of action: 6 hours

examples: eszopiclone (Lunesta)
zolpidem CR (Ambien CR)
? low-dose trazodone (Desyrel)
? low-dose doxepin (Silenor)
? low-dose quetiapine (Seroquel)
? low-dose diphenhydramine (Benadryl)

D

chronically. However, most studies of hypnotics are in primary insomnia, not in insomnia associated with psychiatric disorders, leading to fewer clear guidelines as to how to use hypnotics to treat insomnia in conditions such as depression, anxiety disorders, bipolar disorder, etc.

Investigators are currently beginning to address the appropriate use, including long-term use, of concomitant hypnotics for various psychiatric disorders. For example, recent studies have shown that hypnotics may enhance remission rates both for patients with major depression who have insomnia and for patients with generalized anxiety disorder (GAD) who have insomnia (Figure 11-17). Not only do the symptoms of insomnia improve as expected when patients with GAD or major depression are

Benzo Hypnotics

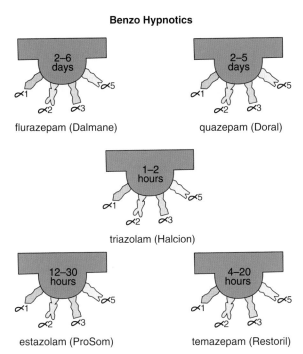

flurazepam (Dalmane)

quazepam (Doral)

triazolam (Halcion)

estazolam (ProSom)

temazepam (Restoril)

Figure 11-14. Benzo hypnotics. Five benzodiazepines that are approved in the United States for insomnia are shown here. These include flurazepam and quazepam, which have ultra-long half-lives; triazolam, which has an ultra-short half-life; and estazolam and temazepam, which have moderate half-lives.

treated with eszopiclone added to an SSRI (e.g., fluoxetine or escitalopram), but so do the other symptoms of GAD or depression, leading to higher remission rates (Figure 11-17). Whether this applies to all Z drugs, or indeed to any hypnotic of any mechanism that is successful in improving insomnia added to any antidepressant for these conditions, is not yet known. Whether treating insomnia will also help prevent future episodes of depression or GAD is also not known, but considering that insomnia is perhaps the most frequent residual symptom after treating depression with an antidepressant (discussed in Chapter 7 and illustrated in Figure 7-5), it makes intuitive sense to utilize hypnotics as augmenting agents to first-line treatments for depression or anxiety disorders, and if necessary to utilize hypnotics chronically to eliminate symptoms of insomnia in these conditions.

Melatonergic hypnotics

Melatonin is the neurotransmitter secreted by the pineal gland, and acts especially in the suprachiasmatic nucleus (SCN) to regulate circadian rhythms (discussed in

Chapter 7 and illustrated in Figures 7-42A through 7-42D). Figures 7-42A and 7-42B show the effects of light and dark, respectively, on melatonin. The melatonergic antidepressant agomelatine (Figures 7-41, 7-42D, 11-18) shifts circadian rhythms in depressed subjects with phase delay (Figure 7-42C). Melatonin itself, as well as selective melatonin receptor agonists such as ramelteon or tasimelteon (Figure 11-18), has similar actions on shifting circadian rhythms in individuals without depression but who have phase delay (many normal teenagers) or phase advance (many normal elderly people), or in those experiencing jet lag from travel-induced shifts in circadian rhythms. It is also known that melatonin and selective melatonin receptor agonists (Figure 11-18) are effective hypnotics for sleep onset. Melatonin is available over the counter in the US, in doses that are not always reliable. Commercially available melatonin in a controlled-release formulation is available outside the US.

Melatonin acts at three different sites, not only melatonin 1 (MT_1) and melatonin 2 (MT_2) receptors, but also at a third site, sometimes called the melatonin 3 site, which is now known to be the enzyme NRH: quinone oxidoreductase 2, and which is probably not involved in sleep physiology (Figure 11-18). MT_1-mediated inhibition of neurons in the SCN could help to promote sleep by decreasing the wake-promoting actions of the circadian "clock" or "pacemaker" that functions there, perhaps by attenuating the SCN's alerting signals, allowing sleep signals to predominate and thus inducing sleep. Phase shifting and circadian rhythm effects of the normal sleep/wake cycle are thought to be primarily mediated by MT_2 receptors which entrain these signals in the SCN.

Ramelteon is an MT_1/MT_2 agonist marketed for insomnia, and tasimelteon, another MT_1/MT_2 agonist, is in clinical testing (Figure 11-18). These agents improve sleep onset, sometimes better when used for several days in a row. They are not known to help sleep maintenance, but will induce natural sleep in those subjects who suffer mostly from initial insomnia.

Serotonergic hypnotics

One of the most popular hypnotics among psychopharmacologists is the antidepressant trazodone. This sedating antidepressant with a half-life of only about 6–8 hours was recognized long ago by clinicians as

Long-Term Effects of Benzo Hypnotics

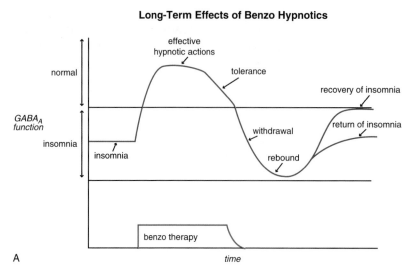

A

Long-Term Effects of GABA_A PAMs ("Z drugs")

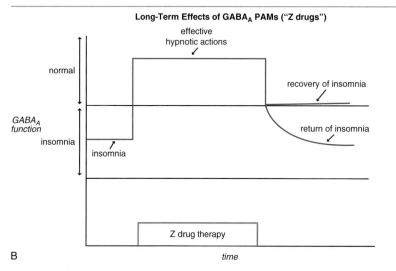

B

Figure 11-15. Long-term effects of hypnotics. (A) Short-term, benzodiazepines can be efficacious for treating insomnia. With long-term use, however, benzodiazepines may cause tolerance and, if discontinued, withdrawal effects that may include rebound insomnia. (B) Positive allosteric modulators (PAMs) at GABA_A receptors are efficacious for insomnia in the short term, and in the long term do not seem to cause tolerance or withdrawal effects.

being highly effective as a hypnotic when given at a lower dose than that used as an antidepressant, and by giving it just once a day at night (see discussion in Chapter 7 and Figures 7-47 through 7-50). In fact, although trazodone was never officially approved as a hypnotic, nor marketed as a hypnotic, it nevertheless accounts for up to half of all prescriptions for hypnotics.

How does trazodone work? In Chapter 7, trazodone's mechanism as an antidepressant is discussed and illustrated (Figures 7-47 through 7-50). It is clear that to act as an antidepressant, the dose of trazodone must be sufficiently high to recruit not only its most potent 5HT$_{2A}$ antagonist properties, but also its serotonin reuptake blocking properties (Figures 7-48 and 7-49). At these doses, trazodone can be quite

sedating, because its H$_1$ antihistamine and α$_1$ antagonist properties are also recruited. Contributions of H$_1$ antagonism and α$_1$-adrenergic antagonism to sedation are discussed in Chapter 5 and illustrated in Figure 5-38.

By trial and error, if not by serendipity, clinicians discovered that trazodone's half-life is actually an advantage when this drug is administered as a hypnotic (Figure 7-50), because its daytime sedating effects, which are so evident when administering high doses twice daily for depression, can be greatly diminished by giving this short-half-life agent only at night and by lowering its dose (Figure 7-48). However, in doing so, trazodone loses its serotonin reuptake blocking properties, and thus its antidepressant actions, yet retains α$_1$ blocking actions, as well as H$_1$ antagonist and 5HT$_{2A}$ antagonist actions (Figure 7-48).

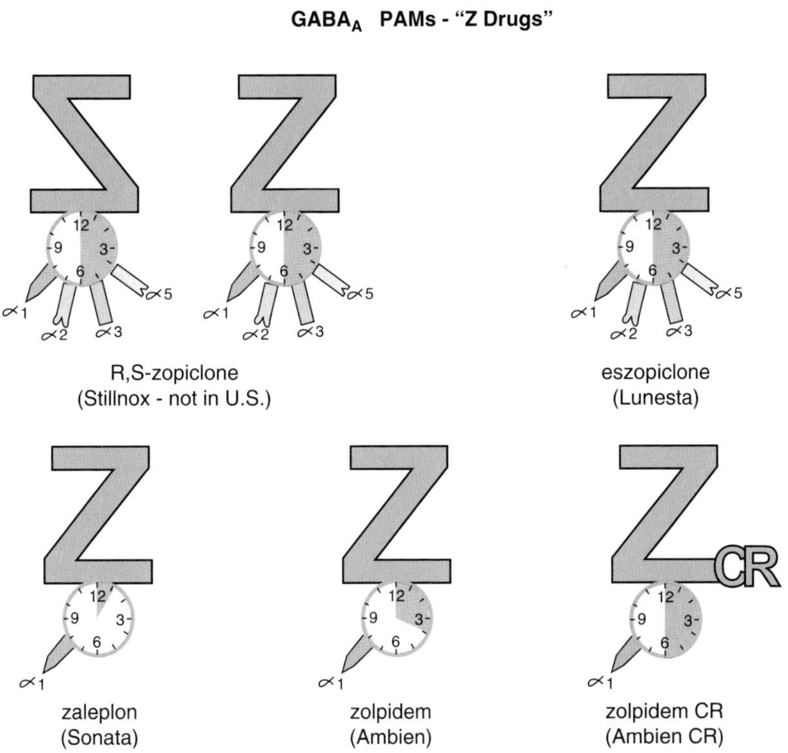

GABA$_A$ PAMs - "Z Drugs"

R,S-zopiclone
(Stillnox - not in U.S.)

eszopiclone
(Lunesta)

zaleplon
(Sonata)

zolpidem
(Ambien)

zolpidem CR
(Ambien CR)

Figure 11-16. GABA$_A$ positive allosteric modulators (PAMs). Several GABA$_A$ PAMs, or "Z drugs," are shown here. These include racemic zopiclone (not available in the United States), eszopiclone, zaleplon, zolpidem, and zolpidem CR. Zaleplon, zolpidem, and zolpidem CR are selective for GABA$_A$ receptors that contain the a_1 subunit; however, it does not appear that zopiclone or eszopiclone have this same selectivity.

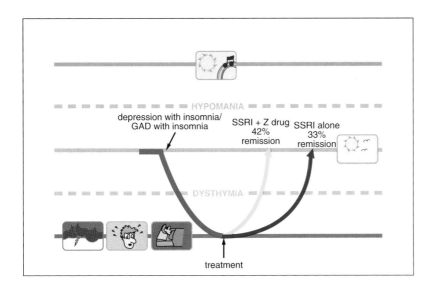

Figure 11-17. Treating psychiatric insomnia. Insomnia is a common residual symptom of psychiatric disorders, including depression and generalized anxiety disorder (GAD). Recent findings suggest that remission rates may be increased in depression or GAD with insomnia when a hypnotic is added to first-line antidepressant treatment, and that this is attributable not only to improvement in insomnia but also to improvement in other symptoms.

Histamine H$_1$ antagonists as hypnotics

It is widely appreciated that antihistamines are sedating. Antihistamines are popular as over-the-counter sleep aids (especially those containing diphenhydramine/ Benadryl or doxylamine) (Figure 11-19). Because antihistamines have been widely used for many years, there is the common misperception that the properties of classic agents such as diphenhydramine apply to any drug with antihistaminic properties. This includes the idea that all antihistamines have "anticholinergic" side effects such as blurred vision, constipation, memory

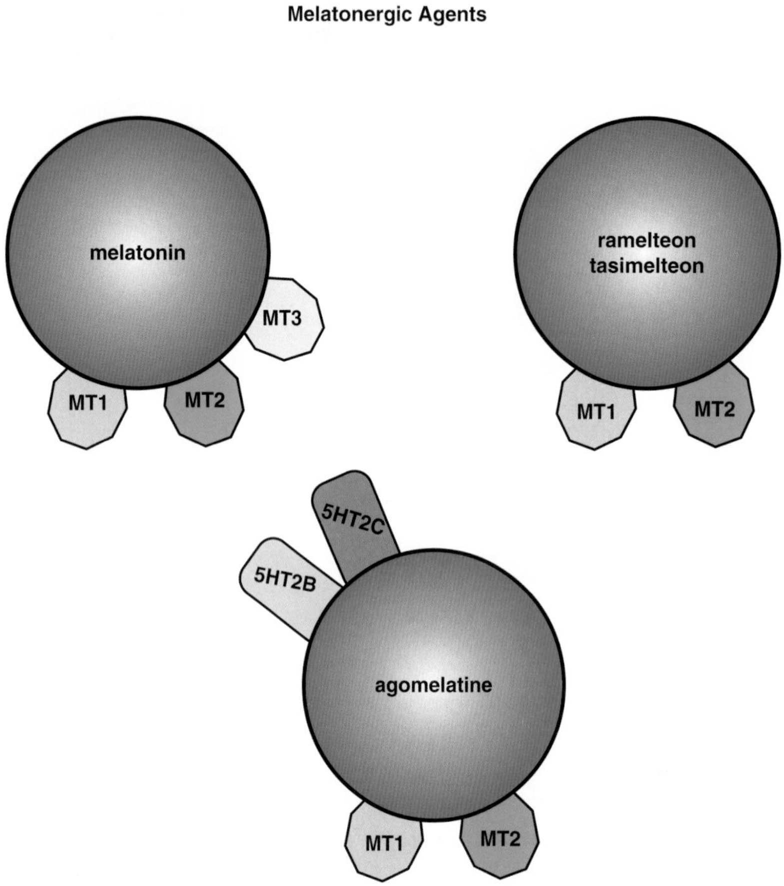

Melatonergic Agents

melatonin

MT3

MT1 MT2

ramelteon
tasimelteon

MT1 MT2

5HT2C

5HT2B

agomelatine

MT1 MT2

Figure 11-18. Melatonergic agents. Endogenous melatonin is secreted by the pineal gland and mainly acts in the suprachiasmatic nucleus to regulate circadian rhythms. There are three types of receptors for melatonin: melatonin 1 and 2 (MT_1 and MT_2), which are both involved in sleep, and melatonin 3, which is actually the enzyme NRH:quinine oxidoreductase 2 and not thought to be involved in sleep physiology. There are several different agents that act at melatonin receptors, as shown here. Melatonin itself, available over the counter, acts at MT_1 and MT_2 receptors as well as at the melatonin 3 site. Both ramelteon and tasimelteon are MT_1 and MT_2 receptor agonists and seem to provide sleep onset though not necessarily sleep maintenance. Agomelatine is not only an MT_1 and MT_2 receptor agonist, but is also a $5HT_{2C}$ and $5HT_{2B}$ receptor antagonist and is available as an antidepressant in Europe.

What Is Diphenhydramine's (Benadryl's) Mechanism as a Hypnotic?

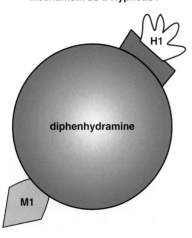

H1

diphenhydramine

M1

Figure 11-19. Diphenhydramine. Diphenhydramine is a histamine 1 receptor antagonist commonly used as a hypnotic. However, this agent is not selective for histamine 1 receptors and thus can also have additional effects. Specifically, diphenhydramine is also a muscarinic 1 receptor antagonist and thus can have anticholinergic effects (blurred vision, constipation, memory problems, dry mouth).

problems, dry mouth; that they cause next-day hangover effects when used as hypnotics at night; that tolerance develops to their hypnotic actions; that they cause weight gain.

It now seems that these ideas about antihistamines arise from the fact that most agents with potent antihistamine properties, from diphenhydramine, to tricyclic antidepressants (discussed in Chapter 7 – see Figures 7-62 through 7-70), mirtazapine (also discussed in Chapter 7 – see Figure 7-45), quetiapine (discussed in Chapter 5 as "baby bear" – see Figures 5-47 through 5-50) and many others, are not selective for H_1 receptors at normal therapeutic doses, and that many of the undesirable properties classically associated with antihistamines are probably due to other receptor actions, not to H_1 antagonism per se. In particular, diphenhydramine and many of the agents classified as antihistamines are also potent antagonists of muscarinic receptors (Figure 11-19), so it is not generally possible to separate the antihistamine

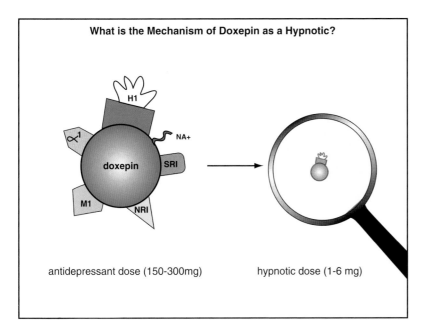

What is the Mechanism of Doxepin as a Hypnotic?

antidepressant dose (150-300mg)   hypnotic dose (1-6 mg)

Figure 11-20. Doxepin. Doxepin is a tricyclic antidepressant (TCA) that, at antidepressant doses (150–300 mg/day), inhibits serotonin and norepinephrine reuptake and is an antagonist at histamine 1, muscarinic 1, and α_1-adrenergic receptors. At low doses (1–6 mg/day), however, doxepin is quite selective for histamine 1 receptors and thus may be used as a hypnotic.

actions of such agents from their antimuscarinic actions in clinical use. The same is true for most tricyclic antidepressants, which have antimuscarinic and α_1-adrenergic blocking properties in addition to their antihistaminic properties (Figures 7-62, 7-68, 7-69).

Some interesting findings are beginning to emerge from clinical investigations of H_1 selective antagonists as hypnotics. The prototype of this approach is very low doses of the tricyclic antidepressant doxepin (Figure 11-20). Because of the very high affinity of doxepin for the H_1 receptor, it is possible to make it into an H_1 selective antagonist just by lowering the dose (Figure 11-20). This agent is so selective at low doses that it is even being used as a PET ligand to label CNS H_1 receptors selectively. At doses a small fraction of those necessary for its antidepressant actions, doxepin can occupy a substantial number of CNS H_1 receptors (e.g., at 1–6 mg of doxepin as a hypnotic compared to 150–300 mg of doxepin as an antidepressant) (Figure 11-20). Furthermore, doxepin is actually a mixture of two chemical forms, one of which (and its active metabolites) has a shorter half-life (8–15 hours) than the other, which has a traditional long tricyclic antidepressant half-life of 24 hours. Functionally, the mixture of the two agents means that nighttime administration yields substantially less residual plasma drug levels in the morning compared to tricyclics with a 24-hour half-life, thus reducing daytime carryover effects.

Although it is not surprising that very low doses of doxepin that selectively antagonize H_1 histamine receptors are effective hypnotics, early clinical testing is revealing that long-term administration of doxepin provides rapid sleep induction with all-night sleep maintenance but without next-day carryover effects, development of tolerance to its hypnotic efficacy, or weight gain. Eliminating α_1-adrenergic and muscarinic cholinergic blockade may explain the lack of anticholinergic side effects, and the lack of development of tolerance to hypnotic actions. Although agents with H_1 antagonist properties can cause weight gain, apparently H_1 selective antagonism without $5HT_{2C}$ antagonism may not be associated with weight gain. These mechanisms are discussed in relation to weight gain in Chapter 5 (illustrated in Figures 5-36 and 5-41 through 5-44) and in Chapter 14 (illustrated in Figure 14-21).

Dopamine agonists and $\alpha_2\delta$ ligands for insomnia associated with restless legs syndrome (RLS)

A common cause of insomnia that is neither primary insomnia nor insomnia secondary to a psychiatric illness is insomnia secondary to restless legs syndrome (Table 11-1). Rather than using traditional sedative hypnotics for insomnia secondary to RLS, first-line treatment is with dopamine agonists such as ropinirole or pramipexole, and second-line treatment

Table 11-1 Restless legs syndrome (RLS) versus periodic limb movement disorder (PLMD)

Clinically diagnosed as urge to move the legs, worse during inactivity, relieved in part by movement, worse in the evening

Can prevent or delay onset of sleep; disrupt sleep if RLS returns; tiredness or sleepiness next day

May be idiopathic or symptomatic (i.e., associated with pregnancy, end-stage renal disease, fibromyalgia, iron deficiency, arthritis, peripheral neuropathy, radiculopathy)

Can be triggered by alcohol, nicotine, caffeine

Majority of RLS patients have PLMD, but only a few PLMD patients have RLS; both may be linked to dopamine or iron deficiency

RLS patients should have iron, iron stores and ferritin levels (ferritin is a cofactor of tyrosine hydroxylase, which synthesizes dopamine)

RLS is not PLMD, which occurs during sleep and is diagnosed by polysomnogram; has no urge sensation to move while awake

Treatments for RLS

Primary

- Dopamine agonists (ropinirole, pramipexole) (may cause somnolence, nausea)
- Iron replacement
- Levodopa (fast onset but short acting – may just delay onset of RLS until later at night unless redosed)

Secondary

- Gabapentin/pregabalin especially if RLS painful; low-potency opioids (propoxyphene, codeine)
- Benzodiazepines or $GABA_A$ PAMs

Table 11-2 Good sleep hygiene

Avoid naps

Use the bed for sleeping, not reading, TV, etc.

Avoid alcohol, caffeine, and nicotine before sleep

Avoid strenuous exercise before sleep

Limit time in bed to sleep time (get up if not asleep within 20 minutes and return to bed when sleepy)

Don't clock-watch

Adopt regular sleep/wake habits

Avoid bright light late at night, and expose self to light in the morning

Table 11-3 Behavioral treatments for insomnia

Stimulus control therapy (go into bedroom only when drowsy)

Progressive muscular relaxation (tense and relax muscles top to bottom of body)

Sleep restriction (consolidate sleep by progressive lengthening of sleep time)

Imagery training (try to stay awake as long as possible)

Biofeedback (learn to recognize arousal with feedback from skin, muscle and brain monitors)

Cognitive therapy (eliminate faulty beliefs and attitudes about sleep)

Sleep hygiene education (understand interaction between lifestyle, environment, and sleep)

is with $\alpha_2\delta$ ligands such as gabapentin or pregabalin (Table 11-1).

Behavioral treatments of insomnia

One should not forget improvement of sleep hygiene (Table 11-2), nor cognitive behavioral approaches (Table 11-3), as adjunctive treatments of insomnia of any cause, and as first-line treatments for primary insomnia, as these can be quite effective in selected patients with various types of insomnia.

Who cares about slow-wave sleep?

The exact function of stage 3 and 4 sleep (delta or slow-wave sleep) remains under active investigation. Not all patients with insomnia have a deficiency of slow-wave sleep, and not all patients with a deficiency of slow-wave sleep have insomnia. However, some empiric clinical observations suggest that a deficiency of slow-wave sleep can contribute to a sense of lack of restorative sleep, and daytime fatigue. Patients with pain syndromes and a deficiency of slow-wave sleep can experience enhanced daytime subjective experience of their pain; patients with depression and a deficiency of slow-wave sleep can have enhanced symptoms of fatigue, apathy, and cognitive dysfunction. Thus, sufficient restorative slow-wave sleep seems intuitively like a good thing to have, but the proof of how much is enough, and what the implications are of too little slow-wave sleep, remain elusive.

Orexin Projections from the Hypothalamus

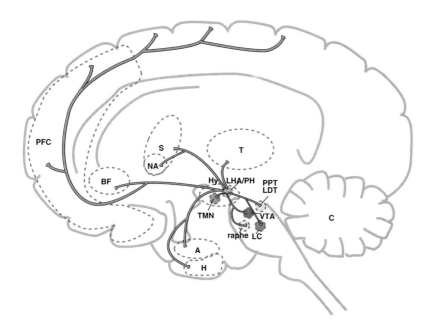

Figure 11-21. Orexin projections from the hypothalamus. The neurotransmitter orexin (also called hypocretin) is made by cells located in the hypothalamus, specifically in the lateral hypothalamic area (LHA) and the perifornical and posterior hypothalamus (PH). Orexin A and orexin B produced by these cells are released at various brain areas, including monoamine neurotransmitter centers in the hypothalamic tuberomammillary nucleus (TMN; for histamine) and in the brainstem such as the ventral tegmental area (VTA; for dopamine), the locus coeruleus (LC; for norepinephrine), the pedunculopontine tegmental and laterodorsal tegmental nuclei (PPT/LDT; for acetylcholine), and raphe nucleus (for serotonin).

Some agents such as serotonergic antidepressants (SSRIs, SNRIs), stimulants, and stimulating antidepressants (e.g., NDRIs) can all interfere with slow-wave sleep, and a limited number of agents are known to enhance slow-wave sleep. These include $\alpha_2\delta$ ligands (e.g., gabapentin and pregabalin), the GABA reuptake inhibitor tiagabine, and $5HT_{2A/2C}$ antagonists including trazodone and GHB (the $GABA_B$-enhancing agent γ-hydroxybutyrate, also known as sodium oxybate). Augmenting the treatment of fatigue and pain with slow-wave sleep-enhancing agents can sometimes reduce these symptoms.

Orexin antagonists as novel hypnotics

Orexin neurons are localized exclusively in certain hypothalamic areas (lateral hypothalamic area, perifornical area, and posterior hypothalamus) (Figure 11-21). These orexin neurons make the neurotransmitters orexin A and orexin B, which are released from their neuronal projections all over the brain, but especially in the monoamine neurotransmitter centers in the brainstem (Figure 11-21). The postsynaptic actions of the orexins are mediated by two receptors called orexin 1 and orexin 2 (Figure 11-22). The neurotransmitter orexin A interacts with both orexin 1 and 2 receptors but orexin B interacts only

with orexin 2 receptors (Figure 11-22). Notably, orexin 1 receptors are particularly highly expressed in the brainstem locus coeruleus, site of noradrenergic neurons; orexin 2 receptors are highly expressed in the TMN (tuberomammillary nucleus), site of histamine neurons. It is believed that the effect of orexin on wakefulness is largely mediated by activation of the TMN histaminergic neurons that express orexin 2 receptors. Presumably orexin 2 receptors therefore play a pivotal role, with orexin 1 receptors playing an additional role in sleep/wake regulation. Orexins mediate behaviors in addition to wakefulness and vigilance; they also regulate feeding behavior and reward, perhaps particularly through orexin 1 receptors.

Lack of orexins is associated with narcolepsy. Pharmacologic blockade of orexin receptors has been investigated not only as a novel hypnotic mechanism, but also for weight loss and to treat drug abuse. Specifically, both the dual orexin receptor antagonists (DORAs) for both orexin 1 and 2 receptors, and single orexin receptor antagonists (SORA1s and SORA2s), selective either for orexin 1 receptors or for orexin 2 receptors, have been developed (Figure 11-23) and are being extensively tested at this time. DORAs such as almorexant, SB-649868, and suvorexant (also known as MK-4305) have

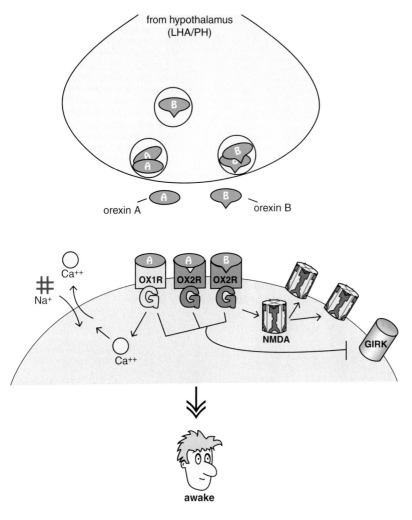

Figure 11-22. Orexin receptors. Orexin neurotransmission is mediated by two types of postsynaptic G-protein-coupled receptors, orexin 1 (Ox1R) and orexin 2 (Ox2R). Orexin A is capable of interacting with both Ox1R and Ox2R, whereas orexin B binds selectively to Ox2R. Binding of orexin A to Ox1R receptors leads to increased intracellular calcium as well as activation of the sodium/calcium exchanger. Binding of orexin A and B to Ox2R leads to increased expression of NMDA (*N*-methyl-D-aspartate) glutamate receptors as well as inactivation of G-protein-regulated inward rectifying potassium channels (GIRK). Ox1R are found particularly highly expressed in the noradrenergic locus coeruleus, whereas Ox2R are highly expressed in the histaminergic tuberomammillary nucleus (TMN).

preliminary evidence of efficacy in the treatment of insomnia, and some are advancing in clinical trials, particularly suvorexant. Other DORAs include MK-6096, DORA 1, DORA 5, and DORA 22, Single-action SORAs are also in development with SORA1 agents (e.g., SB-334867, SB674042, SB408124, SB410220) proving not to be particularly robust in treating insomnia, but with promising preliminary preclinical results for SORA2 agents (e.g., EMPA, JNJ10394049).

Notably, the localization of orexin 1 and 2 receptors, coupled with the lack of preclinical effects of some orexin 1 antagonists on sleep, suggests that the wake-promoting effects of orexins are mediated mainly by orexin 2 receptors or a combination of orexin 1 and 2 receptors (Figure 11-24). Thus, hypnotics are either DORAs targeting both receptors or SORA2s targeting orexin 2 receptors. SORA1s

targeting orexin 1 receptors are in development as possible treatments to reduce craving for drugs or food (see discussion in Chapter 14).

To date, the DORA suvorexant appears to improve both the initiation and maintenance of sleep in human subjects, without the side effects expected of a benzodiazepine or Z-drug hypnotic, namely lacking dependence, withdrawal, rebound, unsteady gait, falls, confusion, amnesia, or respiratory depression (Figures 11-23 and 11-24). So far the theoretical possibility that DORAs could cause a reversible form of narcolepsy with hypnagogic hallucinations, sleep paralysis, and cataplexy has not been observed. It appears that acute, short-lived, and intermittent temporary blockade of orexin receptors is well tolerated without the induction of a narcolepsy-like syndrome.

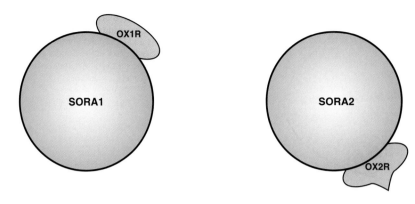

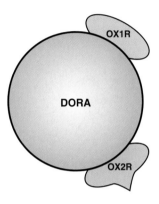

Figure 11-23. Orexin receptor antagonists. Several orexin receptor antagonists are currently in testing as hypnotics. Single orexin receptor antagonists (SORAs) work selectively at orexin 1 receptors (SORA1) or at orexin 2 receptors (SORA2). Dual orexin antagonists (DORAs) that bind both orexin 1 and orexin 2 receptors are also being studied.

Excessive daytime sleepiness (hypersomnia) and wake-promoting agents

What is sleepiness?

Sleepiness is a term that is sometimes used synonymously with hypersomnia. Here we will discuss the symptom of excessive daytime sleepiness, its causes, and especially its treatment with three wake-promoting agents: caffeine, modafinil, and stimulants. The most common cause of sleepiness is sleep deprivation, and the treatment is sleep, not drugs. Other causes of excessive daytime sleepiness are various sleep disorders, psychiatric disorders, medications, and medical disorders (Table 11-4). Although society often devalues sleep and can often imply that only wimps complain of sleepiness, it is clear that excessive daytime sleepiness is not benign, and in fact can even be lethal. That is, loss of sleep causes performance decrements equivalent to intoxication with alcohol and, not surprisingly, traffic accidents and fatalities. Thus, sleepiness is important to assess even though patients often do not complain about it when they have it. Comprehensive assessment of patients with sleepiness requires additional information be obtained from the patient's partner, particularly the bed partner. Most conditions can be evaluated by patient and partner interviews, but sometimes augmented with subjective ratings of sleepiness such as the Epworth Sleepiness Scale, as well as objective evaluations of sleepiness such as overnight polysomnograms, plus next-day multiple sleep latency testing and/or maintenance of wakefulness testing (Table 11-5).

What's wrong with being sleepy?

Patients with excessive daytime sleepiness have problems with cognitive functioning. For example, when patients with narcolepsy or sleep deprivation try to perform cognitive testing, with great effort

465

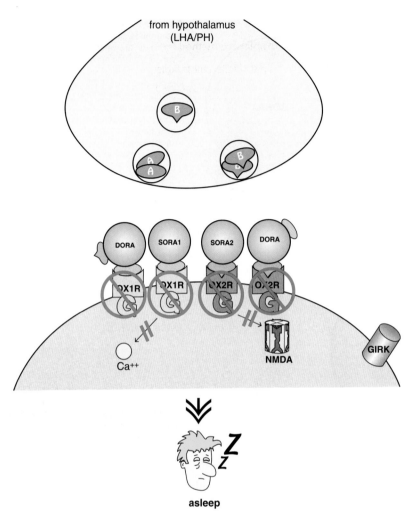

Figure 11-24. Blockade of orexin receptors. Blockade of orexin receptors by SORAs and DORAs is hypothesized to lead to blockade of the excitatory effects of orexin neurotransmitters, thus promoting sleep.

they can often activate their dorsolateral prefrontal cortex (DLPFC) normally, but cannot sustain it, yet when narcoplesy patients take a stimulant or modafinil they are able to sustain the activation of their DLPFC and also to sustain their cognitive performance without decrement. Presumably, this improvement is the result of optimizing and increasing the actions of dopamine in DLPFC brain circuits.

Mechanism of action of wake-promoting agents

Modafinil

This drug is a proven wake-promoting agent whose exact molecular mechanism of action remains debated. It is known to activate relatively selectively neurons in the wake-promoting TMN and the lateral hypothalamus, and this leads to the release of both histamine and orexin. However, the activation of the lateral hypothalamus and release of orexin do not appear to be necessary for the action of modafinil, since modafinil still promotes wakefulness in patients who have loss of hypothalamic orexin neurons in narcolepsy. The activation of TMN and lateral hypothalamic neurons may be secondary and downstream actions resulting from modafinil's effects on dopamine neurons.

The most likely modafinil binding site is probably the dopamine transporter (DAT or DA reuptake pump) (Figure 11-25). Although modafinil is a weak DAT inhibitor, the concentrations of the drug achieved after oral dosing are quite high, and sufficient to have a substantial action on DAT. In fact, the

Table 11-4 What causes sleepiness?

Sleep deprivation

Sleep disorders

Narcolepsy

Obstructive sleep apnea (OSA)

Restless legs

Periodic limb movement disorder (PLMD)

Circadian rhythm disorders (shift work, jet lag, delayed sleep)

Primary hypersomnia

Poor sleep hygiene

Psychiatric illness

Psychiatric and other medications

Substance use/abuse

Medical disorders

Obesity

Insulin resistance/diabetes

Table 11-5 How is sleepiness evaluated?

Subjective method

Epworth Sleepiness Scale

- 8 questions self rated on a 0–3 scale

Objective method

Multiple Sleep Latency Test (MSLT)

- Nocturnal polysomnogram
- Five daytime nap opportunities lying in a quiet, dark room at 2-hour intervals – told not to oppose sleep
- Score time to sleep onset defined by EEG

  - max time 20 minutes
  - wake patient 15 minutes from sleep onset

Maintenance of Wakefulness Test (MWT)

- Nocturnal polysomnogram
- Five daytime nap opportunities lying in a quiet, dark room at 2-hour intervals – instructed to resist sleep
- Often the morning after an overnight polysomnogram

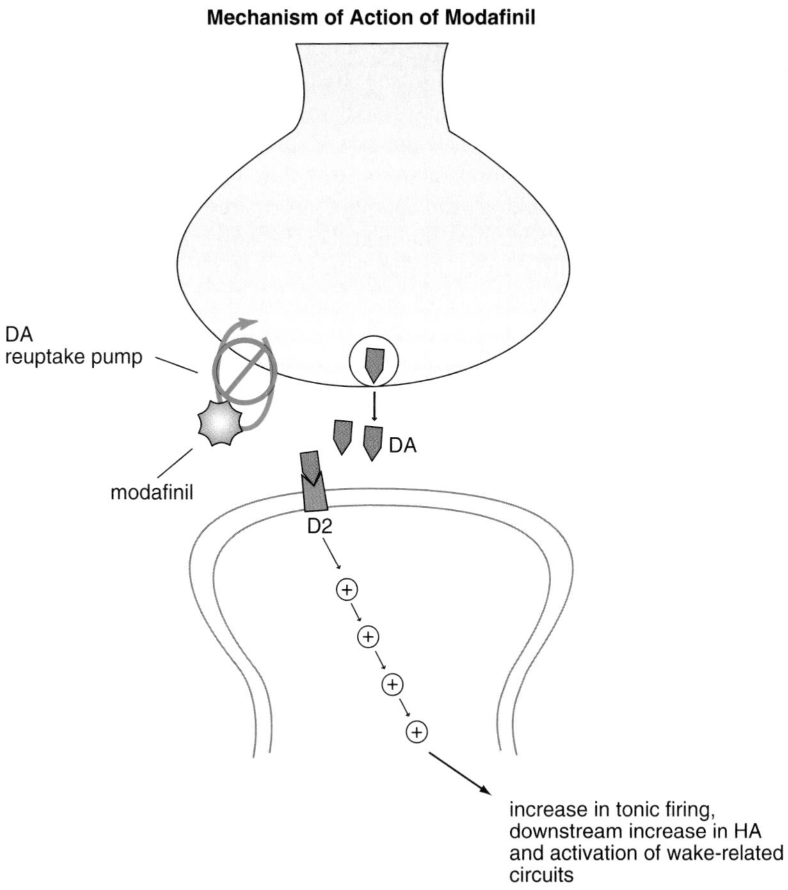

Mechanism of Action of Modafinil

increase in tonic firing, downstream increase in HA and activation of wake-related circuits

Figure 11-25. Modafinil. The precise mechanism of action of modafinil is yet to be fully elucidated. It is known to bind to the dopamine transporter (DAT) and in fact requires its presence. Modafinil's low affinity for the DAT has led some to question whether its binding there is relevant; however, because plasma levels of modafinil are high, this "compensates" for the low binding affinity. It is believed that the increase in synaptic dopamine following blockade of DAT leads to increased tonic firing and downstream effects on neurotransmitters including those involved in wakefulness, such as histamine and orexin/hypocretin.

467

pharmacokinetics of modafinil suggest that this drug acts via a slow rise in plasma levels, sustained plasma levels for 6–8 hours, and incomplete occupancy of DAT, all properties that could be ideal for enhancing tonic dopamine activity to promote wakefulness (Figure 11-25) rather than phasic dopamine activity to promote reinforcement and abuse (see discussion in Chapter 14 on substance abuse). Once dopamine release is activated by modafinil, and the cortex is aroused, this can apparently lead to downstream release of histamine from the TMN and then further activation of the lateral hypothalamus with orexin release to stabilize wakefulness. The same appears to occur after administration of the stimulants amphetamine and methylphenidate.

A newer wake-promoting agent is the R enantiomer of modafinil, called armodafinil (Nuvigil). Armodafinil has a later time to peak levels, a longer half-life, and higher plasma drug levels 6–14 hours after oral administration than the marketed form of modafinil, which is a racemic mixture of R plus S modafinil. The pharmacokinetic properties of armodafinil could theoretically improve the clinical profile of modafinil, with greater activation of phasic dopamine firing, possibly eliminating the need for a second daily dose, as is often required with racemic modafinil.

Stimulants

The two principal stimulants used as wake-promoting agents are methylphenidate and amphetamine, especially *d*-amphetamine. Many forms of these stimulants are now available and are reviewed in detail in Chapter 12 on attention deficit hyperactivity disorder (ADHD) and in Chapter 14 on substance abuse. Amphetamine is known to be a competitive inhibitor and substrate for the dopamine transporter (DAT) and also a dopamine releaser and inhibitor of the vesicular monoamine transporter (VMAT2) within presynaptic dopamine nerve terminals. Methylphenidate is also known to be an inhibitor of DAT which acts not unlike the NDRI (norepinephrine–dopamine reuptake inhibitor) antidepressants discussed in Chapter 7. The mechanism of methylphenidate is also discussed in more detail in Chapter 12. At the doses used to treat sleepiness and ADHD, both of which are much lower than doses used by stimulant addicts, the agents amphetamine and methylphenidate also block the norepinephrine transporter (NET), especially in

controlled-release formulations. Basically, the stimulants as dosed to treat sleepiness or ADHD enhance the synaptic availability of dopamine and norepinephrine, and thereby improve wakefulness.

Caffeine

Caffeine is an incredible over-the-counter drug, popular in many beverages, but how does it work? Originally thought to work as an inhibitor of the enzyme phosphodiesterase, it now appears to act mostly as an antagonist of endogenous neurotransmitters called purines, of which an important one is adenosine, at purine receptors (Figure 11-26). Certain purine receptors are functionally coupled with dopamine receptors such that the actions of dopamine at D_2 receptors (Figure 11-26A) are antagonized when adenosine is binding to its receptor (Figure 11-26B). Not surprisingly, therefore, when an antagonist of adenosine such as caffeine is present, this indirectly promotes the actions of dopamine (Figure 11-26C).

GHB

Gamma-hydroxybutyrate or GHB is also known as sodium oxybate and as Xyrem. This agent is approved for the treatment of excessive daytime sleepiness associated with narcolepsy, as well as for cataplexy. It appears to promote wakefulness by its profound actions on slow-wave sleep at night, making the patient more rested and therefore more alert the next day. Because of its abuse potential and colorful history, it is scheduled as a controlled substance and its supplies are tightly regulated through a central pharmacy in the US. It has been labeled a "date rape" drug by the press, as it has occasionally been used with alcohol for this purpose. Because it profoundly increases slow-wave sleep and the growth hormone surge that accompanies slow-wave sleep, it was used (abused) by athletes as a performance-enhancing drug especially in the 1980s when it was sold over the counter in health-food stores. GHB is used in some European countries as a treatment for alcoholism. Because of the observed enhancement of slow-wave sleep, GHB was recently developed for the treatment of narcolepsy and cataplexy. It is sometimes used "off label" to treat refractory cases of fibromyalgia (see Chapter 10 for discussion of pain syndromes such as fibromyalgia and their treatment).

Mechanism of Action of Caffeine: DA Actions at D2 Receptors

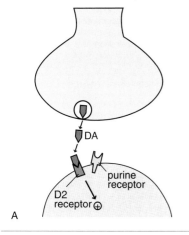

Adenosine and Endogenous Purines Reduce DA Binding

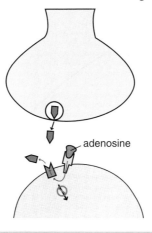

Figure 11-26. Caffeine. Caffeine is an antagonist at purine receptors, and in particular adenosine receptors. (A) These receptors are functionally coupled with certain postsynaptic dopamine receptors, such as dopamine 2 (D_2) receptors, at which dopamine binds and has a stimulatory effect. (B) When adenosine binds to its receptors, this causes reduced sensitivity of D_2 receptors. (C) Antagonism of adenosine receptors by caffeine prevents adenosine from binding there, and thus can enhance dopaminergic actions.

Caffeine Antagonizes Adenosine Binding and Enhances DA Actions

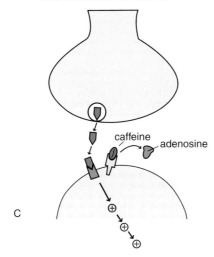

GHB is actually a natural product present in the brain, with its own GHB receptors upon which it acts (Figure 11-27). GHB is formed from the neurotransmitter GABA, and also acts at $GABA_B$ receptors as a partial agonist (Figure 11-27).

Summary

The neurobiology of wakefulness is linked to an arousal system that utilizes the five neurotransmitters histamine, dopamine, norepinephrine, acetylcholine, and serotonin as components of the ascending reticular activating system. Sleep and wakefulness are also regulated by a hypothalamic sleep/wake switch, with wake-promoter neurons in the tuberomammillary nucleus that utilize histamine as neurotransmitter, and sleep-promoter neurons in the ventrolateral preoptic nucleus that utilize GABA as neurotransmitter, both stabilized by the peptide neurotransmitters orexin A and B. The synthesis, metabolism, receptors, and pathways for the neurotransmitter histamine are reviewed in this chapter, as are the pathways for the orexin neurons and the distribution of their receptors. Insomnia is also briefly reviewed, as are the mechanisms of action of several hypnotics, from the benzodiazepines to the popular "Z drugs" that act as positive allosteric modulators or PAMs for $GABA_A$ receptors. Other hypnotics include trazodone, melatonergic hypnotics,

Mechanism of Action of Sodium Oxybate (Xyrem, GHB)

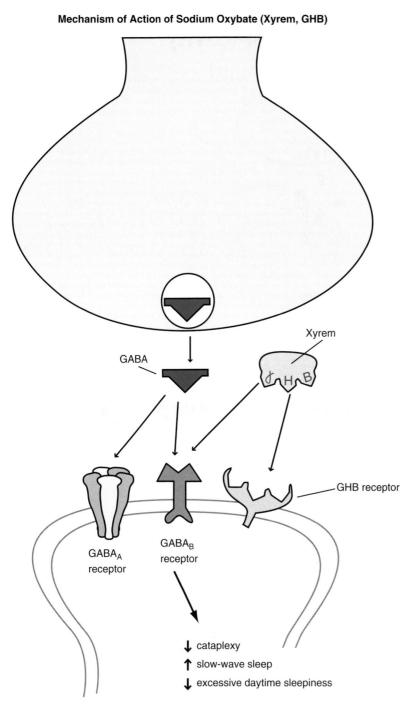

Figure 11-27. Sodium oxybate.
Gamma-hydroxybutyrate (GHB, also called sodium oxybate), is formed from the neurotransmitter GABA and acts as a partial agonist at GABA_B receptors. It is approved for use both in cataplexy and for excessive sleepiness, and appears to enhance slow-wave sleep.

and antihistamines, including novel dual orexin receptor antagonists (DORAs) currently in clinical testing.

Excessive daytime sleepiness is also briefly reviewed, as are the mechanisms of action of the wake-promoting drugs modafinil, caffeine, and stimulants. The actions of GHB (γ-hydroxybutyrate) plus a number of novel sleep- and wake-promoting drugs in clinical development are also reviewed.

12 Attention deficit hyperactivity disorder and its treatment

Attention deficit hyperactivity disorder (ADHD) is increasingly being seen not just as a disorder of attention, nor just as a disorder of children. Paradigm shifts are altering the landscape for treatment options across the full range of ADHD symptoms, from inattention to impulsivity. This chapter will provide an overview of the psychopharmacology of ADHD, including only short discussions of the symptoms of ADHD. The mechanism of action of stimulants and nonstimulants in ADHD will also be explored. Information on the full clinical descriptions and formal criteria for how to diagnose and rate ADHD and its symptoms should be obtained by consulting standard reference sources. The discussion here will emphasize the links between various brain circuits and their neurotransmitters and the various symptoms and comorbidities of ADHD, and how these are linked to effective psychopharmacologic treatments. The goal of this chapter is to acquaint the reader with ideas about the clinical and biological aspects of attention, impulsivity, and hyperactivity, also covering some of the aspects involved in treating adults with this disorder. For details of doses, side effects, drug interactions, and other issues relevant to the prescribing of drugs for ADHD in clinical practice, the reader should consult standard drug handbooks (such as *Stahl's Essential Psychopharmacology: the Prescriber's Guide*).

Symptoms and circuits: ADHD as a disorder of the prefrontal cortex

ADHD is noted for a trio of symptoms: inattention, hyperactivity, and impulsivity (Figure 12-1). It is currently hypothesized that all these symptoms arise in part from abnormalities in various circuits involving the prefrontal cortex (Figures 12-2 through 12-8). Specifically, the most prominent symptoms of inattention in ADHD, better known as executive dysfunction and as the inability to sustain attention and thus to solve problems, are hypothetically linked to inefficient information processing in the dorsolateral prefrontal cortex (DLPFC) (Figures 12-2, 12-3, 12-7). DLPFC is activated by a cognitive task known as the *n*-back test, which can be monitored in living patients doing it while in a functional magnetic resonance imaging (fMRI) brain scanner (explained in Figure 12-3). Problems activating this part of the brain cut across many psychiatric disorders that share the symptom of executive dysfunction, not just ADHD but also including schizophrenia (discussed in Chapter 4), major depression (discussed in Chapter 6), mania (discussed in Chapter 6), anxiety (discussed in

ADHD: Deconstruct the Syndrome into Diagnostic Symptoms

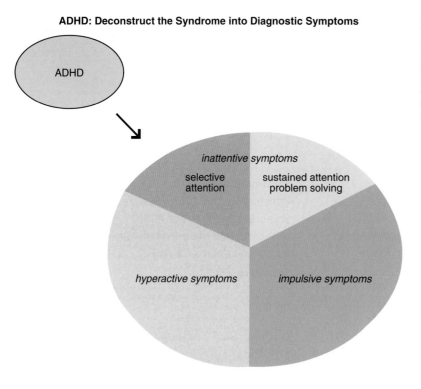

Figure 12-1. Symptoms of ADHD. There are three major categories of symptoms associated with attention deficit hyperactivity disorder (ADHD): inattention, hyperactivity, and impulsivity. Inattention itself can be divided into difficulty with selective attention and difficulty with sustained attention and problem solving.

ADHD: Core Symptoms Hypothetically Linked to Malfunctioning Prefrontal Cortex

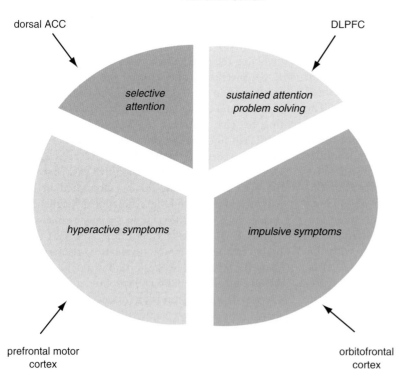

Figure 12-2. Matching ADHD symptoms to circuits. Problems with selective attention are believed to be linked to inefficient information processing in the dorsal anterior cingulate cortex (dACC), while problems with sustained attention are linked to inefficient information processing in the dorsolateral prefrontal cortex (DLPFC). Hyperactivity may be modulated by the prefrontal motor cortex and impulsivity by the orbitofrontal cortex (OFC).

Assessing Sustained Attention and Problem Solving With the *n*-Back Test

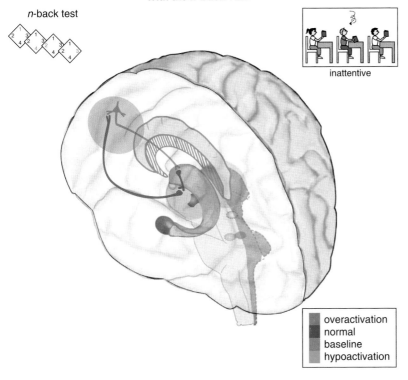

Figure 12-3. Sustained attention and problem solving: the *n*-back test. Sustained attention is hypothetically modulated by a cortico-striato-thalamo-cortical (CSTC) loop that involves the dorsolateral prefrontal cortex (DLPFC) projecting to the striatal complex. Inefficient activation of the DLPFC can lead to difficulty following through or finishing tasks, disorganization, and trouble sustaining mental effort. Tasks such as the *n*-back test are used to measure sustained attention and problem-solving abilities. In the 0-back variant of the *n*-back test, a participant looks at a number on the screen, and presses a button to indicate which number it is. In the 1-back variant, a participant only looks at the first number, and when the second number appears the participant is supposed to press a button corresponding to the first number. Higher *n* values are correlated with increased difficulty in the test.

Assessing Selective Attention With the Stroop Task

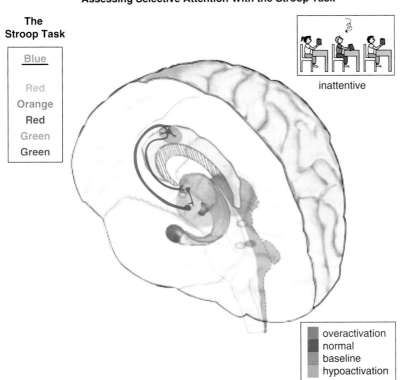

Figure 12-4. Selective attention: the Stroop task. Selective attention is hypothetically modulated by a cortico-striato-thalamo-cortical (CSTC) loop arising from the dorsal anterior cingulate cortex (dACC) and projecting to the striatal complex, then the thalamus, and back to the dACC. Inefficient activation of dACC can result in symptoms such as paying little attention to detail, making careless mistakes, not listening, losing things, being distracted, and forgetting things. An example of a test that involves selective attention, and thus should activate the dACC, is the Stroop task. The Stroop task requires the participants to name the color with which a word is written, instead of saying the word itself. In the present case, for example, the word "blue" is written in orange. The correct answer is therefore "orange," while "blue" is the incorrect choice.

473

Impulsivity is Modulated by the Orbitofrontal Cortex

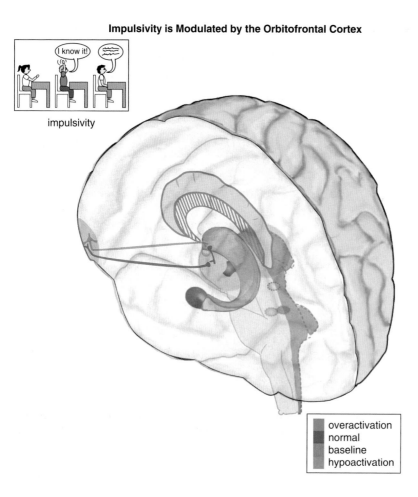

impulsivity

Figure 12-5. Impulsivity. Impulsivity is associated with a cortico-striato-thalamo-cortical (CSTC) loop that involves the orbitofrontal cortex (OFC), the striatal complex, and the thalamus. Examples of impulsive symptoms in ADHD include talking excessively, blurting things out, not waiting one's turn, and interrupting.

overactivation
normal
baseline
hypoactivation

Chapter 9), pain (discussed in Chapter 10), and disorders of sleep and wakefulness (discussed in Chapter 11). One can see how inefficient information processing in this particular DLPFC circuit when put under a cognitive "load" can be associated with the same symptom in many different psychiatric disorders. This is why diagnosis in psychiatry is now moving from describing categorical syndromes that mix together many symptoms (as in the DSM and ICD), towards characterizing single symptom domains such as executive dysfunction that cut across many psychiatric disorders, sometimes called Research Domain Criteria (RDoC) for future diagnostic schemes that are set up to better correlate with neuroimaging and genetic findings.

Another symptom of ADHD is *selective* inattention, or not being able to focus, and thus differing from the executive dysfunction described above.

The symptom of difficulty focusing is hypothetically linked to inefficient information processing in a different brain area, namely the dorsal anterior cingulate cortex (dACC) (Figures 12-2, 12-4, 12-7). The dACC can be activated by tests of selective attention, such as the Stroop test (explained in Figure 12-4). ADHD patients may either fail to activate the dACC when they should be focusing their attention, or they activate this part of the brain very inefficiently and only with great effort and easy fatigability.

Other areas of prefrontal cortex that are hypothetically not functioning efficiently in ADHD are the orbitofrontal cortex (OFC), linked to symptoms of impulsivity (Figures 12-2, 12-5, 12-7) and the supplementary motor area, linked to symptoms of motor hyperactivity (Figures 12-2, 12-6, 12-7). The OFC is hypothetically linked to a wide variety of symptoms

Motor Hyperactivity is Modulated by the Prefrontal Cortex

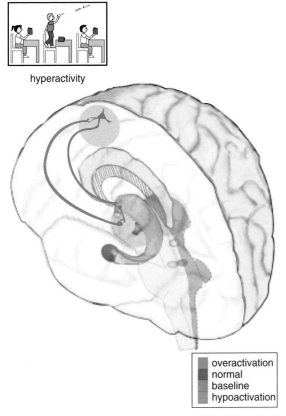

hyperactivity

	overactivation
	normal
	baseline
	hypoactivation

Figure 12-6. Hyperactivity. Motor activity, such as hyperactivity and psychomotor agitation or retardation, can be modulated by a cortico-striato-thalamo-cortical (CSTC) loop from the prefrontal motor cortex to the putamen (lateral striatum) to the thalamus and back to the prefrontal motor cortex. Common symptoms of hyperactivity in children with ADHD include fidgeting, leaving one's seat, running/climbing, being constantly on the go, and having trouble playing quietly.

that cut across several psychiatric conditions, including impulsivity in ADHD (Figures 12-2, 12-5, 12-7), impulsivity and violence in schizophrenia (discussed in Chapter 4), suicidality in depression (discussed in Chapter 6), impulsivity in mania (discussed in Chapter 6), and impulsivity/compulsivity in substance abuse (discussed in Chapter 14). Impulsive symptoms in other psychiatric conditions commonly comorbid with ADHD are also hypothetically related to the orbitofrontal cortex, such as conduct disorder, oppositional defiant disorder, and bipolar disorder (Figure 12-8). Impulsivity is discussed extensively in Chapter 14 (see Tables 14-1 through 14-8 and Figures 14-1 through 14-5).

ADHD as a disorder of inefficient "tuning" of the prefrontal cortex by dopamine and norepinephrine

ADHD patients generally cannot activate prefrontal cortex areas appropriately in response to cognitive tasks of attention and executive functioning. Some studies suggest that this is because dopamine (DA) and norepinephrine (NE) dysregulation in ADHD prevents the normal "tuning" of pyramidal neurons in the prefrontal cortex. In the case of DA and NE neurons, their normal firing at baseline is considered slow and "tonic," stimulating a few receptors on postsynaptic neurons and allowing for optimal signal transmission and downstream neuronal firing (Figure 12-9). Modest levels of NE release will hypothetically improve prefrontal cortical function by stimulating postsynaptic α_{2A} receptors, but high levels of NE release will lead to impaired working memory when α_1 and β_1 receptors are also recruited (Figure 12-9). Similarly, modest levels of DA will first stimulate D_3 receptors, as these are more sensitive to DA than D_1 or D_2 receptors (Figure 12-9). Hypothetically, low to moderate, but not high, levels of D_1 receptor stimulation is beneficial to optimizing prefrontal cortical functioning.

Dopamine neurons in particular can also exhibit bursts of firing, called phasic (Figure 12-10). Phasic DA release is thought to reinforce learning and reward conditioning, providing the motivation to pursue naturally rewarding experiences such as education, recognition, career development, enriching social and family connections, etc. When the phasic DA system is hijacked by drugs, it can induce uncontrolled DA firing that reinforces the reward of drug abuse, and lead to compulsive behaviors such as mindless self-destructive drug seeking (discussed in Chapter 14). Thus, finely tuning the DA reward pathway in the nucleus accumbens and its connections to the amygdala and prefrontal cortex by attaining a low level of phasic firing in relation to tonic firing will theoretically lead to proper functioning of this complex system.

In ADHD, imbalances in NE and DA circuits in the prefrontal cortex hypothetically cause inefficient information processing in prefrontal circuits, and thus the symptoms of ADHD (as shown for *circuits* in Figures 12-2 through 12-8). At the level of NE

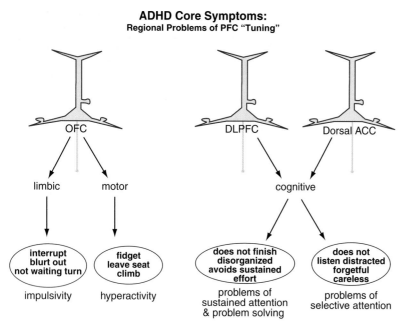

ADHD Core Symptoms:
Regional Problems of PFC "Tuning"

Figure 12-7. ADHD: out-of-tune prefrontal cortex. Different brain areas are hypothetically important in the symptoms of ADHD. Alterations within the orbitofrontal cortex (OFC) are hypothesized to lead to problems with impulsivity or hyperactivity. Inadequate tuning of the DLPFC or the dACC can respectively lead to sustained or selective attentive symptoms. It is becoming increasingly clear that dysfunction in specific brain areas leads to specific symptoms, such that abnormalities in the orbitofrontal–limbic motivation networks have been observed in children with conduct disorder, while aberrations in the dorsolateral cognitive network have been observed in children with problems of sustained attention.

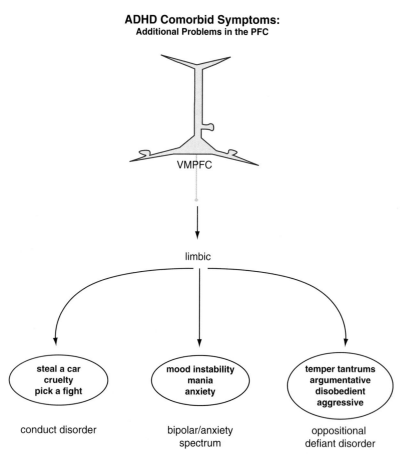

ADHD Comorbid Symptoms:
Additional Problems in the PFC

Figure 12-8. ADHD and comorbid symptoms. The comorbidities associated with ADHD are often the result of similar or additional dysfunctions within the prefrontal cortex–limbic network. Many mood disorders are comorbid with ADHD both in children and in adults, and it has been suggested that the symptoms in adults might be most disabling if the comorbidities were already present in the child. This emphasizes the importance of treating all the symptoms in the younger population of ADHD patients in order to maximize their chances of a "regular" adult life. VMPFC, ventromedial prefrontal cortex.

Baseline NE and DA Neuronal Firing is Tonic

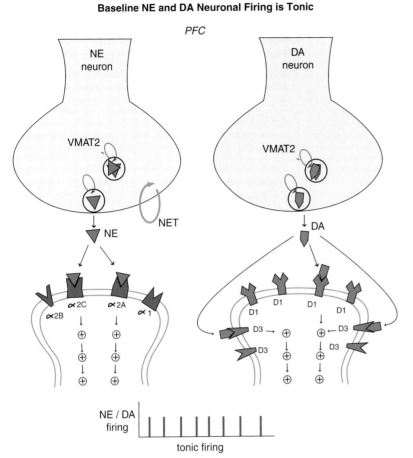

Figure 12-9. Baseline tonic firing. Modulation of prefrontal cortical function, and therefore regulation of attention and behavior, relies on the optimum release of dopamine (DA) and norepinephrine (NE). Under normal conditions, released NE and DA in the prefrontal cortex stimulate a few receptors on postsynaptic neurons allowing for optimal signal transmission and neuronal firing. At modest levels, NE can improve prefrontal cortical function by stimulating postsynaptic α_{2A} receptors, but will lead to impaired working memory at high levels when α_1 and β_1 receptors are also recruited. Similarly, modest levels of DA will first stimulate D_3 receptors as these are more sensitive to DA than D_1/D_2 receptors. Low to moderate, but not high, levels of D_1 receptor stimulation can be beneficial to prefrontal cortical functioning. In the case of both DA and NE systems, moderation is certainly key.

and DA *synapses* in the prefrontal cortex, deficient signaling in prefrontal cortical DA and NE pathways is reflected by decreased neurotransmission and thus reduced stimulation of postsynaptic receptors (Figure 12-11). Agents that can lead to increased release of these two neurotransmitters or increased tonic firing of these neurons will be hypothetically beneficial in patients with ADHD by bringing prefrontal activity back to optimal levels. On the other hand, ADHD can also be hypothetically associated with excessive signaling in prefrontal cortical DA and NE pathways, particularly in adolescents and adults (Figure 12-12). That is, stress can activate NE and DA circuits in the prefrontal cortex, leading to high levels of DA and NE release, and thus cause an excess of phasic NE and DA firing (Figure 12-12). This excessive NE and DA neurotransmission may be the underpinning of the development of drug and alcohol abuse, impulsivity, inattention and anxiety,

all comorbid with ADHD, particularly in adolescents and adults.

So, is the prefrontal cortex out of tune when NE and DA are too high or too low? The answer seems to be that either too much or too little stimulation by NE or DA can cause inefficient information processing, because for the prefrontal cortex to work properly, cortical pyramidal neurons need to be tuned, meaning that moderate stimulation of α_{2A} receptors by NE and D_1 receptors by DA is required, neither too high nor too low. In theory, the role of NE is to increase the incoming signal by allowing for increased connectivity of the prefrontal networks, while the role of DA is to decrease the noise by preventing inappropriate connections from taking place. Pyramidal cell function is optimal at the top of this inverted U-shaped curve, when stimulation of both α_{2A} and D_1 receptors is moderate (Figure 12-13). If stimulation at α_{2A} and D_1 receptors is too low (left side of Figure 12-13), all

Salience Provokes Phasic DA Neuronal Firing in Reward Centers

Nucleus Accumbens

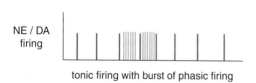

NE / DA firing

tonic firing with burst of phasic firing

Figure 12-10. Salience-provoked phasic firing. While tonic firing, as seen in the prefrontal cortex, is often preferred in neuronal systems, a little bit of phasic firing of DA neurons in the nucleus accumbens can be a good thing. Phasic firing will lead to bursts of DA release, and when this happens in a controlled manner it can reinforce learning and reward conditioning, which can provide the motivation to pursue naturally rewarding experiences (e.g., education, career development, etc). When this system however is out of bounds, it can induce uncontrolled DA firing that reinforces the reward of taking drugs of abuse, for example, in which case the reward circuitry can be hijacked and impulses are followed by the development of uncontrolled compulsions to seek drugs.

incoming signals are the same, preventing a person from focusing on one single task (unguided attention). When stimulation is too high (right side of Figure 12-13) the signals get scrambled as additional receptors are recruited, again misguiding a person's attention. A balanced, moderate stimulation of α_{2A} and D_1 receptors is thus critical for correct interpretation of an incoming signal.

In prefrontal cortex, α_{2A} and D_1 receptors are often located on the spines of cortical pyramidal neurons, and can thus gate incoming signals (Figures 12-14 through 12-18). Alpha-2A receptors are linked to the molecule cyclic adenosine monophosphate (cAMP) via the inhibitory G protein, or Gi (Figure 12-14). D_1 receptors, on the other hand, are linked to the cAMP signaling system via the stimulatory G protein (Gs) (Figure 12-14). In either case, the cAMP molecule links the receptors to the hyperpolarization-activated cyclic nucleotide-gated (HCN) cation channels. An open channel will lead to a low membrane resistance, thus shunting inputs out of the spine. In the presence of an open channel, the signal leaks out and is therefore lost. However, when these channels are closed, the incoming signal survives and can be directed down the neuron to strengthen the network connectivity of similar neurons and lead to the appropriate signal and response.

When NE, or a noradrenergic agonist, binds to an α_{2A} receptor, the activated Gi-linked system inhibits cAMP, thereby closing the HCN channel (Figure 12-15). Closure of the channel allows the signal to go through the spine and down the neuron, thereby strengthening network connectivity with similar neurons (Figure 12-15). So in general, in the prefrontal cortex, stimulation of α_{2A} receptors strengthens an incoming signal.

By contrast, stimulation of D_1 receptors leads to weakening of the signal (Figure 12-16). That is, when DA, or a DA agonist, binds to a D_1 receptor, the activated Gs-linked system will lead to increased stimulation – or opening – of HCN channels. The opening of the HCN channels, especially if excessive, will lead to leakage of the signal, thereby shunting any input out of the spine. So excessive stimulation of D_1 receptors will, in contrast to stimulation of α_{2A} receptors, result in the dissipation and/or weakening of a signal. The mechanism of action of α_{2A} (Figure 12-15) and D_1 receptors (Figure 12-16) explains in general why moderate stimulation of both types of receptors

ADHD and Deficient Arousal:
Weak NE and DA Signals

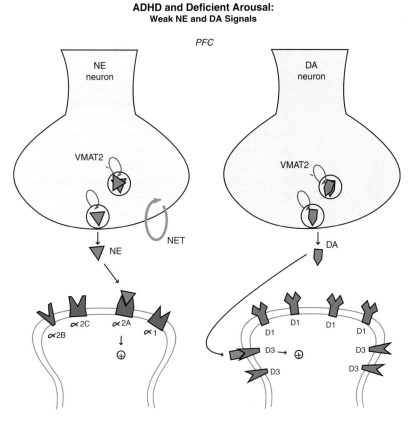

Figure 12-11. ADHD and deficient arousal. Besides being a key player in the arousal pathways, the prefrontal cortex is also the main brain area where imbalances in NE and DA systems hypothetically occur in ADHD. Deficient signaling in prefrontal cortical DA and NE pathways is reflected by reduced stimulation of postsynaptic receptors. Agents that can lead to (1) increased release of these two neurotransmitters, or (2) increased tonic firing of these neurons, will be hypothetically beneficial in patients with ADHD by bringing prefrontal activity back to optimal level.

(Figure 12-14) is preferred in order to strengthen the signal-to-noise ratio in prefrontal cortical neurons (Figure 12-17).

What happens following concurrent stimulation of α_{2A} and D_1 receptors by NE and DA, respectively (Figure 12-17)? While the exact localization and density of α_{2A} and D_1 receptors within various cortical areas are still under intense investigation, it is possible to imagine the same pyramidal neuron receiving NE input from the locus coeruleus (LC) on one spine and DA input from the ventral tegmental area (VTA) on another spine. If the systems are properly "tuned," then D_1 receptor stimulation can reduce the noise and α_{2A} receptor stimulation can increase the signal to result in proper prefrontal cortex functioning (Figure 12-17). Theoretically, this will result in adequate guided attention (Figure 12-13), focus on a specific task, and adequate control of emotions and impulses.

What happens, however, when there is low release of both DA and NE and thus low stimulation

of both D_1 and α_{2A} receptors on the spines of these pyramidal neurons (Figure 12-18)? Deficient DA and NE input will theoretically lead to increased noise and decreased signal, respectively, thus preventing a coherent signal from being sent (Figure 12-18). Hypothetically, this could cause hyperactivity, inattention, impulsivity, or some combination of symptoms, depending upon the localization of the mis-tuned pyramidal neuron in prefrontal cortex (Figures 12-3 through 12-8). Furthermore, if one neurotransmitter is low while the other is high, then a person could be exhibiting a whole different set of symptoms. By knowing both the levels of DA and NE neurotransmission and the specific area of the possible disturbances, it may one day be possible to predict the degree and type of symptoms with which a patient is ailing. With this in mind, Figures 12-7 and 12-8 show how pyramidal neurons in different brain areas may be responsible for the different symptom presentations in ADHD.

ADHD and Excessive Arousal:
Impact of Stress and Comorbidities

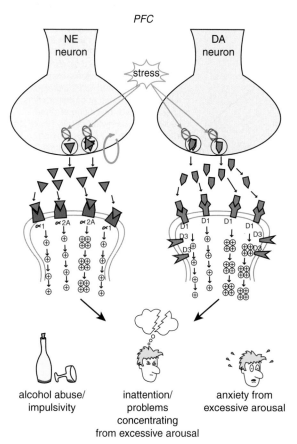

Figure 12-12. ADHD and excessive arousal. Nontreated adults with ADHD can often be stressed as they are trying to deal with their disorder while at the same time attempting to accomplish as much as their peers. Unfortunately, stress can activate NE and DA circuits in the prefrontal cortex, leading to an excess of phasic NE and DA firing. This excessive NE and DA neurotransmission may herald the development of impulsivity, inattention, and comorbidities associated with ADHD such as anxiety and substance abuse. This emphasizes the notion that treatment of all comorbid disorders is necessary to attain good patient outcomes.

Neurodevelopment and ADHD

ADHD has traditionally been considered a childhood disorder, but this perspective is rapidly changing, with ADHD now being seen also as a major psychiatric disorder of adults, with some major differentiating features between ADHD in children and adolescents (Table 12-1). Nevertheless, the classic form of ADHD has onset by age seven, possibly related to abnormalities in prefrontal cortex circuits that begin before age seven but last a lifetime (Figure 12-19). Synapses

rapidly increase in prefrontal cortex by age six, and then up to half of them are rapidly eliminated by adolescence (Figure 12-19). The timing of onset of ADHD suggests that the formation of synapses, and perhaps more importantly the selection of synapses for removal in prefrontal cortex during childhood, may contribute to the onset and lifelong pathophysiology of this condition (Figure 12-19). Those who are able to compensate for these prefrontal abnormalities by new synapse formation may be the ones who "grow out of their ADHD," and this may explain why the prevalence of ADHD in adults is only half that in children and adolescents.

What causes these problems in the circuits of the prefrontal cortex in ADHD? Currently, leading hypotheses propose that neurodevelopmental abnormalities occur in the circuits of the prefrontal cortex in ADHD (Figures 12-2 through 12-8). In fact, genes that code for subtle molecular abnormalities are thought to be just as important to the etiology of ADHD as they are to the etiology of schizophrenia. Many of the ideas about the neurodevelopmental basis of schizophrenia, such as abnormal synapse formation and abnormal synaptic neurotransmission, serve as a conceptual framework and neurobiological model for ADHD as well. The genetic factors linked to schizophrenia are discussed extensively in Chapter 4. The major genes implicated in ADHD are those linked to the neurotransmitter dopamine, although links to the genes for the α_{2A}-adrenergic receptor, serotonin receptors, and some other proteins are also under intense investigation. Environmental factors inevitably contribute to ADHD, as they do to so many other psychiatric disorders. This includes factors such as preterm birth, maternal smoking during pregnancy, and others.

The impact of neurodevelopment on the specific symptom patterns of ADHD is shown in Figure 12-20. Inattentive symptoms are not really seen in preschool children with ADHD, perhaps because they do not have a sufficiently mature prefrontal cortex to manifest this symptom in a manner that is abnormal compared to normal development. Preschool ADHD and its treatment are a current controversial concept in the field, because most studies of stimulants involve children over the age of six. Once inattention becomes a prominent symptom of ADHD, it remains so over the life cycle (Figure 12-20). However, hyperactivity declines notably by adolescence and early adulthood, while recognized comorbidities

Tuning Cortical Pyramidal Neurons in ADHD

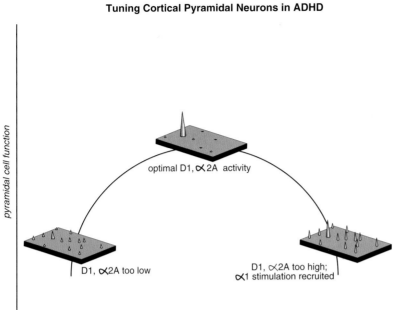

optimal D1, α2A activity

D1, α2A too low

D1, α2A too high;
α1 stimulation recruited

pyramidal cell function

Figure 12-13. ADHD and maladaptive signal-to-noise ratios. In order for the prefrontal cortex to work properly, moderate stimulation of α$_2$ receptors by NE and D$_1$ receptors by DA is required. In theory, the role of NE is to *increase* the incoming *signal* by allowing for increased connectivity of the prefrontal networks, while the role of DA is to *decrease* the *noise* by preventing inappropriate connections from taking place. At the top of the inverted U-shaped curve depicted here, stimulation of both α$_{2A}$ and D$_1$ receptors is moderate and pyramidal cell function is optimal. If stimulation at α$_{2A}$ and D$_1$ receptors is too low (left side), all incoming signals are the same, making it difficult for a person to focus on one single task (unguided attention). If stimulation is too high (right side), incoming signals get jumbled as additional receptors are recruited, resulting in the misdirection of attention.

Signal Distribution in a Dendritic Spine

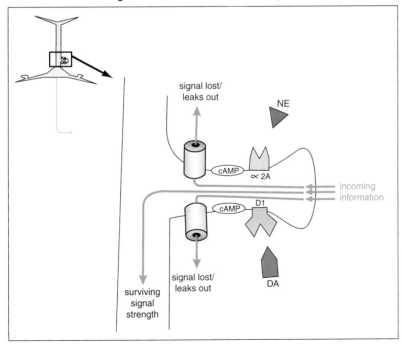

signal lost/
leaks out

NE

cAMP

α 2A

cAMP

D1

incoming
information

signal lost/
leaks out

DA

surviving
signal
strength

Figure 12-14. Signal distribution in a dendritic spine. The location of α$_{2A}$ and D$_1$ receptors on dendritic spines of cortical pyramidal neurons in the prefrontal cortex allows them to gate incoming signals. Both α$_{2A}$ and D$_1$ receptors are linked to the molecule cyclic adenosine monophosphate (cAMP). The effects on cAMP from NE and DA binding at their respective receptors are opposite (inhibitory in the case of NE and excitatory in the case of DA). In either case the cAMP molecule links the receptors to the hyperpolarization-activated cyclic nucleotide-gated (HCN) cation channels. When HCN channels are open, incoming signals leak out before they can be passed along. However, when these channels are closed, the incoming signal survives and can be directed down the neuron.

NE Actions at Alpha 2A Receptors Strengthen Signal

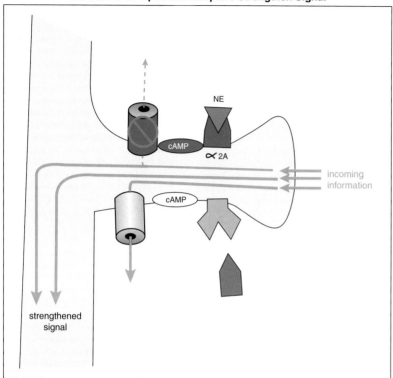

Figure 12-15. Norepinephrine actions at α₂ₐ receptors strengthen the incoming signal. Alpha$_{2A}$ receptors are linked to cAMP via an inhibitory G protein (Gi). When NE occupies these $α_{2A}$ receptors, the activated Gi-linked system inhibits cAMP and the HCN channel is closed, preventing loss of the incoming signal.

DA Actions at D1 Receptors Weaken Signal

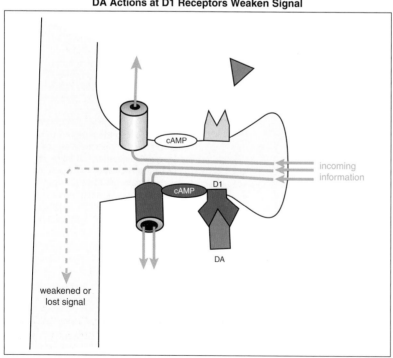

Figure 12-16. Dopamine actions at D₁ receptors weaken the incoming signal. D1 receptors are linked to cAMP via a stimulatory G protein (Gs). When DA occupies these D_1 receptors, the activated Gs-linked system activates cAMP, leading to opening of HCN channels. The opening of the HCN channels, especially if excessive, will lead to loss of the incoming signal before it can be passed along.

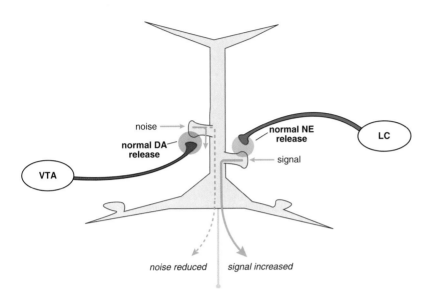

How DA and NE Hypothetically "Tune" the PFC:
Signal Increased and Noise Reduced

Figure 12-17. Dopamine and norepinephrine "tune" the PFC. The same pyramidal neuron may receive NE input from the locus coeruleus (LC) on one spine and DA input from the ventral tegmental area (VTA) on another spine. When properly "tuned," D_1 receptor stimulation will reduce the noise while $α_{2A}$ receptor stimulation will increase the signal, resulting in appropriate prefrontal cortex functioning, guided attention, focus on a specific task, and control of emotions and impulses.

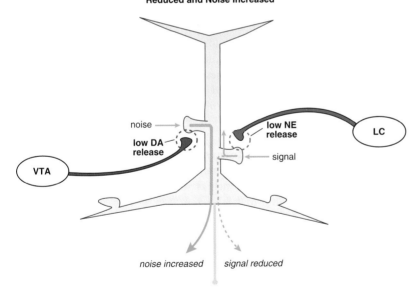

How DA and NE Hypothetically "Tune" the PFC:
Low NE and Low DA: ADHD With Signals Reduced and Noise Increased

Figure 12-18. Dopamine and norepinephrine improperly "tune" the PFC in ADHD. Deficient DA will theoretically lead to increased noise, whereas deficient NE input will cause a decrease in the incoming signal. Hypothetically, this improper tuning of the PFC by DA and NE can lead to hyperactivity, or inattention, or both. Depending on the relative levels of both DA and NE, a person could display a wide range of clinical symptoms.

skyrocket in frequency as ADHD patients enter adulthood (Figure 12-20).

The prevalence of ADHD in adults may be only about half of that in children, but it is not recognized nearly as often as it is in children, possibly because it is much harder to diagnose and its symptoms are very often not treated. Whereas half of all children or adolescents with ADHD are thought to be diagnosed and treated, less than one in five adults with ADHD is thought to be diagnosed and treated (Table 12-1). The reasons for this are multiple, starting with the diagnostic requirement that ADHD symptoms must begin by age seven. Adults often have difficulty making accurate retrospective diagnoses, especially if the

Table 12-1 Differences in ADHD in adults versus children and adolescents

Children 6–12 / Adolescents 13–17	Adults > 18
7–8% prevalence	4–5% prevalence
Easy to diagnose	Hard to diagnose • Inaccurate retrospective recall of onset • Onset by age 7 too stringent • Late onset, same genetics, comorbidity, and impairment
Diagnosed by pediatricians, child psychiatrists, child psychologists	Diagnosed by adult psychiatrists, adult mental/medical health professionals
High levels of identification and treatment: > 50% treated	Low levels of identification and treatment: < 20% treated
Stimulants prescribed first- and second-line	Nonstimulants often prescribed first-line
2/3 of stimulant use is under age 18, most of this under age 13	1/3 of stimulant use is age 18 or over
1/3 of atomoxetine use is under age 18, most of this over age 12	2/3 of atomoxetine use is age 18 or over

condition was not identified and treated as a child. Furthermore, many experts now question whether it is appropriate to exclude from the diagnosis of ADHD those adults whose ADHD symptoms started after age seven, so-called late-onset ADHD. Many cases have onset up to the age of 12 and some up to the age of 45. Do these patients have ADHD? Genetic studies suggest that full syndrome ADHD with onset after age seven has similar psychiatric comorbidity, functional impairment, and familial transmission to ADHD with onset by age seven. Thus, there is a movement to consider the age of onset in some diagnostic criterion as too stringent for the diagnosis of ADHD in adults.

Differences in diagnostic rates in children versus adults may also be due to differences in referral patterns and in the specialties of practitioners who treat children versus those who treat adults. Most children with ADHD are diagnosed and treated by pediatricians, child psychiatrists, and child psychologists and are referred by parents and teachers with a high degree of suspicion for the diagnosis, generally requesting a trial of a stimulant, and usually these are patients without comorbidity. On the other hand, most adults with ADHD are self-referred and seen by psychiatrists and adult mental and medical health professionals; adult cases mostly have a comorbid condition that is the focus of treatment, not their ADHD. Thus, adult practitioners may prioritize the treatment of these other conditions over ADHD (see

Figure 12-21) to the extent that ADHD is never formally diagnosed, nor is it specifically targeted for treatment.

There are also many differences in how ADHD is treated in children and adolescents compared to adults (Table 12-1). For example two-thirds of all stimulant use for ADHD is in patients under the age of 18, most of these under the age of 13. Stimulant use falls off in adolescents and then falls way off in adults. Only one-third of all stimulant use for ADHD is in adults. On the other hand, two-thirds of all atomoxetine use is in adults, one-third in those under the age of 18, mostly in adolescents (Table 12-1). Why these differences? One reason could be that many adult practitioners do not like to prescribe controlled substances such as stimulants. Another reason could be due to the differences in the rates of comorbidity of children versus adults with ADHD, and in the types of comorbid conditions of children versus adults with ADHD. Thus, the frequent comorbidities of substance abuse, anxiety disorders, and bipolar or mixed states can limit the utility and tolerability of stimulants in the typical adult ADHD patient with these comorbidities. Augmenting antidepressants and anxiolytics with nonstimulants can therefore be preferable. There is also much more off-label use of the NDRI antidepressant bupropion, the various SNRIs, and the wake-promoting agents modafinil and armodafinil in adults than in children, often as augmenting agents in comorbid adult ADHD.

Synaptogenesis in Prefrontal Cortex and the Development of Executive Functions

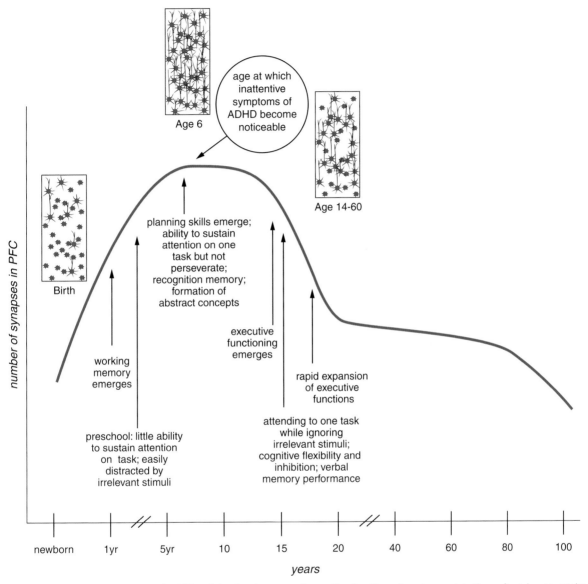

Figure 12-19. Synaptogenesis in the PFC and the development of executive functions. Synaptogenesis in the prefrontal cortex might be responsible for altered connections that could prime the brain for ADHD. Specifically, executive function develops throughout adolescence. At one year of age, working memory emerges. Around three to four years of age, children do not yet have the capability to sustain attention for long periods of time, and can be easily distracted. By age six to seven, this changes; attention can be sustained and planning can take place. This age is also characterized by "synaptic pruning," a process during which overproduced or "weak" synapses are "weeded out," thus allowing for the child's cognitive intelligence to mature. Errors in this process could hypothetically affect the further development of executive function and be one of the causes of ADHD. This timeline also represents when symptoms of ADHD often become noticeable, which is around the age of six.

Impact of Development on ADHD

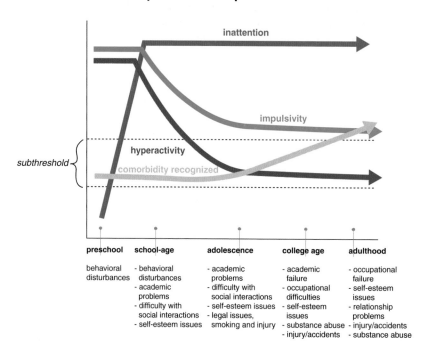

Figure 12-20. Impact of development on ADHD. The evolution of symptoms across the ages shows that although hyperactivity and impulsivity are key symptoms in childhood, inattention becomes prevalent as the patient ages. Additionally, the rates of recognized comorbidities increase over time. This could be due to the fact that the comorbidities were overlooked in children with ADHD, or because ADHD was never diagnosed in some patients presenting with anxiety or learning disabilities. One could say that "the jury is still out" on this issue.

What Should be Treated First?

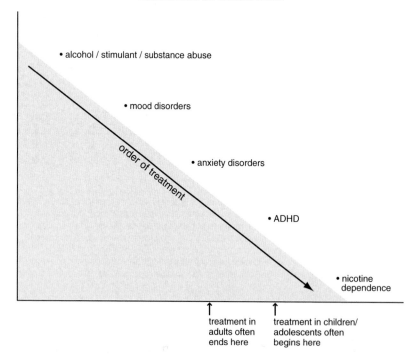

Figure 12-21. ADHD and comorbidities: what should be treated first? What should a psychopharmacologist do with a patient with ADHD and comorbid disorders? Once the proper diagnosis has been reached, it is imperative to treat all disorders appropriately, and in terms of highest degree of impairment. This might mean that in one patient it is necessary to first stabilize the alcohol abuse, while in another patient the symptoms of ADHD might be more impairing than the underlying anxiety disorder. Additionally, some medications used to treat these disorders could exacerbate the comorbid ailment. Thus, care needs to be taken when choosing the appropriate treatment. An individualized treatment plan should therefore be established for each patient, depending on his/her symptomatic portfolio.

Currently, the recognition and treatment of ADHD in adults, tailoring the diagnostic and psychopharmacologic considerations to the unique features of this illness in adults, is increasing at a rapid pace. Thus, there is a call for more recognition that ADHD is only half the problem in mostly comorbid adults, and that treatment of ADHD in adults generally means concomitant treatment of ADHD with one or more additional disorders, and generally with a combination of drugs for the different conditions. It is increasingly recognized that atomoxetine (or another NET inhibitor) augmentation of antidepressants and anxiolytics can not only improve cognitive symptoms of ADHD, but has the potential of improving anxiety symptoms, depressive symptoms, and perhaps even heavy drinking. It is possible that the α_{2A} selective adrenergic agonist guanfacine ER, approved for use in children, may also be useful for off-label treatment of adults. Long-acting stimulants may also be useful in adults, not just those stimulants specifically approved in adults, but also those newer agents first tested and approved for use in children which can be used for off-label treatment of adults.

Treatment

Which symptoms should be treated first?

It can be helpful in managing ADHD to prioritize which symptoms to target first with psychopharmacological treatments, even at the expense of delaying treatment for a while for some conditions, or even making some of these comorbid conditions transiently worse while other symptoms are targeted for improvement first (Figure 12-21). Although there are no definitive studies on this approach, clinical experience from many experts suggests that in such complex cases it can be very difficult to make any therapeutic progress if the patient continues to abuse alcohol or stimulants; thus substance-abuse problems must be managed top line (Figure 12-21). Treating ADHD may also have to await improvement from mood and anxiety disorder treatments, with ADHD seen as more of a fine-tune adjustment to a patient's symptom portfolio (Figure 12-21).

There are problems, however, with this approach of setting priorities of which symptoms and disorders to treat first. For example, many children are treated for their ADHD first, and perhaps in isolation, without necessarily evaluating possible comorbidities until they fail to respond robustly to stimulant treatment

(Figure 12-21). In adults it can be so difficult to treat substance abuse, mood disorders, and anxiety disorders that the focus of therapeutic attention never gets to ADHD or certainly to nicotine dependence. Once the mood or anxiety disorder is improving, treatment can plateau or stop. Too often the focus of psychopharmacological management is the mood or anxiety disorder to the exclusion of any comorbid ADHD (or nicotine dependence). That is, ADHD can be considered a mere afterthought to be addressed if cognitive symptoms do not remit once the primary focus of therapeutic attention, namely the mood or anxiety disorder, is treated. It is interesting that ADHD is not often the focus of treatment in adults unless it presents with no comorbid conditions. Since lack of comorbidity in adults with ADHD is rare, this may explain why the majority of adults with ADHD are not treated.

The modern, sophisticated psychopharmacologist keeps a high index of suspicion for the presence of ADHD in mood and anxiety and substance-abuse disorders especially in adults, always aiming for complete symptomatic remission in patients under treatment. In practice, this means exploring the use of ADHD treatments as augmenting agents to first-line treatments of mood, anxiety, and substance-abuse disorders, rather than the other way around. It also means for long-term management of ADHD to eventually address the treatment of nicotine dependence once the ADHD symptoms are under control (Figure 12-21). Adults with ADHD smoke as frequently as adults with schizophrenia, about twice the rate of the normal adult population in the US. This may be due to the fact that nicotine subjectively improves ADHD symptoms, especially in patients who are not treated for their ADHD. Nicotine enhances DA release and enhances arousal, so it is not surprising that it may be subjectively effective for ADHD symptoms. Nicotine dependence and psychopharmacological treatments for smoking cessation are discussed in more detail in Chapter 14 on drug abuse.

Stimulant treatment of ADHD
General principles

As discussed above, and as illustrated in Figures 12-11 and 12-13, when both DA and NE are too low the strength of output in the prefrontal cortex is also too low, thus leading to reduced signal and increased

Importance of NE and DA Levels in PFC in ADHD

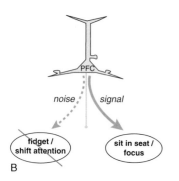

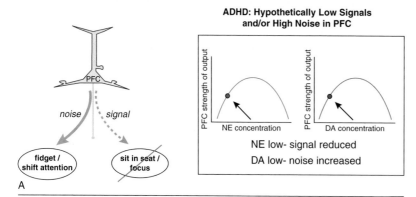

Figure 12-22. The importance of NE and DA levels in the PFC in ADHD. When both DA and NE are too low, i.e., on the left side of the inverted U-shaped curve, the strength of output in the prefrontal cortex is too low, leading to reduced signal and increased noise (A, right side). Inability to sit still and focus are often clinical manifestations of this imbalanced signal-to-noise ratio (A, left side). In order to treat these symptoms, it is necessary to increase strength output by dialing up (B, right side, toward the right on the U-shaped curve) the concentrations of both DA and NE until they reach the optimal dose (top of the inverted U-shaped curve).

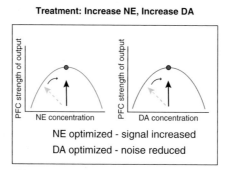

noise (Figure 12-22A). Behaviorally, this could translate into a person not being able to sit in his/her seat and focus, and fidgeting and shifting attention (Figure 12-22A). In order to treat these symptoms, it is necessary to increase signal strength output by dialing up the release of both DA and NE until they reach the optimal levels (Figure 12-22B). This can be done both by stimulants and by some noradrenergic agents, as discussed below. Strengthening prefrontal cortical output is hypothesized to be beneficial in restoring a patient's ability to tease out important signals from unimportant ones, and to manage to sit still and focus.

What if NE and DA signals are excessive? Excessive as well as deficient activation of NE and DA in the prefrontal cortex can lead to ADHD as discussed above, namely by increasing the noise and decreasing the signal (Figure 12-13). The theory is that at first the added stress of suffering from ADHD, plus other stressors from the environment, can even further dial up the noise and reduce the signal, resulting in high NE and DA release, yet causing reduced signals and

inefficient information processing (Figure 12-23A). As stress becomes chronic, however, NE and DA levels eventually plummet due to depletion over time, but with no relief in terms of poor signal output (Figure 12-23B). Ultimately the appropriate treatment is to increase NE and DA concentrations to allow for normalization of behavior (Figure 12-23C: noise is reduced and signal is increased).

Experienced clinicians are well aware that such patients with too much DA and NE (represented in Figure 12-23A), too little DA and NE (represented in Figure 12-23B), or a combination of these in different pathways, can be very difficult to treat. For example, in children, the combination of tics generally representing excessive DA activation in striatum may require DA-blocking antipsychotics, and it can be very difficult to treat simultaneously in patients with ADHD who have deficient DA activation in cortex and require DA-enhancing stimulants. Stimulants may help the ADHD symptoms but make the tics much worse. Children and adolescents who have conduct disorder, oppositional disorders, psychotic

Effects of Chronic Stress in ADHD

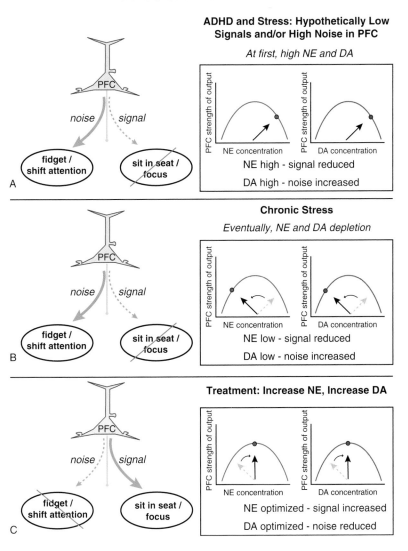

ADHD and Stress: Hypothetically Low Signals and/or High Noise in PFC

At first, high NE and DA

NE high - signal reduced

DA high - noise increased

A

Chronic Stress

Eventually, NE and DA depletion

NE low - signal reduced

DA low - noise increased

B

Treatment: Increase NE, Increase DA

NE optimized - signal increased

DA optimized - noise reduced

C

Figure 12-23. Chronic stress in ADHD. Excessive activation of NE and DA in prefrontal cortex (PFC) can lead to ADHD by increasing the noise and decreasing the signal. At first, the added stress of suffering from the disorder can further dial up the noise and reduce the signal (A: high NE and DA concentration leading to decreased output). As chronic stress sets in, NE and DA levels plummet (B: low NE and DA concentration also leading to decreased output), but with no relief in terms of signal output. Treatments that increase NE and DA concentrations may normalize behavior (C: noise is reduced and signal is increased).

disorders, and/or bipolar mania or mixed conditions (theoretically associated with excessive DA activation in some prefrontal circuits: Figure 12-8) comorbid with ADHD (theoretically associated with deficient DA activation in other prefrontal circuits: Figure 12-7) are among the most challenging patients for clinicians treating young patients.

Conditions of excessive DA activation suggest treatment with an atypical antipsychotic, yet ADHD suggests treatment with a stimulant. Can these two agents be combined? In fact, in heroic cases stimulants can be combined with atypical antipsychotics. The rationale for this combination exploits the fact that atypical antipychotics simultaneously release DA in prefrontal cortex to stimulate D_1 receptors there while acting in limbic areas to block D_2 receptors there. This mechanism of action of atypical antipsychotics is discussed extensively in Chapter 5. In patients who may require atypical antipsychotic treatment for psychotic or manic symptoms, yet still have ADHD, it is sometimes possible to augment the atypical antipsychotic cautiously with a stimulant, thereby increasing DA release to an even greater extent to act at D_1 receptors in prefrontal cortex, hopefully reducing ADHD symptoms while blocking DA stimulation at D_2 receptors sufficiently in limbic areas to prevent worsening of mania or psychosis. Such an approach is controversial and best left to experts for difficult patients who fail to improve adequately on monotherapies.

For adults with ADHD and anxiety, it can be difficult or even self-defeating to try to treat anxiety with SSRIs/SNRIs or benzodiazepines while simultaneously administering a stimulant to improve the ADHD, only to cause the anxiety to worsen. For adults with ADHD and substance abuse, it makes little sense to give stimulants to drug abusers in order to treat their ADHD. In these cases, augmenting antidepressant or anxiolytic therapies with a tonic activator of DA and/or NE systems such as a long-lasting NET inhibitor (norepinephrine reuptake inhibitors, NRIs), or an α_{2A}-adrenergic agonist rather than a stimulant, can be an effective long-term approach for comorbid anxiety, depression, or substance abuse with ADHD. Some studies of NET inhibitors report improvement in both ADHD and anxiety symptoms, and other studies report improvement in both ADHD and heavy drinking. Further controlled trials are needed to clarify the responsiveness of both ADHD and comorbid conditions to treatment with NET inhibitors or α_{2A}-adrenergic agonists.

Methylphenidate

The mechanism of action of the stimulants is shown in Figures 12-24 through 12-31. Oral administration of clinically approved doses of the stimulant methylphenidate blocks the transporters for both NE and DA (NET and DAT) (Figures 12-25, 12-30, 12-31). Normally, dopamine is released (arrow 1 in Figure 12-25A), and then taken back up into the dopaminergic neuron by DAT (arrows 2 in Figure 12-25A), and finally stored in the synaptic vesicle by VMAT (arrows 3 in Figure 12-25A). Methylphenidate blocks DAT and NET allosterically, stopping the reuptake of dopamine via DAT (Figure 12-25B) and norepinephrine via NET (Figure 12-25C), with no actions on VMAT (Figures 12-25B and 12-25C). Methylphenidate blocks NET and DAT in much the same way as antidepressants block them (see discussion in Chapter 7 and Figure 7-36), namely by binding to NET and DAT at sites *distinct* from where monoamines bind NET and DAT, i.e., allosterically. Thus, methylphenidate stops the reuptake pumps so that no methylphenidate is transported into the presynaptic neuron (Figures 12-25B and 12-25C). Methylphenidate has a *d*- and an *l*-isomer (Figure 12-24), with the *d*-isomer being much more potent than the *l*-isomer

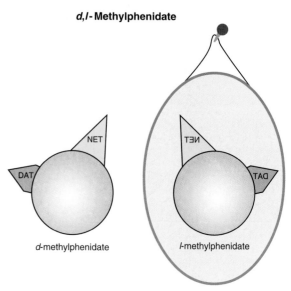

d,l-Methylphenidate

d-methylphenidate   *l*-methylphenidate

Figure 12-24. d,l-Methylphenidate. The racemic form of methylphenidate includes both the *d*- and the *l*-isomers. *d,l*-Methylphenidate will lead to increased release of DA in the nucleus accumbens and NE and DA in the prefrontal cortex by blocking the reuptake pumps, DAT and NET. The same effects are caused by *d*-methylphenidate. Methylphenidate comes in many different formulations, such as regular and chewable immediate-release tablets, new and old sustained-release tablets, new sustained-release capsules, and oral solutions, as well as a transdermal patch. The transdermal formulation may not only confer lower abuse potential but may also enhance adherence.

on both NET and DAT binding (Figure 12-30). Methylphenidate is available as the single enantiomer *d*-methylphenidate in both immediate-release and controlled-release preparations.

Amphetamine

Oral administration of clinically approved doses of the stimulant amphetamine, like methylphenidate, also blocks the transporters both for NE and DA (NET and DAT), but in a different manner (Figures 12-26, 12-27, 12-28, 12-30, 12-31). Unlike methylphenidate and antidepressants, amphetamine is a competitive inhibitor and pseudosubstrate for NET and DAT (Figure 12-28), binding at the *same* site that the monoamines bind to the transporter, thus inhibiting NE and DA reuptake (Figure 12-28). At the doses of amphetamine used for the treatment of ADHD, the clinical differences in the actions of amphetamine versus methylphenidate can be relatively small. However, at the high doses of amphetamine used by stimulant addicts, additional pharmacologic actions of amphetamine are triggered. Following competitive

Regulation of the Transport and Availability of Synaptic DA

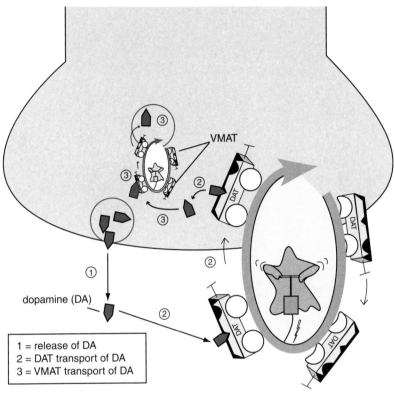

1 = release of DA
2 = DAT transport of DA
3 = VMAT transport of DA

Figure 12-25A. Regulation of transport and availability of synaptic dopamine. To understand how stimulants work, it is necessary to know how DA is cleared from the synaptic cleft and stored. The regulation of synaptic DA is dependent upon proper functioning of two transporters, namely the dopamine transporter (DAT) and the vesicular monoamine transporter (VMAT). After DA is released (1) it can act at postsynaptic receptors or it can be transported back into the terminal via DAT (2). Once inside the terminal, DA is "encapsulated" into vesicles via VMAT (3). These DA-filled vesicles can then merge with the membrane and lead to more DA release. This finely tuned machinery ensures that DA levels never reach toxic levels in the synapse, nor in the DA terminal. By "engulfing" DA into vesicles it is possible for the DA neuron to ensure the viability of DA.

inhibition of DAT (Figure 12-28A) amphetamine is actually transported as a hitchhiker into the presynaptic DA terminal, an action not shared by methylphenidate or antidepressants (Figure 12-28A). Once there in sufficient quantities, such as occurs with doses taken for abuse, amphetamine is also a competitive inhibitor of the vesicular transporter (VMAT2) for both DA and NE (Figure 12-28B). Once amphetamine hitchhikes another ride into synaptic vesicles, it displaces DA there, causing a flood of DA release (Figure 12-28C). As DA accumulates in the cytoplasm of the presynaptic neuron, it causes the DAT to reverse directions, spilling intracellular DA into the synapse, and also opening presynaptic channels to further release DA in a flood into the synapse (Figure 12-28D). These pharmacologic actions of high-dose amphetamine are not linked to any therapeutic action in ADHD but to reinforcement, reward, euphoria, and continuing abuse. Actions of high-dose amphetamine, methamphetamine, and cocaine, given orally in immediate-release formulations or intranasally, intravenously, or smoked, are discussed further in Chapter 14 on drug abuse.

Amphetamine has a *d*- and an *l*-isomer (Figures 12-26, 12-27, 12-30). The *d*-isomer is more potent than the *l*-isomer for DAT binding, but *d*- and *l*-amphetamine isomers are more equally potent in their actions on NET binding. Thus, *d*-amphetamine preparations will have relatively more action on DAT than NET; mixed salts of both *d*- and *l*-amphetamine will have relatively more action on NET than *d*-amphetamine but overall still more action on DAT than NET (see Figure 12-30). These pharmacological mechanisms of action of the stimulants come into play particularly at lower therapeutic doses utilized for the treatment of ADHD. *d*-Amphetamine also comes in a formulation linked to the amino acid lysine (Figure 12-27) which is not absorbed until slowly cleaved into active *d*-amphetamine in the stomach, and slowly, rather than rapidly, absorbed.

Slow-release versus fast-release stimulants and the mysterious DAT

Rapid and high degrees of DAT occupancy by stimulants may cause euphoria and lead to abuse, whereas slow onset and lower degrees of DAT occupancy

Mechanism of Action of Methylphenidate

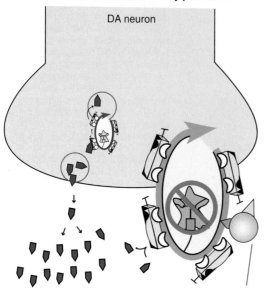

Figure 12-25B. Mechanism of action of methylphenidate: dopaminergic neurons. Methylphenidate works at DAT similar to how selective serotonin reuptake inhibitors (SSRIs) work at the serotonin transporter (SERT), namely by blocking the reuptake of DA into the terminal. Methylphenidate basically freezes the transporter in time, preventing DA reuptake and thus leading to increased synaptic availability of DA. Unlike amphetamine, methylphenidate is not itself taken up into the DA terminal via the transporter.

Mechanism of Action of Methylphenidate

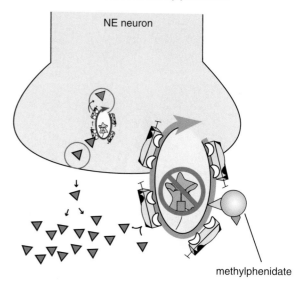

Figure 12-25C. Mechanism of action of methylphenidate: noradrenergic neurons. Methylphenidate works at NET in a manner similar to its actions at DAT, namely by blocking the reuptake of NE into the terminal. Methylphenidate freezes the transporter in time, preventing NE reuptake and thus leading to increased synaptic availability of NE. Unlike amphetamine, methylphenidate is not itself taken up into the NE terminal via the transporter.

may be consistent with antidepressant actions and improvement in attention in ADHD. The DAT appears therefore to be a somewhat mysterious target for drugs, giving one set of responses if occupancy by a given stimulant is rapid, saturating, and short-acting (namely, resulting in "highs" and reinforcement and eventually compulsive use) (Figure 12-30), and a completely different set of responses if occupancy by that same stimulant of that very same DAT target ramps up slowly, has incomplete target saturation, and lasts a long time (resulting in therapeutic actions in ADHD and depression without "highs" or abuse) (Figure 12-31). Thus, pharmacokinetic considerations seem to be just as important to the actions of stimulants in general, and in ADHD in particular, as their pharmacodynamic mechanisms.

Clinicians, parents, and patients often ask if there is a difference between the use of stimulants in the treatment of ADHD and the abuse of stimulants in substance-use disorders. The difference lies less in the mechanism of action, but more in the nature of the

mysterious DAT, which has very different clinical responses to different routes of administration and doses, and thus how quickly, how strongly, and how completely DAT is blocked. When using stimulants to treat a patient it may be preferable to obtain a slow-rising, constant, steady-state level of the drug (Figure 12-29A). Under those circumstances the firing pattern of DA will be tonic, regular, and not at the mercy of fluctuating levels of DA. Some pulsatile firing is fine, especially when involved in reinforcing learning and salience (Figure 12-10). However, as seen in Figure 12-13, DA stimulation follows an inverted U-shaped curve, such that too much DA will mimic the actions of DA in stress (Figure 12-12) at higher doses, or mimic drug abuse at the highest doses (Figure 12-29B). Thus a pulsatile drug administration that causes intermittent release of DA, unlike constant release, will lead to the highly reinforcing pleasurable effects of drugs of abuse.

The past several years have seen a flurry of new drug development activities aimed at optimizing the drug delivery characteristics of stimulants for ADHD. These are not mere patent extension gimmicks, nor

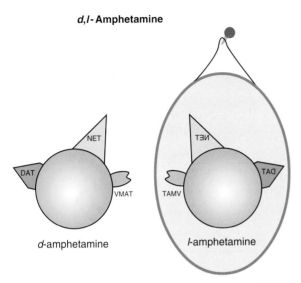

Figure 12-26. *d,l*-Amphetamine. *d,l*-Amphetamine includes both *d*- and *l*-enantiomers. Similar to *d*-amphetamine, *d,l*-amphetamine is a competitive inhibitor of DAT, NET, and VMAT. There are, however, subtle differences. For example the *d*-isomer is more potent for DAT binding, and both *d*- and *l*-isomers are equipotent for NET binding. This translates to the following actions of these compounds: *d*-amphetamine will have relatively more action on DAT than NET, while the mixed salts of both *d*- and *l*-amphetamine will have relatively more action on NET than the *d*-isomer, but overall still more action on DAT than NET. These small differences are especially noticeable at the lower doses of both *d*-amphetamine and *d,l*-amphetamine and in some individual patients. Different formulations of *d,l*-amphetamine are approved for the treatment of ADHD in children and adults.

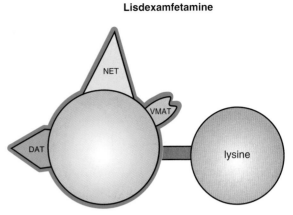

Figure 12-27. Lisdexamfetamine. Lisdexamfetamine is the prodrug of *d*-amphetamine, linked to the amino acid lysine. It is only centrally active as *d*-amphetamine once it has been cleaved in the stomach into the active compounds *d*-amphetamine plus free L-lysine.

mere convenience features, although it is certainly an advantage for a child not to have to take a second dose of a stimulant in the middle of the day at school. More importantly, the "slow-dose" stimulants, shown in Figure 12-30, optimize the rate, the amount, and the length of time that a stimulant occupies NET and DAT for therapeutic use in ADHD. Optimization for ADHD means occupying enough of the NET in prefrontal cortex at a slow enough onset and long enough duration of action to enhance tonic NE signaling there via α_{2A} receptors and to increase tonic DA signaling there via D_1 receptors, yet occupying little enough of the DAT in nucleus accumbens so as not to increase phasic signaling there via D_2 receptors (Figure 12-30). It appears that ADHD patients have their therapeutic improvement by stimulants at the mercy of how fast, how much, and for how long stimulants occupy NET and DAT. When this is done in an ideal manner with slow onset, robust but subsaturating drug levels, and long duration of action before declining and wearing off, the patient benefits

with improved ADHD symptoms, hours of relief, and no euphoria (Figure 12-30). Tonic drug delivery of stimulants amplifies the desired tonic increases in DA and NE action for ADHD improvement for several hours. On the other hand, Figure 12-31 shows how *not* to treat ADHD with stimulants: namely by frequent high-dose and pulsatile delivery of short-acting stimulants, which approximates very closely the best way to use these agents for euphoria and reinforcement with amplifying phasic NE and DA signals (Figure 12-31).

Noradrenergic treatment of ADHD

Atomoxetine

Atomoxetine is a selective norepinephrine reuptake inhibitor or selective NRI. Sometimes called NET inhibitors, the selective NRIs have known antidepressant properties (discussed in Chapter 7). In terms of their mechanism of therapeutic action in ADHD, since the prefrontal cortex lacks high concentrations of DAT, DA is inactivated in this part of the brain by NET. Thus, inhibiting NET increases both DA and NE in prefrontal cortex (Figures 12-32 and 12-33; see also discussion in Chapter 7 and Figure 7-34). However, since there are few NE neurons and NETs in nucleus accumbens, inhibiting NET does not lead to an increase in either NE or DA there (Figure 12-32). For this reason, in ADHD patients with weak NE and DA signals in prefrontal cortex, a selective NRI such as atomoxetine increases both NE and DA in

Mechanism of Action of Amphetamine:
The Yin and the Yang

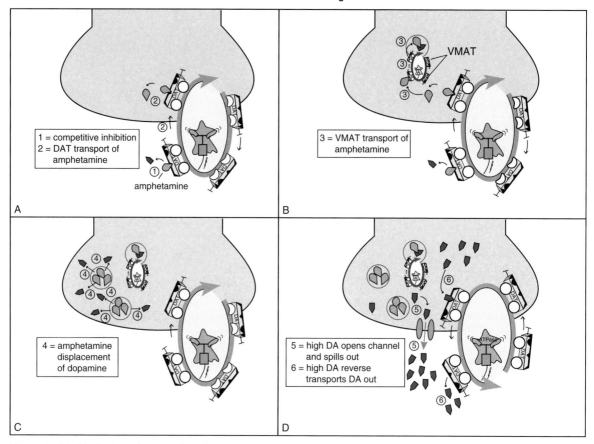

Figure 12-28. Mechanism of action of amphetamine: the yin and the yang. The yin – therapeutic and controlled drug delivery causes tonic-like increases; the yang – abusive doses and pulsatile drug delivery cause phasic-like increases. Shown here is amphetamine acting as a competitive inhibitor at DAT, thus competing with DA (1), or NE at NET (not shown). This is unlike methylphenidate's actions at DAT and NET, which are not competitive. Additionally, since amphetamine is also a competitive inhibitor of VMAT (a property that methylphenidate lacks) it is actually taken into the DA terminal via DAT (2), where it can then also be packaged into vesicles (3). At high levels, amphetamine will lead to the displacement of DA from the vesicles into the terminal (4). Furthermore, once a critical threshold of DA has been reached, DA will be expelled from the terminal via two mechanisms: the opening of channels to allow for a massive dumping of DA into the synapse (5) and the reversal of DAT (6). This fast release of DA will lead to the euphoric effect experienced after amphetamine use.

prefrontal cortex, enhancing tonic signaling of both, but increases neither NE nor DA in accumbens. Therefore, atomoxetine has no abuse potential.

Atomoxetine is the only such agent approved for use in ADHD, but several other agents have NRI actions, including the approved (outside of the US) antidepressant and selective NRI reboxetine (Figure 7-38), and the various SNRIs, which not only have NRI actions but also serotonin reuptake inhibiting properties (Figures 7-30 through 7-34).

Bupropion is a weak NRI and also a weak DAT inhibitor known as a norepinephrine–dopamine reuptake inhibitor (NDRI). Figure 12-34 compares

the actions of bupropion and atomoxetine (also discussed in Chapter 7: see Figures 7-35 through 7-37). Several tricyclic antidepressants have notable NRI actions, such as desipramine and nortriptyline. All of these agents with NRI properties have been utilized in the treatment of ADHD, with varying amounts of success, but only atomoxetine is well investigated and approved for this use in children and adults.

Atomoxetine's hypothetical actions in ADHD patients with stress and comorbidity states presumably linked to excessive and phasic DA and NE release are shown conceptually by comparing the untreated states in Figure 12-12 with the changes that

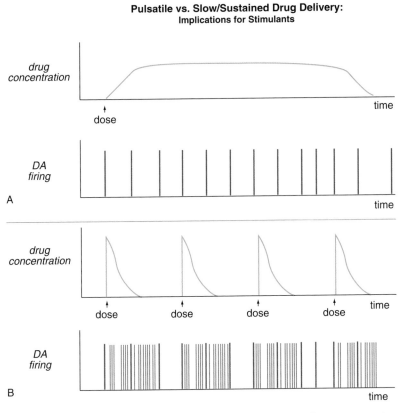

Pulsatile vs. Slow/Sustained Drug Delivery:
Implications for Stimulants

Figure 12-29. Pulsatile versus slow and sustained drug delivery. The difference between stimulants as treatments and stimulants as drugs of abuse lies less in their mechanism of action than in the route of administration and dose, and thus how fast, how completely, and for how long DAT is blocked. When using stimulants to treat a patient it may be preferable to obtain a slow-rising, constant, steady-state level of the drug (A). Under those circumstances the firing pattern of DA will be tonic, regular, and not at the mercy of fluctuating levels of dopamine. While some pulsatile firing can be beneficial, especially when involved in reinforcing learning and salience, higher doses of DA will mimic the actions of DA in stress and mimic drug abuse at the highest doses (B). Unlike a constant administration of DA, pulsatile administration of DA may lead to the highly reinforcing pleasurable effects of drugs of abuse, and to compulsive use and addiction.

theoretically follow chronic treatment with atomoxetine in Figure 12-33. That is, ADHD linked to conditions that are associated with chronic stress and comorbidities is theoretically caused by overly active NE and DA circuits in prefrontal cortex causing an excess of phasic NE and DA activity (Figure 12-12). When slow-onset, long-duration, and essentially perpetual NET inhibition occurs in prefrontal cortex due to atomoxetine, this theoretically restores tonic postsynaptic D_1 and α_{2A}-adrenergic signaling, downregulates phasic NE and DA actions, and desensitizes postsynaptic NE and DA receptors. The possible consequences of this are to reduce chronic HPA axis overactivation and thereby potentially reverse stress-related brain atrophy and even induce neurogenesis that could protect the brain. Such biochemical and molecular changes could be associated with decreases in ADHD symptoms, reduction of relapse, and decreases in anxiety, depression, and heavy drinking. Unlike stimulant use, where the therapeutic actions are at the mercy of plasma drug levels and momentary NET/DAT occupancies, actions from long-term NRI actions give 24-hour symptom relief, in much the same manner as do SSRIs and SNRIs for the treatment of

depression and anxiety. Such possibilities are already indicated by early clinical investigations of this mechanism of selective NRI action in ADHD, but much further work is necessary to establish with certainty the long-term effects of selective NRI action, the differences of outcomes if any compared to long-term stimulant actions, and the best ADHD patient profile to choose for the selective NRI mechanism. Selective NRIs generally have smaller effect sizes for reducing ADHD symptoms than stimulants in short-term trials, especially in patients without comorbidity. However, NRIs are not necessarily inferior in ADHD patients who have not been previously treated with stimulants, or in ADHD patients who have been treated long-term (longer than 8–12 weeks). NRIs may actually be preferred to stimulants in patients with complex comorbidities.

Alpha-2A-adrenergic agonists

Norepinephrine receptors are discussed in Chapter 6 and illustrated in Figures 6-27 through 6-30. There are numerous subtypes of α-adrenergic receptors, from presynaptic autoreceptors, generally of the α_{2A} subtype (Figures 6-27, 6-28, 6-29) to postsynaptic α_{2A}, α_{2B}, α_{2C}, and α_1 subtypes (Figure 6-27). Alpha-2A receptors are

"Slow-Dose" Stimulants Amplify Tonic NE and DA Signals

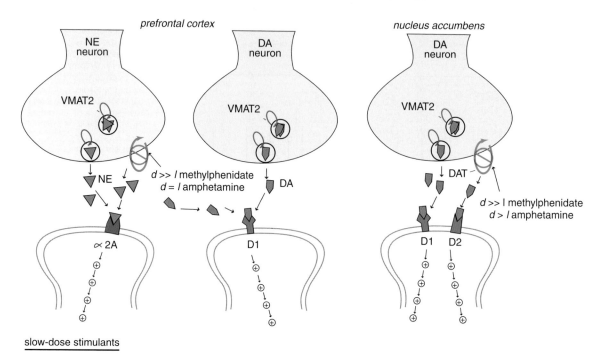

slow-dose stimulants

OROS - methylphenidate, LA - methylphenidate, XR - *d*-methylphenidate, transdermal methylphenidate *d*-amphetamine spansules. XR - *d,l* mixed amphetamine salts, XXR - *d,l* mixed amphetamine salts prodrug *d*-amphetamine (lisdexamfetamine)

Figure 12-30. Slow-dose stimulants amplify tonic norepinephrine and dopamine signals. Hypothetically, whether a drug has abuse potential depends on how it affects the DA pathway. In other words, the pharmacodynamic and pharmacokinetic properties of stimulants affect their therapeutic as well as their potential abuse profiles. Extended-release formulations of oral stimulants, the transdermal methylphenidate patch, and the new prodrug lisdexamfetamine are all considered "slow-dose" stimulants and may amplify tonic NE and DA signals, presumed to be low in ADHD. These agents block the norepinephrine transporter (NET) in the prefrontal cortex and the DA transporter (DAT) in the nucleus accumbens. Hypothetically, the "slow-dose" stimulants occupy NET in the prefrontal cortex with slow enough onset, and for long enough duration, that they enhance tonic NE and DA signaling via α_{2A} and D_1 postsynaptic receptors, respectively, but they do not occupy DAT quickly or extensively enough in the nucleus accumbens to increase phasic signaling via D_2 receptors. The latter hypothetically suggests reduced abuse potential.

widely distributed throughout the CNS, with high levels in the cortex and locus coeruleus. These receptors are thought to be the primary mediators of the effects of NE in prefrontal cortex regulating symptoms of inattention, hyperactivity, and impulsivity in ADHD. Alpha-2B receptors are in high concentrations in the thalamus and may be important in mediating sedating actions of NE, while α_{2C} receptors are densest in striatum. Alpha-1 receptors generally have opposing actions to α_2 receptors, with α_2 mechanisms predominating when NE release is low or moderate (i.e., for normal attention), but with α_1 mechanisms predominating at NE synapses when NE release is high (e.g., associated with stress and comorbidity)

and contributing to cognitive impairment. Thus, selective NRIs at low doses will first increase activity at α_{2A} postsynaptic receptors to enhance cognitive performance, but at high doses may swamp the synapse with too much NE and cause sedation, cognitive impairment or both. Patients with these responses to selective NRIs may benefit from lowering the dose. Alpha-2-adrenergic receptors are present in high concentrations in the prefrontal cortex, but only in low concentrations in the nucleus accumbens.

There are two direct-acting agonists for α_2 receptors used to treat ADHD, guanfacine (Figure 12-35) and clonidine (Figure 12-36). Guanfacine is relatively more selective for α_{2A} receptors (Figure 12-35).

Pulsatile Stimulants Amplify Tonic and Phasic NE and DA Signals

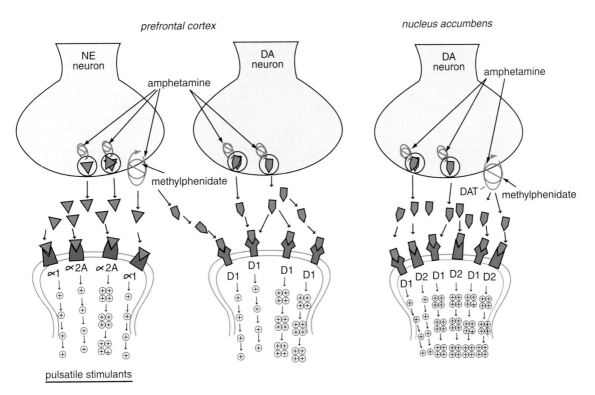

pulsatile stimulants

oral immediate-release, intravenous, intranasal, smoked, *d*-amphetamine,

d,l amphetamine salts, methylphenidate, *d*-methylphenidate, cocaine,

methamphetamine

Figure 12-31. Pulsatile stimulants amplify tonic and phasic norepinephrine and dopamine signals. Immediate-release oral stimulants – similarly to intravenous, smoked, or snorted stimulants (which are considered pulsatile stimulants) – lead to a rapid increase in NE and DA levels. Rapidly amplifying the phasic neuronal firing of DA and NE is associated with euphoria and abuse. While methylphenidate and amphetamine have slightly different mechanisms of action, both medications can lead to massive release of DA. This increased release of DA may also contribute to the abuse potential of immediate-release formulations of stimulants, due to increased phasic as well as tonic DA signaling.

Recently, guanfacine has been formulated into a controlled-release product, guanfacine ER, that allows once-daily administration, and lower peak-dose side effects than immediate-release guanfacine. Only the controlled-release version of guanfacine is approved for treatment of ADHD.

Clonidine is a relatively nonselective agonist at α_2 receptors, with actions on α_{2A}, α_{2B}, and α_{2C} receptors (Figure 12-36). In addition, clonidine has actions on imidazoline receptors, thought to be responsible for some of clonidine's sedating and hypotensive actions (Figure 12-37). Although the actions of clonidine at

α_{2A} receptors exhibit therapeutic potential for ADHD, its actions at other receptors may increase side effects. Clonidine is approved for the treatment of hypertension, but not for the treatment of ADHD, conduct disorder, oppositional defiant disorder, or Tourette's syndrome, for which it is often used "off-label."

By contrast, the selective α_{2A} receptor agonist guanfacine is 15–60 times more selective for α_{2A} receptors than for α_{2B} and α_{2C} receptors. Additionally, guanfacine is 10 times weaker than clonidine at inducing sedation and lowering blood pressure, yet it is 25 times more potent in enhancing prefrontal

497

Atomoxetine in ADHD With Weak Prefrontal NE and DA Signals

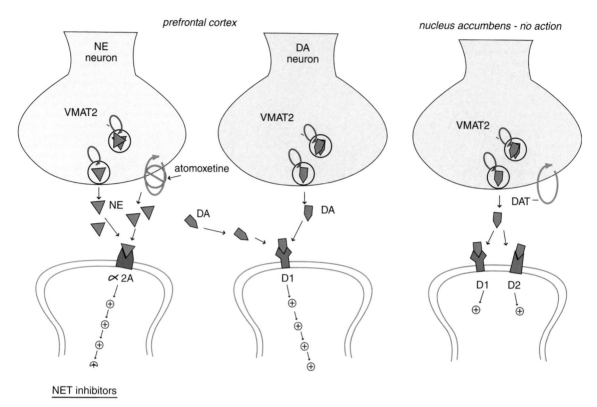

NET inhibitors

atomoxetine, reboxetine, bupropion (NDRI), venlafaxine (SNRI),
duloxetine (SNRI), desvenlafaxine (SNRI), milnacipran (SNRI),
desipramine (TCA), nortriptyline (TCA)

Figure 12-32. Atomoxetine in ADHD with weak prefrontal norepinephrine and dopamine signals. It has been suggested that atomoxetine can have therapeutic effects in ADHD without abuse potential. As a norepinephrine reuptake blocker, atomoxetine causes NE and DA levels to increase in the prefrontal cortex, where inactivation of both of these neurotransmitters is largely due to NET (on the left). At the same time, the relative lack of NETs in the nucleus accumbens prevents atomoxetine from increasing NE or DA levels in that brain area, thus reducing the risk of abuse (on the right). Thus, as shown in Figure 12-22, by increasing NE and DA levels to their optimal levels in the prefrontal cortex (top of the inverted U-shaped curve), atomoxetine may be able to increase attention and decrease hyperactivity in patients with ADHD.

cortical function. Thus, it can be said that guanfacine exhibits therapeutic efficacy with a reduced side-effect profile compared to clonidine. The therapeutic benefits of guanfacine are related to the direct effects of the drug on postsynaptic receptors in the PFC, which lead to the strengthening of network inputs, and to behavioral improvements as seen in Figures 12-38 and 12-39.

Who are the best candidates for monotherapy with guanfacine ER? Hypothetically, the symptoms of ADHD could be caused in some patients by NE levels being low in the prefrontal cortex, without additional impairments in DA neurotransmission (Figure 12-38). This would lead to scrambled signals lost within the background noise, which could be seen behaviorally as hyperactivity, impulsivity, and inattention (Figure 12-38A). In this instance, treatment with a selective α_{2A} agonist would lead to increased signal via direct stimulation of postsynaptic receptors, and this would translate into the patient being able to focus, sit still, and behave adequately (Figure 12-38B). There is currently no way to identify these patients in advance, other than by an empiric trial of guanfacine ER.

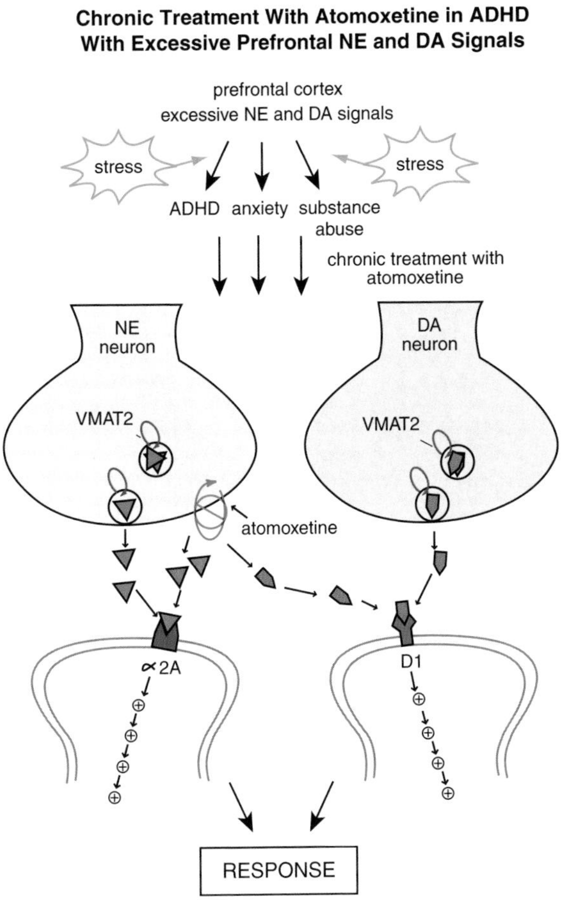

Chronic Treatment With Atomoxetine in ADHD With Excessive Prefrontal NE and DA Signals

Figure 12-33. Chronic treatment with atomoxetine in ADHD. Stress combined with excessive NE and DA signaling can lead to ADHD, anxiety, or substance abuse. One way to reduce excessive stimulation could be to desensitize postsynaptic DA and NE receptors, and thus allow the neurons to return to normal tonic firing over time. By continuously blocking NET, atomoxetine has the capability of doing this. The "big picture" ramification of such a treatment could be decreased anxiety, decreased heavy drinking, and a reduction in relapses of substance abuse.

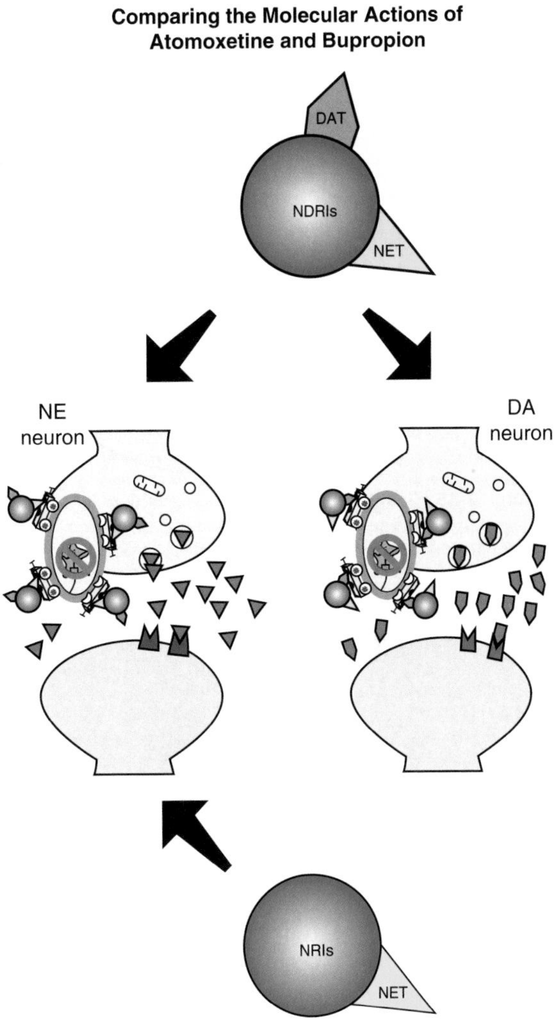

Comparing the Molecular Actions of Atomoxetine and Bupropion

Figure 12-34. Comparing the molecular actions of atomoxetine and bupropion. Atomoxetine is a selective norepinephrine reuptake inhibitor or NRI, while bupropion is a norepinephrine–dopamine reuptake inhibitor or NDRI. Both agents have some pharmacological properties in common, and both of these drugs can have therapeutic effects in the treatment of ADHD.

Patients suffering from ADHD and oppositional symptoms can be argumentative, disobedient, aggressive, and exhibit temper tantrums (Figures 12-8 and 12-39). These behaviors are hypothetically linked to very low levels of NE and low levels of DA in the ventromedial prefrontal cortex (VMPFC), thus leading to much reduced signal and increased noise (Figure 12-39A). While treatment with a stimulant will improve the situation by reducing the noise, it will not solve the strong NE deficiencies (Figure 12-39B), therefore only partially improving

behavior. Augmenting a stimulant with an α_{2A} agonist (Figure 12-39C) will hypothetically solve the problem by optimizing the levels of NE, thus enhancing the signal, in the presence of an already optimized DA output. Behaviorally, this can result in a patient cooperating and behaving appropriately. Guanfacine ER has been approved as an augmenting agent for patients inadequately responsive to stimulants, and may be especially helpful in patients with oppositional symptoms.

guanfacine

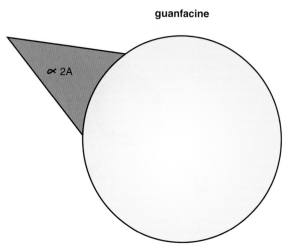

Figure 12-35. Guanfacine. Guanfacine is much more selective for α_{2A} receptors than clonidine and also exhibits therapeutic efficacy with a reduced side-effect profile compared to clonidine. The therapeutic benefits of guanfacine are related to its enhancement of prefrontal cortical functioning, which leads to behavioral improvements. Tolerability and convenience are also enhanced by once-daily oral controlled-release formulation.

clonidine

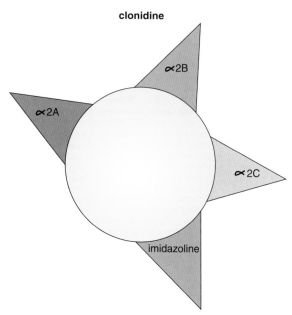

Figure 12-36. Clonidine. The nonselective α_2-adrenergic agonist clonidine binds to α_{2A}, α_{2B}, and α_{2C} receptors. Moreover, clonidine also binds to imidazoline receptors, which contribute to its sedating and hypotensive effects. Clonidine is approved for the treatment of hypertension but is often used "off-label" for the treatment of ADHD, conduct disorder, oppositional defiant disorder, and Tourette's syndrome.

Future treatments for ADHD

Several new mechanisms being targeted for the symptoms of ADHD also are being targeted for cognitive symptoms in other disorders including schizophrenia and Alzheimer's dementia. Enhancing prefrontal cortex histamine actions by blocking its presynaptic H_3 autoreceptor is discussed in Chapter 11 and illustrated in Figure 11-11. Several **H_3 antagonists** are in testing to boost cognitive function in ADHD.

Boosting acetylcholine function in prefrontal cortex is another pro-cognitive approach. Muscarinic agonists tend to be poorly tolerated, but there are several emerging approaches to stimulating nicotinic cholinergic receptors. Several **α_7-nicotinic receptor agonists** are being tested (e.g., EVP-6124, TC5619, DMXB-A/GTS21, MEM3454, R4996/MEM63908, AZD0328, ABT560, JN403, RG3487), some with promising early clinical results in ADHD. Ongoing investigations are dealing with the possible development of tolerance to full agonists without allosteric actions, insufficient efficacy in partial agonists, and how to treat smokers who are already stimulating their nicotinic receptors. One multifunctional agent is RG3487, which is both an α_7-nicotinic partial agonist and a **$5HT_3$ antagonist**, the latter

mechanism discussed in Chapter 7 and illustrated in Figure 7-46 as a mechanism to raise acetylcholine levels in the cortex. Vortioxetine, a novel multifunctional antidepressant with $5HT_3$ antagonist, SERT inhibition, and multiple other pharmacologic actions, discussed in Chapter 7 and illustrated in Figure 7-89, also raises acetylcholine levels in experimental models and has theoretical appeal as a pro-cognitive agent not only in depression but also in other disorders such as ADHD. Agonists for a different nicotinic receptor, the **$\alpha_4\beta_2$-nicotinic receptor**, are discussed in Chapter 14 on substance abuse, and are being tested as well for potential precognitive actions (e.g., varenicline, ABT560, also an $\alpha_4\beta_2$ agonist).

Other early-stage pro-cognitive mechanisms being tested in ADHD and other disorders are **AMPAkines**, boosting glutamate neurotransmission at AMPA receptors (e.g., CX1739, CS717, LY451395), **$5HT_6$ antagonists** (e.g., PRX03140, PRX07034, SAM-315, SAM-531, SB742457, SYN114, SYN120), and phosphodiesterase 4 **(PDE$_4$) inhibitors** (e.g., HT0712).

The Mechanism of Action of Clonidine and Guanfacine and How They Affect the Three Alpha-2 Receptors

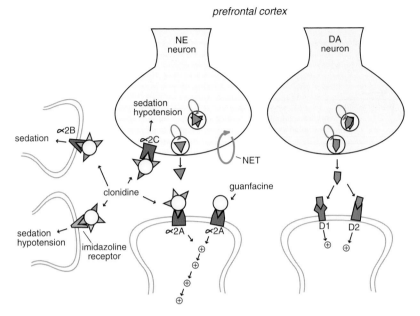

Figure 12-37. Mechanism of action of clonidine and guanfacine. Alpha-2-adrenergic receptors are present in high concentrations in the prefrontal cortex (PFC), but only in low concentrations in the nucleus accumbens. Alpha-2 receptors come in three flavors: α_{2A}, α_{2B}, and α_{2C}. The most prevalent subtype in the prefrontal cortex is the α_{2A} receptor, and these apparently mediate the inattentive, hyperactive, and impulsive symptoms of ADHD by regulating the PFC. Alpha-2B receptors are mainly located in the thalamus and are associated with sedative effects. Alpha-2C receptors are located in the locus coeruleus, with few in the PFC. Besides being associated with hypotensive effects, they also have sedative actions. In ADHD, clonidine and guanfacine – by stimulating postsynaptic receptors – can increase NE signaling to normal levels. The lack of action at postsynaptic DA receptors parallels their lack of abuse potential.

Effects of an Alpha-2A Agonist in ADHD

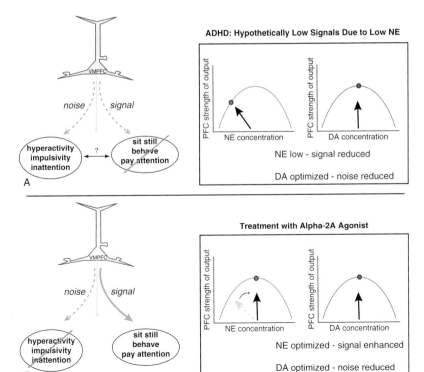

Figure 12-38. Effects of an α_{2A} agonist in ADHD. The symptoms of ADHD could hypothetically be due to low NE levels in the PFC, without additional impairments in DA neurotransmission. The resulting scrambled signals may manifest as hyperactivity, impulsivity, and inattention (A). Treatment with a selective α_{2A} agonist (B) would lead to increased signal via direct stimulation of postsynaptic receptors, resulting in increased ability to sit still and focus.

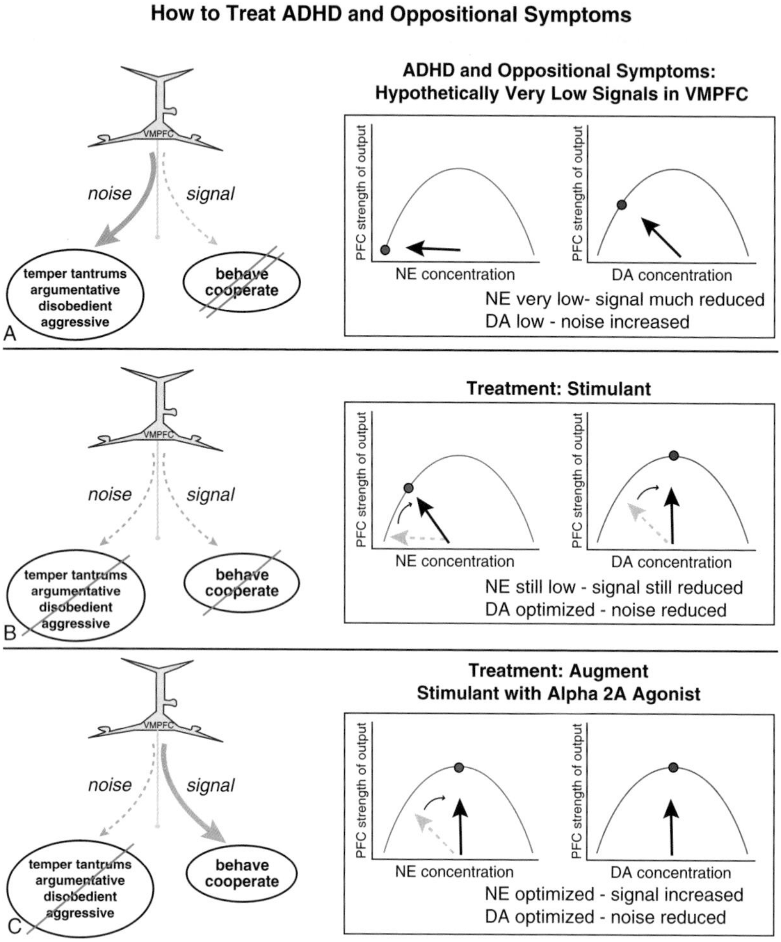

How to Treat ADHD and Oppositional Symptoms

Figure 12-39. How to treat ADHD and oppositional symptoms. Argumentative, disobedient, and aggressive behaviors are often seen in patients suffering from ADHD and oppositional symptoms. These behaviors could theoretically be due to low levels of DA and extensively low levels of NE in the VMPFC in some patients, thus leading to much reduced signal and increased noise (A). While treatment with a stimulant may reduce the noise, it will not solve the strong NE deficiencies (B), therefore only partially improving behavior. The augmentation of a stimulant with an α_{2A} agonist (C) could optimize the levels of NE, thus enhancing the signal, in the presence of an already optimized DA output.

Summary

Attention deficit hyperactivity disorder (ADHD) has core symptoms of inattentiveness, impulsivity, and hyperactivity, linked theoretically to specific malfunctioning neuronal circuits in prefrontal cortex. ADHD can also be conceptualized as a disorder of dysregulation of norepinephrine (NE) and dopamine (DA) in the prefrontal cortex, including some patients with deficient NE and DA and others with excessive NE and DA. Treatments theoretically return patients to normal efficiency of information processing in the prefrontal circuits. Differences exist between children and adults with ADHD, and the special considerations for adults, such as treating comorbidities and using nonstimulants, are receiving increasing attention in psychopharmacology. The mechanisms of action, both in terms of pharmacodynamics and pharmacokinetics, for stimulant treatments of ADHD are discussed in detail. The goal is to amplify tonic but not phasic norepinephrine and dopamine actions in ADHD by controlling the rate of stimulant drug delivery, the degree of transporter occupancy, and the duration of transporter occupancy by stimulants. Theoretical mechanisms of action of selective norepinephrine reuptake inhibitors such as atomoxetine and their possible advantages in adults with chronic stress and comorbidities are discussed. Actions of a novel α_{2A}-adrenergic agonist, guanfacine ER, are also introduced.

Chapter 13

Dementia and its treatment

This chapter will provide a brief overview of the various causes of dementias and their pathologies, including the most recent diagnostic criteria and the emerging integration of biomarkers into clinical practice for Alzheimer's disease. Full clinical descriptions and formal criteria for how to diagnose the numerous known dementias should be obtained by consulting standard reference sources. The discussion here will emphasize the links between various pathological mechanisms, brain circuits, and neurotransmitters and the various symptoms of dementia, with an emphasis on Alzheimer's disease. The goal of this chapter is to acquaint the reader with ideas about the clinical and biological aspects of dementia and its currently approved treatments as well as new treatments that are on the horizon. The emphasis here is on the biological basis of symptoms of dementia and

of their relief by psychopharmacologic agents, as well as on the mechanism of action of drugs that treat these symptoms. For details of doses, side effects, drug interactions, and other issues relevant to the prescribing of these drugs in clinical practice, the reader should consult standard drug handbooks (such as *Stahl's Essential Psychopharmacology: the Prescriber's Guide*).

Causes, pathology, and clinical features of dementia

Dementia consists of memory impairment (amnesia) plus deficits in either language (aphasia), motor function (apraxia), recognition (agnosia), or executive function such as working memory and problem solving. Personality changes can also be present,

Table 13-1 Pathological features of selected degenerative dementias

Disorder	Pathology
Alzheimer's disease	Amyloid/tau pathology
Dementia with Lewy bodies Parkinson's dementia Multisystem atrophy	Alpha-synuclein pathology
Frontotemporal dementia Progressive supranuclear palsy Corticobasilar degeneration	Tau pathology
Huntington's disease Spinocerebellar ataxia	Trinucleotide repeat
Wilson's disease (copper) Hallervorden–Spatz disease (iron)	Toxic/metabolic
Metachromatic leukodystrophy	Leukodystrophy
Creutzfeldt–Jakob disease Variant Creutzfeldt–Jakob disease (bovine spongiform encephalopathy) Gerstmann–Sträussler–Scheinker disease Fatal familiar insomnia (thalamic dementia)	Prion-related dementias

Table 13-2 Not all memory disturbance is Alzheimer's disease: clinical features of selected degenerative dementias

Dementia	Clinical features
Alzheimer's disease	Memory deficit Aphasia Apraxia Agnosia
Dementia with Lewy bodies	Memory deficit Fluctuating attention Extrapyramidal signs Psychosis (hallucinations)
Frontotemporal dementia	Memory deficit Speech/language disorders Disinhibition Hyperorality
Huntington's disease	Memory deficit Executive dysfunction Chorea
Creutzfeldt–Jakob disease	Memory deficit Ataxia Myoclonus Language disturbance

sometimes even before memory impairment begins. There are many causes of dementia (Tables 13-1 through 13-3), and the unique pathologies associated with some of the major dementias are listed in Table 13-1. Knowing the pathology does not mean that a treatment is available, as it is often not evident how to translate information about brain pathology into pharmacological treatments. The best hope currently is in the area of amyloid pathology, where new treatments under investigation are attempting to interfere with amyloid processing in Alzheimer's disease, as will be discussed later in this chapter.

Just because a patient develops memory disturbance does not mean it is Alzheimer's disease (Table 13-2). Alzheimer's dementia is perhaps the best-known and commonest dementia, but it is often the other symptoms associated with memory loss that help make the diagnosis clinically (Table 13-2). Just to complicate things, many patients have mixed types of dementia, particularly Alzheimer's dementia plus dementia with Lewy bodies, or Alzheimer's dementia plus vascular dementia (Figure 13-1). Such cases

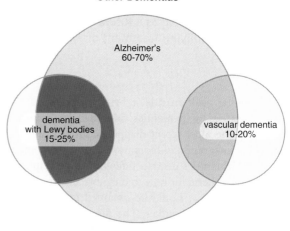

Mixed Dementia: Overlap of Alzheimer's Disease with Other Dementias

Figure 13-1. Mixed dementia. There are several types of dementia, of which Alzheimer's disease is the most common. They are distinguished by their underlying pathologies. It is possible to have more than one dementia, and in fact many patients have both Alzheimer's disease and either dementia with Lewy bodies or vascular dementia.

are complicated to diagnose clinically, and definitive diagnosis sometimes must await autopsy. Most dementias are really pathological diagnoses, not clinical diagnoses.

Table 13-3 Nondegenerative dementias

Vascular	Multi-infarct dementia
	Strategic single-infarct dementia
	Small vessel disease
	Watershed area hypoperfusion
Infectious	HIV dementia
	Neurosyphilis
	Whipple's disease
	Progressive multifocal
	leukoencephalopathy
	Tuberculosis
	Fungal/protozoal
	Sarcoidosis
Demyelinating	Multiple sclerosis
Endocrine	Hypothyroidism
	Cushing's syndrome
	Adrenal insufficiency
	Hypoparathyroidism
	Hyperparathyroidism
Brain injuries	Post-anoxic
	Post-encephalitic
	Chronic subdural hematoma
Vitamin deficiency	B_{12}, B_1, folate, niacin
Vasculitides	Lupus erythematosus
	Sjögren's disease
Toxicities	Heavy metal (storage) disorders (arsenic, mercury, lead)
	Industrial/environmental toxins (fertilizers, pesticides)
	Medications
	Chronic alcohol/drug abuse
	Wernicke–Korsakoff syndrome
	Marchiafava–Bignami disease
Organ failure	Hepatic encephalopathy
	Uremic encephalopathy
	Pulmonary insufficiency
Other causes	Dementia syndrome of depression
	Normal pressure hydrocephalus
	Nonconvulsive status epilepticus
	Acute intermittent poyphyria

A wide variety of dementias are considered nondegenerative, and these are listed in Table 13-3. Many of these are treatable upon discovering the underlying cause, but others are not. Extensive clinical evaluation and laboratory testing must rule out these causes prior to concluding that a case of dementia is due to Alzheimer's disease.

Alzheimer's disease: β-amyloid plaques and neurofibrillary tangles

Without the introduction of disease-modifying treatments, Alzheimer's disease is poised for an exponential increase throughout the world, with projections that it will quadruple over the next 40 years to affect 1 in every 85 people on earth: over 100 million people by 2050. Fortunately, new treatments are being designed to interfere with various known pathological processes, particularly the formation of amyloid plaques, in an attempt to halt or slow disease progression in Alzheimer's disease before neurons are irretrievably lost. To understand the current diagnostic criteria for Alzheimer's disease, how and why biomarkers are being integrated into the diagnosis of this disorder, and the rationale behind the hot pursuit of new therapeutics, it is necessary to understand how the two hallmarks of this disorder, amyloid plaques and neurofibrillary tangles, are thought to be formed in the brain in Alzheimer's disease.

The amyloid cascade hypothesis

The leading contemporary theory for the biological basis of Alzheimer's disease centers around the formation of toxic amyloid plaques from peptides due to the abnormal processing of amyloid precursor protein (APP) into toxic forms of Abeta (Aβ) peptides (Figures 13-2 through 13-9). Why do we make Aβ in the first place? Although this is not fully understood, nontoxic Aβ peptides have antioxidant properties, can chelate metal ions, regulate cholesterol transport, and may be involved in blood vessel repair, as a sealant at sites of injury or leakage, possibly protecting from acute brain injury. Hypothetically, Alzheimer's disease is a disorder in which toxic Aβ peptides are formed, leading to deposition of amyloid plaque in the brain, with the ultimate destruction of neurons diffusely throughout the brain, somewhat analogous to how the abnormal deposition of cholesterol in blood vessels causes atherosclerosis.

Thus, Alzheimer's disease may be essentially a problem of too much formation of Aβ amyloid-forming peptides, or too little removal of them. One idea is that neurons in some patients destined to have Alzheimer's disease have abnormalities either in genes that code for a protein called amyloid precursor protein (APP), or in the enzymes that cut this precursor into smaller peptides, or in the mechanisms of removal of these peptides from the brain and from the body. APP is a

Processing of Amyloid Precursor Protein into Soluble Peptides

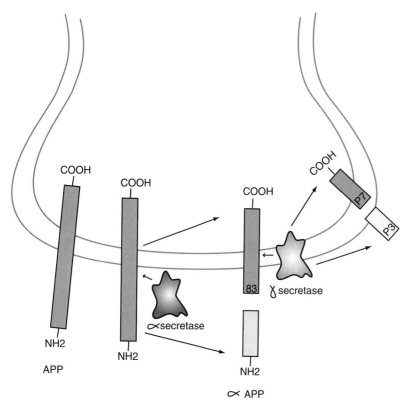

Figure 13-2. Processing of amyloid precursor protein into soluble peptides. The way in which amyloid precursor protein (APP) is processed may help determine whether an individual develops Alzheimer's disease or not. A nontoxic pathway for APP processing is shown here. APP is a transmembrane protein with the C-terminal inside the neuron and the N-terminal outside the neuron. The enzyme α-secretase cuts APP close to where it comes out of the membrane to form two peptides: α-APP, which is soluble, and an 83-amino-acid peptide that remains in the membrane. A second enzyme, γ-secretase, cuts the embedded peptide into two smaller peptides, p7 and p3, which are not "amyloidogenic" and thus are not toxic.

transmembrane protein with the C-terminal inside the neuron and the N-terminal outside the neuron. One pathway for APP processing does not produce toxic peptides and involves the enzyme α-secretase (Figure 13-2). Alpha-secretase cuts APP close to the area where the protein comes out of the membrane, forming two peptides: a soluble fragment known as α-APP and a smaller 83-amino-acid peptide that remains embedded in the membrane until it is further cleaved by a second enzyme acting within the neuronal membrane, called γ-secretase (Figure 13-2). That enzyme produces two smaller peptides, p7 and p3, which are apparently not "amyloidogenic" and therefore not toxic (Figure 13-2).

Another pathway for APP processing can produce toxic peptides that form amyloid plaques (i.e., "amyloidogenic" peptides). In this case a different enzyme, β-secretase, cuts APP a little bit further away from the area where APP comes out of the membrane, forming two peptides: a soluble fragment known as β-APP and a smaller 91-amino-acid peptide that remains embedded in the membrane until it is

further cleaved by γ-secretase within the membrane (Figure 13-3). This releases Aβ peptides of 40, 42 or 43 amino acids that are "amyloidogenic," especially Aβ42 (Figure 13-3).

In Alzheimer's disease, genetic abnormalities may produce an altered APP that, when processed by this second pathway involving β-secretase, produces smaller peptides that are especially toxic. Individuals who do not get Alzheimer's disease may produce peptides that are not very toxic, or may have highly efficient removal mechanisms that prevent neuronal toxicity from developing. The amyloid cascade hypothesis of Alzheimer's disease therefore begins with an APP that is hypothetically genetically abnormal, or genetically or environmentally abnormal in the way it is processed, so that when it is cut into smaller peptide fragments too many toxic peptides are made, accumulate, and form neuron-destroying amyloid plaques, i.e., amyloidosis, and neurofibrillary tangles. Hypothetically, this process triggers a lethal chemical cascade that ultimately results in Alzheimer's disease (Figures 13-3 through 13-8).

Processing of Amyloid Precursor Protein into Aβ peptides

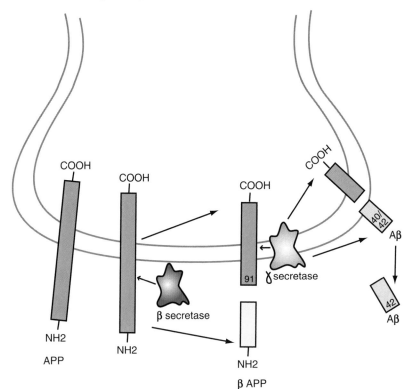

Figure 13-3. Processing of amyloid precursor protein into Aβ peptides. The way in which amyloid precursor protein (APP) is processed may help determine whether an individual develops Alzheimer's disease or not. A toxic pathway for APP processing is shown here. APP is a transmembrane protein with the C-terminal inside the neuron and the N-terminal outside the neuron. The enzyme β-secretase cuts APP at a spot outside the membrane to form two peptides: β-APP, which is soluble, and a 91-amino-acid peptide that remains in the membrane. Gamma-secretase then cuts the embedded peptide; this releases Aβ peptides of 40, 42, or 43 amino acids. These toxic (amyloidogenic) peptides form amyloid plaques.

Specifically, abnormal genes or other influences cause the formation of an altered APP, or altered processing into too many toxic Aβ42 peptides (Figure 13-4). Next, the Aβ42 peptides form oligomers (a collection of a few copies of Aβ42 assembled together: Figure 13-5). These oligomers can interfere with synaptic functioning and neurotransmitter actions such as those of acetylcholine, but they are not necessarily lethal to the neurons at first. Eventually, Aβ42 oligomers form amyloid plaques, which are even larger clumps of Aβ42 peptides stuck together with a number of other molecules (Figure 13-6). A number of nasty biochemical events then occur, including inflammatory responses, activation of microglia and astrocytes, and release of toxic chemicals including cytokines and free radicals (Figure 13-6). These chemical events then hypothetically trigger the formation of neurofibrillary tangles within neurons by altering the activities of various kinases and phosphatases, causing hyperphosphorylation of tau proteins, and converting neuronal

Amyloid Cascade Hypothesis, Part One - Increased Production of Aβ42

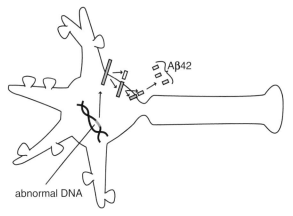

Figure 13-4. Amyloid cascade hypothesis, part 1: increased production of Aβ42. One theory for the pathophysiology of Alzheimer's disease is that there are genetic abnormalities in amyloid precursor protein (APP), so that when it is processed by the pathway involving β-secretase, it produces smaller, toxic peptides (especially Aβ42, as shown here).

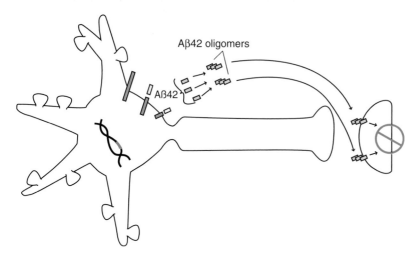

**Amyloid Cascade Hypothesis, Part Two -
Aβ42 Oligomers Form and Interfere with Synaptic Function**

Figure 13-5. Amyloid cascade hypothesis, part 2: Aβ42 oligomers form and interfere with synaptic function. Aβ42 peptides assemble together to form oligomers, which interfere with synaptic functioning and neurotransmitter actions but are not necessarily lethal to neurons.

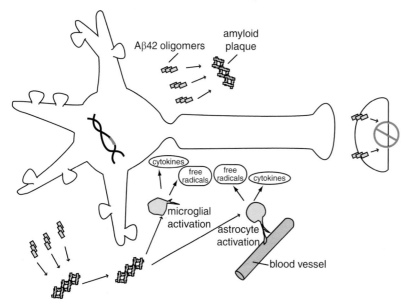

**Amyloid Cascade Hypothesis, Part Three -
Formation of Amyloid Plaques Causing Inflammation**

Figure 13-6. Amyloid cascade hypothesis, part 3: formation of amyloid plaques causing inflammation. Aβ42 oligomers clump together along with other molecules to form amyloid plaques. These plaques can cause inflammatory responses, activation of microglia and astrocytes, and release of toxic chemicals such as cytokines and free radicals.

microtubules into tangles (Figure 13-7). Finally, widespread synaptic dysfunction from Aβ42 oligomers, neuronal dysfunction and death from formation of amyloid plaques outside of neurons and neurofibrillary tangles within neurons leads to diffuse neuronal death (Figure 13-8) and regional expansion of neuronal destruction in the cortex, causing the relentless progression of Alzheimer's symptoms of amnesia, aphasia, agnosia, apraxia, and executive dysfunction. Some investigators believe that Alzheimer's disease may spread from neuron to neuron, with pathological phosphorylated tau transported down axons, released at synapses and then taken up by neighboring cells. Pathological tau possibly then latches onto normal tau in the connected neurons, triggering the formation of new pathological mis-folded tau, from one affected neuron to the next.

**Amyloid Cascade Hypothesis, Part Four-
Amyloid Plaque Induces Formation of Tangles**

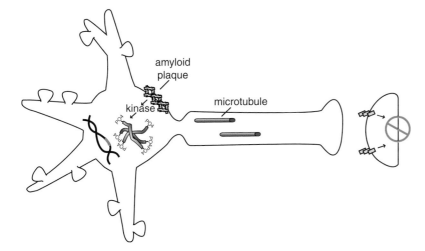

Figure 13-7. Amyloid cascade hypothesis, part 4: amyloid plaque induces formation of tangles. Amyloid plaques and the chemical events they cause activate kinases, cause phosphorylation of tau proteins, and convert microtubules into tangles within neurons.

Support for the amyloid cascade hypothesis comes from genetic studies of those relatively rare inherited autosomal dominant forms of Alzheimer's disease. Sporadic (i.e., noninherited) cases account for the vast majority of Alzheimer's disease cases, but inherited cases can provide clues for what is wrong in the usual sporadic cases of Alzheimer's disease. Rare familial cases of Alzheimer's disease have an early onset (i.e., before age 65) and have been linked to mutations in at least three different chromosomes: 21, 14, and 1. The mutation on chromosome 21 codes for a defect in APP, leading to increased deposition of β-amyloid. Recall that Down's syndrome is also a disorder of this same chromosome (i.e., trisomy 21), and virtually all such persons develop Alzheimer's disease if they live past age 50. A different mutation on chromosome 14 codes for an altered form of a protein called presenilin 1, a component of the γ-secretase enzyme complex. A third mutation, on chromosome 1, codes for an altered form of presenilin 2, a component of a different form of γ-secretase. It is not yet clear what if anything these three mutations in the rare familial cases tell us about the pathophysiology of the usual sporadic, nonfamilial, and late-onset cases of Alzheimer's disease. However, they all point to abnormal processing of APP into amyloidogenic β-amyloid peptides as a cause for the dementia, consistent with the amyloid cascade hypothesis. Theoretically, different abnormalities in amyloid processing may occur in sporadic Alzheimer's disease from those identified in inherited cases, and there

may even be multiple abnormalities that could be responsible for sporadic Alzheimer's disease as a final common pathway, but the evidence nevertheless implicates something in the amyloid cascade that goes wrong in Alzheimer's disease. If so, this implies that preventing the formation of amyloidogenic peptides could prevent Alzheimer's disease.

ApoE and risk of Alzheimer's disease

A corollary to the amyloid cascade hypothesis is the possibility that something may be wrong with a protein that binds to amyloid peptides in order to remove them (Figure 13-9). This protein is called apolipoprotein E (ApoE). In the case of "good" ApoE, it binds to β-amyloid peptides and removes them, hypothetically preventing the formation of Alzheimer's disease and dementia (Figure 13-9A). In the case of "bad" ApoE, a genetic abnormality in the formation of ApoE causes it to be ineffective in how it binds to β-amyloid peptides. This causes amyloid plaques to be formed and deposited around neurons, which goes on to damage neurons and cause Alzheimer's disease (Figure 13-9B).

Genes coding for ApoE are associated with different risks for Alzheimer's disease. There are three alleles (or variants) of this gene coding for this apolipoprotein called E2, E3, and E4, and everyone has two alleles. The E4 variant on chromosome 19 ("bad" ApoE) is linked to many cases of late-onset Alzheimer's disease, the usual form of this

509

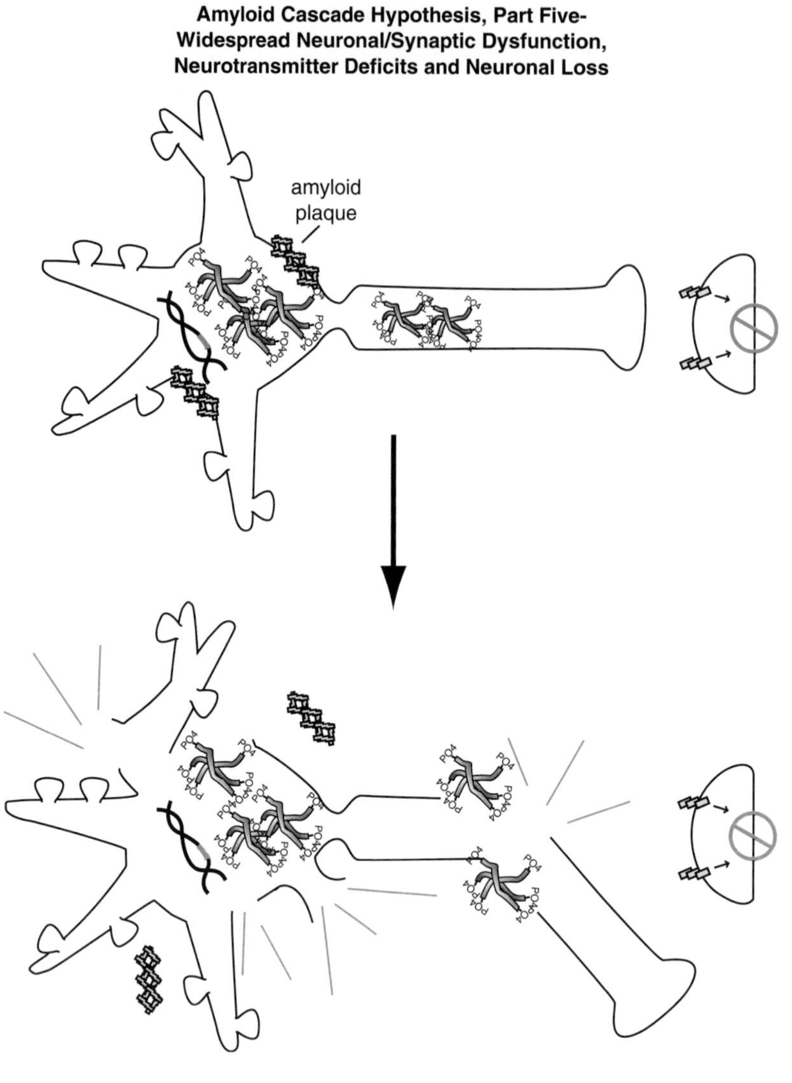

Amyloid Cascade Hypothesis, Part Five-Widespread Neuronal/Synaptic Dysfunction, Neurotransmitter Deficits and Neuronal Loss

amyloid plaque

Figure 13-8. Amyloid cascade hypothesis, part 5: neuronal dysfunction and loss. The effects of amyloid plaques and the build-up of neurofibrillary tangles can ultimately lead to neuronal dysfunction and death.

illness. ApoE is associated with cholesterol transport and involved with other neuronal functions including repair, growth, and maintenance of myelin sheaths and cell membranes. Having one or two copies of E4 increases the risk of getting Alzheimer's disease. In fact, some studies show that you have a 50–90% chance of developing Alzheimer's disease by age 85 if you are an E4 homozygote (i.e., you have two copies of E4); a 45% chance if you are a heterozygote for E4, versus the risk in the general population at 20%. Alzheimer's patients with the E4 gene also have more amyloid deposits and progress more rapidly to dementia than those without the E4 gene. The E2 variant may actually be somewhat protective.

Three stages of Alzheimer's disease

The old way of diagnosing Alzheimer's dementia was neurological and neuropsychological testing for the tentative clinical diagnosis of possible or probable Alzheimer's disease and then postmortem evaluation for confirmation of an actual diagnosis of Alzheimer's disease. In 2011, the diagnostic criteria were revised in two major ways: firstly, they expanded the notion of Alzheimer's disease into three stages to reflect the current dynamic sequence model of structural and functional brain changes over time in elderly people who are first cognitively normal, then have mild cognitive changes, and finally develop Alzheimer's disease (Figure 13-10). Secondly, the new diagnostic

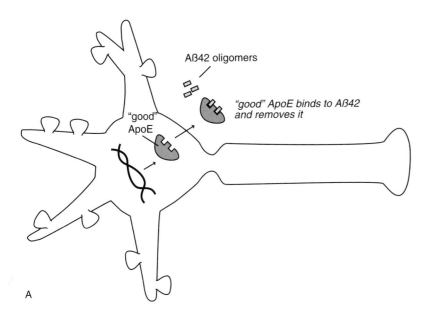

A

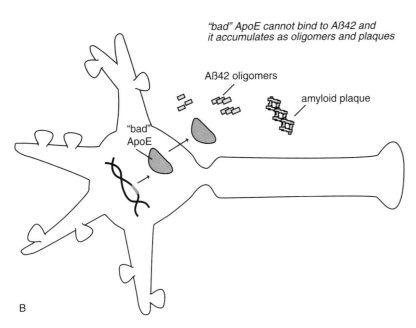

B

Figure 13-9. ApoE and Alzheimer's disease. Another version of the amyloid cascade hypothesis is the possibility that something is wrong with the protein apolipoprotein E (ApoE). (A) Properly functioning ("good") ApoE binds to β-amyloid and removes it, thus preventing development of Alzheimer's disease and dementia. (B) An abnormality in DNA could lead to the formation of a defective or "bad" version of the ApoE protein, such that it cannot effectively bind to amyloid. This would prevent removal of amyloid, allowing it to accumulate and damage neurons, so that Alzheimer's disease develops.

criteria have incorporated biomarkers. The five biomarkers in the new Alzheimer's dementia criteria include both biomarkers of amyloidosis/amyloid accumulation and biomarkers of neurodegeneration (Table 13-4).

First stage of Alzheimer's disease: preclinical (asymptomatic amyloidosis)

It seems obvious that the dementia of Alzheimer's disease does not occur as soon as the first amyloid plaque arrives in the brain. Early plaques in fact seem to be relatively asymptomatic, but somewhere along the way, sufficient accumulation of them seems to trigger the neurodegeneration, or at least is associated with the neurodegeneration, that leads to dementia. It is not clear whether amyloid is an epiphenomenon of the neurodegenerative process, or whether amyloid drives the neurodegenerative process. Amyloid biomarkers are certainly assisting in the diagnostic process for identifying early

Three Stages of Alzheimer's Disease

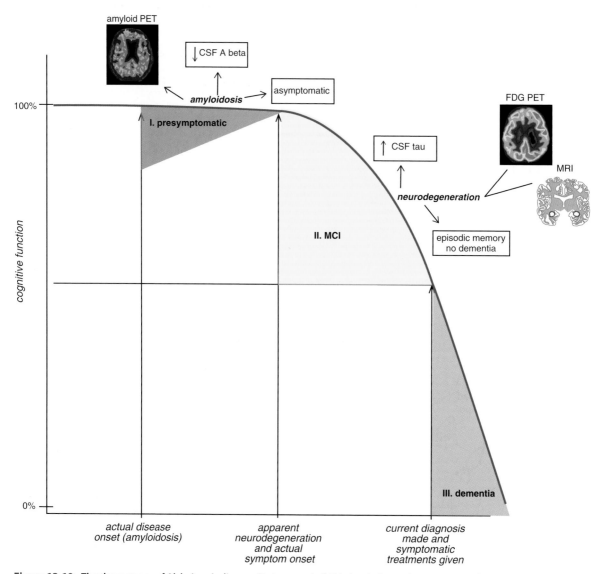

Figure 13-10. The three stages of Alzheimer's disease. During stage I of Alzheimer's disease (presymptomatic), cognition is intact despite elevated levels of brain amyloid as evidenced by both positive amyloid positron emission tomography (PET) and reduced levels of Aβ toxic peptides in cerebrospinal fluid (CSF). Clinical signs of cognitive impairment in the form of episodic memory deficits begin to manifest during stage II (mild cognitive impairment, MCI). The onset of clinical symptoms in stage II appears to be correlated with neurodegeneration, as evidenced by elevated CSF tau, brain glucose hypometabolism on fluorodeoxyglucose PET (FDG-PET) scans and volume loss in key brain regions on magnetic resonance imaging (MRI) scans. During stage III of Alzheimer's disease (dementia), cognitive deficits can be severe. Currently, treatment of Alzheimer's symptoms does not typically begin until stage III, long after the actual disease onset.

stages of Alzheimer's disease. Therapeutics, discussed below, includes many agents in clinical testing that interfere with amyloid accumulation, hypothesizing that amyloid drives neurodegeneration, and that interfering with amyloidosis will halt or delay the progress of Alzheimer's disease. However, the lack of convincing evidence of clinical benefit of this approach to date suggests that another process may be the culprit causing neurodegeneration while amyloid is accumulating.

Table 13-4 Biomarkers integrated into the diagnostic criteria for Alzheimer's disease

Biomarkers of amyloid accumulation	Biomarkers of neurodegeneration
Abnormal radioactive tracer retention on amyloid PET scans	Elevated CSF tau (total and phosphorylated tau)
Low CSF amyloid levels of Aβ42	Decreased FDG uptake on PET
	Atrophy on structural magnetic resonance imaging • hippocampal atrophy • ventricular enlargement • cortical thinning

CSF, cerebrospinal fluid; FDG, fluorodeoxyglucose; PET, positron emission tomography.

Here we will discuss how amyloid imaging is enhancing the diagnostic accuracy of Alzheimer's disease in its early stages. The first stage of Alzheimer's disease is now considered to be preclinical and silent, but trouble is brewing (Figures 13-10 and 13-11). That trouble is the slow, relentless deposition of Aβ peptides into the brain rather than their elimination via the CSF, plasma, and liver. This presymptomatic stage can now be identified with biomarkers (Table 13-4; Figures 13-10 and 13-11): for example, CSF levels of Aβ are *low* because Aβ is being deposited in the brain instead of leaving the brain. Furthermore, amyloidosis is detectable with PET scans at the presymptomatic stage using radioactive neuroimaging tracers that label amyloid plaques (Figure 13-11). Tracers bind to the fibrillar form of amyloid and thus label mature neuritic plaques which can be seen on PET scans after administering a radioactive chemical that binds to amyloid.

Interestingly, amyloid is rarely detected in the brains of individuals under the age of 50, even those with the high-risk E4 genotype. Although most cognitively normal healthy elderly people show no evidence of amyloid deposition (13-11A), about a quarter of cognitively normal elderly controls are amyloid positive (Figure 13-11B), and are thus considered to have presymptomatic Alzheimer's disease (Figure 13-10). About half of patients with MCI show no evidence of amyloid deposition (Figure 13-11C), but the other half do show either

moderate (Figure 13-11D) or severe amyloid deposition (Figure 13-11E). Almost 100% of patients with clinically probable Alzheimer's disease show heavy amyloid deposition (Figure 13-11F).

Thus, Aβ amyloid pathology is not specific for the dementia phase of Alzheimer's disease, but may mean that the fuse is already lit in the presymptomatic phase. Serial amyloid scans show an annual increase of up to 4% of amyloid in patients with probable Alzheimer's disease. Although amyloid can be seen in the presymptomatic stage of Alzheimer's disease, by definition, clinical changes are not detectable at this stage, presumably because there is not much neurodegeneration yet. It is not the amyloid plaques per se, but the neurodegeneration with which they are later associated, that seems to correlate with the onset of symptoms in the second and third stages of Alzheimer's disease.

Most worrisome for the eventual progression of presymptomatic Alzheimer's disease to the MCI symptomatic stage of illness is that some studies suggest that Aβ deposition in the preclinical stage is already associated with some degree of gray-matter atrophy in the hippocampus and the posterior cingulate gyrus that can be demonstrated with structural MRI scanning (Figure 13-12). Cognitively normal elderly adults with the E4 genotype have greater hippocampus volume loss than do cognitively normal adults without E4. Furthermore, those cognitively normal elderly adults with the E4 genotype exhibit faster atrophy, so both elevated Aβ levels and the E4 genotype are associated with gray-matter atrophy in subjects even without cognitive impairment. Reliable atrophy and cortical thinning are identifiable in the hippocampus and in entorhinal, temporal, and parietal cortices in asymptomatic individuals nearly a decade before the onset of dementia.

Now that biomarkers are clarifying this first stage of presymptomatic Alzheimer's disease, it has come to be viewed as the leading edge of a continuum of a process of formation of plaques and tangles causing a relentless march towards dementia. Since some patients may develop amyloid plaques but do not progress to neurodegeneration or dementia, the notion of a preclinical stage is intended for research purposes at this time in order to sort out more reliably who is destined to progress (and thus possibly who to treat at this stage with anti-amyloid therapies on the horizon) and who is not. Early brain changes at

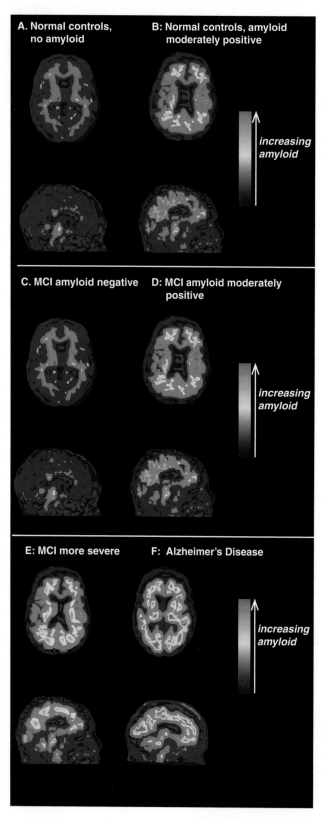

A. Normal controls, no amyloid

B: Normal controls, amyloid moderately positive

increasing amyloid

C. MCI amyloid negative

D: MCI amyloid moderately positive

increasing amyloid

E: MCI more severe

F: Alzheimer's Disease

increasing amyloid

Figure 13-11. Amyloid PET imaging. Positron emission tomography (PET) using amyloid tracers can be used to detect the presence of amyloid during the progression of Alzheimer's disease. In cognitively normal controls (A), amyloid PET imaging shows the absence of amyloid. Individuals who are cognitively normal but have moderate accumulation of amyloid (B) are likely in the presymptomatic first stage of Alzheimer's disease. Although mild cognitive impairment (MCI) is often present in the prodromal second stage of Alzheimer's disease, not all patients with MCI have brain amyloid deposition (C). In such cases, the clinical presence of cognitive impairments is likely attributable to a cause other than Alzheimer's disease. Unfortunately, MCI is often a harbinger of impending Alzheimer's dementia. In these cases (D), amyloid deposition accompanies cognitive impairments and both amyloid accumulation and clinical symptoms of MCI worsen as Alzheimer's disease progresses (E). In the third and final stage of Alzheimer's disease, when full-blown dementia is clinically evident, a large accumulation of brain amyloid can readily be seen (F).

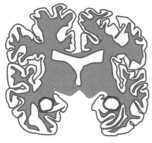

hippocampal atrophy

A

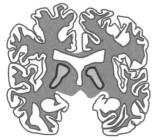

ventricular enlargement

B

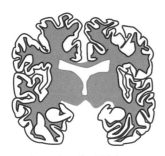

loss of cortical thickness

C

Figure 13-12. Structural MRI. Although hippocampal atrophy (A) and ventricular enlargement (B) are seen with normal aging, the progression of this volume loss is significantly more rapid in patients with Alzheimer's disease. The brains of patients with Alzheimer's disease also show a progressive thinning of the cortex (C).

Risk factors at this presymptomatic stage of illness that may hasten the pace or increase the likelihood of progressing to dementia include depression, type 2 diabetes, ApoE4 genotype, and vascular disease, particularly cerebral emboli. Some experts even wonder whether the effects of type 2 diabetes in the brain can be called "type 3 diabetes," since toxic amyloid peptides are overexpressed in the fat cells of obese individuals, and in the brains of Alzheimer's patients with dementia insulin concentrations, insulin-like growth factor, and insulin receptors are decreased by up to 80%. Since insulin modulates neurotransmitter release, tubulin activity, neuronal survival, and synaptic plasticity, losing your insulin from diabetes does not look like a good idea if you want to prevent Alzheimer's dementia. Thus factors that prevent type 2 diabetes may also help prevent the progression of preclinical Alzheimer's disease to dementia, but that is still a matter of investigation – although it does seem like a matter of common sense. Other common-sense factors that may promote healthy brain aging but are not yet proven to slow the progression of preclinical Alzheimer's disease to dementia include:

- a healthy diet
- adequate sleep
- daily exercise
- active, socially integrated lifestyle
- leisure activities
- cognitive stimulation
- optimized treatment of depression and other mental illnesses
- meditation and other mindfulness strategies (e.g., yoga)
- spiritual activities
- controlling vascular risk factors (hypertension, diabetes, dyslipidemia, obesity)

Second stage of Alzheimer's disease: mild cognitive impairment (MCI) (symptomatic, predementia stage of amyloidosis plus some neurodegeneration)

Patients with mild cognitive impairment (MCI) have mild cognitive symptoms but not dementia. Some call this stage of disease "predementia Alzheimer's disease," or "MCI due to Alzheimer's disease" or even "prodromal Alzheimer's disease." However, this

the preclinical stage that herald clinical progression to Alzheimer's dementia is consistent with the current amyloid cascade hypothesis, but at this point it is not proven for whom this is true, nor how to apply an individual patient's biomarker results to make an accurate prognosis for that individual. A major research question remains as to whether there is a threshold level of Aβ deposition at which brain atrophy occurs, or whether there is another process occurring later and then in parallel that causes the brain atrophy. The exact definition of pathological levels of Aβ deposition (Figure 13-11) remains open, which is why this presymptomatic stage of Alzheimer's disease with amyloidosis but no symptoms is a research diagnosis now.

diagnosis of MCI does not yet mean that Alzheimer's disease pathology has necessarily caused the symptoms or even that MCI patients will inevitably progress to dementia. In fact, there is great debate about what is MCI versus what is "normal aging." Hopefully, the study of biomarkers will be able to settle this in the future. From a purely clinical perspective, over half of elderly residents living in the community complain of memory impairment. They have four common complaints: compared to their functioning of 5–10 years ago, they experience diminished ability (1) to remember names, (2) to find the correct word, (3) to remember where objects are located, and (4) to concentrate. When such complaints occur in the absence of overt dementia, depression, anxiety disorder, sleep/wake disorder, pain disorder, or ADHD (attention deficit hyperactivity disorder) it is called MCI. As already mentioned, the new diagnostic criteria, coupled with biomarkers, are attempting to make the distinction among those with normal aging, those with reversible conditions, and those with MCI destined to progress to the dementia stage of Alzheimer's disease. On clinical grounds alone and without biomarkers, studies show that between 6% and 15% of MCI patients convert to a diagnosis of dementia every year; after 5 years about half meet the criteria for dementia; after 10 years or autopsy, up to 80% will prove to have Alzheimer's disease. Also, MCI patients who have depression exhibit more neurodegeneration and brain atrophy than MCI patients without depression.

Biomarker studies seek to determine who among these MCI patients are destined to progress inevitably to Alzheimer's dementia and who are the lucky ones with a benign and nonprogressive condition. Already foreseen is the need to identify the high-risk group of MCI patients in order to be able to treat them to *prevent* dementia rather than to treat them as we are doing now, *after* the brain has already degenerated and the third stage of Alzheimer's disease has been reached. Also, there is the need to identify those with benign conditions or conditions other than those linked to neurodegeneration associated with amyloidosis, so that they are not needlessly treated with amyloid-targeted therapies which may be both expensive and have side effects.

Only a subset of MCI patients display measurable amyloidosis (Figure 13-11C, D, and E) and only a small proportion (about 10%) of MCI patients without amyloid progress to dementia. However, in those MCI patients with both cognitive symptoms and amyloidosis, the assumption is that they have progressed beyond a presumed earlier state of presymptomatic and silent amyloidosis without damage to the brain (Table 13-4: positive amyloid PET scans and low CSF Aβ levels) to early neurodegeneration (Table 13-4: high CSF tau levels plus structural neuroimaging abnormalities) (Figure 13-10). About half of amyloid-positive MCI patients progress to dementia within a year, and 80% may progress to dementia within 3 years, with MCI patients having the E4 genotype progressing even more rapidly. Those MCI patients who convert to dementia have higher amyloid loads, and the utility of amyloid PET to identify Alzheimer's pathology in the setting of clinical MCI is becoming increasingly convincing. Impairment in episodic memory (the ability to learn and retain new information) is the cognitive symptom most commonly seen in those MCI patients who eventually progress to Alzheimer's dementia. Those MCI patients with the E4 genotype have acceleration of the time to progression from MCI to dementia, so that amyloid imaging, plus testing of episodic memory, plus genetic determination of E4 may currently be the most valuable way to predict higher risk of progression to dementia from the MCI stage.

However, as already mentioned, brain amyloidosis alone does not appear sufficient to produce cognitive decline. Rather, neurodegeneration must occur as the probable direct substrate of cognitive impairment, with the rate of cognitive decline being driven by the rate of neurodegeneration, not by the rate of amyloid deposition. Neurodegenerative atrophy on structural magnetic resonance imaging (MRI) scans both precedes and parallels cognitive decline. The new diagnostic criteria for Alzheimer's disease suggest that it is important to determine whether an MCI patient with impairment of episodic memory has neurodegeneration (as well as amyloidosis and the E4 genotype), to help distinguish MCI that is destined to progress to dementia from nonprogressive MCI and normal aging. Thus, the MCI stage of Alzheimer's disease by definition not only has amyloidosis and cognitive symptoms, but also biomarker evidence of neurodegeneration (Table 13-4; Figures 13-10 through 13-13).

One biomarker for neurodegeneration is the presence of elevated cerebrospinal fluid (CSF) tau (including phospho-tau), thought to be associated with neuronal loss in the brains of Alzheimer's

FDG PET

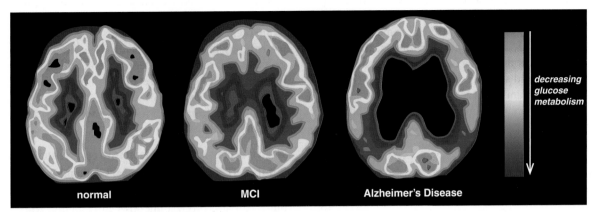

Figure 13-13. Glucose hypometabolism in Alzheimer's disease. The brains of normal, healthy controls show robust glucose metabolism throughout the brain using fluorodeoxyglucose positron emission tomography (FDG-PET). During the early, prodromal stage of Alzheimer's disease, when mild cognitive impairment (MCI) is present, there is a reduction in brain glucose metabolism in more posterior brain regions such as temporoparietal cortex. As the disease progresses to full-blown Alzheimer's dementia, brain glucose hypometabolism becomes evident on FDG-PET. The worsening of glucose metabolism with the progression of Alzheimer's disease is believed to reflect accumulating neurodegeneration, especially in key brain areas such as temporoparietal cortices.

disease patients because it is also elevated in other neurodegenerative diseases such as stroke and Creutzfeldt–Jakob disease (Table 13-4). Numerous neuroimaging biomarkers of neurodegeneration also are available, from single photon emission computerized tomography (SPECT) and fluorodeoxyglucose positron emission tomography (FDG-PET) scans (Figure 13-13), to structural magnetic resonance imaging (MRI) of hippocampal atrophy and of cortical thinning (Figure 13-12), to functional MRI and beyond.

Neurodegeneration and MRI

MRI is more widely available than PET scanning and has numerous structural techniques including volumetric MRI, diffusion-weighted MRI, diffusion tensor imaging (DTI), and magnetization transfer ratio (MTR), and functional techniques such as perfusion MRI, arterial spin labeling (ASL), and fMRI (functional MRI). Some fMRI studies show decreased activation in the hippocampus during episodic memory tasks in dementia.

Among all the MRI techniques, volumetric MRI is generally the method of choice as a biomarker for staging Alzheimer's disease, for measuring disease progression serially over time, and for clinical trials attempting to detect disease-modifying treatments (Figure 13-12). MRI machines are widely available and have good test/retest reliability, and there is a good correlation between MRI measures of atrophy and neuronal cell loss.

Hippocampal atrophy (Figure 13-12A) identifies patients with Alzheimer's dementia, and atrophy in this region progresses more rapidly in patients with Alzheimer's dementia (about 5% per year) compared to healthy elderly controls without cognitive symptoms (about 1.5% per year). Ventricular enlargement (Figure 13-12B) is about 1.3 cm^3 per year in healthy elderly patients without cognitive problems, about 2.5 cm^3 per year in MCI patients, and about 7.7 cm^3 per year in those with Alzheimer's dementia. Alzheimer's disease is also associated with progressive cortical thinning (Figure 13-12C), reflecting loss of brain substance in the cortex, and this cortical thinning can distinguish between Alzheimer's dementia and normal healthy elderly people without cognitive impairment.

The signature pattern of brain atrophy is medial temporal cortex (14% cortical thinning), temporal cortex (11%), parietal cortex (9.6%), and frontal cortex (7.8%) in mild Alzheimer's dementia compared to normal healthy controls. This same topographical pattern is detected in patients with MCI and in normal elderly people with positive amyloid PET scans. Interestingly, autopsy studies of Alzheimer's patients with whole-brain atrophy measured by MRI show that atrophy is related both to cognitive decline and to the amount of neurofibrillary tangles, but not

517

to the amount of amyloid plaques. Since increased brain amyloid and decreased CSF Aβ levels are associated with hippocampal and other brain area atrophy in MCI by volumetric MRI in some but not all MCI patients, as previously mentioned, the working hypothesis is that those MCI patients with increased brain amyloid and decreased CSF Aβ levels (i.e., those who have amyloidosis) (Figure 13-11) and who also have brain atrophy on structural MRI scans (Figure 13-12, i.e., those with documented neurodegeneration) are defined not only as those who are at the MCI stage of Alzheimer's disease (Figure 13-10), but also as those at the highest risk for progressing to the dementia stage of Alzheimer's disease.

Neurodegeneration and FDG-PET

FDG-PET measures synaptic activity, so low amounts of FDG uptake, called hypometabolism, indicate synaptic dysfunction. SPECT imaging provides data similar to FDG-PET, if less spatial resolution, with evidence of reduced activity in temporoparietal cortex in Alzheimer's dementia. Hypometabolism on FDG-PET is also seen mostly in temporoparietal region of the cortex (Figure 13-13), and the lower the metabolism in these areas on FDG-PET scans, the greater the amount of amyloid deposition seen in these same brain areas on amyloid PET scans in patients with Alzheimer's dementia. However, FDG-PET is not abnormal in cognitively normal subjects with amyloidosis on amyloid PET scans, suggesting no neurodegeneration has yet occurred in these subjects. On the other hand, some studies show hypometabolism on FDG-PET scans in normal cognitively functioning elderly if they have the E4 genotype. The hypometabolic FDG-PET pattern is also seen in MCI subjects, with some studies predicting progression from MCI to dementia of 80–90% within 1–1.5 years, a rate that is even faster in subjects who have the E4 genotype. Amyloid PET scans and hippocampal MRI volume provide complementary information for diagnosis of dementia along with FDG-PET scans, and the best predictors of progression of MCI to dementia might include right entorhinal cortical thickness and right hippocampal volume. However, MCI patients who have the combination of gray-matter atrophy on MRI plus hypometabolism of posterior cingulate on FDG-PET also have a higher risk of progression to dementia than those MCI patients with either finding alone. There is a fourfold risk of conversion of MCI to dementia within 2 years if the patient has abnormal episodic memory alone, but there is a 12-fold risk if the patient is abnormal on both FDG and episodic memory in MCI. Thus, combinations of abnormal biomarkers in MCI enhance the odds that such a patient may progress to dementia. The findings suggest that it is really neurodegeneration and not amyloidosis that drives the onset of symptoms at the MCI stage of Alzheimer's disease as well as the progression of symptoms from the MCI stage to the dementia stage of this illness.

When is depression a major depressive episode and when is it the MCI prodrome of Alzheimer's dementia?

Depression can not only be mistaken for dementia, but it can also precede the onset of dementia and be associated with a twofold increase in the risk of developing cognitive impairment or dementia. When depression occurs in late life, whether it is a recurrent episode in a patient with a lifetime of episodes, or a first episode in late life, a major depressive episode can actually present with prominent cognitive symptoms, especially apathy, lack of interest, and slowing of information processing, rather than depressed mood and sadness. Depression with lack of interest or sadness can also occur in patients with established dementia, in patients whose depression may represent the MCI prodrome to dementia, and even in patients who ultimately prove to have reversible cognitive impairments from "pseudodementia" or the "dementia of depression." It remains controversial whether depression reflects a causative factor for MCI or dementia, is part of MCI, or shares neuropathological features with the dementia stage of Alzheimer's disease. Hopefully, studies of biomarkers in elderly patients with depression with or without the MCI prodrome will help sort this out. CSF Aβ peptides are low in cognitively intact elderly with major depressive disorder (MDD) similar to individuals with MCI or Alzheimer's dementia. Other studies suggest that there are increased amyloid plaques in cognitively intact elderly patients with major depression (i.e., similar to the findings at the preclinical asymptomatic stage of Alzheimer's disease), and that depressive symptoms in the symptomatic MCI stage without dementia predict greater brain atrophy in those patients with both depression and MCI. Some experts believe that depressive symptoms associated with MCI are an ominous combination, with depression being a prodromal manifestation of dementia. Thus, depression that begins in late life may possibly represent an Alzheimer's disease symptomatic pro-drome, whereas recurrent depression with another episode in late life may be related either to vascular dementia or to no dementia at all.

Third and final stage of Alzheimer's disease: dementia (amyloidosis with neurodegeneration plus cognitive decline)

The final stage of Alzheimer's disease is dementia, which applies to those who develop cognitive or behavioral problems that interfere with function at work or in everyday activities. Similar to the old guidelines, the new criteria classify patients into "probable" and "possible" Alzheimer's dementia, with no change in those with probable Alzheimer's dementia. However, the new criteria include two new categories: probable and possible Alzheimer's dementia *with evidence of the Alzheimer's pathophysiological process*. These new criteria are for research purposes.

To diagnose probable Alzheimer's dementia, one must first diagnose dementia itself (see Table 13-5 for the core clinical criteria for "all-cause" dementia). Patients who meet these criteria for all-cause dementia have probable Alzheimer's dementia when they also meet the core clinical criteria outlined in Table 13-6. Briefly, patients with probable Alzheimer's disease have dementia which is insidious in onset, clearly has demonstrated worsening of cognition over time, and has either an amnestic (problems with learning and recall) or a nonamnestic presentation (language, visuospatial, or executive dysfunction). Probable Alzheimer's dementia *with increased level of certainty* can be diagnosed pre-mortem when the patient meets the core criteria (Table 13-6) and also has formal documented cognitive decline on neuropsychological testing or has been proven to be a carrier of a causative Alzheimer's disease genetic mutation (in the genes for APP, presenilin 1, or presenilin 2). Despite many ominous associations with neuroimaging biomarkers, the E4 allele of ApoE is not sufficiently specific to be considered in this category.

The new research category of probable Alzheimer's dementia with evidence of the Alzheimer's pathophysiological process includes patients with probable Alzheimer's disease (Table 13-6) who have *clearly positive* biomarker evidence either of brain amyloid deposition/amyloidosis (Figure 13-11) or of downstream neuronal degeneration (Figures 13-12 and 13-13). (In these cases, results from biomarker

Table 13-5 Core clinical criteria for all-cause dementia

Dementia is diagnosed when there are cognitive or behavioral symptoms that:

1. Interfere with the ability to function at work or at usual activities; and
2. Represent a decline from previous levels of functioning and performing; and
3. Are not explained by delirium or major psychiatric disorder.
4. Cognitive impairment is detected and diagnosed through a combination of (1) history-taking from the patient and a knowledgeable informant and (2) an objective cognitive assessment, either a "bedside" mental status examination or neuropsychological testing. Neuropsychological testing should be performed when the routine history and bedside mental status examination cannot provide a confident diagnosis.
5. The cognitive or behavioral impairment involves a minimum of two of the following domains:

   a. Impaired ability to acquire and remember new information – symptoms include: repetitive questions or conversations, misplacing personal belongings, forgetting events or appointments, getting lost on a familiar route.
   b. Impaired reasoning and handling of complex tasks, poor judgment – symptoms include: poor understanding of safety risks, inability to manage finances, poor decision-making ability, inability to plan complex or sequential activity.
   c. Impaired visuospatial ability – symptoms include: inability to recognize faces or common objects or to find objects in direct view despite good acuity, inability to operate simple implements or orient clothing to the body.
   d. Impaired language functions (speaking, reading, writing) – symptoms include: difficulty thinking of common words while speaking; hesitation; speech, spelling, and writing errors.
   e. Changes in personality, behavior or comportment – symptoms include: uncharacteristic mood fluctuations such as agitation, impaired motivation or initiative, apathy, loss of drive, social withdrawal, decreased interest in previous activities, loss of empathy, compulsive or obsessive behaviors, socially unacceptable behaviors.

Table 13-6 Core clinical criteria for probable Alzheimer's dementia

Probable Alzheimer's dementia is diagnosed when the patient:

Meets criteria for dementia (Table 13-5) and in addition, has the following characteristics:

1. Insidious onset. Symptoms have a gradual onset over months to years, not sudden over hours or days
2. Clear-cut history of worsening of cognition by report or observations
3. The initial and most prominent cognitive deficits are evident on history and examination in one of the following categories:
   i. Amnestic presentation. It is the most common syndromic presentation of Alzheimer's dementia. The deficits should include impairment in learning and recall of recently learned information. There should also be evidence of cognitive dysfunction in at least one other cognitive domain, as defined earlier in the text.
   ii. Nonamnestic presentations:
      1. Language presentation: the most prominent deficits are in word-finding, but deficits in other cognitive domains should be present.
      2. Visuospatial presentation: the most prominent deficits are in spatial cognition, including object agnosia, impaired face recognition, simultanagnosia, and alexia. Deficits in other cognitive domains should be present.
      3. Executive dysfunction: the most prominent deficits are impaired reasoning, judgment, and problem solving. Deficits in other cognitive domains should be present.
4. The diagnosis of probable Alzheimer's dementia should not be applied when there is evidence of:
   i. Substantial concomitant cerebrovascular disease defined by a history of a stroke temporally related to the onset or worsening of cognitive impairment; or the presence of multiple or extensive infarcts or severe white-matter hyperintensity burden; or
   ii. Core features of dementia with Lewy bodies other than dementia itself; or
   iii. Prominent features of semantic variant primary progressive aphasia or nonfluent/agrammatic variant primary progressive aphasia; or
   iv. Evidence for another concurrent, active neurological disease, or a non-neurological medical comorbidity or use of medication that could have a substantial effect on cognition.

studies can be judged to be clearly positive, clearly negative, or indeterminate.) The new research category of possible Alzheimer's dementia with evidence of the Alzheimer's pathophysiological process is for persons who meet clinical criteria for a dementia other than Alzheimer's disease but who have clearly positive biomarker evidence (pre-mortem) or neuropathological evidence (postmortem) of the Alzheimer's pathophysiological process, including both evidence of amyloidosis and evidence of neuronal degeneration. This does not preclude that a second pathophysiological condition may also be present.

Targeting amyloid as a future disease-modifying treatment of Alzheimer's disease

The likely fate of subjects with asymptomatic amyloidosis (stage I presymptomatic Alzheimer's disease) or cognitive changes with early neurodegeneration (stage II Alzheimer's disease, MCI) means it is becoming ever more urgent to intervene in this disorder at an earlier and earlier time, when brain changes are present without any overt cognitive decline, or certainly before dementia sets in. Since nearly all current Alzheimer's drug development candidates target some aspect of the amyloid cascade, biomarkers have the potential to work hand-in-glove not only with making an early diagnosis potentially in the first or second stage of this disease to therefore identify which patients to treat with a specific agent of a given mechanism of action, but also to demonstrate objectively whether disease progression is slowed, halted, or even reversed by novel treatments that interfere with amyloidosis. From the point of view of current clinical practice, the value of the information that biomarkers can provide has to be balanced against their costs, the side effects of radioactivity, the invasiveness of lumbar puncture, the availability of specialized technology, and of course the psychological costs of learning about Alzheimer's brain pathology and possible clinical prognosis at a time when there is no cure or even any therapy to halt or slow the progression of this disorder. Thus the main current utility of biomarker-enhanced early detection of Alzheimer's disease is to identify those with high risk of progression to dementia, for participation in clinical trials of new drug testing, and especially of new drug testing of various anti-amyloid therapies.

Aβ Immunizations as Potential Disease-Modifying Treatments for Alzheimer's Disease

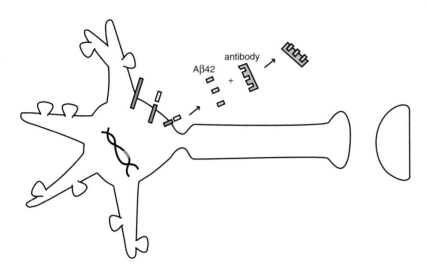

Figure 13-14. Future treatments: β-amyloid immunizations. One potential future treatment for Alzheimer's disease is a vaccine that immunizes against β-amyloid, which could not only slow cognitive decline but also perhaps remove already formed plaques.

Vaccines and immunotherapy

The quest for an Alzheimer's vaccine has great appeal, but its clinical development has had its ups and downs. Immunizing the body to β-amyloid could in concept not only slow or stop progression of cognitive decline but, by removal of plaques already formed, potentially improve cognitive function. Positive tests of amyloid vaccines in animals led to early clinical trials that showed evidence not only of stabilization of memory in Alzheimer's patients but, perhaps more importantly, that amyloid plaques were removed (Figure 13-14). However, the first vaccine to the Aβ peptide (AN1792) caused brain inflammation (meningoencephalitis) in 6% of cases in phase II, and the trials had to be stopped. Other immunotherapy trials include passive immunization with antibodies against Aβ peptide. However, results with bapineuzumab (humanized mouse monoclonal antibody against terminal portion of Aβ), solanezumab (humanized mouse monoclonal antibody against the midportion of Aβ), and others (crenezumab) have so far yielded disappointing results in clinical trials. There are also clinical trials of passive immunization with intravenous immunoglobulin (IVIG) in the hopes that it might contain naturally occurring antibodies against β-amyloid and promote the clearance of β-amyloid from the brain. Some surprisingly positive results in stopping decline in cognitive function with IVIG have been reported, with further testing required to follow this up.

Gamma-secretase inhibitors

Another strategy to block amyloid plaque formation is to inhibit the enzyme γ-secretase (Figure 13-15). Several γ-secretase inhibitors (GSIs) are in clinical development. Notably, however, semagacestat (LY450139) was terminated from clinical trials for safety reasons, namely that this agent actually impaired cognition and function *more* than placebo did, and also increased the occurrence of skin cancer. The future of this approach is now in doubt. What is confusing about the semagacestat findings is that it was shown to successfully target the enzyme γ-secretase and to reduce Aβ production in a dose-dependent manner, yet this did not translate into a clinical benefit. One mechanism of toxicity for semagacestat may be the fact that many GSIs also inhibit other proteases, especially one called Notch, which is involved in cell fate pathways in rapidly dividing cells, which may have caused the skin-cancer side effect. Future GSIs selective for γ-secretase and not for Notch may be necessary to move this target forward in Alzheimer's disease.

521

Gamma-Secretase Inhibitors and Gamma-Secretase Modulators (Selective Amyloid-Lowering Agents) as Potential Disease-Modifying Treatments for Alzheimer's Disease

Figure 13-15. Gamma-secretase inhibitors and modulators. The way in which amyloid precursor protein (APP) is processed may help determine whether an individual develops Alzheimer's disease. Thus a drug that affects this process could prevent or treat Alzheimer's disease. The enzyme γ-secretase cleaves embedded peptides, which in some cases leads to release of toxic peptides (particularly Aβ42). Inhibition of this enzyme could therefore prevent formation of toxic peptides, and so could modulation of this enzyme with selective amyloid-lowering agents (SALAs).

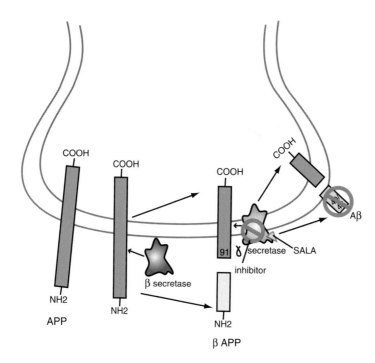

Beta-secretase inhibitors

Inhibitors of the β-secretase enzyme have been difficult to synthesize, but compounds such as SCH 1381252, CTS21666, and others are moving forward in clinical development, and their results are eagerly awaited because of their theoretical promise as a mechanism of preventing β-amyloid formation (Figure 13-16).

Targeting acetylcholine as a current symptomatic treatment of Alzheimer's disease

Acetylcholine and the pharmacologic basis of cholinesterase treatments for dementia

Many of the current approved agents used to treat symptoms of dementia in Alzheimer's disease are based upon boosting the availability of the neurotransmitter acetylcholine. Prior to discussing these treatments, we will review the pharmacology of acetylcholine.

Acetylcholine is formed in cholinergic neurons from two precursors: choline and acetyl coenzyme A (AcCoA) (Figure 13-17). Choline is derived from dietary and intraneuronal sources, and AcCoA is made from glucose in the mitochondria of the neuron. These two substrates interact with the synthetic enzyme choline acetyl-transferase (CAT) to produce the neurotransmitter acetylcholine (ACh).

ACh's actions are terminated by one of two enzymes, either acetylcholinesterase (AChE) or butyrylcholinesterase (BuChE), sometimes also called "pseudocholinesterase" or "nonspecific cholinesterase" (Figure 13-18). Both enzymes convert ACh into choline, which is then transported back into the presynaptic cholinergic neuron for resynthesis into ACh (Figure 13-18). Although both AChE and BuChE can metabolize ACh, they are quite different in that they are encoded by separate genes and have different tissue distributions and substrate patterns. There may be different clinical effects of inhibiting these two enzymes as well. High levels of AChE are present in brain, especially in neurons that receive ACh input

Beta-Secretase Inhibitors as Potential Disease-Modifying Treatments for Alzheimer's Disease

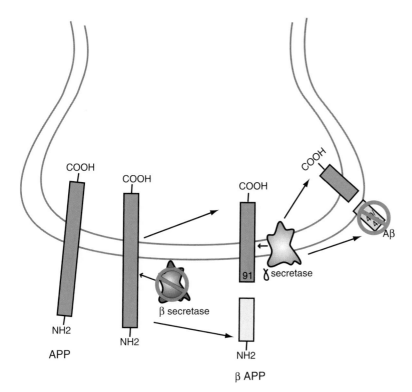

Figure 13-16. Beta-secretase inhibitors. The way in which amyloid precursor protein (APP) is processed may help determine whether an individual develops Alzheimer's disease. Thus a drug that affects this process could prevent or treat Alzheimer's disease. The enzyme β-secretase cuts APP at a spot outside the membrane to form two peptides: β-APP, which is soluble, and a 91-amino-acid peptide that remains in the membrane. Gamma-secretase then cuts the embedded peptide; this releases Aβ peptides of 40, 42, or 43 amino acids, which are toxic. Thus inhibition of β-secretase could prevent the formation of toxic peptides.

(Figure 13-18). BuChE is also present in brain, especially in glial cells (Figure 13-18). As will be discussed below, some cholinesterase inhibitors specifically inhibit AChE, whereas others inhibit both enzymes. It is AChE that is thought to be the key enzyme for inactivating ACh at cholinergic synapses, although BuChE can take on this activity if ACh diffuses to nearby glia. AChE is also present in the gut, skeletal muscle, red blood cells, lymphocytes, and platelets. BuChE is also present in the gut, plasma, skeletal muscle, placenta, and liver. BuChE may be present in some specific neurons, and it may also be present in amyloid plaques.

ACh released from CNS neurons is destroyed too quickly and too completely by AChE to be available for transport back into the presynaptic neuron, but the choline that is formed by the breakdown of ACh is readily transported back into the presynaptic cholinergic nerve terminal by a transporter similar to the transporters for other neurotransmitters already discussed earlier in relation to norepinephrine, dopamine, and serotonin neurons. Once back in the

presynaptic nerve terminal, it can be recycled into new ACh synthesis (Figure 13-18). Once synthesized in the presynaptic neuron, ACh is stored in synaptic vesicles after being transported into these vesicles by the vesicular transporter for ACh (VAChT), analogous to the vesicular transporters for the monoamines and other neurotransmitters.

There are numerous receptors for ACh (Figures 13-19 and 13-20). The major subtypes are nicotinic and muscarinic subtypes of cholinergic receptors. Classically, muscarinic receptors are stimulated by the mushroom alkaloid muscarine and nicotinic receptors by the tobacco alkaloid nicotine. Nictotinic receptors are all ligand-gated, rapid-onset, and excitatory ion channels blocked by curare. Muscarinic receptors, by contrast, are G-protein-linked, can be excitatory or inhibitory, and many are blocked by atropine, scopolamine, and other well-known so-called "anticholinergics" discussed throughout this text. Both nicotinic and muscarinic receptors have been further subdivided into numerous receptor subtypes.

Acetylcholine is Produced

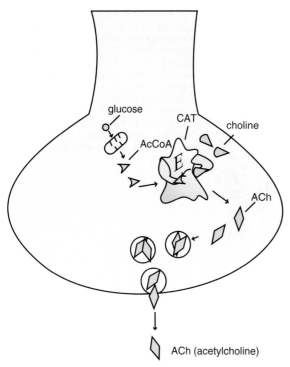

Figure 13-17. Acetylcholine is produced. Acetylcholine is formed when two precursors – choline and acetyl coenzyme A (AcCoA) – interact with the synthetic enzyme choline acetyl-transferase (CAT). Choline is derived from dietary and intraneuronal sources, and AcCoA is made from glucose in the mitochondria of the neuron.

Subtypes of muscarinic receptors include the well-known postsynaptic M_1 subtype, which appears to be key to the regulation of some of the memory functions of ACh acting at cholinergic synapses (Figure 13-19). The M_2 subtype is presynaptic, and serves as an autoreceptor, blocking the further release of ACh when it is activated by the build-up of synaptic levels of ACh (Figure 13-19). The functions of other muscarinic receptor subtypes are still under investigation, including some, such as the M_3 subtype, which are also expressed outside of the brain and may mediate some of the peripheral side effects of some anticholinergics.

A number of nicotinic receptor subtypes also exist in the brain, with different subtypes outside the brain in skeletal muscle and ganglia. Two of the most important CNS nicotinic cholinergic receptors are the subtype with all α_7 subunits, and the subtype with α_4 and β_2 subunits (Figure 13-20). The $\alpha_4\beta_2$ subtype is postsynaptic and plays an important role in regulating

dopamine release in the nucleus accumbens. It is thought to be a primary target of nicotine in cigarettes, and to contribute to the reinforcing and addicting properties of tobacco. The $\alpha_4\beta_2$ subtypes of nicotinic cholinergic receptors are discussed in further detail in Chapter 14 on drug abuse.

Alpha-7-nicotinic cholinergic receptors can be either presynaptic or postsynaptic (Figures 13-20 and 13-21). When they are postsynaptic, they may be important mediators of cognitive functioning in the prefrontal cortex. When they are presynaptic and on cholinergic neurons, they appear to mediate a "feed-forward" release process where ACh can facilitate its own release by occupying presynaptic α_7-nicotinic receptors (Figure 13-20). Furthermore, α_7-nicotinic receptors are present on neurons that release other neurotransmitters, such as dopamine and glutamate neurons (Figure 13-21). When ACh diffuses away from its synapse to occupy these presynaptic heteroreceptors, it facilitates the release of the neurotransmitter there (e.g., dopamine or glutamate) (Figure 13-21).

Just as described for other ligand-gated ion channels such as the $GABA_A$ receptor and the NMDA receptor, it appears that ligand-gated nicotinic cholinergic receptors are also regulated by allosteric modulators (Figure 13-22). Positive allosteric modulators (PAMs) have been identified for nicotinic receptors in brain; indeed, the cholinesterase inhibitor galantamine has a second therapeutic mechanism as a PAM for nicotinic receptors, as described for this agent below.

The principal cholinergic pathways are illustrated in Figures 13-23 and 13-24. Cell bodies of some cholinergic pathways arise from the brainstem and project to many brain regions, including prefrontal cortex, basal forebrain, thalamus, hypothalamus, amygdala, and hippocampus (Figure 13-23). Other cholinergic pathways have their cell bodies in the basal forebrain, project to prefrontal cortex, amygdala, and hippocampus, and are thought to be particularly important for memory (Figure 13-24). Additional cholinergic fibers in the basal ganglia are not illustrated.

The cholinergic deficiency hypothesis of amnesia in Alzheimer's disease and other dementias

Numerous investigators have shown that a deficiency in cholinergic functioning is linked to a disruption in memory, particularly short-term

Acetylcholine Action is Terminated

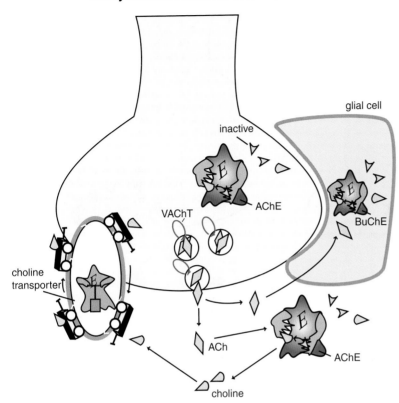

Figure 13-18. Acetylcholine's action is terminated. Acetylcholine's action can be terminated by two different enzymes: acetylcholinesterase (AChE), which is present both intra- and extracellularly, and butyrylcholinesterase (BuChE), which is particularly present in glial cells. Both enzymes convert acetylcholine into choline, which is then transported out of the synaptic cleft and back into the presynaptic neuron via the choline transporter. Once inside the presynaptic neuron, choline can be recycled into acetylcholine and then packaged into vesicles by the vesicular transporter for acetylcholine (VAChT).

memory. For example, blockers of muscarinic cholinergic receptors (such as scopolamine) can produce a memory disturbance in normal human volunteers that has similarities to the memory disturbance in Alzheimer's disease. Boosting cholinergic neurotransmission with cholinesterase inhibitors not only reverses scopolamine-induced memory impairments in normal human volunteers, but also enhances memory functioning in patients with Alzheimer's disease. Both animal and human studies have demonstrated that the nucleus basalis of Meynert in the basal forebrain is the major brain center for cholinergic neurons that project throughout the cortex (Figure 13-24). These neurons have the principal role in mediating memory formation. It is suspected that the short-term memory disturbance of Alzheimer's patients is due to degeneration of these particular cholinergic neurons. Other cholinergic neurons, such as those in the striatum and those projecting from the lateral tegmental area, are not involved in the memory disorder of Alzheimer's disease.

Cholinesterase inhibitors
General

The most successful approach to boosting cholinergic functioning in patients with Alzheimer's disease and improving memory has been to inhibit ACh destruction by blocking the enzyme acetylcholinesterase (Figure 13-18). This causes the build-up of ACh because it can no longer be destroyed by acetylcholinesterase. The enhanced availability of acetylcholine can impact the clinical outcome in Alzheimer's disease, from enhancing memory in some patients, to slowing the decline in function of Alzheimer's patients for several months, rather than improving their memory. Since cholinergic agents require postsynaptic cholinergic receptors to mediate the benefits of the enhanced cholinergic input, they may be most effective in the early stages of Alzheimer's disease, while postsynaptic cholinergic targets are still present. However, late in the illness, degeneration of neurons that have postsynaptic ACh receptors means that the drug may lose its benefits.

Muscarinic Acetylcholine Receptors

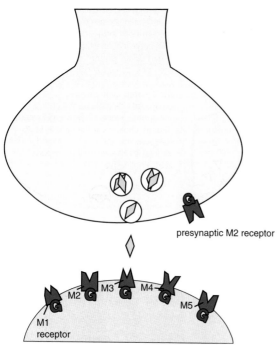

Figure 13-19. Muscarinic acetylcholine receptors.
Acetylcholine neurotransmission can be regulated by G-protein-linked muscarinic acetylcholine receptors, shown here. Muscarinic 1 (M_1) receptors are postsynaptic and important for regulation of memory. Muscarinic 2 (M_2) receptors exist both presynaptically as autoreceptors and postsynaptically. Other postsynaptic muscarinic receptors include M_3, M_4, and M_5.

Nicotinic Acetylcholine Receptors

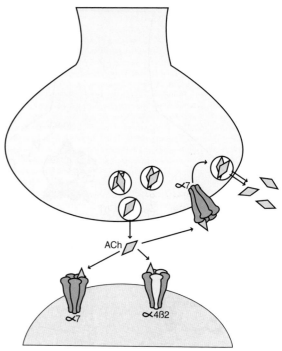

Figure 13-20. Nicotinic acetylcholine receptors. Acetylcholine neurotransmission can be regulated by ligand-gated excitatory ion channels known as nicotinic acetylcholine receptors, shown here. There are multiple subtypes of these receptors, defined by the subunits they contain. Two of the most important are those that contain all α_7 subunits and those that contain α_4 and β_2 subunits. The α_7 receptors can exist presynaptically, where they facilitate acetylcholine release, or postsynaptically, where they are important for regulating cognitive function. The $\alpha_4\beta_2$ receptors are postsynaptic and regulate release of dopamine in the nucleus accumbens.

Donepezil

Donepezil is a reversible, long-acting, selective inhibitor of acetylcholinesterase (AChE) without inhibition of butyrylcholinesterase (BuChE) (Figure 13-25). Donepezil inhibits AChE in pre- and postsynaptic cholinergic neurons, and in other areas of the CNS outside of cholinergic neurons where this enzyme is widespread (Figure 13-25A). Its CNS actions boost the availability of ACh at the remaining sites normally innervated by cholinergic neurons, but which are now suffering from a deficiency of ACh as cholinergic neurons die off (Figure 13-25A). Donepezil also inhibits AChE in the periphery, where its actions in the gastrointestinal (GI) tract can produce GI side effects (Figure 13-25B). Donezezil is easy to dose and has mostly gastrointestinal side effects, which are mostly transient.

Rivastigmine

Rivastigmine (Figure 13-26) is "pseudoirreversible" (which means it reverses itself over hours), intermediate-acting, and not only selective for AChE

over BuChE, but perhaps for AChE in the cortex and hippocampus over AChE in other areas of brain (Figure 13-26A). Rivastigmine also inhibits BuChE within glia, which may contribute somewhat to the enhancement of ACh levels within the CNS (Figure 13-26A). Inhibition of BuChE within glia may be even more important in patients with Alzheimer's disease as they develop gliosis when cortical neurons die, because these glia contain BuChE, and inhibition of this increased enzyme activity may have a favorable action on increasing the availability of ACh to cholinergic receptors via this second mechanism. Rivastigmine appears to have comparable safety and efficacy to donepezil, although it may have more gastrointestinal side effects when given orally (Figure 13-26B), perhaps due to its pharmacokinetic profile, and perhaps due to inhibition of both AChE and BuChE in the periphery (Figure 13-26C). However, there is now a

Presynaptic Nicotinic Heteroreceptors Facilitate Dopamine and Glutamate Release

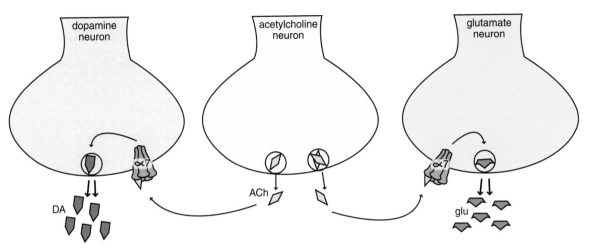

Figure 13-21. Presynaptic nicotinic heteroreceptors facilitate dopamine and glutamate release. Acetylcholine (ACh) that diffuses away from the synapse can bind to presynaptic α_7-nicotinic receptors on dopamine and glutamate neurons, where it stimulates release of these neurotransmitters.

transdermal formulation of rivastigmine available that greatly reduces the peripheral side effects of oral rivastigmine, probably by optimizing drug delivery and reducing peak drug concentrations.

Galantamine

Galantamine is a very interesting cholinesterase inhibitor found in snowdrops and daffodils! It has a dual mechanism of action, matching AChE inhibition with positive allosteric modulation (PAM) of nicotinic cholinergic receptors (Figure 13-27). Theoretically, the inhibition of AChE (Figure 13-27A) could be enhanced when joined by the second action of galantamine at nicotinic receptors (Figure 13-27B). Thus, raising ACh levels at nicotinic cholinergic receptors by AChE inhibition could be boosted by the PAM actions of galantamine (Figure 13-27B). However, it has not been proven that this theoretically advantageous second action as a nicotinic PAM translates into clinical advantages.

Targeting glutamate

The glutamate hypothesis of cognitive deficiency in Alzheimer's disease

Glutamate has been hypothesized to be released in excess during Alzheimer's disease, perhaps in part triggered by neurotoxic amyloid plaques and

neurofibrillary tangles (Figure 13-28). In the resting state, glutamate is normally quiet, and the NMDA receptor is physiologically blocked by magnesium ions (Figure 13-28A). When normal excitatory neurotransmission comes along, a flurry of glutamate is released (Figure 13-28B). The postsynaptic NMDA receptor is a "coincidence detector" and allows inflow of ions if three things happen at the same time: neuronal depolarization, often from activation of nearby AMPA receptors; glutamate occupying its binding site on the NMDA receptor; and the cotransmitter glycine occupying its site on the NMDA receptor (Figure 13-28B). If plaques and tangles cause a steady "leak" of glutamate, this would theoretically interfere with the fine-tuning of glutamate neurotransmission, and possibly interfere with memory and learning but not necessarily damaging neurons (Figure 13-28C). Hypothetically, as the disease progresses, glutamate release could be increased to a level that is tonically bombarding the postsynaptic receptor, eventually killing off dendrites and then killing off full neurons due to excitotoxic cell death (Figure 13-28C).

Memantine

The rationale for the use of memantine, a type of NMDA antagonist, is to reduce abnormal activation of glutamate neurotransmission and thus interfere

527

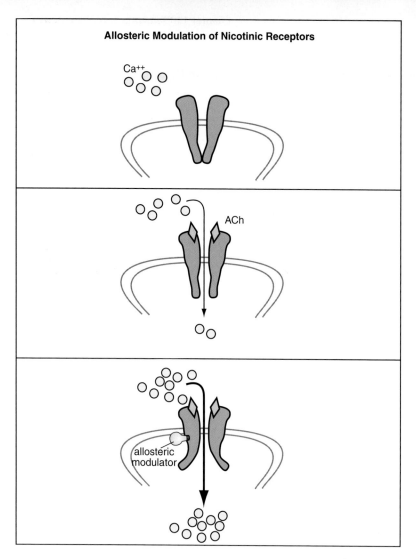

Figure 13-22. Allosteric modulation of nicotinic receptors. Nicotinic receptors can be regulated by allosteric modulators. These ligand-gated ion channels control the flow of calcium into the neuron (top panel). When acetylcholine (ACh) is bound to these receptors, it allows calcium to pass into the neuron (middle panel). A positive allosteric modulator bound in the presence of acetylcholine increases the frequency of opening of the channel and thus can allow for more calcium to pass into the neuron (bottom panel).

Cholinergic Projections from Basal Forebrain

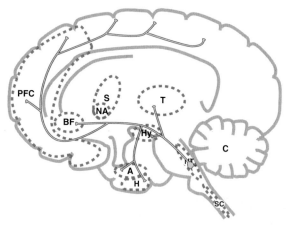

Figure 13-23. Cholinergic projections from the brainstem. The cell bodies of cholinergic neurons can be found in the brainstem and project to many different brain areas including prefrontal cortex (PFC), basal forebrain (BF), thalamus (T), hypothalamus (Hy), amygdala (A), and hippocampus (H).

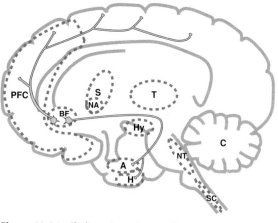

Figure 13-24. Cholinergic projections from the basal forebrain. Other cholinergic neurons project from the basal forebrain (BF) to prefrontal cortex (PFC), amygdala (A), and hippocampus (H). They are thought to be important for memory.

Donepezil Actions: CNS

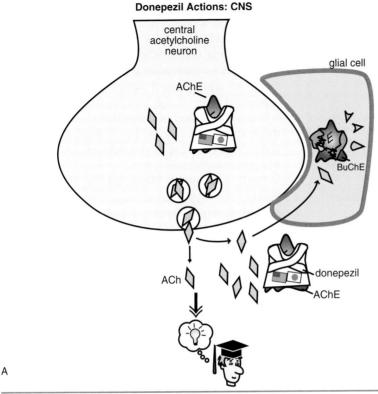

Figure 13-25. Donepezil actions. Donepezil inhibits the enzyme acetylcholinesterase (AChE), which is present both in the central nervous system (CNS) and peripherally. (A) Central cholinergic neurons are important for regulation of memory; thus in the CNS, the boost of acetylcholine caused by AChE blockade contributes to improved cognitive functioning. (B) Peripheral cholinergic neurons in the gut are involved in gastrointestinal effects; thus the boost in peripheral acetylcholine caused by AChE blockade may contribute to gastrointestinal side effects. *Donepezil is represented here by a straitjacket icon with the American and Japanese flags (the countries of its manufacturers).*

Donepezil Actions: Peripheral

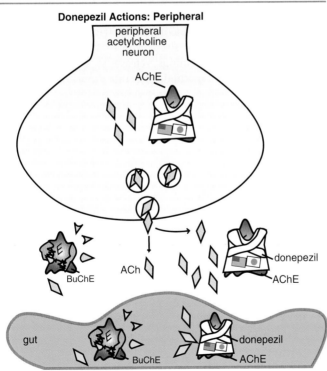

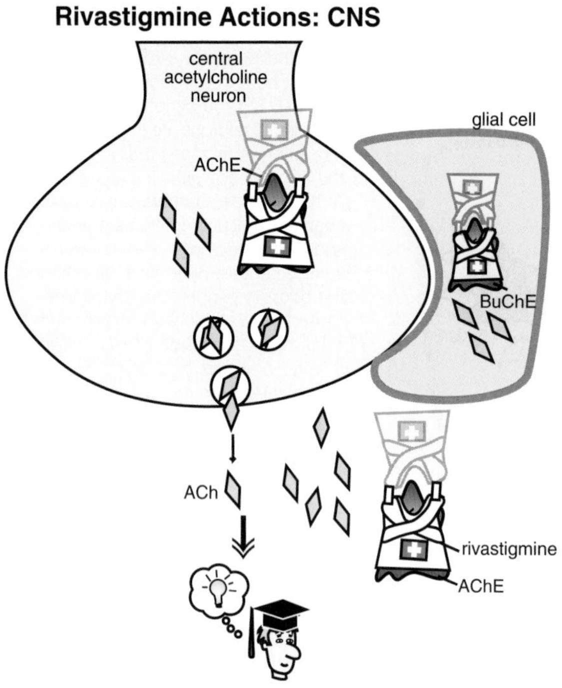

Rivastigmine Actions: CNS

Figure 13-26A. Rivastigmine actions, part 1. Rivastigmine inhibits the enzymes acetylcholinesterase (AChE) and butyrylcholinesterase (BuChE), which are present both in the central nervous system (CNS) and peripherally. Central cholinergic neurons are important for regulation of memory; thus in the CNS the boost of acetylcholine caused by AChE blockade contributes to improved cognitive functioning. In particular, rivastigmine appears to be somewhat selective for AChE in the cortex and hippocampus – two regions important for memory – over other areas of the brain. Rivastigmine's blockade of BuChE in glia may also contribute to enhanced acetylcholine levels. *Rivastigmine is represented here by two straitjacket icons end-to-end, one for acetylcholinesterase and another for butyrylcholinesterase, with the Swiss flag indicating the country of its manufacturer.*

with the pathophysiology of Alzheimer's disease, improve cognitive function, and slow the rate of decline over time. Blocking NMDA receptors chronically would interfere with memory formation and neuroplasticity. So what do you do to decrease the excessive and sustained but low level of excitotoxic activation of NMDA receptors yet not interfere with learning, memory, and neuroplasticity, and without inducing a schizophrenia-like state?

The answer seems to be that you interfere with NMDA-mediated glutamatergic neurotransmission with a weak (low-affinity) NMDA antagonist that works at the same site plugging the ion channel where the magnesium ion normally blocks this channel at rest. That is, memantine is an uncompetitive

open-channel NMDA receptor antagonist with low to moderate affinity, voltage dependence, and fast blocking and unblocking kinetics. That is a fancy way of saying that it only blocks the ion channel of the NMDA receptor when it is open. This is why it is called an open-channel antagonist and why it is dependent upon voltage: namely, to open the channel. It is also a fancy way of saying that memantine blocks the open channel quickly, but is readily and quickly reversible if a barrage of glutamate comes along from normal neurotransmssion.

This concept is illustrated in Figure 13-29. Firstly, the hypothetical state of the glutamate neuron during Alzheimer's excitotoxicity is shown in Figure 13-29A. Here, steady, tonic and excessive amounts of glutamate are continuously released in a manner that interferes with the normal resting state of the glutamate neuron (Figure 13-28A), and in a manner that interferes with established memory functions, new learning, and normal neuronal plasticity. Eventually, this leads to the activation of intracellular enzymes that produce toxic free radicals that damage the membranes of the postsynaptic dendrite and eventually destroy the entire neuron (Figure 13-29A). When memantine is given, it blocks this tonic glutamate release from having downstream effects, thus returning the glutamate neuron to a new resting state despite the continuous release of glutamate (Figure 13-29B). Hypothetically, this stops the excessive glutamate from interfering with the resting glutamate neuron's physiological activity, therefore improving memory; it also hypothetically stops the excessive glutamate from causing neurotoxicity, therefore slowing the rate of neuronal death and also the associated cognitive decline that this causes in Alzheimer's disease (Figure 13-29B).

However, at the same time, memantine is not so powerful a blocker of NMDA receptors that it stops all neurotransmission at glutamate synapses (Figure 13-29C). That is, when a phasic burst of glutamate is transiently released during normal glutamatergic neurotransmission, this causes a depolarization that is capable of reversing the memantine block, until the depolarization goes away (Figure 13-29C). For this reason, memantine does not have the psychotomimetic actions of other more powerful NMDA antagonists such as PCP (phencyclidine) and ketamine, and does not shut down new learning or the ability of normal neurotransmission to occur when necessary

Rivastigmine Actions: Gliosis

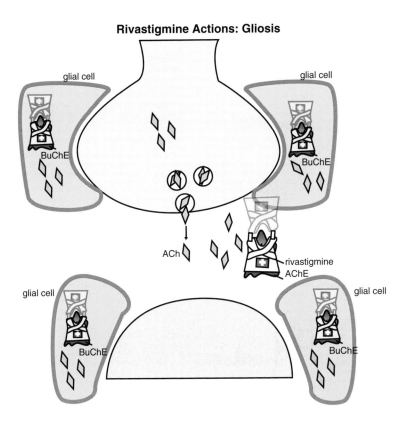

Figure 13-26B. Rivastigmine actions, part 2. Rivastigmine inhibits the enzymes acetylcholinesterase (AChE) and butyrylcholinesterase (BuChE), which are present both in the central nervous system (CNS) and peripherally. Inhibition of BuChE may be more important in later stages of disease, because as more cholinergic neurons die and gliosis occurs, BuChE activity increases.

Rivastigmine Actions: Peripheral

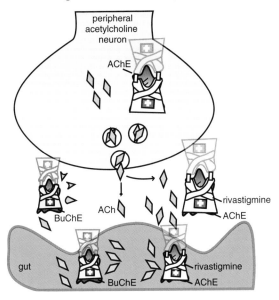

Figure 13-26C. Rivastigmine actions, part 3. Rivastigmine inhibits the enzymes acetylcholinesterase (AChE) and butyrylcholinesterase (BuChE), which are present both in the central nervous system (CNS) and peripherally. Peripheral cholinergic neurons in the gut are involved in gastrointestinal effects; thus the boost in peripheral acetylcholine caused by AChE and BuChE blockade may contribute to gastrointestinal side effects.

(Figure 13-29C). The blockade of NMDA receptors by memantine can be seen as a kind of "artificial magnesium," more effective than physiological blockade by magnesium, which is overwhelmed by excitotoxic glutamate release, but less effective than PCP or ketamine so that the glutamate system is not entirely shut down. Sort of like having your cake and eating it, too.

Memantine also has σ antagonist properties and weak $5HT_3$ antagonist properties, but it is not clear what these contribute to the actions of this agent in Alzheimer's disease. Since its mechanism of action in Alzheimer's disease is so different from cholinesterase inhibition, memantine is usually given concomitantly with a cholinesterase inhibitor to exploit the potential of both of these approaches and to get additive results in patients.

Treatments for psychiatric and behavioral symptoms in dementia

Dementia is not just a disturbance of memory, as many patients have a variety of behavioral and emotional symptoms as well. Treatment of agitation and aggression in dementia is a very controversial area, due to the potential for misuse of antipsychotics as "chemical straightjackets" to over-tranquilize patients, and also safety concerns about cardiovascular

Galantamine Actions

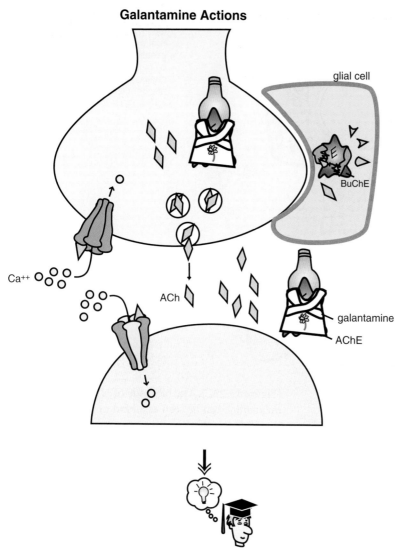

Figure 13-27A. Galantamine actions, part 1. Galantamine inhibits the enzyme acetylcholinesterase (AChE). Central cholinergic neurons are important for regulation of memory, and thus in the CNS the boost of acetylcholine caused by AChE blockade contributes to improved cognitive functioning. *Galantamine is represented here by a straitjacket icon with a lightbulb on top. The straitjacket has a daffodil on front, since galantamine was originally extracted from daffodils; the light bulb represents a second mechanism of action of galantamine, namely positive allosteric modulation of nicotinic receptors.*

events and death from these drugs. Antipsychotics are thus not recommended for use for agitation and behavioral symptoms of Alzheimer's disease, because there is little evidence of efficacy from controlled trials and also because there are demonstrated safety concerns that antipsychotics cause increased cardiovascular events and increased mortality in elderly patients with dementia. At this time, no antipsychotic is FDA-approved for this use and all carry warnings about the risk of cardiovascular events and increased mortality in this population. Because, in the real world, there are also risks of nontreatment, including early institutionalization and the dangers of agitated and psychotic behaviors to the patient and others around them, some patients will nevertheless require

treatment with an atypical antipsychotic. In this case, risperidone is often a preferred agent at very low doses. Clinicians should be alerted to the need to distinguish Alzheimer's disease from dementia with Lewy bodies prior to prescribing an antipsychotic. Patients with dementia with Lewy bodies can look psychotic, with their prominent behavioral symptoms, dramatic fluctuations, and visual hallucinations, but are exquisitely sensitive to extrapyramidal side effects even of the atypical antipsychotics, which can result in very severe and potentially life-threatening reactions to such drugs. An agent approved for treatment of the behavioral symptoms of dementia would be a welcome solution to a huge unmet need for these patients.

Galantamine Actions: Nicotinic Allosteric Modulation

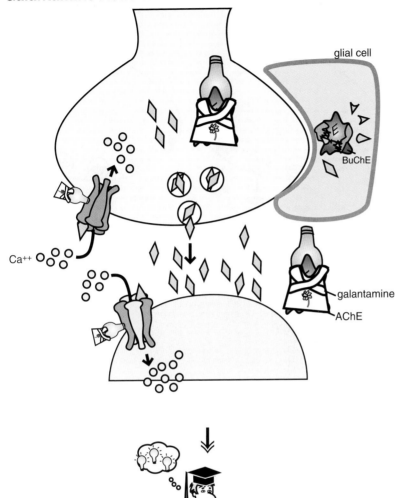

Figure 13-27B. Galantamine actions, part 2. Galantamine is unique among cholinesterase inhibitors in that it is also a positive allosteric modulator (PAM) at nicotinic cholinergic receptors, which means it can boost the effects of acetylcholine at these receptors. Thus galantamine's second action as a PAM at nicotinic receptors could theoretically enhance its primary action as a cholinesterase inhibitor.

glial cell

BuChE

Ca++

galantamine

AChE

Before using medications at all, reversible precipitants of agitation in dementia should be managed: pain, nicotine withdrawal, medication side effects, undiagnosed medical and neurological illnesses, and provocative environments that are either too stimulating or not stimulating enough. When use of medications is necessary, cholinesterase inhibitors may be effective in some patients and are a first-line consideration in Alzheimer's disease, but might work better for prevention of these symptoms than for their treatment once they have emerged. Also, frontotemporal dementia patients may be more likely to benefit from SSRIs (e.g., citalopram or escitalopram) or SNRIs. In general, first-line treatment of agitation and aggression in dementia is SSRI/SNRI therapy. Second-line treatments that may help to avoid use of atypical antipsychotics can also include β blockers, valproate, gabapentin, pregabalin, and selegilene. Others may respond to carbamazepine, oxcarbazepine, benzodiazepines, buspirone, or trazodone.

Other proposed targets for dementia

A number of psychopharmacological agents have been tested for their potential as treatments in Alzheimer's disease, but none has yet proven effective. This includes various antioxidants, anti-inflammatory agents, statins, vitamin E, estrogen, the MAO inhibitor selegiline, the antidiabetic agent rosiglitazone and other peroxisome proliferator-activated receptor gamma (PPARγ)

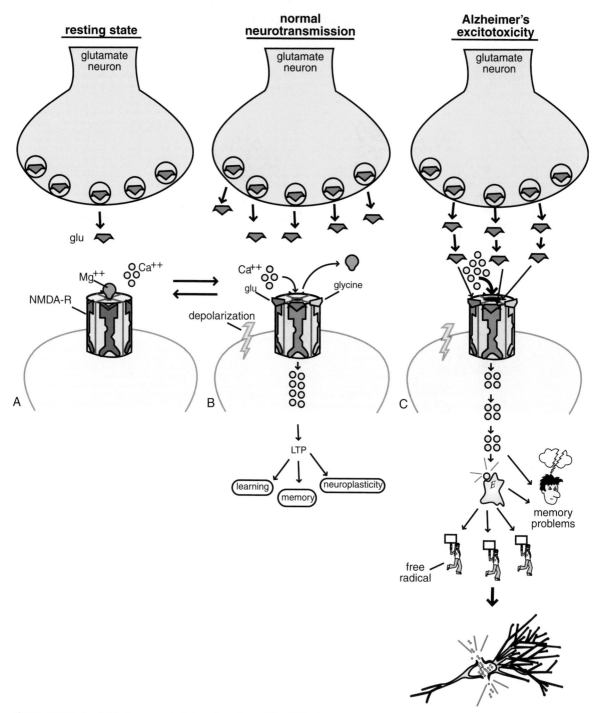

Figure 13-28. Amyloid plaques and glutamate excitotoxicity. (A) In the resting state glutamate is quiet and *N*-methyl-D-aspartate (NMDA) receptors are blocked by magnesium. (B) With normal neurotransmission, glutamate binds to NMDA receptors and, if the postsynaptic receptor is depolarized and glycine is simultaneously bound to the NMDA receptors, the channel opens and allows ion influx. (C) If amyloid's synaptic effects include downregulating the glutamate transporter, inhibiting glutamate reuptake, or enhancing glutamate release, this could cause a steady leak of glutamate and result in excessive calcium influx in postsynaptic neurons, which in the short term may cause memory problems and in the long term may cause accumulation of free radicals and thus destruction of neurons.

Mechanism of Action of Memantine

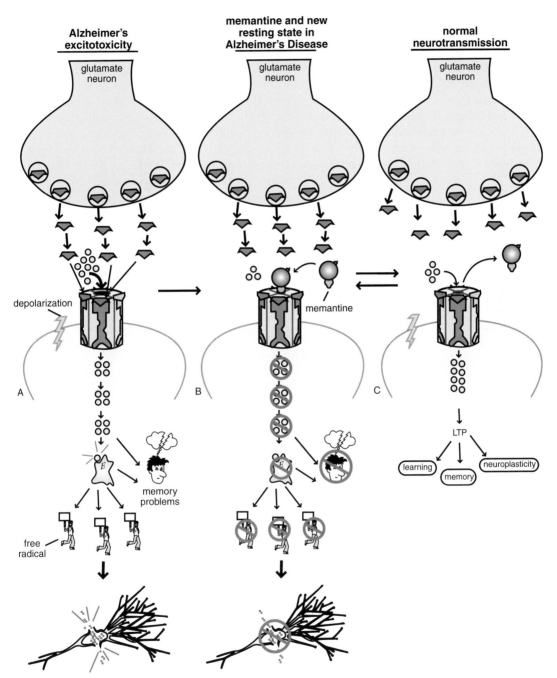

Figure 13-29. Memantine actions. Memantine is a noncompetitive low-affinity *N*-methyl-D-aspartate (NMDA) receptor antagonist that binds to the magnesium site when the channel is open. (A) If amyloid's synaptic effects lead to a steady (tonic) leak of glutamate and result in excessive calcium influx in postsynaptic neurons, this could cause memory problems and, in the long term, accumulation of free radicals and thus destruction of neurons. (B) Memantine blocks the downstream effects of tonic glutamate release by "plugging" the NMDA ion channel and thus may improve memory and prevent neurodegeneration. (C) Because memantine has low affinity, when there is a phasic burst of glutamate and depolarization occurs, this is enough to remove memantine from the ion channel and thus allow normal neurotransmission.

agonists, lithium and other glycogen synthase kinase (GSK) inhibitors, agents that attempt to block tau phosphorylation, and phosphodiesterase inhibitors.

Many of the same agents proposed as pro-cognitive in ADHD and discussed in Chapter 12, and as pro-cognitive in schizophrenia and discussed in Chapter 5, have also been studied in Alzheimer's disease as potential symptomatic treatments, from H_3 histamine antagonists, to AMPAkines, to nicotinic cholinergic agonists, $5HT_6$ antagonists, phosphodiesterase inhibitors, metabotropic glutamate receptor agents, and others, but not with robust promise at the present time.

Summary

The most common dementia is Alzheimer's disease, and the leading theory for its etiology is the amyloid cascade hypothesis. Other dementias are briefly discussed as well, as are their differing pathologies. New diagnostic criteria now propose that there are three stages of Alzheimer's disease. The first stage is preclinical, asymptomatic but with amyloid accumulation; the second stage is mild cognitive impairment, with both amyloid accumulation and biomarker evidence of neurodegeneration in the presence of memory problems; and the last stage, dementia. Major research efforts are attempting to find disease-modifying treatments that could halt or even reverse the course of this illness by interfering with amyloid accumulation in the brain. Leading treatments for Alzheimer's disease today include the cholinesterase inhibitors, based upon the cholinergic hypothesis of amnesia, and memantine, an NMDA antagonist, based upon the glutamate hypothesis of cognitive decline.

Impulsivity, compulsivity, and addiction

Recent advances in understanding the neurocircuitry of impulsivity and compulsivity has led to the notion that many different psychiatric disorders share these two dimensions of psychopathology. Here we take a look not only at drug addiction, the best-known set of disorders in this category, but also briefly at other "impulsive–compulsive disorders" including obsessive–compulsive disorder (OCD), trichotillomania, gambling, aggression, obesity, and other disorders thought to be related in part to inefficient information processing in prefrontal cortex/striatal circuitry (Figure 14-1 and Table 14-1). Earlier chapters have already touched upon impulsivity in attention deficit hyperactivity disorder (ADHD, discussed in Chapter 12) and in bipolar mania (discussed in Chapters 6 and 7), and the discussion in this chapter applies to impulsivity in these disorders as well.

Here we review the hypothetical shared neurobiology of impulsive–compulsive disorders and discuss the treatments that are available for some of these conditions. Although serotonergic treatments of OCD are well known, psychopharmacologists have generally been reluctant to embrace therapeutics for substance abuse, whereas family physicians

and subspecialty substance abuse experts use the available psychopharmacological treatments more frequently. Perhaps the lack of highly effective psychopharmacologic treatments for many impulsive–compulsive disorders has led to a certain amount of therapeutic nihilism towards psychopharmacologic approaches to these conditions. Nevertheless, an explosion of neurobiological understanding of the symptom dimensions of impulsivity and compulsivity now sets the stage for novel therapeutic interventions to be discovered in the future, making it worthwhile understanding contemporary neurobiological formulations of addiction, compulsions, and impulsivity. Full clinical descriptions and formal criteria for how to diagnose the numerous known diagnostic entities should be obtained by consulting standard reference sources.

Overview of impulsive–compulsive disorders

Impulsivity and compulsivity are proposed as *endophenotypes*, namely symptoms linked to specific brain circuits and that are present trans-diagnostically as a dimension of psychopathology that cuts across

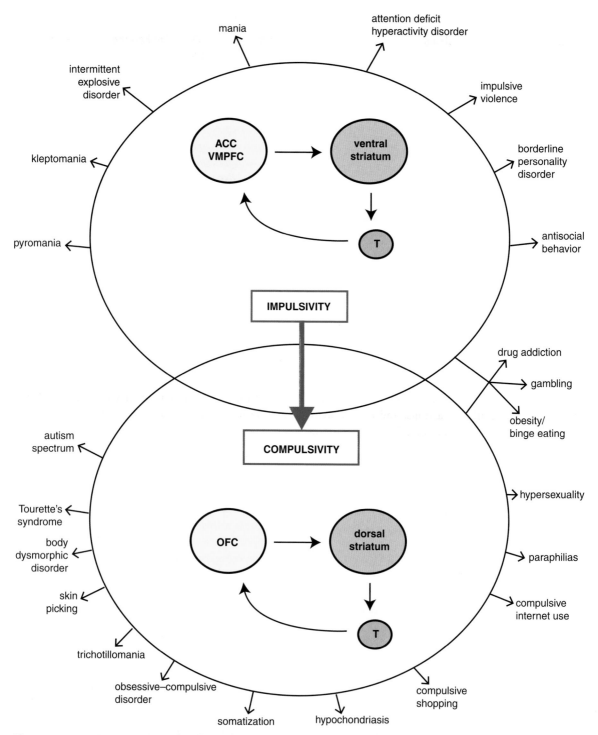

Figure 14-1. Impulsive–compulsive disorder construct. Impulsivity and compulsivity are seen in a wide variety of psychiatric disorders. Impulsivity can be thought of as the inability to stop the initiation of actions and involves a brain circuit centered on the ventral striatum, linked to the thalamus (T), to the ventromedial prefrontal cortex (VMPFC), and to the anterior cingulate cortex (ACC). Compulsivity can be thought of as the inability to terminate ongoing actions and hypothetically is centered on a different brain circuit, namely the dorsal striatum, thalamus (T), and orbitofrontal cortex (OFC). Impulsive acts such as drug use, gambling, and obesity can eventually become compulsive due to neuroplastic changes that engage the dorsal habit system and theoretically cause impulses in the ventral loop to migrate to the dorsal loop.

Table 14-1 Possible categorization of impulsivity and compulsivity endophenotypes as impulsive–compulsive disorders

Obsessive–compulsive related spectrum disorders	Substance/behavioral addictions	Disruptive/impulse control	Sexual
Obsessive–compulsive disorder (OCD)	Drug addiction	Pyromania	Hypersexual
Hair pulling (trichotillomania; TTM)	Gambling	Kleptomania	Paraphilias
Skin picking	Internet addiction	Intermittent explosive disorder	
Body dysmorphic disorder (BDD)	Food addiction (binge eating, obesity)	Impulsive violence	
Hoarding	Compulsive shopping	Borderline personality disorder	
Tourette's syndrome/tic disorders		Self harm/parasuicidal behavior	
Stereotyped movement disorders		Antisocial behavior	
Autism spectrum disorders		Conduct disorder	
Hypochondriasis		Oppositional defiant disorder	
Somatization		Mania	
		ADHD	

many psychiatric disorders (Table 14-1, Figure 14-1). Simply put, impulsivity and compulsivity are both symptoms that result from the brain having a hard time saying "no." In fact, these two symptom constructs can perhaps be best differentiated by how they both fail to control responses: impulsivity as the inability to stop *initiating* actions, and compulsivity as the inability to *terminate* ongoing actions. Both impulsivity and compulsivity are therefore forms of cognitive inflexibility.

More precisely, **impulsivity** is defined as acting without forethought; the lack of reflection on the consequences of one's behavior; the inability to postpone reward with preference for immediate reward over more beneficial but delayed reward; a failure of motor inhibition, often choosing risky behavior; or (less scientifically) lacking the willpower not to give in to temptations (see definitions in Table 14-2).

On the other hand, **compulsivity** is defined as actions inappropriate to the situation but which nevertheless persist, and which often result in undesirable consequences. In fact, compulsions are characterized by the inability to adapt behavior after negative feedback. *Habits* are a type of compulsion, and can be seen as responses triggered by environmental stimuli regardless of the current desirability of the consequences of that response (Table 14-2). Habits can be seen as *conditioned responses* (such as drug seeking, food seeking, gambling) to a conditioning stimulus (such as being around people or places or items associated with drugs, food, or

gambling in the past) that have been reinforced and strengthened either by past experience with reward (positive reinforcement) or with the omission of an aversive event (loss of the negative reinforcement that comes from withdrawal or craving). Whereas goal-directed behavior is mediated by knowledge of and desire for the consequences, in contrast, habits are controlled by external stimuli through stimulus–response associations that are stamped into brain circuits through behavioral repetition and formed after considerable training, can be automatically triggered by stimuli, and are defined by their insensitivity to their outcomes. Given that goal-directed actions are relatively cognitively demanding, for daily routines it can be adaptive to rely on habits that can be performed with minimal conscious awareness. However, habits can also represent severely maladaptive perseveration of behaviors (Figure 14-1, Table 14-1).

Neurocircuitry and the impulsive–compulsive disorders

Why can't impulses and compulsions be stopped in various psychiatric disorders (Table 14-1, Figure 14-1)? The answer may lie in a problem in cortical circuits that normally suppress these behaviors. An oversimplification of this notion is that impulsivity and compulsivity are hypothetically neurobiological drives that are "bottom-up," with impulsivity coming from the ventral striatum, compulsivity coming from

Table 14-2 Definitions of key terms

Abuse	Self-administration of any drug in a culturally disapproved manner that causes adverse consequences.
Addiction	A behavioral pattern of drug abuse characterized by overwhelming involvement with the use of a drug (compulsive use), the securing of its supply, and a high tendency to relapse after discontinuation.
Compulsivity	Repetitive actions inappropriate to the situation that persist, that have no obvious relationship to the overall goal, and that often result in undesirable consequences; behavior that results in perseveration in responding in the face of adverse consequences; perseveration in responding in the face of incorrect responses in choice situations or persistent reinitiation of habitual acts.
Cross-tolerance and cross-dependence	The ability of one drug to suppress the manifestations of physical dependence produced by another drug and to maintain the physically dependent state.
Dependence	The physiological state of adaptation produced by repeated administration of certain drugs such as alcohol, heroin, and benzodiazepines when they are abruptly discontinued, and are associated with physical drug withdrawal distinct from the motivational changes of acute withdrawal and protracted abstinence, which is part of addiction.
Habit	Responses triggered by environmental stimuli regardless of the current desirability of the consequences. This conditioned response to a stimulus has been reinforced and strengthened either by past experience with reward (positive reinforcement) or by the omission of an aversive event (negative reinforcement).
Impulsivity	The tendency to act prematurely without foresight; actions which are poorly conceived, prematurely expressed, unduly risky, or inappropriate to the situation and that often result in undesirable consequences; predisposition toward rapid, unplanned responses to internal and external stimuli without regard for the negative consequences of those reactions to themselves or others. Impulsivity is often measured in two domains: the choice of a small, immediate reward over a larger delayed reward, or the inability to inhibit behavior to change the course of action or to stop a response once it is initiated.
Rebound	The exaggerated expression of the original condition sometimes experienced by patients immediately after cessation of an effective treatment.
Reinforcement	The tendency of a pleasure-producing drug to lead to repeated self-administration.
Relapse	The reoccurrence, upon discontinuation of an effective medical treatment, of the original condition from which the patient suffered.
Tolerance	Tolerance has developed when, after repeated administration, a given dose of a drug produces a decreased effect, or, conversely, when increasingly larger doses must be administered to obtain the effects observed with the original use.
Withdrawal	The psychologic and physiologic reactions to abrupt cessation of a dependence-producing drug.

the dorsal striatum, and different areas of prefrontal cortex acting "top-down" to suppress these drives (Figures 14-1 through 14-3). Inhibitory volitional control is thus exerted top-down by cortical mechanisms, implying that impulsivity and compulsivity could result from a relaxation of this control. According to this formulation of impulsivity and compulsivity, behavioral output is thus controlled by a balance between dual and sometimes competing neurobehavioral systems. What actually happens depends upon the balance between "top-down" and "bottom-up," with both impulsivity and compulsivity being either caused by a failure of response inhibition systems (i.e., inadequate top-down cognitive control: Figures 14-1 through 14-3) or the result of too much pressure coming bottom-up from the ventral striatum

Impulsivity and Reward

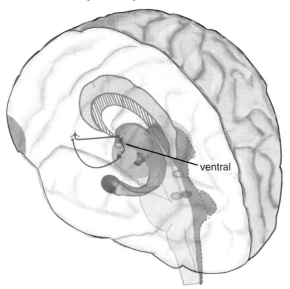

Figure 14-2. Circuitry of impulsivity and reward. The "bottom-up" circuit that drives impulsivity (shown in pink) is a loop with projections from the ventral striatum to the thalamus, from the thalamus to the ventromedial prefrontal cortex (VMPFC), and from the VMPFC back to the ventral striatum. This circuit is usually modulated "top-down" from the prefrontal cortex (PFC). If this top-down response inhibition system is inadequate or is overcome by activity from the bottom-up ventral striatum, impulsive behaviors may result.

Compulsivity and Motor Response Inhibition

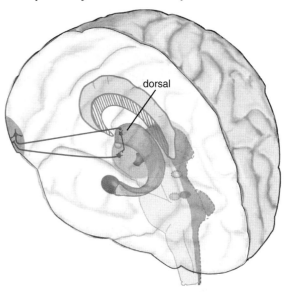

Figure 14-3. **Circuitry of compulsivity and motor response inhibition.** The "bottom-up" circuit that drives compulsivity (shown in pink) is a loop with projections from the dorsal striatum to the thalamus, from the thalamus to the orbitofrontal cortex (OFC), and from the OFC back to the dorsal striatum. This habit circuit can be modulated "top-down" from the OFC, but if this top-down response inhibition system is inadequate or is overcome by activity from the bottom-up dorsal striatum, compulsive behaviors may result.

for impulsivity (Figure 14-2) or from the dorsal striatum for compulsivity (Figure 14-3).

Neuroanatomically, impulsivity and compulsivity are seen as engaging different neuronal loops: impulsivity as an action–outcome ventrally dependent learning system (Figure 14-2) and compulsivity a habit system that is dorsal (Figure 14-3). Many behaviors start out as impulses in the ventral loop of reward and motivation (Figure 14-2). Over time, however, some of these behaviors migrate dorsally (Figure 14-3) due to a cascade of neuroadaptations and neuroplasticity that engage the habit system by means of which an impulsive act eventually becomes compulsive (Figure 14-1). These spirals of information from one neuronal loop to another also appear to involve regulatory input from hippocampus and amygdala and other areas of prefrontal cortex (Figure 14-4).

A well-known example of ventral to dorsal migration is drug addiction. Although initial drug use is thought to be voluntary and linked to trait impulsivity, drug abusers gradually lose control over drug-seeking and drug-taking behavior, which becomes compulsive (Figure 14-5). Impulses to take drugs or

to perform certain behaviors initially give a "high" or at least great pleasure and satisfaction (Figure 14-5). If this happens infrequently enough so as *not* to trigger neuroplastic cascades from ventral to dorsal, this remains under relative control, and can be seen as being occasionally "naughty" (Figure 14-5). However, impulsive drug use or impulsive behaviors repeated too often may progress to compulsive use driven by a desire to reduce the distressing symptoms of withdrawal that develop over time as the drug/behavior is repeated many times (Figure 14-5). Individuals with drug or behavioral addictions experience tension and arousal in anticipation of performing the behavior but dysphoric mood (but no physiological withdrawal) when prevented from performing the behavior or taking the drug. The pleasure and gratification that the drug/behavior initially causes, however, diminish over time, perhaps requiring increasing doses (e.g., gambling higher dollar amounts, more amounts or frequency of drug ingestion) in order to achieve the same effects (akin to tolerance) (Figure 14-5).

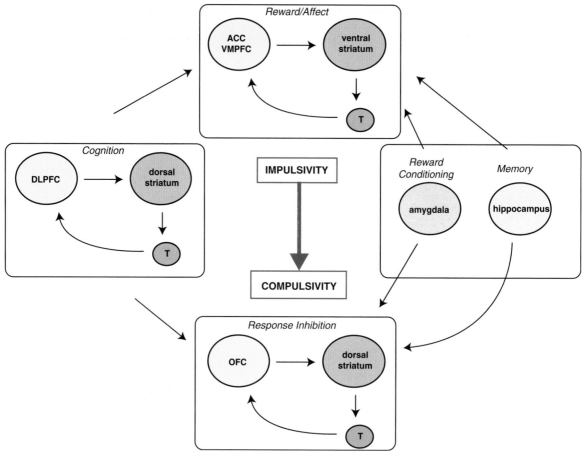

Figure 14-4. Spiraling circuits of impulsivity and compulsivity. The progression from occasional, impulsive drug use to compulsive use and addiction involves both the dysregulation of bottom-up reward circuits and insufficient top-down inhibition of these circuits. The amygdala and hippocampus provide regulatory input to this system as well. ACC, anterior cingulate cortex; DLPFC, dorsolateral prefrontal cortex; OFC, orbitofrontal cortex; T, thalamus; VMPFC, ventromedial prefrontal cortex.

Maybe the first dose of any drug will always be the best one, most reinforcing and without penalty. However, individuals do not usually just take one dose of a drug, or perform satisfying behaviors just once. High impulsivity predisposes to the development of compulsions and is predictive of over-reliance on habit learning. Accelerated habit formation may underlie the transition in individuals who have high impulsivity to compulsions and habits. Compulsivity is clearly a maladaptive perseveration of behavior. This is not so much being naughty and giving into temptations (Figure 14-5) as being more like one of Pavlov's dogs with a mindless involuntary conditioned compulsive response, with willpower being totally inadequate to interrupt the potentially destructive perseverations of behavior once they have become compulsive habits (Table 14-2 and Figure 14-5).

The mesolimbic dopamine circuit as the final common pathway of reward

All drugs that can lead to addiction increase dopamine (DA) in ventral striatum, also called the nucleus accumbens. This area of the brain is familiar to readers, as it is the same area discussed in Chapter 4 on psychosis and also known as the mesolimbic dopamine pathway hypothesized to be overly active in psychosis and to mediate the positive symptoms of schizophrenia (see Figures 4-12, 4-13, 4-30, 4-31). The final common pathway of reinforcement and reward in the brain is also hypothesized to be this same mesolimbic dopamine pathway (Figure 14-6). Some even consider this to be the "center of hedonic pleasure" of the brain and dopamine to be the "neurotransmitter of hedonic pleasure." There are many

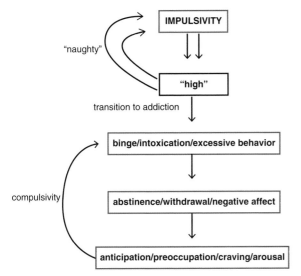

Figure 14-5. Shifting from impulsivity to compulsivity. Drug addiction provides a good example of the shift from impulsivity to compulsivity that comes with migration from ventral to dorsal circuits. The impulse to take a drug initially leads to great pleasure and satisfaction (a "high"). If this happens infrequently, the behavior may be a bit "naughty" but will not necessarily progress to compulsivity. With chronic substance use, compulsivity may develop as an individual's drive turns from seeking pleasure to seeking relief from distressing symptoms of withdrawal and anticipation of obtaining the drug.

natural ways to trigger your mesolimbic dopamine neurons to release dopamine, ranging from intellectual accomplishments to athletic accomplishments, to enjoying a good symphony, to experiencing an orgasm. These are sometimes called "natural highs" (Figure 14-6). The inputs to the mesolimbic pathway that mediate these natural highs include a most incredible "pharmacy" of naturally occurring substances ranging from the brain's own morphine/heroin (endorphins), to the brain's own marijuana (anandamide), to the brain's own nicotine (acetylcholine), to the brain's own cocaine and amphetamine (dopamine itself) (Figure 14-7).

The numerous psychotropic drugs of abuse also have a final common pathway of causing the mesolimbic pathway to release dopamine, often in a manner more explosive and pleasurable than that which occurs naturally. Also, it now appears that potentially maladaptive behaviors as well as drugs can result in the release of dopamine that in turn stimulates the reward system (Figure 14-7). These are included in the impulsive–compulsive disorder construct (Figure 14-1) and include behaviors such as gambling, using the internet, shopping, and even eating. Drugs bypass the brain's own neurotransmitters and directly

stimulate the brain's own receptors for these drugs, causing dopamine to be released. Since the brain already uses neurotransmitters that resemble drugs of abuse, it is not necessary to earn your reward naturally since you can get a much more intense reward in the short run and upon demand from a drug of abuse than you can from a natural high with the brain's natural system. However, unlike a natural high, a drug-induced reward can start a cascade of neuroadaptation in the ventral striatum loop that migrates to the dorsal striatal loop (Figure 14-1), such that the initial high caused by impulsive early use of a drug leads to withdrawal, craving, and pre-occupation with finding drug, thus beginning a vicious cycle of abuse, addiction, dependence, and withdrawal (Figure 14-5).

Substance addictions

Not everyone who takes a drug once gets addicted to it. Why? For one thing, some drugs seem to be intrinsically more addicting than others (Table 14-3). For another, some individuals may be more impulsive by nature or have a genetically dysfunctional reward system. It seems that impulsive traits and a dysfunctional reward system may confer a propensity towards drug use and abuse, and when drugs are ingested frequently, impulsive drug use can recruit the involvement of the habit system perhaps in some individuals more readily than in others, triggering neuroplasticity in the compulsivity circuit, which hypothetically is the means by which drug ingestion eventually becomes compulsive in some individuals (Figures 14-1 and 14-5).

Stimulants

The speed with which a drug enters the brain dictates the degree of the subjective "high" (Figure 14-8). This may be the reason why drugs that are inhaled, snorted, or injected, thus entering the brain in a sudden explosive manner, are usually much more reinforcing than when those same drugs are taken orally, where speed of entry to the brain is considerably slowed by the process of gastrointestinal absorption. Cocaine is not even active orally, so users have learned over the years to take it intranasally – where the drug rapidly enters the brain directly, bypassing the liver, and thus can have a more rapid onset this way than even with intravenous administration. The most rapid and robust way to deliver drugs to

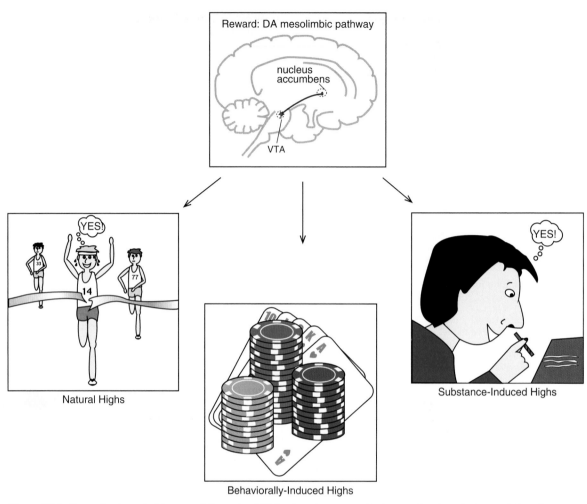

Figure 14-6. Dopamine is central to reward. Dopamine (DA) has long been recognized as a major player in the regulation of reinforcement and reward. Specifically, the mesolimbic pathway from the ventral tegmental area (VTA) to the nucleus accumbens seems to be crucial for reward. Naturally rewarding activities, such as achieving major accomplishments or enjoying a good meal, can cause fast and robust increases in DA in the mesolimbic pathway. Drugs of abuse also cause DA release in the mesolimbic pathway. In fact, drugs of abuse can often increase dopamine in a manner that is more explosive and pleasurable than that which occurs naturally. Unfortunately, unlike a natural high, the activation caused by drugs of abuse can eventually cause changes in reward circuitry that are associated with a vicious cycle of drug preoccupation, craving, addiction, dependence, and withdrawal. This conceptualization has similarities to many impulsive–compulsive disorders such as pathological gambling. That is, individuals with these disorders experience tension and arousal in anticipation of performing the behavior and dysphoric mood (but no physiological withdrawal) when prevented from performing the behavior. In addition, the pleasure and gratification that is initially experienced when performing the behavior seems to diminish over time, perhaps requiring increasing "doses" (e.g., gambling higher dollar amounts) in order to achieve the same effects (akin to tolerance).

the brain is to smoke those that are compatible with this route of administration, as this avoids first-pass metabolism through the liver and is somewhat akin to giving the drug by intra-arterial/intra-carotid bolus via immediate absorption across the massive surface area of the lung. The faster the drug's entry into the brain, the stronger are its reinforcing effects, probably because this form of drug delivery triggers phasic DA firing, the type

associated with reward and saliency (see Chapter 12 for discussion, and Figures 12-10, 12-29, and 12-31).

On the other hand, some of these very same stimulants taken at low doses orally, especially within controlled-release formulations that minimize peak absorption, slow the rate of absorption, and prolong the duration of drug exposure, are not particularly reinforcing, but instead are therapeutic agents for treating ADHD, as discussed in Chapter 12 and

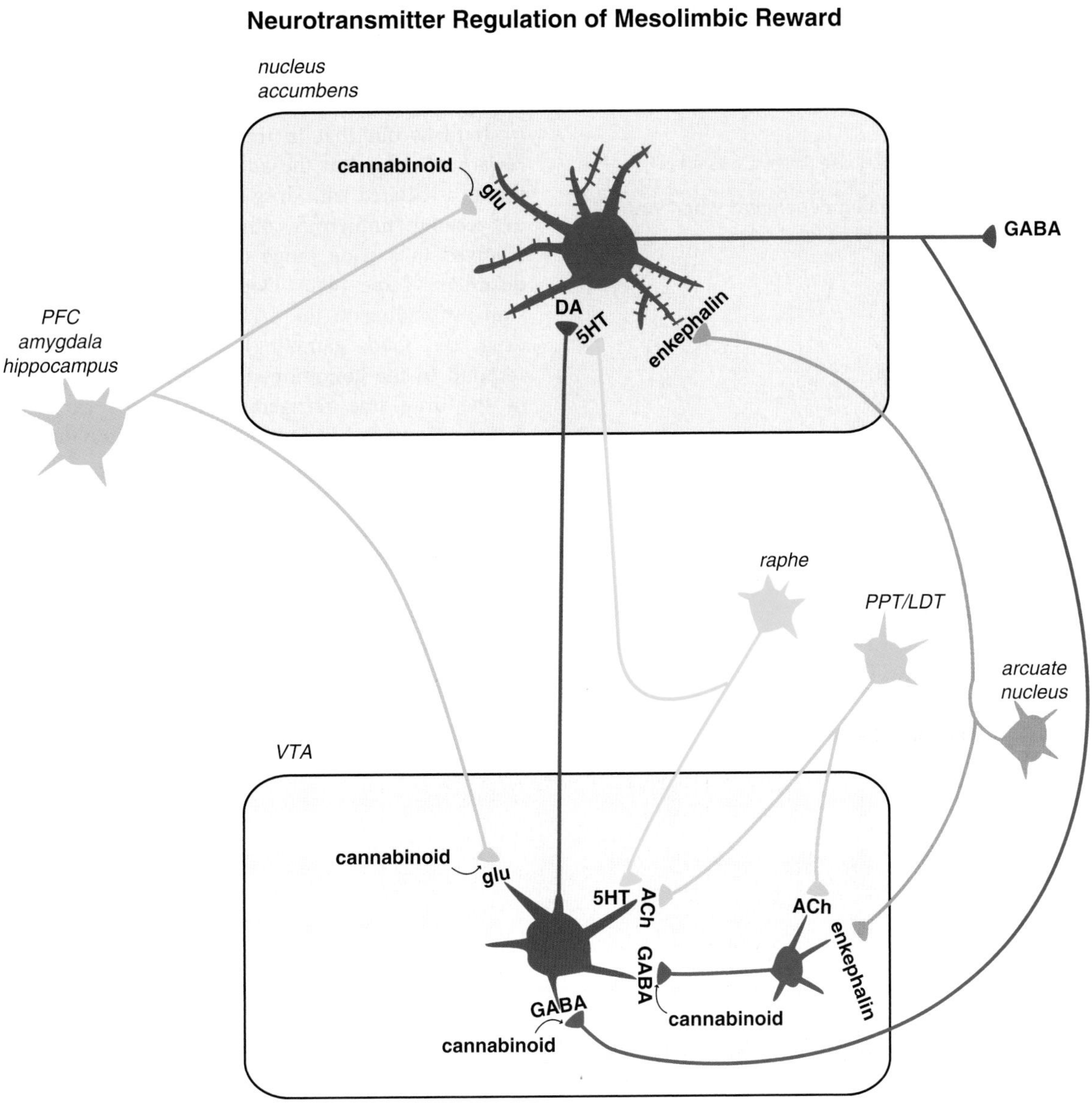

Neurotransmitter Regulation of Mesolimbic Reward

Figure 14-7. Neurotransmitter regulation of mesolimbic reward. The final common pathway of reward in the brain is hypothesized to be the mesolimbic dopamine pathway. This pathway is modulated by many naturally occurring substances in the brain in order to deliver normal reinforcement to adaptive behaviors (such as eating, drinking, sex) and thus to produce "natural highs," such as feelings of joy or accomplishment. These neurotransmitter inputs to the reward system include the brain's own morphine/heroin (i.e., endorphins such as enkephalin), the brain's own cannabis/marijuana (i.e., anandamide), the brain's own nicotine (i.e., acetylcholine), and the brain's own cocaine/amphetamine (i.e., dopamine itself), among others. The numerous psychotropic drugs of abuse that occur in nature bypass the brain's own neurotransmitters and directly stimulate the brain's receptors in the reward system, causing dopamine release and a consequent "artificial high." Thus alcohol, opioids, stimulants, marijuana, benzodiazepines, sedative hypnotics, hallucinogens, and nicotine all affect this mesolimbic dopaminergic system. PFC, prefrontal cortex; PPT/LDT, pedunculopontine tegmental and laterodorsal tegmental nuclei.

illustrated in Figures 12-29 and 12-30. As discussed in Chapter 12, hypothetically, stimulants administered in this slow-release manner act to "tune" inefficient brain circuits by targeting the prefrontal cortex, enhancing tonic dopamine firing for motivation and attention, and reducing impulses and hyperactivity, while allowing sufficient phasic dopamine firing for learning and for facilitating appropriate goal-directed behaviors/reward (Figures 12-10 through 12-31). Although *therapeutic* actions of stimulants are thought to be directed at the prefrontal cortex to enhance both norepinephrine and dopamine neurotransmission there (Figures 12-13 through 12-18; Figure 12-31), the *reinforcing effects* and *abuse* of

stimulants are thought to be directed at reward circuits, especially at dopamine release from mesolimbic dopamine neurons in the nucleus accumbens (Figure 12-31).

It turns out that in the long run it is not the reward of drug, but the anticipation of the reward, that is associated with drug seeking, or food seeking, or seeking numerous other types of situations involved in a wide range of impulsive–compulsive disorders (Table 14-1). Dopamine neurons actually stop responding to the primary reinforcer (i.e., the drug, the food, gambling) and instead begin to respond to the conditioned stimulus (i.e., the sight of the drug, the refrigerator door, the gambling casino). Conditioned responses underlie craving and compulsive use, and the increased dopamine migrates to the dorsal striatum (Figures 14-1 and 14-4). Drugs and behaviors may initially lead to dopamine increase in the ventral striatum and reward (Figures 14-1, 14-2, 14-4, 14-6, 14-7), but with repeated administration, as habits develop, dopamine increases shift

Table 14-3 How addicting are different substances?

Probability of becoming dependent when you have tried a substance at least once	
Tobacco	32%
Heroin	23%
Cocaine	17%
Alcohol	15%
Stimulants	11%
Anxiolytics	9%
Cannabis	9%
Analgesics	8%
Inhalants	4%

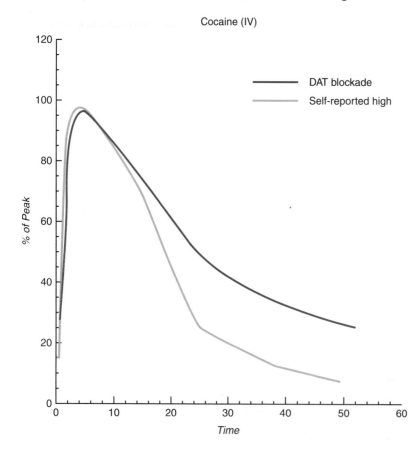

Dopamine, Pharmacokinetics, and Reinforcing Effects

Cocaine (IV)

— DAT blockade
— Self-reported high

Figure 14-8. Dopamine, pharmacokinetics, and reinforcing effects. Acute drug use causes dopamine (DA) release in the striatum. However, the reinforcing effects of the drug are largely determined not only by the presence of DA but also by the rate at which DA increases in the brain, which in turn is dictated by the speed at which the drug enters and leaves the brain, in this case targeting the dopamine transporter (DAT). An abrupt and large increase in DA (such as that caused by drugs of abuse that block DAT) mimic the phasic DA firing associated with conveying information about reward and saliency. The rate of drug uptake is subject to the route of administration, with intravenous administration and inhalation producing the fastest drug uptake, followed by snorting. In addition, different drugs of abuse have different "reward values" (i.e., different rates at which they increase DA) based on their individual mechanisms of action.

from the drug/behavior to the conditioned response/ environmental trigger, as the dopamine increases shift from the ventral striatum/nucleus accumbens (Figure 14-2) to the dorsal striatum (Figure 14-3).

Dopamine is associated with motivation, and the motivation to procure drugs is the hallmark of addiction. Drug seeking and drug taking become the main motivational drive when one is addicted, and thus the addicted subject is aroused and motivated when seeking to procure the drug, but is withdrawn and apathetic when exposed to non-drug-related activities (Figures 14-5 and 14-8). What starts out as increased DA release leading to increased ventral striatum and anterior cinguluate cortex (ACC) activity with reward may end up as a compulsive drive with escalating dosing in an attempt to get increased reward stimulation to restore a resultant DA deficiency. The discrepancy between expectation for drug effects and the blunted DA effects maintains drug taking in an attempt to achieve the expected reward. High doses of stimulants can cause tremor, emotional lability, restlessness, irritability, panic, and repetitive stereotyped behavior. At even higher repetitive doses, stimulants can induce paranoia and hallucinations, with hypertension, tachycardia, ventricular irritability, hyperthermia, and respiratory depression. In overdose, stimulants can cause acute heart failure, stroke, and seizures.

Not only methylphenidate and amphetamines, but also cocaine are all inhibitors of the dopamine transporter (DAT) and the norepinephrine transporter (NET) (see discussion in Chapter 12, and Figures 12-25 and 12-28). Cocaine also inhibits the serotonin transporter (SERT) and is also a local anesthetic, which Freud himself exploited to help dull the pain of his cancer of the jaw and mouth. He may have also exploited the second property of the drug, which is to produce euphoria, reduce fatigue, and create a sense of mental acuity due to inhibition of dopamine reuptake at the dopamine transporter, at least for a while, until drug-induced reward is replaced by drug-induced compulsivity.

Although there are no approved treatments for stimulant addicts, in the future there may be a cocaine vaccine that removes the drug before it reaches the brain so there are no more reinforcing effects that accompany drug ingestion. Theoretically, it may also be possible to administer intravenously a long-acting form of the enzyme cocaine esterase that destroys cocaine before it can exert its reinforcing effects, as has been shown in animal models. Naltrexone, a μ-opioid antagonist approved for the treatment of both opioid and alcohol addiction, is also being investigated for patients with stimulant addiction, particularly for those patients with polydrug dependence on both the opioid heroin and the stimulant amphetamine. Buprenorphine, a synthetic opioid used for treatment of pain and for opioid addiction, stimulates as a partial agonist both μ- and κ-opioid receptors, and can decrease cocaine use in opioid addicts. It is also being studied in combination with naltrexone for cocaine addicts who do not have opioid addiction. The combination results in stimulation only of κ-opioid receptors and not of μ-opioid receptors and may decrease compulsive cocaine self-administration in animals without producing opioid addiction – suggesting that, at least in this case, three drugs might be better than one!

Nicotine

How common is smoking in clinical psychopharmacology practices? Some estimates are that more than half of all cigarettes are consumed by patients with a concurrent psychiatric disorder, and that smoking is the most common comorbidity among seriously mentally ill patients. It is estimated that about 20% of the general population (in the US) smoke, about 30% of people who regularly see general physicians smoke, but that 40–50% of patients in a psychopharmacology practice smoke, including 60–85% of patients with ADHD, schizophrenia, and bipolar disorder. Unfortunately, histories of current smoking are often not carefully taken nor recorded as one of the diagnoses for smokers in mental health practices, and only about 10% of smokers report being offered treatment proactively by psychopharmacologists and other clinicians.

Nicotine acts directly upon nicotinic cholinergic receptors in reward circuits (Figure 14-7). Cholinergic neurons and the neurotransmitter acetylcholine are discussed in Chapter 13 and illustrated in Figures 13-17 through 13-24. Nicotinic receptors are illustrated in Figures 13-20 through 13-22. There are two major subtypes of nicotinic receptors that are known to be present in the brain, the $\alpha_4\beta_2$ subtype and the α_7 subtype (discussed in Chapter 13 and illustrated in Figure 13-20). Nicotine's actions in the ventral tegmental area are those that are theoretically linked to addiction, namely at $\alpha_4\beta_2$-nicotinic postsynaptic receptors on dopamine neurons, leading to dopamine release in the nucleus accumbens, and at α_7-nicotinic presynaptic receptors on glutamate neurons, which causes glutamate release, and in turn dopamine release in the nucleus accumbens (Figure 14-9). The release-promoting

Detail of Nicotine Actions

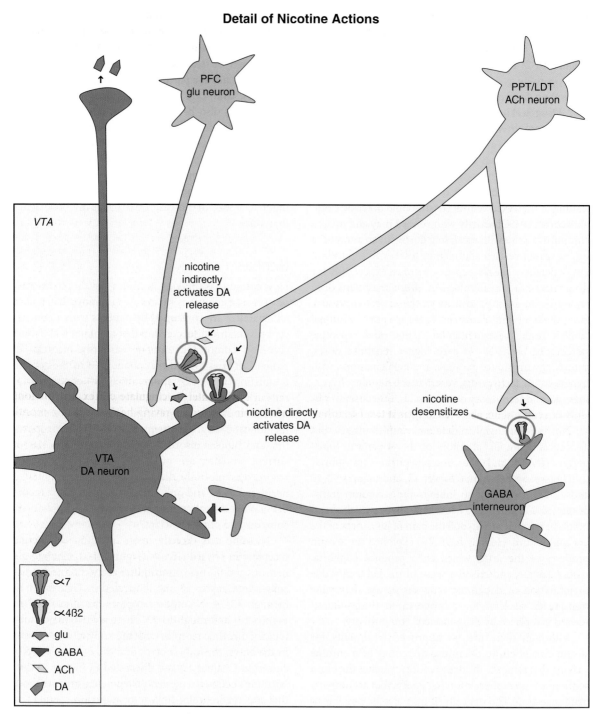

Figure 14-9. Actions of nicotine. Nicotine directly causes dopamine release in the nucleus accumbens by binding to $\alpha_4\beta_2$-nicotinic postsynaptic receptors on dopamine neurons in the ventral tegmental area (VTA). In addition, nicotine binds to α_7-nicotinic presynaptic receptors on glutamate neurons in the VTA, which in turn leads to dopamine release in the nucleus accumbens. Nicotine also seems to desensitize $\alpha_4\beta_2$ postsynaptic receptors on GABA interneurons in the VTA; the reduction of GABA neurotransmission disinhibits mesolimbic dopamine neurons and thus is a third mechanism for enhancing dopamine release in the nucleus accumbens. PFC, prefrontal cortex; PPT/LDT, pedunculopontine tegmental and laterodorsal tegmental nuclei.

actions of presynaptic α_7-nicotinic receptors on glutamate neurons are discussed in Chapter 13 and illustrated in Figure 13-20. Nicotine also appears to desensitize $\alpha_4\beta_2$ postsynaptic receptors on inhibitory GABAergic interneurons in the VTA (Figure 14-9); this also leads to DA release in nucleus accumbens by disinhibiting dopaminergic mesolimbic neurons. Actions of nicotine on postsynaptic α_7-nicotinic receptors in the prefrontal cortex may be linked to the pro-cognitive and mentally alerting actions of nicotine, but not to addictive actions.

The $\alpha_4\beta_2$-nicotinic receptors adapt to the chronic intermittent pulsatile delivery of nicotine in a way that leads to addiction (Figure 14-10). That is, initially these receptors in the resting state are opened by delivery of nicotine, which in turns leads to dopamine release and reinforcement, pleasure, and reward (Figure 14-10A). By the time the cigarette is finished, these receptors become desensitized, so that they cannot function temporarily and thus cannot react either to acetylcholine or to nicotine (Figure 14-10A). In terms of obtaining any further reward, you might as well stop smoking at this point. An interesting question to ask is: how long does it take for the nicotinic receptors to desensitize? The answer seems to be: about as long as it takes to inhale all the puffs of a standard cigarette and burn it down to a butt. Thus, it is probably not an accident that cigarettes are the length that they are. Shorter does not maximize the pleasure. Longer is a waste since by then the receptors are all desensitized anyway (Figure 14-10A).

The problem for the smoker is that when the receptors resensitize to their resting state, this initiates craving and withdrawal due to the lack of release of further dopamine (Figure 14-10A). Another interesting question is: how long does it take to resensitize nicotinic receptors? The answer seems to be: about the length of time that smokers take between cigarettes. For the average one pack per day smoker awake for 16 hours, that would be about 45 minutes, possibly explaining why there are 20 cigarettes in a pack (i.e., enough for an average smoker to keep his or her nicotinic receptors completely desensitized all day long).

Putting nicotinic receptors out of business by desensitizing them causes neurons to attempt to overcome this lack of functioning receptors by upregulating the number of receptors (Figure 14-10B). That, however, is futile, since nicotine just desensitizes

all of them the next time a cigarette is smoked (Figure 14-10C). Furthermore, this upregulation is self-defeating because it serves to amplify the craving that occurs when the extra receptors are resensitizing to their resting state (Figure 14-10C).

From a receptor point of view, the goal of smoking is to desensitize all nicotinic $\alpha_4\beta_2$ receptors, get the maximum dopamine release at first, but eventually mostly to prevent craving. Positron emission tomography (PET) scans of $\alpha_4\beta_2$-nicotinic receptors in human smokers confirm that nicotinic receptors are exposed to just about enough nicotine for just about long enough from each cigarette to accomplish this. Craving seems to be initiated at the first sign of nicotinic receptor resensitization. Thus, the bad thing about receptor resensitization is craving. The good thing from a smoker's point of view is that as the receptors resensitize, they are available to release more dopamine and cause pleasure or suppress craving and withdrawal again.

Treating nicotine dependence is not easy. There is evidence that nicotine addiction begins with the first cigarette, with the first dose showing signs of lasting a month in experimental animals (e.g., activation of the anterior cingulate cortex for this long after a single dose). Craving begins within a month of repeated administration. Perhaps even more troublesome is the finding that the "diabolical learning" that occurs from substance abuse of all sorts including nicotine may be very, very long-lasting once exposure to nicotine is stopped. Some evidence suggests that these changes even last a lifetime, with a form of "molecular memory" to nicotine, even in long-term abstinent former smokers. One of the first successful agents proven to be effective is nicotine itself, but in a route of administration other than smoking: gums, lozenges, nasal sprays, inhalers, and transdermal patches. Delivering nicotine by these other routes does not attain the high levels or the pulsatile blasts that are delivered to the brain by smoking, so they are not very reinforcing. However, these alternative forms of nicotine delivery can help to reduce craving due to a steady amount of nicotine that is delivered, presumably desensitizing an important number of resensitizing and craving nicotinic receptors.

Another treatment for nicotine dependence is varenicline, a selective $\alpha_4\beta_2$-nicotinic acetylcholine receptor partial agonist (Figures 14-11 and 14-12). Figure 14-11 contrasts the effects of nicotinic partial agonists (NPAs) with nicotinic full agonists and

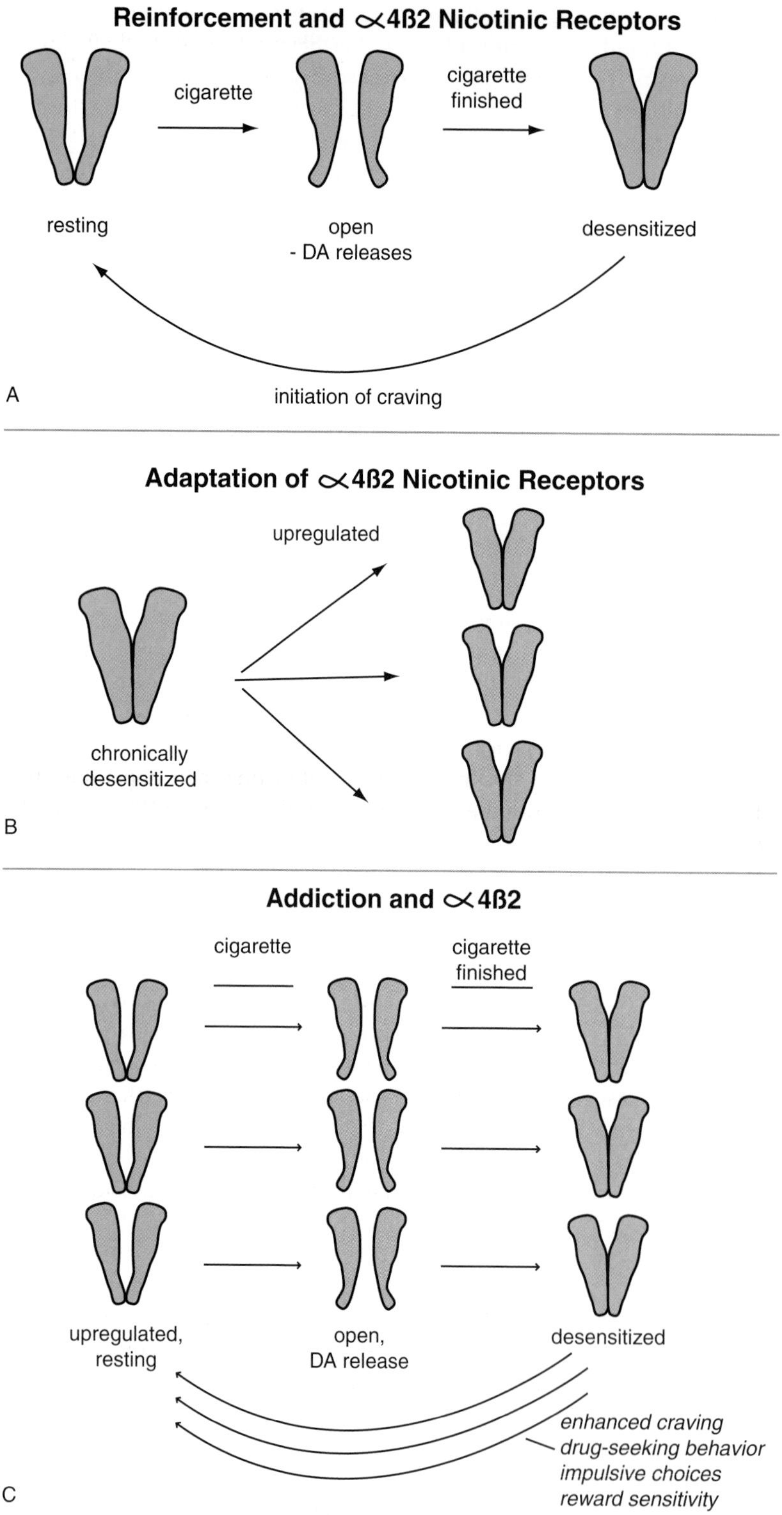

Reinforcement and α4ß2 Nicotinic Receptors

resting   open - DA releases   desensitized

A   initiation of craving

Adaptation of α4ß2 Nicotinic Receptors

upregulated

chronically desensitized

B

Addiction and α4ß2

upregulated, resting   open, DA release   desensitized

enhanced craving
drug-seeking behavior
impulsive choices
reward sensitivity

C

Figure 14-10. Reinforcement and $\alpha_4\beta_2$ nicotinic receptors. (A) In the resting state $\alpha_4\beta_2$ nicotinic receptors are closed (left). Nicotine administration, as by smoking a cigarette, causes the receptor to open, which in turn leads to dopamine release (middle). Long-term stimulation of these receptors leads to their desensitization, such that they temporarily can no longer react to nicotine (or to acetylcholine); this occurs in approximately the same length of time it takes to finish a single cigarette (right). As the receptors resensitize, they initiate craving and withdrawal due to the lack of release of further dopamine. (B) With chronic desensitization, $\alpha_4\beta_2$ receptors upregulate to compensate. (C) If one continues smoking, however, the repeated administration of nicotine continues to lead to desensitization of all of these $\alpha_4\beta_2$ receptors, and thus the upregulation does no good. In fact, the upregulation can lead to amplified craving as the extra receptors resensitize to their resting state.

Molecular Actions of a Nicotinic Partial Agonist (NPA)

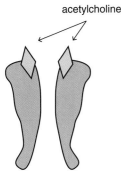
acetylcholine

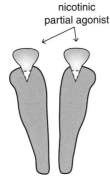
nicotinic
partial agonist

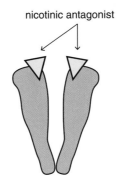
nicotinic antagonist

Figure 14-11. Molecular actions of a nicotinic partial agonist (NPA). Full agonists at $\alpha_4\beta_2$ receptors, such as acetylcholine and nicotine, cause the channels to open frequently (left). In contrast, antagonists at these receptors stabilize them in a closed state, such that they do not become desensitized (right). Nicotinic partial agonists (NPAs) stabilize the channels in an intermediate state, causing them to open less frequently than a full agonist but more frequently than an antagonist (middle).

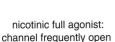

nicotinic full agonist:
channel frequently open

nicotinic partial agonist (NPA):
stabilizes channel in less
frequently open state,
not desensitized

nicotinic antagonist:
stabilizes channel in closed
state, not desensitized

nicotinic antagonists on the cation channel associated with nicotinic cholinergic receptors. Nicotinic full agonists include acetylcholine, a short-acting full agonist, and nicotine, a long-acting full agonist. They open the channel fully and frequently (Figure 14-11, left). By contrast, nicotinic antagonists stabilize the channel in the closed state, but do not desensitize these receptors (Figure 14-11, right). NPAs stabilize nicotinic receptors in an intermediate state which is not desensitized and where the channel is open less frequently than with a full agonist, but more frequently than with an antagonist (Figure 14-11, middle).

How addicting is tobacco, and how well do NPAs work to achieve cessation of smoking? About two-thirds of smokers want to quit, one-third try, but only 2–3% succeed long-term. Of all the substances of abuse, some surveys show that tobacco has the highest probability of making you become dependent when you have tried a substance at least once (Table 14-3). It could be argued, therefore, that nicotine might be the most addicting substance known. The good news is that the NPA varenicline triples or quadruples the 1-month, 6-month, and 1-year quit rates compared to placebo; the bad news is that this means only about 10% of smokers who have taken varenicline are still abstinent a year later. Many of these patients are prescribed varenicline for only 12 weeks, which might be far too short a period of time for maximal effectiveness.

Another approach to the treatment of smoking cessation is to try to reduce the craving that occurs during abstinence by boosting dopamine with the norepinephrine–dopamine reuptake inhibitor (NDRI) bupropion (see Chapter 7, and Figures 7-35 through 7-37). The idea is to give back some of the dopamine downstream to the craving postsynaptic D_2 receptors in the nucleus accumbens while they are readjusting to the lack of getting their dopamine "fix" from the recent withdrawal of nicotine (Figure 14-13). Thus, while smoking, dopamine is happily released in the nucleus accumbens because of the actions of nicotine on $\alpha_4\beta_2$ receptors on the VTA dopamine neuron (Figure 14-13A). During smoking cessation, resensitized nicotinic receptors no longer receiving nicotine are craving due to an absence of dopamine release in the nucleus accumbens ("where's my dopamine?" – Figure 14-13B). When the NDRI bupropion is administered, theoretically a bit of dopamine is now released in the nucleus accumbens, making the craving less but usually not eliminating it (Figure 14-13C). How effective is bupropion in smoking cessation? Quit rates for bupropion are about half that of the NPA varenicline. Quit rates for nicotine in alternative routes of administration such as transdermal patches are similar to those of bupropion. Novel approaches to treating nicotine addiction include the investigation of nicotine vaccines and other direct-acting nicotinic cholinergic agents.

Alcohol

The famous artist Vincent van Gogh reportedly drank ruinously, some speculating that he self-medicated his bipolar disorder this way, a notion reinforced by

551

Varenicline Actions on Reward Circuits

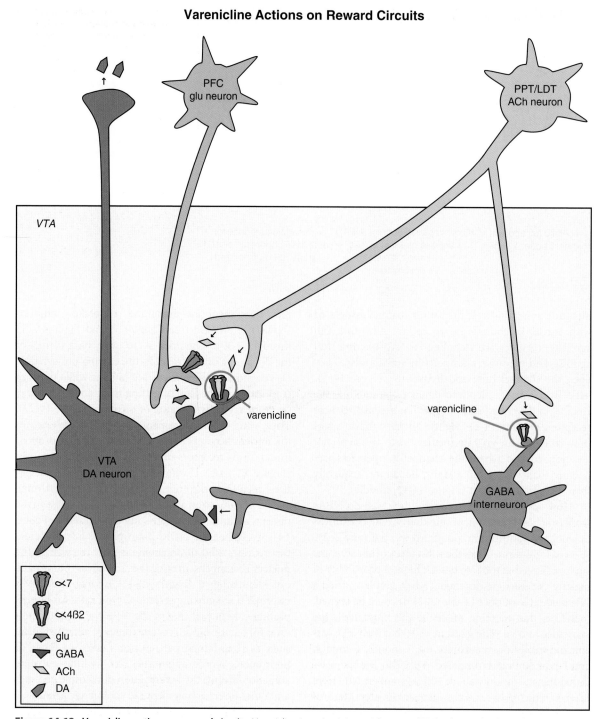

Figure 14-12. Varenicline actions on reward circuits. Varenicline is a nicotinic partial agonist (NPA) selective for the $\alpha_4\beta_2$ receptor subtype. Its actions at $\alpha_4\beta_2$-nicotinic receptors – located on dopamine neurons and GABA interneurons in the VTA – are all shown. PFC, prefrontal cortex; PPT/LDT, pedunculopontine tegmental and laterodorsal tegmental nuclei.

Mechanism of Action of Bupropion in Smoking Cessation

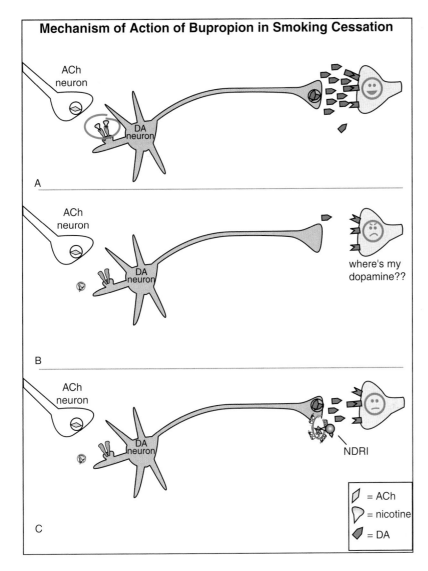

Figure 14-13. Mechanism of action of bupropion in smoking cessation. (A) A regular smoker delivers reliable nicotine (circle), releasing dopamine in the limbic area at frequent intervals, which is rewarding to the limbic dopamine D_2 receptors on the right. (B) However, during attempts at smoking cessation, dopamine will be cut off when nicotine no longer releases it from the mesolimbic neurons. This upsets the postsynaptic D_2 limbic receptors and leads to craving and what some call a "nicotine fit." (C) A therapeutic approach to diminishing craving during the early stages of smoking cessation is to deliver a bit of dopamine itself by blocking dopamine reuptake directly at the nerve terminal with bupropion. Although not as powerful as nicotine, it does take the edge off and can make abstinence more tolerable.

his explanation, "If the storm within gets too loud, I take a glass too much to stun myself." Alcohol may stun but it does not treat psychiatric disorders adaptively long term. Unfortunately, many alcoholics who have comorbid psychiatric disorders continue to self-medicate with alcohol rather than seeking treatment to receive a more appropriate psychopharmacologic agent. In addition to frequent comorbidity with psychiatric disorders, it is estimated that 85% of alcoholics also smoke.

An oversimplified view of alcohol's mechanism of action is that it enhances inhibition at GABA synapses and reduces excitation at glutamate synapses. Alcohol actions at GABA synapses enhance

GABA release via blocking presynaptic $GABA_B$ receptors, and also directly stimulate postsynaptic $GABA_A$ receptors, especially those of the δ subtype that are responsive to neurosteroid modulation but not to benzodiazepine modulation, either via direct actions or by releasing neurosteroids (Figure 14-14). Delta subtypes of $GABA_A$ receptors are discussed in Chapter 9 and illustrated in Figure 9-21. Alcohol also acts at presynaptic metabotropic glutamate receptors (mGluRs) and presynaptic voltage-sensitive calcium channels (VSCCs) to inhibit glutamate release (Figure 14-15). mGluRs are introduced in Chapter 4 and illustrated in Figures 4-22 and 4-23. VSCCs and their role in glutamate release

Binding Sites for Sedative Hypnotic Drugs

Figure 14-14. Binding sites for sedative hypnotic drugs. (A) Benzodiazepines (BZs) and barbiturates both act at GABA$_A$ receptors, but at different binding sites. Benzodiazepines do not act at all GABA$_A$ receptors; rather, they are selective for the α_1, α_2, α_3, and α_5 subtypes of receptors that also contain γ but not δ subunits. (B) General anesthetics, alcohol, and neurosteroids may bind to other types of GABA$_A$ receptors, particularly those containing δ subunits.

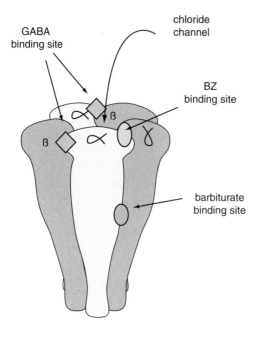

A   benzodiazepine receptors: α1, α2, α3, α5 subtypes

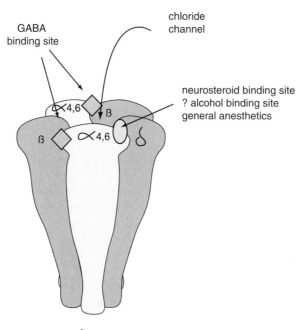

B   benzodiazepine receptors: δ subtypes (alpha 4, alpha 6)

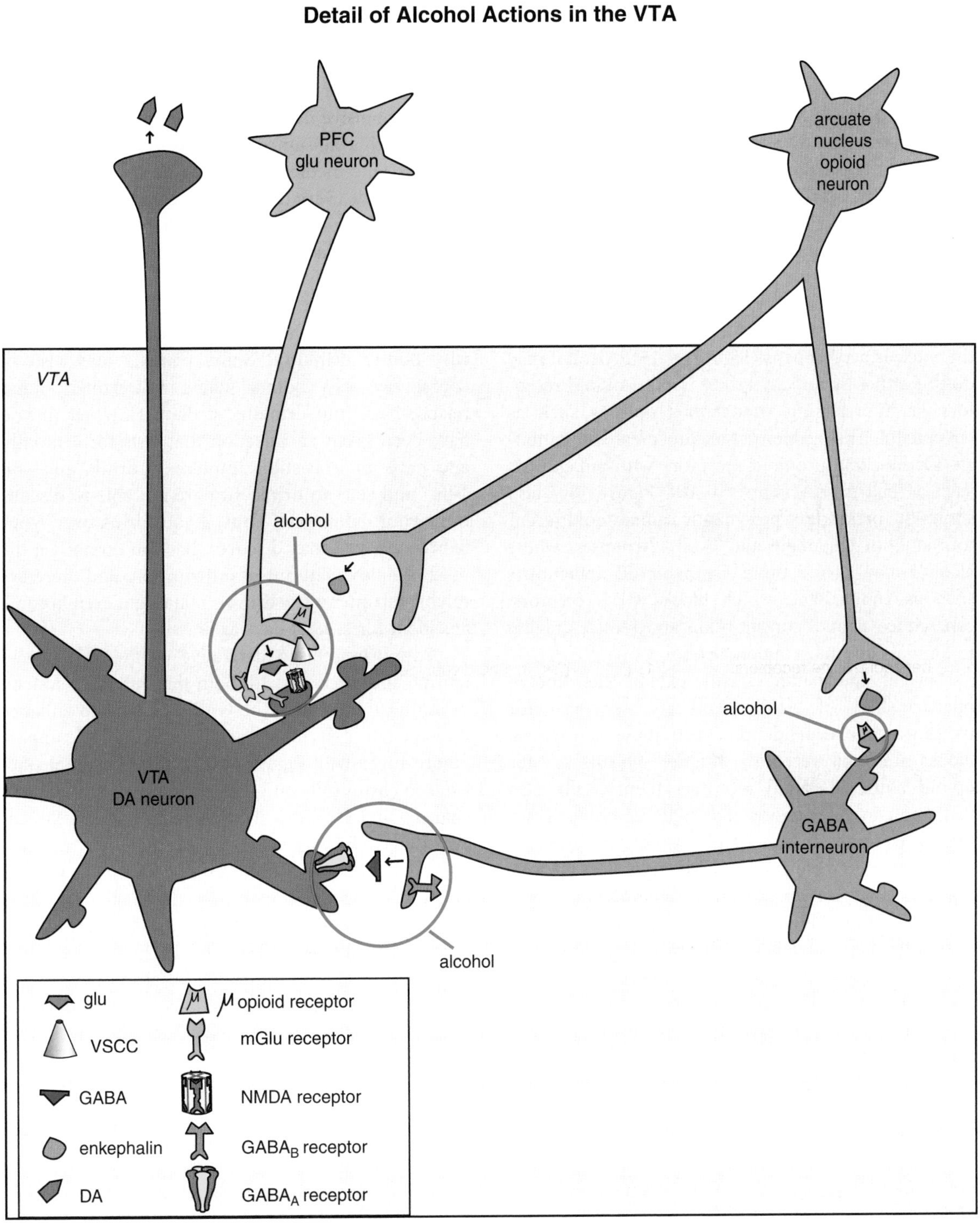

Detail of Alcohol Actions in the VTA

Figure 14-15. Actions of alcohol in the ventral tegmental area (VTA). Opioid neurons synapse in the VTA with GABAergic interneurons and with presynaptic nerve terminals of glutamate neurons. Inhibitory actions of opioids at μ-opioid receptors there cause disinhibition of dopamine release in the nucleus accumbens. Alcohol either directly acts upon μ receptors or causes release of endogenous opioids such as enkephalin. Alcohol also acts at presynaptic metabotropic glutamate receptors (mGluRs) and presynaptic voltage-sensitive calcium channels (VSCCs) to inhibit glutamate release. Finally, alcohol enhances GABA release by blocking presynaptic GABA_B receptors and through direct or indirect actions at GABA_A receptors.

are introduced in Chapter 3 and illustrated in Figures 3-22 through 3-24. Alcohol may also have some direct or indirect effects on reducing the actions of glutamate at postsynaptic NMDA receptors and at postsynaptic mGluR receptors (Figure 14-15). Alcohol's reinforcing effects are theoretically mediated not only by its effects at GABA and glutamate synapses but also by actions at opioid synapses within mesolimbic reward circuitry (Figure 14-15). Opioid neurons arise in the arcuate nucleus and project to the VTA, synapsing on both glutamate and GABA neurons. The net result of alcohol actions on opioid synapses is thought to be the release of dopamine in the nucleus acccumbens (Figure 14-15). Alcohol may do this either by directly acting upon μ-opioid receptors or by releasing endogenous opioids such as enkephalin. These actions of alcohol create the rationale for blocking μ-opioid receptors with antagonists such as naltrexone (Figure 14-16). Figure 14-7 also shows the presence of presynaptic cannabinoid receptors at both glutamate and GABA synapses, where alcohol may have actions. Cannabinoid antagonists such as rimonabant, which blocks CB_1 receptors, can reduce alcohol consumption and reduce craving in animals dependent upon alcohol.

Several therapeutic agents exploit the known pharmacology of alcohol and are approved for treating alcohol dependence. One of these, naltrexone, blocks μ-opioid receptors (Figure 14-16). As for opioid abuse, μ-opioid receptors theoretically also contribute to the euphoria and "high" of heavy drinking. It is therefore not surprising that a μ-opioid antagonist would block the enjoyment of heavy drinking and increase abstinence by its actions upon reward circuitry (Figure 14-16). This theory is supported by clinical trials, which show that naltrexone not only increases the chances of attaining complete abstinence from alcohol, but also reduces "heavy drinking" (defined as five or more drinks per day for a man and four or more for a woman).

Outcomes for patients with alcohol dependence who take naltrexone may be more favorable when the form of naltrexone that is administrated is given once monthly by intramuscular injection, called XR-naltrexone. This may be due to the fact that this method of drug administration forces compliance for at least a month. Monthly rather than daily drug administration may be just what the reward circuitry needs for someone with a substance-abuse problem. As discussed earlier in this chapter, patients addicted

to various substances lose their ability to make rational decisions, and instead respond immediately and impulsively to the desire to seek drugs, and have vast capacity for denial of the maladaptive nature of their compulsive decisions. It is hard enough to get a patient with a substance-abuse disorder to enter treatment or take medications at all, let alone make that person decide every day not only to stay abstinent but also to take a medication. Addiction and human nature being what they are, it is not surprising that patients frequently drop out of treatment and resume substance abuse. If you drink when you take naltrexone, the opioids released do not lead to pleasure, so why bother drinking? Some patients may also of course say, why bother taking naltrexone? – and relapse back into drinking alcohol. However, if you have been given an injection that lasts for a month, and have an irresistible impulse to drink, and you "slip" and start to drink, you are not able to discontinue your naltrexone. Thus, if you "drink over" your naltrexone, you may discover that you do not get the buzz or enjoyment out of intoxication, and therefore might stop after a few drinks. You might even become abstinent for several days again.

Acamprosate is a derivative of the amino acid taurine and interacts with both the glutamate system, to inhibit it, and with the GABA system, to enhance it, a bit like a form of "artificial alcohol" (compare Figure 14-15 with Figure 14-17). Thus, when alcohol is taken chronically and then withdrawn, the adaptive changes that it causes in both the glutamate system and the GABA system create a state of glutamate overexcitement and even excitotoxicity as well as GABA deficiency. Too much glutamate can cause neuronal damage, as discussed in Chapter 13 and illustrated in Figures 13-28 and 13-29. To the extent that acamprosate can substitute for alcohol in patients during withdrawal, the actions of acamprosate mitigate the glutamate hyperactivity and the GABA deficiency (Figure 14-17). This occurs because acamprosate appears to have direct blocking actions on certain glutamate receptors, particularly mGlu receptors (specifically mGluR5 and perhaps mGluR2). One way or another, acamprosate apparently reduces the glutamate release associated with alcohol withdrawal (Figure 14-17). Actions, if any, at NMDA receptors may be indirect, as are actions at GABA systems, both of which may be secondary downstream effects from acamprosate's actions on mGlu receptors (Figure 14-17).

Actions of Naltrexone in the VTA: Reducing the Reward Associated with Drinking

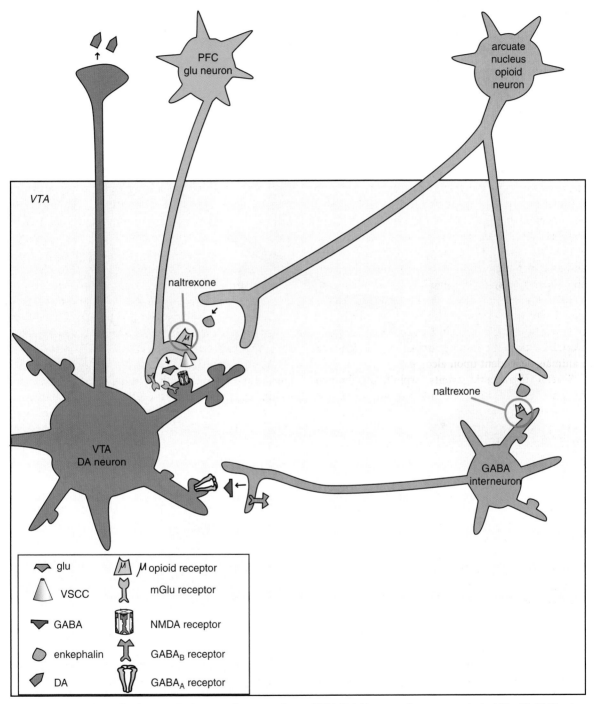

Figure 14-16. Actions of naltrexone in the ventral tegmental area (VTA). Opioid neurons form synapses in the VTA with GABAergic interneurons and with presynaptic nerve terminals of glutamate neurons. Alcohol either acts directly upon μ receptors or causes release of endogenous opioids such as enkephalin; in either case, the result is increased dopamine release to the nucleus accumbens. Naltrexone is a μ-opioid receptor antagonist; thus it blocks the pleasurable effects of alcohol mediated by μ-opioid receptors.

Actions of Acamprosate in the VTA:
Reducing Excessive Glutamate Release to Relieve Withdrawal

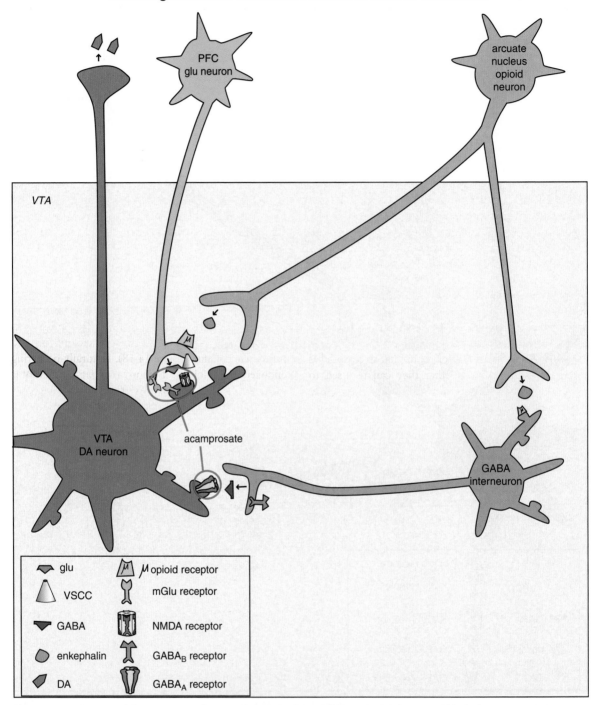

Figure 14-17. Actions of acamprosate in the ventral tegmental area (VTA). Acamprosate seems to block glutamate receptors, particularly metabotropic glutamate receptors (mGluRs) and perhaps also *N*-methyl-ᴅ-aspartate (NMDA) receptors. When alcohol is taken chronically and then withdrawn, the adaptive changes that it causes in both the glutamate system and the GABA system create a state of glutamate overexcitation as well as GABA deficiency. By blocking glutamate receptors, acamprosate may thus mitigate glutamate hyperexcitability during alcohol withdrawal.

Disulfiram is the classic drug for treating alcoholism. It is an irreversible inhibitor of aldehyde dehydrogenase and, when alcohol is ingested, results in the build-up of toxic levels of acetaldehyde. This creates an aversive experience with flushing, nausea, vomiting, and hypotension, hopefully conditioning the patient to a negative rather than positive response to drinking. Obviously, compliance is a problem with this agent, and its aversive reactions are occasionally dangerous.

Experimental agents that show some promise in treating alcohol dependence include the anticonvulsant topiramate (discussed in more detail below in the section on obesity), the $5HT_3$ antagonists (mechanism discussed in Chapter 7 and illustrated in Figure 7-46), and cannabinoid CB_1 receptor antagonists. New opioid antagonists such as nalmefene (Selinco) are also in late-stage clinical testing. The subject of how to treat alcohol abuse and dependence is obviously complex, and the psychopharmacological treatments are most effective when integrated with structured therapies such as 12-step programs, a topic which is beyond the scope of this text. Hopefully, clinicians will learn how to better leverage the various treatments for alcoholism that are available today, and determine whether they can be used to treat this devastating illness to attain far better outcomes than are available when no treatment is provided, accepted, or sustained.

Sedative hypnotics

Sedative hypnotics include barbiturates and related agents such as ethchlorvynol and ethinamate, chloral hydrate and derivatives, and piperidinedione derivatives such as glutethimide and methyprylon. Experts often include alcohol, benzodiazepines (discussed in Chapter 9), and Z-drug hypnotics (discussed in Chapter 11) in this class as well. The mechanism of action of sedative hypnotics is basically the same as those described in Chapter 9 and illustrated in Figure 9-23 for the action of benzodiazepines: namely, they are positive allosteric modulators (PAMs) for $GABA_A$ receptors. Actions of sedative hypnotics are at $GABA_A$ receptor sites in reward circuits (Figure 14-7). Molecular actions of all sedative hypnotics are similar, but benzodiazepines and barbiturates seem to work at different sites from each other, and also only on some $GABA_A$ receptor subtypes, namely those with α_1, α_2, α_3, or α_5 subunits (Figure 14-14). Barbiturates

are much less safe in overdose than benzodiazepines, cause dependence more frequently, are abused more frequently, and produce much more dangerous withdrawal reactions. Apparently, the receptor site at $GABA_A$ receptors mediating the pharmacologic actions of barbiturates is even more readily desensitized with even more dangerous consequences than the benzodiazepine receptor (Figure 14-14). The barbiturate site must also mediate a more intense euphoria and a more desirable sense of tranquility than the benzodiazepine receptor site. Since benzodiazepines are generally an adequate alternative to barbiturates, psychopharmacologists can help to minimize abuse of barbiturates by prescribing them rarely if ever. In the case of withdrawal reactions, reinstituting and then tapering the offending barbiturate under close clinical supervision can assist the detoxification process.

Opioids

Opioids act as neurotransmitters released from neurons that arise in the arcuate nucleus and project both to the VTA and to the nucleus accumbens, and release enkephalin (Figure 14-18). Naturally occurring endogenous opioids act upon a variety of receptor subtypes. The three most important receptor subtypes are the μ-, δ-, and κ-opioid receptors (Figure 14-18). The brain makes a variety of its own endogenous opioid-like substances, sometimes referred to as the "brain's own morphine." These are all peptides derived from precursor proteins called pro-opiomelanocortin (POMC), proenkephalin, and prodynorphin (Figure 14-18). Parts of these precursor proteins are cleaved off to form endorphins, enkephalins, or dynorphins, stored in opioid neurons, and presumably released during neurotransmission to mediate endogenous opioid-like actions, including a role in mediating reinforcement and pleasure in reward circuitry (Figure 14-7).

Exogenous opioids in the form of pain relievers (such as oxycodone, hydrocodone, and many others) or drugs of abuse (such as heroin) are also thought to act as agonists at μ-, δ-, and κ-opioid receptors, particularly at μ sites. At and above pain-relieving doses, the opioids induce euphoria, which is the main reinforcing property of the opioids. Opioids can also induce a very intense but brief euphoria, sometimes called a "rush," followed by a profound sense of tranquility which may last several hours, followed in

Endogenous Opioid Neurotransmitters

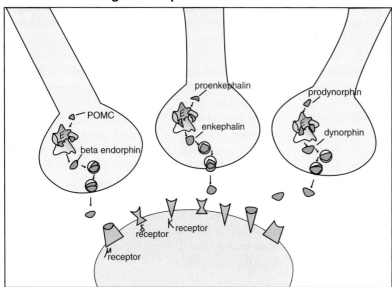

Figure 14-18. Endogenous opioid neurotransmitters. Opioid drugs act on a variety of receptors called opioid receptors, the most important of which are μ, δ, and κ. Endogenous opioid-like substances are peptides derived from precursor proteins called POMC (pro-opiomelanocortin), proenkephalin, and prodynorphin. Parts of these precursor proteins are cleaved off to form endorphins, enkephalins, or dynorphins, which are then stored in opioid neurons and presumably released during neurotransmission to mediate reinforcement and pleasure.

turn by drowsiness ("nodding"), mood swings, mental clouding, apathy, and slowed motor movements. In overdose, these same agents act as depressants of respiration, and can also induce coma. The acute actions of opioids can be reversed by synthetic opioid antagonists, such as naloxone and naltrexone, which compete as antagonists at opioid receptors.

When given chronically, opioids readily cause both tolerance and dependence. Adaptation of opioid receptors occurs quite readily after chronic opioid administration. The first sign of this is the need of the patient to take a higher and higher dose of opioid in order to relieve pain or to induce the desired euphoria. Eventually, there may be little room between the dose that causes euphoria and that which produces toxic effects of an overdose. Another sign that dependence has occurred and that opioid receptors have adapted by decreasing their sensitivity to agonist actions is the production of a withdrawal syndrome once the chronically administered opioid wears off. The opioid antagonists, such as naloxone, can precipitate a withdrawal syndrome in opioid-dependent persons. The opioid withdrawal syndrome is characterized by the patient feeling dysphoria, craving another dose of opioid, being irritable, and having signs of autonomic hyperactivity such as tachycardia, tremor, and sweating. Pilo-erection ("goose-bumps") is often associated with opioid

withdrawal, especially when drug is stopped suddenly ("cold turkey"). This is so subjectively horrible that the opioid abuser will often stop at nothing in order to get another dose of opioid to relieve symptoms of withdrawal. Thus, what may have begun as a quest for euphoria may end up as a quest to avoid withdrawal. Clonidine, an α2-adrenergic agonist, can reduce signs of autonomic hyperactivity during withdrawal and aid in the detoxification process.

Opioid receptors can readapt to normal if given a chance to do so in the absence of additional intake of an opioid. This may be too difficult to tolerate, so reinstituting another opioid, such as methadone, which can be taken orally and then slowly tapered, may assist in the detoxification process. A partial μ-opioid agonist, buprenophine, now available in a sublingual dosage formulation combined with naloxone, can also substitute for stronger full agonist opioids, and then be tapered. It is combined with the opioid antagonist naloxone, which does not get absorbed orally or sublingually, but prevents intravenous abuse, since injection of the combination of buprenorphine plus naloxone results in no high and may even precipitate withdrawal. Agonist substitution treatments are best used in the setting of a structured maintenance treatment program that includes random urine drug screening and intensive psychological, medical, and vocational services. For those who can stop taking opioids for at least 7–10 days so that serious withdrawal symptoms do not occur, long-acting injectable naltrexone can be a highly effective therapy for opioid addicts, since this drug blocks any "cheating" for a month, and prevents the pharmacologic actions of abused opioids at the μ-opioid site, allowing detoxification to proceed even if the patient tries to take an opioid. This is the same drug in the same formulation discussed above and approved for treatment of alcohol abuse.

Not all who abuse opioids are the stereotypical addict who smokes or injects drugs, lives on the streets, and supports himself with crime. There also is a current serious epidemic of oral abuse of prescription opioids by those who are employed or students, and who obtain these drugs either from prescribers or from drug dealers who procure them from prescribers, pharmacies, or online.

Marijuana

You can indeed get stoned without inhaling! Actions of marijuana and its active ingredient Δ9-tetrahydrocannabinol (THC) on reward circuits are at cannabinoid receptors, shown in Figure 14-7, which are the sites where endogenous cannabinoids are utilized naturally as retrograde neurotransmitters. Cannabis preparations are smoked in order to deliver cannabinoids that interact with the brain's own cannabinoid receptors to trigger dopamine release from the mesolimbic reward system (Figure 14-7). There are two known cannabinoid receptors, CB_1 (in brain, coupled via G proteins and modulate adenylate cyclase and ion channels) and CB_2 (predominantly in the immune system). CB_1 receptors may mediate not only marijuana's reinforcing properties, but also those of alcohol and to some extent those of other psychoactive substances (including possibly some foods). Anandamide is one of the endocannabinoids and a member of a chemical class of neurotransmitter that is not a monoamine, not an amino acid, and not a peptide: it is a lipid, specifically a member of a family of fatty acid ethanolamides. Anandamide shares most but not all of the pharmacologic properties of THC, since its actions at brain cannabinoid receptors are mimicked not only by THC but are antagonized in part by the selective brain cannabinoid CB_1 receptor antagonist rimonabant.

In usual intoxicating doses, marijuana produces a sense of well-being, relaxation, a sense of friendliness,

a loss of temporal awareness, including confusing the past with the present, slowing of thought processes, impairment of short-term memory, and a feeling of achieving special insights. At high doses, marijuana can induce panic, toxic delirium, and, rarely, psychosis. One complication of long-term use is the "amotivational syndrome" in frequent users. This syndrome is seen predominantly in heavy daily users and is characterized by the emergence of decreased drive and ambition, thus "amotivational." It is also associated with other socially and occupationally impairing symptoms, including a shortened attention span, poor judgment, easy distractibility, impaired communication skills, introversion, and diminished effectiveness in interpersonal situations. Personal habits may deteriorate, and there may be a loss of insight, and even feelings of depersonalization. Another downside to marijuana is that individuals vulnerable to schizophrenia might precipitate this illness, make its onset earlier, or exacerbate established illness when abusing marijuana, and to a greater extent than with any other abusable drug.

Hallucinogens

The hallucinogens are a group of agents that act at serotonin synapses in the reward system (Figure 14-19). They produce intoxication, sometimes called a "trip" associated with changes in sensory experiences, including visual illusions and hallucinations, an enhanced awareness of external stimuli and an enhanced awareness of internal thoughts and stimuli. These hallucinations are produced with a clear level of consciousness and a lack of confusion and may be both *psychedelic* and *psychotomimetic*. *Psychedelic* is the term for the subjective experience that, due to heightened sensory awareness, one's mind is being expanded or that one is in union with mankind or the universe and having some sort of a religious experience. *Psychotomimetic* means that the experience mimics a state of psychosis, but the resemblance between a trip and psychosis is superficial at best. The stimulants cocaine and amphetamine and the club drug phencyclidine (PCP) much more genuinely mimic psychosis (see discussion in Chapter 4). Hallucinogen intoxication includes visual illusions; visual "trails" where the image smears into streaks of its image as it moves across a visual trail; macropsia and micropsia; emotional and mood lability; subjective slowing of time;

Mechanism of Hallucinogens at 5HT2A receptors

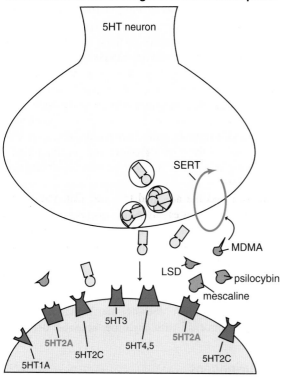

Figure 14-19. Mechanism of hallucinogens at 5HT$_{2A}$ receptors. The primary action of hallucinogenic drugs such as LSD, mescaline, psilocybin, and MDMA are shown here: namely, agonism of 5HT$_{2A}$ receptors. Hallucinogens may have additional actions at other serotonin receptors (particularly 5HT$_{1A}$ and 5HT$_{2C}$) and at other neurotransmitter systems, and MDMA in particular also blocks the serotonin transporter (SERT).

the sense that colors are heard and sounds are seen; intensification of sound perception; depersonalization and derealization; yet retaining a state of full wakefulness and alertness. Other changes may include impaired judgment, fear of losing one's mind, anxiety, nausea, tachycardia, increased blood pressure, and increased body temperature. Not surprisingly, hallucinogen intoxication can cause what is perceived as a panic attack, often called a "bad trip." As intoxication escalates, one can experience an acute confusional state called delirium where the abuser is disoriented and agitated. This can evolve further into frank psychosis with delusions and paranoia.

Common hallucinogens include two major classes of agents. The first class of agents resemble serotonin (indole-alkylamines) and include the classical hallucinogens D-lysergic acid diethylamide (LSD), psilocybin, and dimethyltryptamine (DMT) (Figure 14-19). The second class of agents resemble

norepinephrine and dopamine and are also related to amphetamine (phenylalkylamines) and include mescaline, 2,5-dimethoxy-4-methylamphetamine (DOM) and others. More recently, synthetic chemists have come up with some new "designer drugs" such as 3,4-methylenedioxymethamphetamine (MDMA) and "Foxy" (5-methoxy-diisopropyltryptamine). These are either stimulants or hallucinogens and produce a complex subjective state sometimes referred to as "ecstacy," which is also what abusers call MDMA itself. MDMA produces euphoria, disorientation, confusion, enhanced sociability, and a sense of increased empathy and personal insight.

Hallucinogens have rather complex interactions at neurotransmitter systems, but one of the most prominent is a common action as agonists at 5HT$_{2A}$ receptor sites (Figure 14-19). Hallucinogens certainly have additional effects at other 5HT receptors (especially 5HT$_{1A}$ somatodendritic autoreceptors and 5HT$_{2C}$ postsynaptic receptors) and also at other neurotransmitter systems, especially norepinephrine and dopamine, but the relative importance of these other actions is less well known. MDMA also appears to be a powerful inhibitor of the serotonin transporter (SERT) and is also a releaser of serotonin. MDMA and several other drugs structurally related to it may even destroy serotonin axon terminals. However, the action that appears to explain a common mechanism for most of the hallucinogens is the stimulation of 5HT$_{2A}$ receptors.

Hallucinogens can produce incredible tolerance, sometimes after a single dose. Desensitization of 5HT$_{2A}$ receptors is hypothesized to underlie this rapid clinical and pharmacological tolerance. Another unique dimension of hallucinogen abuse is the production of "flashbacks," namely the spontaneous recurrence of some of the symptoms of intoxication that lasts from a few seconds to several hours but in the absence of recent administration of the hallucinogen. This occurs days to months after the last drug experience, and can apparently be precipitated by a number of environmental stimuli. The psychopharmacological mechanism underlying flashbacks is unknown, but its phenomenology suggests the possibility of a neurochemical adaptation of the serotonin system and its receptors related to reverse tolerance that is incredibly long-lasting. Alternatively, flashbacks could be a form of emotional conditioning embedded in the amygdala and then triggered when a later emotional experience while not taking a hallucinogen nevertheless reminds one of experiences that occurred when intoxicated with a hallucinogen. This could precipitate a whole cascade of feelings that occurred while intoxicated with a hallucinogen. This is analogous to the types of re-experiencing flashbacks that occur without drugs in patients with posttraumatic stress disorder.

Club drugs and others

Phencyclidine (PCP) and ketamine both have actions at glutamate synapses within the reward system (Figure 14-7 and Figure 7-91). They both act as antagonists of NMDA receptors, binding to a site in the calcium channel (see discussion in Chapter 4 and Figure 4-28). Both were originally developed as anesthetics. PCP proved to be unacceptable for this use because it induces a unique psychotomimetic/hallucinatory experience very similar to schizophrenia. The NMDA receptor hypoactivity that is caused by PCP has become a model for the same neurotransmitter abnormalities postulated to underlie schizophrenia (see discussion in Chapter 4 and Figure 4-28). PCP causes intense analgesia, amnesia, delirium, stimulant as well as depressant actions, staggering gait, slurred speech, and a unique form of nystagmus (i.e., vertical nystagmus). Higher degrees of intoxication can cause catatonia (excitement alternating with stupor and catalepsy), hallucinations, delusions, paranoia, disorientation, and lack of judgment. Overdose effects can include coma, extremely high temperature, seizures, and muscle breakdown (rhabdomyolysis).

PCP's structurally related and mechanism-related analog ketamine is still used as an anesthetic, but causes far less of the psychotomimetic/hallucinatory experience. Nevertheless, some people do abuse ketamine, one of the "club drugs," and it is sometimes called "special K." Interestingly, subanesthetic infusions of ketamine have been repeatedly shown to reduce symptoms of depression in unipolar treatment-resistant depression and in bipolar depression and to decrease suicidal thoughts (see discussion in Chapter 7 and Figures 7-90 through 7-93).

Gamma-hydroxybutyrate (GHB) is discussed in Chapter 11 as a treatment for narcolepsy/cataplexy. It is sometimes also abused by individuals wanting to get high or by predators to intoxicate their dates (GHB is one of the "date rape" drugs). The mechanism of action of GHB is as an agonist at its own GHB receptors and at $GABA_B$ receptors (illustrated in Figure 11-27).

Inhalants such as toluene are thought to be direct releasers of dopamine in the nucleus accumbens. **"Bath salts"** are synthetic stimulants that commonly include the active ingredient methylenedioxypyrovalerone (MDPV) but may also contain mephedrone or mehylone. They are also called "plant food" and like other stimulants can have reinforcing effects but also cause agitation, paranoia, hallucinations, suicidality, and chest pain.

Obesity as an impulsive–compulsive disorder

Can you become addicted to food? Can your brain circuits make you eat it? Although food addiction is not yet accepted as a formal diagnosis, it does appear that when external stimuli are triggers for maladaptive eating habits that are performed despite apparent satiety and adverse health consequences, this does define a compulsion and a habit, with the formation of aberrant eating behaviors in a manner that parallels drug addiction (Table 14-4). Compulsive eating in

Table 14-4 Food addiction: is obesity an impulsive–compulsive disorder?

Obesity, appetite, eating and the dimensions of impulsivity/compulsivity

Enhanced reward of food/enhanced motivation and drive to consume food

Increasing amounts of food to maintain satiety, tolerance

Lack of control over eating – cannot stop

Great deal of time spent eating

Conditioning and habits to food and food cues

Distress and dysphoria when dieting

Eating too rapidly or too much when not hungry, to the point of being uncomfortably full

Overeating maintained despite knowledge of adverse physical and psychological consequences caused by excessive food consumption

Eating alone, feeling disgusted with oneself, guilty, or depressed

Binge eating can occur with or without purging

Bulimia is binge eating with self-disgust and purging leading to attempts to prevent weight gain by excessive exercise, induced vomiting, abuse of laxatives, enemas, or diuretics

obesity, and in binge eating disorder and bulimia, can be mirrored by compulsive rejection of food as in anorexia nervosa. This chapter does not provide a comprehensive explanation of eating disorders but addresses only aspects of obesity that may in some cases fit with the construct of an impulsive–compulsive disorder and how some of the new treatments for obesity may help such cases.

When is the way you eat a lifestyle choice and when is it an impulsive–compulsive disorder? Obesity is defined by one's body mass index (BMI ≥ 30), and not by any associated behaviors. Not everyone who is obese has an eating compulsion, since obesity is also related to genetic and lifestyle factors such as exercise, caloric intake, and the foods eaten and their specific content (fat, carbohydrates, vitamins, and other components). It is only those forms of obesity apparently driven by excessive motivational drive for food and mediated by reward circuitry that might be considered impulsive–compulsive disorders (Table 14-4). When exposed to food cues, obese individuals exhibit increased brain activation (compared to lean individuals) in anatomic areas that process palatability, and decreased activation of reward circuits during actual food consumption, analogous to what happens in drug addiction.

Appetite/motivation for eating, and the actual amount of food consumed, can both be influenced by centrally active psychopharmacologic agents in many individuals. For example, several known drugs of abuse reduce appetite, especially stimulants and nicotine. Bupropion, naltrexone, topiramate, and zonisamide have all been observed anecdotally to cause weight loss in patients taking these agents for other reasons. By contrast, marijuana and some atypical antipsychotics (see Chapter 5 and Figure 5-41) actually stimulate appetite and cause weight gain. The neurobiological basis of eating and appetite are clearly linked to the hypothalamus (Figures 14-20A through 14-20G), and to the connections that hypothalamic circuits make to reward pathways (Figures 14-2 through 14-4). Current research is attempting to

Peptides Regulate Appetite in the Hypothalamus

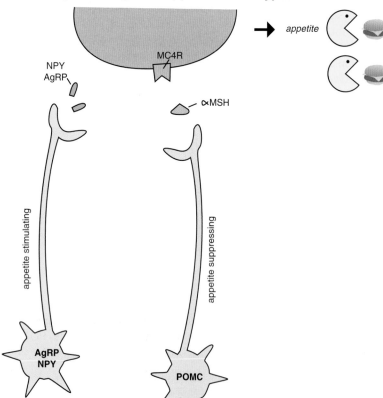

Figure 14-20A. Peptides regulate appetite in the hypothalamus. Appetite is regulated by the balance between an *appetite-stimulating pathway* (on the left) that releases agouti-related peptide (AgRP) and neuropeptide Y (NPY), and an *appetite-suppressing pathway* (on the right) that releases α-melanocyte-stimulating hormone (α-MSH). The appetite-suppressing neurons make the precursor pro-opiomelanocortin (POMC), which is broken down into α-MSH, which in turn binds to melanocortin 4 receptors (MC4R) to suppress appetite. Shown here is no occupancy of MC4R by α-MSH, and thus stimulation of appetite.

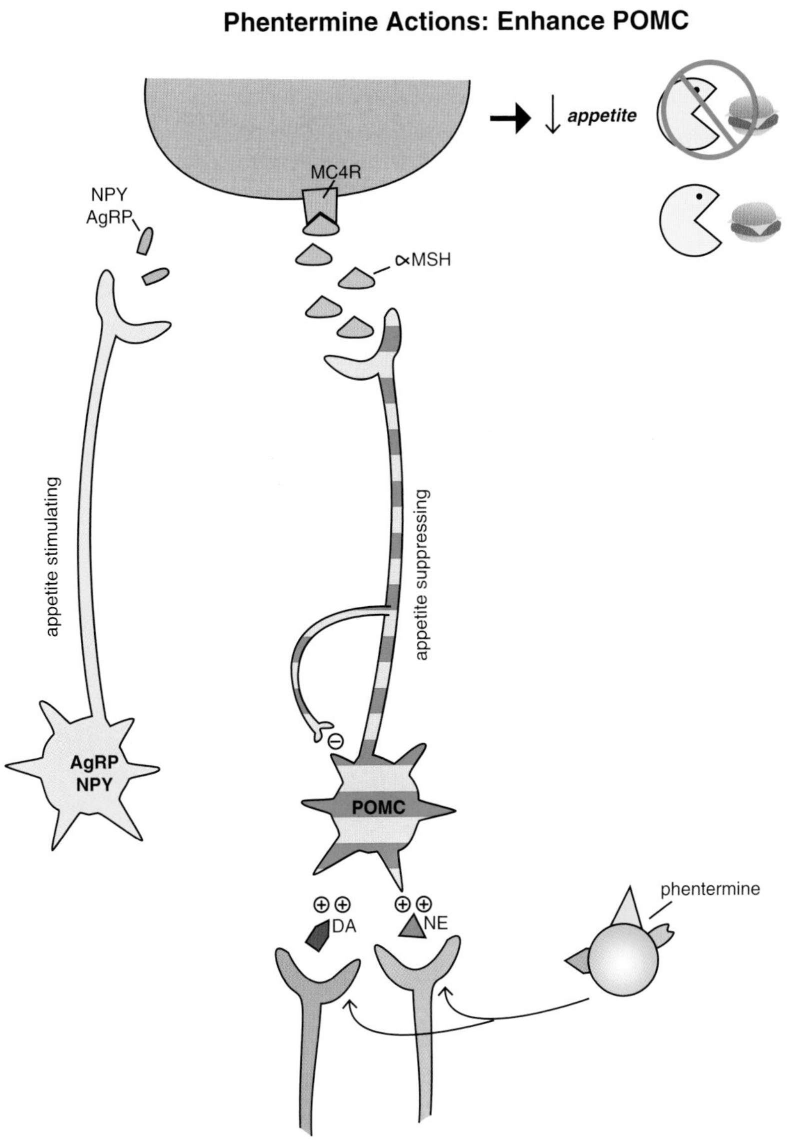

Phentermine Actions: Enhance POMC

Figure 14-20B. Actions of **phentermine.** Phentermine increases dopamine (DA) and norepinephrine (NE) in the hypothalamus by blocking both the norepinephrine and dopamine reuptake transporters (NET and DAT, respectively). The increased input of DA and NE onto pro-opiomelanocortin (POMC) neurons in the *appetite-suppressing pathway* partially activates the POMC neurons (shown as a hatched color on the right), causing an increase in α-melanocyte-stimulating hormone (α-MSH) release, which binds to melanocortin 4 receptors (MC4R) to suppress appetite partially.

clarify the role of a long list of key hypothalamic regulators in the control of eating: orexin (which also regulates sleep and is discussed in Chapter 11 and illustrated in Figures 11-21 through 11-23), α-melanocyte-stimulating hormone (α-MSH), neuropeptide Y, agouti-related peptide (all illustrated in Figures 14-20A through 14-20G), and many more including leptin, ghrelin, adiponectin, melanin-concentrating hormone, cholecystokinin, insulin, glucagon, cytokines, cocaine- and amphetamine-regulated transcript (CART) peptides, galanin, and others.

The hypothalamus thus serves as the brain center that controls appetite by utilizing a complex set of circuits and regulators. One formulation of how the hypothalamus does this is the notion that there is a major *appetite-stimulating pathway* whose actions are mediated by two peptides (neuropeptide Y and agouti-related protein) (Figure 14-20A). Opposing this is a major *appetite-suppressing pathway* whose actions are mediated by pro-opiomelanocortin (POMC) neurons that make the peptide POMC; POMC can be broken down into either β-endorphin or α-melanocyte-stimulating hormone (α-MSH). α-MSH interacts with melanocyte 4 receptors (MC4Rs) to suppress appetite (Figure 14-20A). Weight gain could occur either by excessive activity

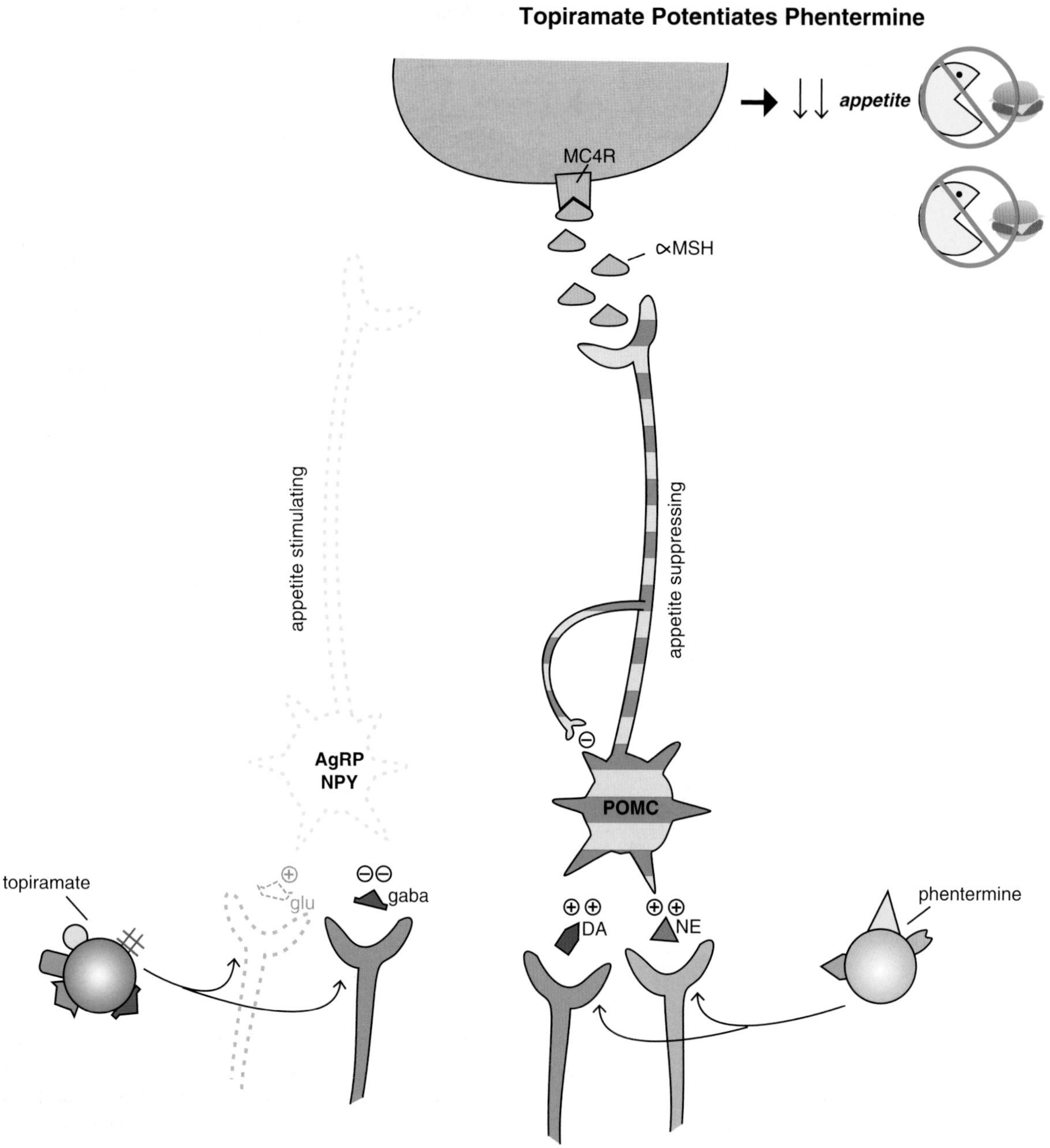

Figure 14-20C. Topiramate potentiates the actions of phentermine. Topiramate hypothetically inhibits the *appetite-stimulating pathway* on the left by reducing excitatory glutamatergic input and by increasing inhibitory GABA-ergic input (shown as faded neurons on the left). Combining this with phentermine's actions on the right that stimulate the *appetite-suppressing pathway* (shown as a hatched color and also shown in Figure 14-20B), this results in a synergistic and enhanced effect on appetite and on weight loss, allowing lower, more tolerable doses of both phentermine and topiramate to be used.

of the appetite-stimulating pathway, by deficient activity of the appetite-suppressing pathway, or both.

Several new treatments for obesity, defined as BMI ≥ 30 (or for being overweight, with a BMI ≥ 27 plus diabetes, hypertension, or dyslipidemia), and not defined by compulsive/addictive behaviors, are now approved or in late-stage clinical testing. One novel obesity treatment that targets

Bupropion Actions: Enhance POMC

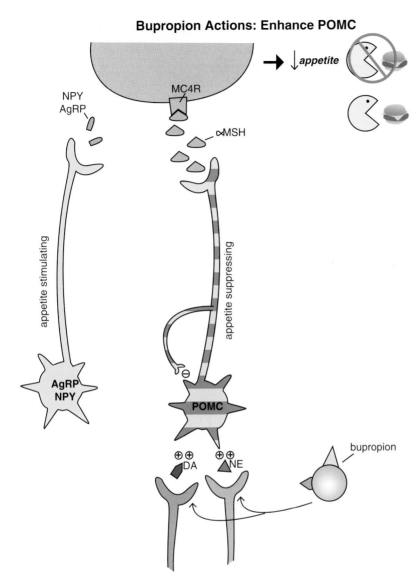

Figure 14-20D. Actions of bupropion. The antidepressant and smoking cessation aid bupropion is thought to have effects in the appetite center of the hypothalamus as well. Bupropion increases dopamine (DA) and norepinephrine (NE) in the hypothalamus by blocking both the norepinephrine and dopamine reuptake transporters (NET and DAT, respectively), just as shown in Figure 14-20B, but perhaps less robustly. The increased input of DA and NE onto pro-opiomelanocortin (POMC) neurons in the *appetite-suppressing pathway* partially activates the POMC neurons (shown as a hatched color on the right) causing an increase in α-melanocyte-stimulating hormone (α-MSH) release, which binds to melanocortin 4 receptors (MC4R) to suppress appetite partially (compare with Figure 14-20B). The actions of bupropion on the appetite-suppressing pathway, however, are mitigated because stimulation of POMC neurons also activates an endorphin/endogenous-opioid-mediated negative feedback loop (also with phentermine and shown in Figure 14-20B).

multiple sites within these hypothalamic appetite pathways is the combination of the stimulant phentermine, already approved as a monotherapy for the treatment of obesity, with the anticonvulsant topiramate (**phentermine/topiramate ER, or Qsymia**). Phentermine acts much like amphetamine, blocking both the dopamine transporter (DAT) and the norepinephrine transporter (NET) and, at high doses, the vesicular monoamine transporter (VMAT) (see discussion of amphetamine's mechanism of action in Chapter 12 and illustrated in Figures 12-28 through 12-31). When stimulants like phentermine increase dopamine and norepinephrine in the hypothalamus, they reduce appetite and cause weight loss. One

hypothesis is that they do this by stimulating POMC neurons to release α-MSH in the hypothalamus (Figure 14-20B). However, when given by itself in doses adequate to suppress appetite (Figure 14-20B), there are limitations to the use of phentermine. For example, tolerance for phentermine usually develops over time, and the weight often returns. Also, phentermine simultaneously targets dopamine in reward circuits and risks causing abuse or addiction. Additional dose-related noradrenergic effects of phentermine can increase pulse rate and blood pressure and cause cardiovascular complications, especially in vulnerable obese patients with cardiovascular disease.

Naltrexone Potentiates Bupropion

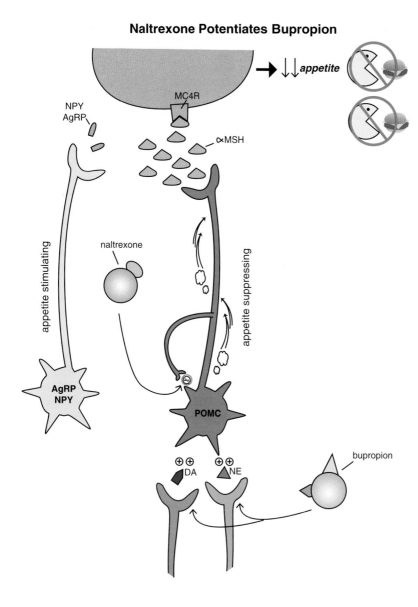

Figure 14-20E. Naltrexone potentiates the actions of bupropion. Both naltrexone and bupropion alone can lead to some weight loss by themselves. However, the combination of naltrexone and bupropion has a synergistic effect on weight loss that surpasses monotherapy with either agent by dual pharmacologic actions on the *appetite-suppressing pathway*. That is, naltrexone blocks the endorphin/ endogenous-opioid-mediated negative feedback loop that normally limits the activation of pro-opiomelanocortin (POMC) neurons in the appetite-suppressing pathway (shown in Figure 14-20D with only a hatched neuron on the right). With this negative feedback removed by administration of naltrexone, bupropion can more readily increase firing of POMC neurons (shown here as a red-hot neuron on the right), leading to highly elevated levels of α-melanocyte-stimulating hormone (α-MSH), which binds more robustly to melanocortin 4 receptors (MC4R) to more potently suppress appetite and cause weight loss.

One solution to these limitations of phentermine monotherapy has been to lower the dose of phentermine yet enhance its actions by adding the agent topiramate. In the combination product phentermine/topiramate ER, the phentermine dose is only about a quarter to half of what is usually prescribed when phentermine is given as a monotherapy for the treatment of obesity. This mitigates potential cardiovascular and reinforcing side effects. By combining it with topiramate, the efficacy of low-dose phentermine is not lost, and in fact it is enhanced because of synergy with topiramate's mechanisms (Figure 14-20C). Topiramate, observed to reduce weight as a

"side effect" when prescribed for the approved treatments of epilepsy or migraine, does so by poorly understood mechanisms, probably related to both boosting inhibitory GABA actions and reducing excitatory glutamate actions via more direct actions on various voltage-gated ion channels (Figure 14-20C). Topiramate also inhibits the enzyme carbonic anhydrase, although what contribution this makes to topiramate's therapeutic actions in obesity remains unclear. Theoretically, topiramate may act to reduce glutamatergic stimulation and to enhance GABAergic inhibition in the appetite-stimulating pathway (Figure 14-20C), resulting in net *inhibition* of this

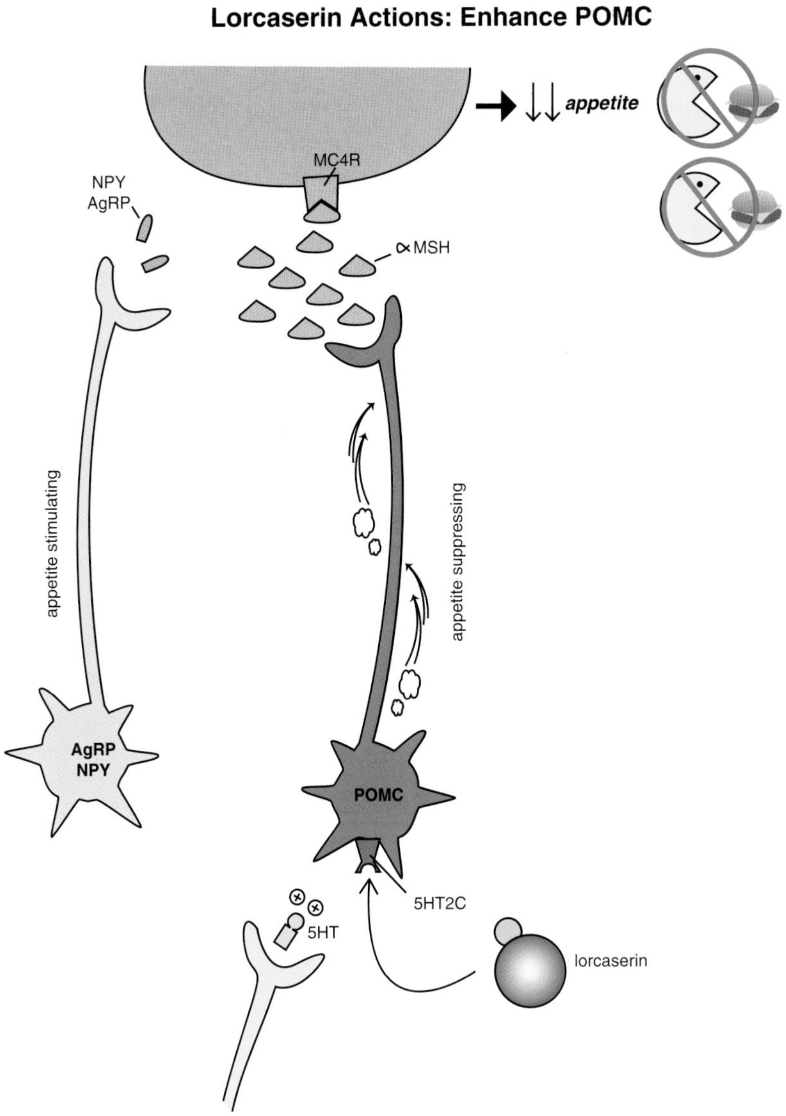

Lorcaserin Actions: Enhance POMC

Figure 14-20F. Actions of lorcaserin. The serotonin 5HT$_{2C}$ agonist lorcaserin has recently been approved for the treatment of obesity. Lorcaserin hypothetically binds to 5HT$_{2C}$ receptors on pro-opiomelanocortin (POMC) neurons in the *appetite-suppressing pathway*, activating POMC neurons and leading to release of α-melanocyte-stimulating hormone (α-MSH), which binds to melanocortin 4 receptors (MC4R) to robustly suppress appetite.

pathway. Such an action would synergize with simultaneous *activation* of the appetite suppressing pathway by phentermine (Figures 14-20B and 14-20C), to produce a more robust and long-lasting result on appetite suppression than with either drug alone. So far, that seems to be the case. Also, the tolerability of topiramate is enhanced by lowering its dose below that used for epilepsy or migraine, or even for its off-label use as a monotherapy for weight loss. Furthermore, topiramate is administered in a controlled-release formulation so that peak plasma drug levels and thus sedation are reduced.

Phentermine/topiramate ER in clinical trials showed dose-related weight loss, from 6% to 9% over placebo, with about two-thirds of obese patients losing at least 5% of their weight (only 20% of obese patients lost this much on placebo) by 12 weeks. Some patients do not respond, of course, and the weight loss can be modest, and long-term outcomes are not known. Also the topiramate component is potentially teratogenic to pregnant patients. However, this combination promises to be very useful in the management of obesity.

Another combination product that targets multiple simultaneous psychopharmacological mechanisms for obesity is **bupropion/naltrexone** (**Contrave**), in late

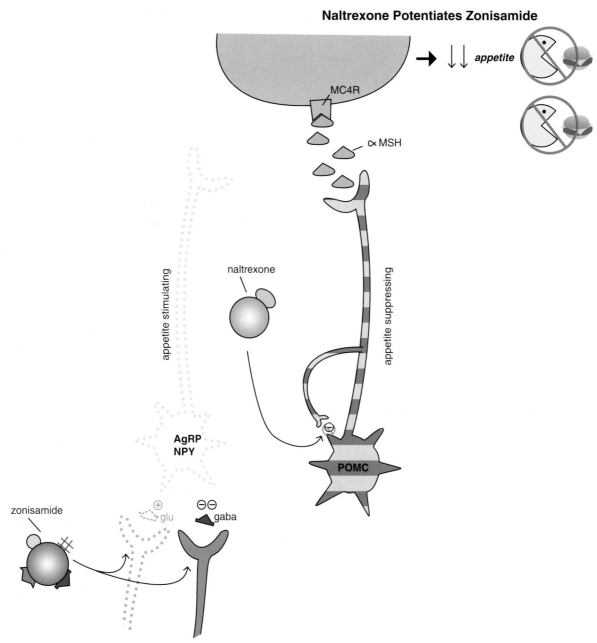

Figure 14-20G. Naltrexone potentiates the actions of zonisamide. The anticonvulsant zonisamide has actions in the appetite center of the hypothalamus that are similar to those of topiramate (Figure 14-20C). Zonisamide hypothetically both reduces excitatory glutamatergic input and increases inhibitory GABAergic input onto neurons in the *appetite-stimulating pathway*, leading to less output of neuropeptide Y (NPY) and agouti-related peptide (AgRP), and decreased appetite stimulation. Naltrexone removes the endorphin/endogenous-opioid-mediated negative feedback that limits activation of pro-opiomelanocrtin (POMC) neurons in the *appetite-suppressing pathway* (Figure 14-20E). With this negative feedback removed, α-melanocyte-stimulating hormone (α-MSH) levels are increased (i.e., disinhibited), leading to appetite suppression. The combination of naltrexone and zonisamide is currently under investigation as a potential treatment for obesity and impulsive–compulsive eating disorders.

clinical testing as of this writing. Bupropion alone has long been observed anecdotally to cause weight loss in some patients (Figure 14-20D). Bupropion is not only a proven antidepressant (see Chapter 7 and Figures 7-35 through 7-37) but is also a proven treatment for smoking cessation (see discussion earlier in this chapter and Figure 14-13), suggesting that bupropion's therapeutic actions are occurring at least in part within reward pathways. It is thus not surprising that bupropion could have therapeutic actions in disorders related to nicotine addiction, including possibly obesity and food addiction.

Bupropion acts as a norepinephrine–dopamine reuptake inhibitor (NDRI, Chapter 7, Figures 7-35 through 7-37). This mechanism is similar but less robust compared to amphetamine (Chapter 12, Figures 12-28 to 12-31; and also Figure 14-20D) or phentermine. When these NDRI actions of bupropion occur in the hypothalamus, this hypothetically enhances POMC-neuron-mediated appetite suppression. However, it also activates a β-endorphin/endogenous-opioid-mediated negative feedback pathway that mitigates how much bupropion can activate the POMC neuron (Figure 14-20D).

Preclinical studies show that addition of naltrexone can remove this negative opioid feedback and potentiate bupropion's ability to increase POMC neuron firing. These observations provide the rational explanation for the synergistic pharmacologic actions on appetite suppression and weight loss that have been observed both in animals and in clinical trials of obesity when naltrexone is combined with bupropion (Figure 14-20E). Naltrexone alone causes a small amount of weight loss in patients taking it for its approved uses for alcohol and opioid addiction. However, when a dose of naltrexone lower than that generally used to treat alcohol or opioid addiction is combined in obese subjects with a dose of bupropion in the general range used to treat depression or for smoking cessation, the combination treatment produces greater weight loss than either monotherapy alone. Notably, subjects treated with the combination appeared to exhibit continued weight loss through week 24, in contrast to an earlier plateau in patients receiving bupropion alone. Further investigation of the safety of this combination is under way, with the possibility that it will be approved soon for the treatment of obesity.

Another recently approved treatment for obesity is the serotonin $5HT_{2C}$ agonist **lorcaserin (Belviq)** (Figures 14-20F and 14-21). $5HT_{2C}$ receptors have long been linked to appetite, food intake, and weight,

and $5HT_{2C}$ antagonists are associated with weight gain, especially if they are given simultaneously with H_1 antihistamines (which is the case for many atypical antipsychotics and some antidepressants) (Figure 14-21; see also the discussion in Chapter 5 on antipsychotics and Figures 5-29, 5-39, 5-41 through 5-43, and the discussion in Chapter 7 on antidepressants and Figures 7-45, 7-66, 7-67). Consistent with the formulation that blockade of $5HT_{2C}$ receptors is associated with weight gain is the observation that experimental animals whose $5HT_{2C}$ receptors are "knocked out" are also obese. It would follow that the opposite action on $5HT_{2C}$ receptors, namely stimulation of them with an agonist, would be associated with reduced appetite, reduced food intake, and weight loss. SSRIs that increase serotonin at all its receptors, including the $5HT_{2C}$ receptor, can be associated with weight loss and can be effective in bulimia. Lorcaserin, a selective and well-characterized $5HT_{2C}$ agonist, may work by activating the POMC appetite-suppressing pathway (Figures 14-20F and 14-21B). Lorcaserin has robust weight-reducing actions in clinical trials with long-term studies up to 2 years in duration. The average weight loss for obese patients taking lorcaserin was 3–4% over those taking placebo. In obese patients who did not have type 2 diabetes, about half of them lost at least 5% of their weight, compared to about a quarter of those treated with placebo.

Future treatments for obesity and impulsive–compulsive eating disorders might include another combination product, namely the anticonvulsant zonisamide plus naltrexone (Figure 14-20G), which combines some of the mechanisms already discussed, as zonisamide has some of the same pharmacologic properties as topiramate. Direct-acting MC4R agonists (Figure 14-20) are also in testing for obesity but may be associated with hypothalamic-related side effects, and the efficacy of this single-mechanism approach, like some other single mechanisms for the treatment of obesity, may not be sufficiently robust. Triple reuptake inhibitors of serotonin, norepinephrine, and dopamine such as tasofensine are associated with weight loss and are in clinical testing for obesity. Some medications approved for diabetes have promise for the treatment of obesity, including metformin.

One available treatment for obesity – orlistat – works peripherally to inhibit fat absorption and not on reward circuitry except to the extent that it causes an aversive response to eating fatty foods (diarrhea and flatus). However, orlistat is not highly utilized nor highly palatable to many patients. Bariatric surgery of

Histamine H1 Antagonism Combined with Serotonin 2C Antagonism Stimulates Appetite

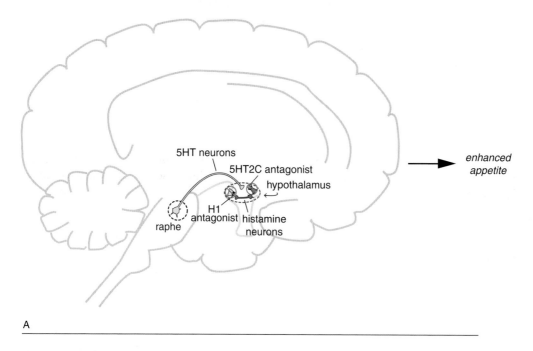

A

Serotonin 2C Agonist Lorcaserin Suppresses Appetite

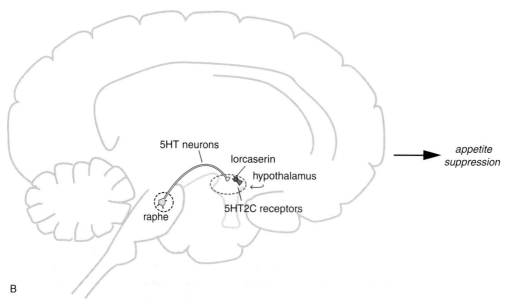

B

Figure 14-21. Serotonin 5HT$_{2C}$ and appetite. The combination of histamine H$_1$ antagonism and serotonin 5HT$_{2C}$ antagonism (A) (present in many atypical antipsychotics) may lead to enhanced appetite and consequential weight gain. Conversely, the actions of a 5HT$_{2C}$ agonist, such as lorcaserin (B), lead to appetite suppression and weight loss.

various types is also effective, particularly for morbid obesity, and is increasingly utilized in obesity in general, but is risky and costly. Several other treatments for obesity have been withdrawn from the market, including various stimulants, such as ephedrine (hypertension and stroke), and the halogenated amphetamine derivative fenfluramine (and dexfenfluramine). Fenfluramine was originally used as a prescription monotherapy, and then later combined with phentermine and widely used for a while in a combination known as phen-fen. However, fenfluramine was pulled from the market after the discovery of cardiac valvular and pulmonary toxicity. Sibutramine (an SNRI at low doses and a triple reuptake inhibitor at high doses) was also withdrawn from the market because of hypertension and cardiac problems. Some stimulants are still available as controlled substances (phentermine, diethylpropion) but are not associated with sustained weight loss in most individuals as monotherapies, and also have side effects from hypertension to abuse potential in monotherapy doses.

Impulsive–compulsive disorders of behavior

The current conceptualization of impulsivity and compulsivity as dimensions of psychopathology that cut across many psychiatric disorders suggests that behaviors themselves may be reinforcing and addicting. Rewarding behaviors and addictions to certain behaviors hypothetically share the same underlying circuitry as drug addiction (Figures 14-1 through 14-7). Impulsivity/compulsivity cannot explain all the aspects of these various and sundry conditions, and discussing how this construct could apply to each of them risks oversimplifying some very complex and very different disorders (Table 14-1; Tables 14-4 through 14-8). Furthermore, the discussion in this chapter does not address the many other unique aspects of these disorders, their current diagnostic criteria, the ongoing debates on their evolving diagnostic criteria, or even whether some conditions are disorders at all. Instead we look here at psychiatric conditions which exhibit behaviors that are either impulsive (meaning that they are difficult to prevent because short-term reward is chosen over long-term gain) or compulsive (meaning that an originally rewarding behavior becomes a habit which is difficult to stop because it reduces tension and withdrawal effects).

Many impulses can become an impulsive–compulsive disorder when done to excess, and several are listed in Table 14-5. Some experts believe **gambling disorder** should be classified along with drug

Table 14-5 When does an impulse become an impulsive–compulsive disorder?

Gambling disorder
Internet addiction
Pyromania
Kleptomania
Paraphilias
Hypersexual disorder

addiction as the only nonsubstance disorder in that category. Gambling disorder is characterized by repeated unsuccessful efforts to stop despite adverse consequences, tolerance (gambling higher and higher dollar amounts), psychological withdrawal when not gambling, and relief when reinitiating gambling. **Internet addiction**, **pyromania**, and **kleptomania** are not considered actual disorders by many, but they can involve an inability to stop the designated behavior (i.e., time on the internet, setting fires, stealing upon impulse), show the development of tolerance and withdrawal, and demonstrate relief when reinitiating the behavior. **Paraphilias**, considered to be psychiatric disorders, and **hypersexual disorder**, under consideration as a psychiatric disorder, all have these same characteristics of impulsivity transitioning to compulsivity for a variety of sexual behaviors.

Many disorders considered to be neurodevelopmental have impulsivity/compulsivity as a symptom dimension. This includes notably **ADHD**, discussed extensively in Chapter 12 (see circuits associated with impulsivity in Figures 12-2, 12-5, 12-7, 12-8 and 14-1, 14-2, 14-4). ADHD is an impulsive–compulsive disorder in which treatments may be effective for the impulsivity. Whereas increasing dopamine in the nucleus accumbens of the ventral striatum with high-dose rapidly administered stimulants can *enhance* impulsive action, increasing dopamine in orbitofrontal cortex (OFC) circuits with low-dose and slow-release stimulants can *decrease* impulsivity and enhance the individual's ability to say no to an impulsive temptation. Impulsivity can also occur in **mania** and is particularly difficult to treat when it accompanies ADHD, especially in children. **Autism** and related spectrum disorders may be associated with impulsivity but also compulsive, stereotyped behaviors. **Tourette's syndrome** and related **tic disorders** and **stereotyped movement disorders** may be forms mostly of compulsivity (Table 14-6).

Table 14-6 Are there neurodevelopmental impulsive–compulsive disorders?

Attention deficit hyperactivity disorder (ADHD)

Autism spectrum disorders

Tourette's syndrome and tic disorders

Stereotyped movement disorders

Table 14-8 OCD or ICD? Are obsessive–compulsive spectrum disorders also impulsive–compulsive disorders?

Obsessive–compulsive disorder (OCD)

Body dysmorphic disorder (BDD)

Hoarding

Trichotillomania (TTM)

Skin picking

Compulsive shopping

Hypochondriasis

Somatization

Table 14-7 Can violence be an impulsive–compulsive disorder?

Intermittent explosive disorder

Impulsive violence in psychosis, mania, and borderline personality disorder

Self-harm and parasuicidal behaviors/violence against self

Oppositional defiant disorder

Conduct disorder

Dyssocial personality disorder

Antisocial personality disorder

Psychopathy

Aggression and violence have long been controversial issues in psychiatry (Table 14-7). When violence is premeditated, callous, and calculated, it may be criminal, psychopathic, and predatory – and this type of violence would be neither impulsive nor compulsive. However, aggression and violence, both to others and to oneself, are associated with many psychiatric disorders (Table 14-7), and especially when aggression and violence are impulsive, and are readily and inappropriately provoked, these behaviors are increasingly being considered an impulsive dimension of psychopathology. Impulsive violence can occur in **psychotic disorders** of many types, including **drug-induced psychosis**, **schizophrenia** and **bipolar mania**, as well as in **borderline personality disorder**. Treatment of the underlying condition, often with antipsychotics, can be helpful. Aggression and violence in such disorders can be considered an imbalance between top-down "stop" signals and bottom-up drives and "go" signals, just as in other impulsive–compulsive disorders (Figures 14-1, 14-2, 14-3). Sometimes aggression becomes increasingly compulsive, rather than manipulative and planned, as in some cases of repetitive self-harm in borderline personality disorder, especially in institutional settings. There is renewed interest in the condition known as **intermittent explosive disorder** as an impulsive–compulsive disorder of aggression. It may be described as repeated reactions to frustration with irritability, temper tantrums, and destructive behavior that is not premeditated and not committed to achieve a tangible objective (e.g., money, power, intimidation), in the absence of another psychiatric disorder that could explain the impulsive aggression. Because individuals with **antisocial personality disorder**, **dyssocial personality disorder**, **psychopathic traits**, and **conduct disorder** can all have a mixture of manipulative and planned aggression as well as impulsive aggression, the cause of a given episode of violence can be very difficult to determine. **Oppositional defiant disorder** in children is often associated with impulsive acts, including impulsive and oppositional verbalizations.

Obsessive–compulsive disorder

Obsessive–compulsive disorder (OCD) in many ways is the prototypical impulsive–compulsive disorder, although it has often been considered to be an anxiety disorder (Table 14-8). In OCD, many patients experience an intense urge to perform stereotypic, ritualistic acts despite having full insight into how senseless and excessive these behaviors are, and having no real desire for the outcome of these actions. The most common types of compulsions are checking and cleaning. For OCD, a general propensity towards habit may be expressed solely as avoidance, deriving from the comorbid anxiety that they report. In the context of high anxiety, superstitious avoidance responses may offer relief, which reinforces the behavior. Stress and anxiety may enhance the formation of habits, whether positively or negatively motivated. However, as the habit becomes progressively compulsive, the experience of relief may no longer be the driving force, and instead the behavior comes under external control as a conditioned response.

Excessive inflexible behaviors are often thought to be carried out in order to neutralize anxiety or distress evoked by particular obsessions. Paradoxically, although OCD patients feel compelled to perform these behaviors, they are often aware that they are more disruptive than helpful. So why do they do them? Rather than conceptualizing compulsive behaviors as goal-directed to reduce anxiety, these rituals might be better understood as habits provoked mindlessly from a stimulus in the environment.

Such hypothesized habit learning can be reduced or reversed with exposure and response prevention, involving graded exposure to anxiety-provoking stimuli/situations, and prevention of the associated avoidance compulsions. This type of cognitive behavioral therapy is thought to have its therapeutic effect by breaking the pattern of compulsive avoidance that confers dominant control to the external environment (such that, for example, the sight of a door elicits checking) and also maintains inappropriate anxiety. Instead of considering compulsions as behavioral reactions to abnormal obsessions, the reverse may be true: obsessions in OCD may in fact be post hoc rationalizations of otherwise inexplicable compulsive urges. OCD patients have demonstrated lack of efficient information processing in their OFC and lack of cognitive flexibility, and thus cannot inhibit their compulsive responses/habits.

First-line treatment of OCD is specifically with one of the SSRIs. Although second-line treatments with one of the tricyclic antidepressants with serotonergic properties, clomipramine, with SNRIs or with MAO inhibitors are all worthy of consideration, the best option for a patient who has failed several SSRIs is often to consider very high doses with an SSRI or augmentation of an SSRI with an atypical antipsychotic. The mechanisms of action of all of these agents are covered in detail in Chapter 7. Augmentation of an SSRI with a benzodiazepine, lithium, or buspirone can also be considered. An experimental treatment for OCD is deep brain stimulation, discussed in Chapter 7 for depression and illustrated in Figure 7-76.

Many conditions related to OCD are listed in Table 14-8. These include **hoarding** and **compulsive shopping** (not necessarily considered a disorder). **Compulsive hair pulling (trichotillomania)**, and **compulsive skin picking** are conditions that are often much more compulsive than impulsive. **Body dysmorphic disorder** is preoccupation with perceived defects or flaws in appearance that cause repetitive behavior such as looking in the mirror, grooming, and reassurance seeking. Even preoccupations with health, body function, and pain such as exist in **hypochondriasis** and **somatization** can be considered types of obsessions.

Summary

We have discussed the current conceptualization of impulsivity and compulsivity as dimensions of psychopathology that cut across many psychiatric disorders. Rewarding behaviors and addiction to drugs or behaviors hypothetically share the same underlying circuitry with impulsivity – defined as behaviors that are difficult to prevent because short-term reward is chosen over long-term gain – mapped onto a prefrontal ventral striatal reward circuit, and compulsivity – defined as an originally rewarding behavior becoming a habit which is difficult to stop because it reduces tension and withdrawal effects – mapped onto a prefrontal dorsal motor response inhibition circuit. Hypothetically, failure of the balance between top-down inhibition and bottom-up drives is the common underlying neurobiological mechanism of impulsivity and compulsivity.

Both drugs and behaviors can be associated with impulsivity/compulsivity and are dimensions of psychopathology for a wide range of drug addictions and psychiatric disorders. The chapter discusses the psychopharmacology of reward and the brain circuitry that regulates reward. We have attempted to explain the psychopharmacological mechanisms of actions of various drugs of abuse, from nicotine to alcohol, and also opioids, stimulants, sedative hypnotics, marijuana, hallucinogens, and club drugs. In the case of nicotine and alcohol, various novel psychopharmacological treatments are discussed, including the $\alpha_4\beta_2$ selective nicotine partial agonist (NPA) varenicline for smoking cessation, naltrexone for opioid and alcohol addiction, and acamprosate for alcohol addiction. Obesity and its relationship to food addiction and impulsive–compulsive disorders is discussed along with numerous new treatments, including lorcaserin, phentermine/topiramate ER, and bupropion/naltrexone. Finally, a number of behavioral disorders are discussed as potential impulsive–compulsive disorders or even as behavioral addictions, including gambling, ADHD, impulsive violence, borderline personality disorder, obsessive–compulsive disorder, and many more.

Suggested reading and selected references

General references: textbooks

Brunton LL (ed) (2011) *Goodman and Gilman's The Pharmacological Basis of Therapeutics*, 12th edn. New York, NY: McGraw-Hill Medical.

Schatzberg AF, Nemeroff CB (eds.) (2009) *Textbook of Psychopharmacology*, 4th edn. Washington, DC: American Psychiatric Publishing.

General references: textbooks in the *Essential Psychopharmacology* series

Beyer CE, Stahl SM (eds.) (2010) *Next Generation Antidepressants*. Cambridge: Cambridge University Press.

Kalali A, Preskorn S, Kwentus J, Stahl SM (eds.) (2012) *Essential CNS Drug Development*. Cambridge: Cambridge University Press.

Silberstein SD, Marmura MJ, Stahl SM (2010) *Essential Neuropharmacology: the Prescriber's Guide*. Cambridge: Cambridge University Press.

Smith H, Pappagallo M, Stahl SM (2012) *Essential Pain Pharmacology*. Cambridge: Cambridge University Press.

Stahl SM (2009) *Stahl's Illustrated Antidepressants*. Cambridge: Cambridge University Press.

Stahl SM (2009) *Stahl's Illustrated Chronic Pain and Fibromyalgia*. Cambridge: Cambridge University Press.

Stahl SM (2009) *Stahl's Illustrated Mood Stabilizers*. Cambridge: Cambridge University Press.

Stahl SM (2011) *Case Studies: Stahl's Essential Psychopharmacology*. Cambridge: Cambridge University Press.

Stahl SM (2011) *Essential Psychopharmacology: the Prescriber's Guide*, 4th edn. Cambridge: Cambridge University Press.

Stahl SM (2012) *Stahl's Self-Assessment Examination in Psychiatry: Multiple Choice Questions for Clinicians*. Cambridge: Cambridge University Press.

Stahl SM, Davis RL (2011) *Best Practices in Medical Teaching*. Cambridge: Cambridge University Press.

Stahl SM, Grady MM (2010) *Stahl's Illustrated Anxiety, Stress, and PTSD*. Cambridge: Cambridge University Press.

Stahl SM, Grady MM (2012) *Stahl's Illustrated Substance Use and Impulsive Disorders*. Cambridge: Cambridge University Press.

Stahl SM, Mignon L (2009) *Stahl's Illustrated Attention Deficit Hyperactivity Disorder*. Cambridge: Cambridge University Press.

Stahl SM, Mignon L (2010) *Stahl's Illustrated Antipsychotics: Treating Psychosis, Mania and Depression*. Cambridge: Cambridge University Press.

Stein DJ, Lerer B, Stahl SM (eds.) (2012) *Essential Evidence-Based Psychopharmacology*, 2nd edn. Cambridge: Cambridge University Press.

Chapters 1–3 (basic neuroscience): textbooks

Iversen LL, Iversen SD, Bloom FE, Roth RH (2009) *Introduction to Neuropsychopharmacology*. New York, NY: Oxford University Press.

Meyer JS, Quenzer LF (2005) *Psychopharmacology: Drugs, the Brain, and Behavior*. Sunderland, MA: Sinauer Associates.

Nestler EJ, Hyman SE, Malenka RC (2009) *Molecular Neuropharmacology: a Foundation for Clinical Neuroscience*, 2nd edn. New York, NY: McGraw-Hill Medical.

Shepherd GM (ed) (2004) *The Synaptic Organization of the Brain*, 5th edn. New York, NY: Oxford University Press.

Squire LR, Bloom FE, McConnell SK, *et al.* (eds.) (2003) *Fundamental Neuroscience*, 2nd edn. San Diego, CA: Academic Press.

Chapters 4 (psychosis and schizophrenia) and 5 (antipsychotic agents), including glutamate

Alphs LD, Summerfelt A, Lann H, Muller RJ (1989) The negative symptom assessment: a new instrument to assess negative symptoms of schizophrenia. *Psychopharmacology Bulletin* 25: 159–163.

Benes FM (2010) Amygdalocortical Circuitry in Schizophrenia: From Circuits to Molecules. (2010) *Neuropsychopharmacology* 35: 239–257.

Citrome L (2009) Asenapine for schizophrenia and bipolar disorder: a review of the efficacy and safety profile for this newly approved sublingually absorbed second-generation antipsychotic. *International Journal of Clinical Practice* **63**: 1762–1784.

Citrome L, Meng X, Hochfeld M, Stahl SM (2012) Efficacy of iloperidone in the short-term treatment of schizophrenia: a *post hoc* analysis of pooled patient data from four phase III, placebo- and active-controlled trials. *Human Psychopharmacology* **27**: 24–32.

Conn PJ, Lindsley CW, Jones CK (2009) Activation of metabotropic glutamate receptors as a novel approach for the treatment of schizophrenia. *Trends in Pharmacological Science* **30**: 25–31.

Cruz DA, Weaver CL, Lovallo EM, Melchitzky DS, Lewis DA (2009) Selective alterations in postsynaptic markers of chandelier cell inputs to cortical pyramidal neurons in subjects with schizophrenia. *Neuropsychopharmacology* **34**: 2112–2124.

Curley AA, Arion D, Volk DW, *et al.* (2011) Cortical deficits of glutamic acid decarboxylase 67 expression in schizophrenia: clinical, protein, and cell type-specific features. *American Journal of Psychiatry* **158**: 921–929.

Dragt S, Nieman DH, Schultze-Lutter F, *et al.* (2012) Cannabis use and age at onset of symptoms in subjects at clinical high risk for psychosis. *Acta Psychiatrica Scandinavica* **125**: 45–53.

D'Souza DC, Singh N, Elander J, *et al.* (2012) Glycine transporter inhibitor attenuates the psychotomimetic effects of ketamine in healthy males: preliminary evidence. *Neuropsychopharmacology* **37**: 1036–1046.

Eisenberg DP, Berman KF (2010) Executive function, neural circuitry, and genetic mechanisms in schizophrenia. *Neuropsychopharmacology* **35**: 258–277.

Enomoto T, Tse MT, Floresco SB (2011) Reducing prefrontal gamma-aminobutyric acid activity induces cognitive, behavioral, and dopaminergic abnormalities that resemble schizophrenia. *Biological Psychiatry* **69**: 432–441.

Fleischhacker WW, Gopal S, Lane R, *et al.* (2012) A randomized trial of paliperidone palmitate and risperidone long-acting injectable in schizophrenia. *International Journal of Neuropsychopharmacology* **15**: 107–118.

Foti DJ, Kotov R, Guey LT, Bromet EJ (2010) Cannabis use and the course of schizophrenia: 10-year follow-up after first hospitalization. *American Journal of Psychiatry* **167**: 987–993.

Fusar-Poli P, Bonoldi I, Yung AR, *et al.* (2012) Predicting psychosis: meta-analysis of transition outcomes in individuals at high clinical risk. *Archives of General Psychiatry* **69**: 220–229.

Hall J, Whalley HC, McKirdy JW, *et al.* (2008) Overactivation of fear systems to neutral faces in schizophrenia. *Biological Psychiatry* **64**: 70–73.

Howes OD, Montgomery AJ, Asselin MC, *et al.* (2009) Elevated striatal dopamine function linked to prodromal signs of schizophrenia. *Archives of General Psychiatry* **66**: 13–20.

Jensen NH, Rodriguiz RM, Caron MG, *et al.* (2008) N-Desalkylquetiapine, a potent norepinephrine reuptake inhibitor and partial 5-HT$_{1A}$ agonist, as a putative mediator of quetiapine's antidepressant activity. *Neuropsychopharmacology* **33**: 2303–2312.

Kane JM, Sanches R, Perry PP, *et al.* (2012) Aripiprazole intramuscular depot as maintenance treatment in patients with schizophrenia: a 52-week, multicenter, randomized, double-blind, placebo-controlled study. *Journal of Clinical Psychiatry* **73**: 617–624.

Karlsgodt KH, Robleto K, Trantham-Davidson H, *et al.* (2011) Reduced dysbindin expression mediates N-methyl-D-aspartate receptor hypofunction and impaired working memory performance. *Biological Psychiatry* **69**: 28–34.

Kegeles LS, Mao X, Stanford AD, *et al.* (2012) Elevated prefrontal cortex γ-aminobutyric acid and glutamate-glutamine levels in schizophrenia measured in vivo with proton magnetic resonance spectroscopy. *Archives of General Psychiatry* **69**: 449–459.

Large M, Sharma S, Compton MT, Slade T, Nielssen O (2011) Cannabis use and earlier onset of psychosis. *Archives of General Psychiatry* **68**: 555–561.

Lewis DA, Gonzalez-Burgos G (2008) Neuroplasticity of neocortical circuits in schizophrenia. *Neuropsychopharmacology* **33**: 141–165.

Lodge DJ, Grace AA (2011) Hippocampal dysregulation of dopamine system function and the pathophysiology of schizophrenia. *Trends in Pharmacological Science* **32**: 507–513.

Mechelli A, Riecher-Rossler A, Meisenzahl EM, *et al.* (2011) Neuroanatomical abnormalities that pre-date the onset of psychosis. *Archives of General Psychiatry* **68**: 489–495.

Meltzer HY, Cucchiaro J, Silva R, *et al.* (2011) Lurasidone in the treatment of schizophrenia: a randomized, double-blind, placebo- and olanzapine-controlled study. *American Journal of Psychiatry* **168**: 957–967.

Meyer JM, Stahl SM (2009) The metabolic syndrome and schizophrenia. *Acta Psychiatrica Scandinavica* **119**: 4–14.

Nicodemus KK, Law AJ, Radulescu E, *et al.* (2010) Biological validation of increased schizophrenia risk with NRG1, ERBB4, and AKT1 epistasis via functional neuroimaging in healthy controls. *Archives of General Psychiatry* **67**: 991–1001.

Patil ST, Zhang L, Martenyi F, *et al.* (2007) Activation of mGlu 2/3 receptors as a new approach to treat schizophrenia: a randomized phase 2 clinical trial. *Nature Medicine* **13**: 1102–1107.

Perkins DO, Gu H, Boteva K, Lieberman JA (2005) Relationship between duration of untreated psychosis and outcome in first episode schizophrenia: a critical review and meta-analysis. *American Journal of Psychiatry* **162**: 1785–1804.

Pinkham AE, Loughead J, Ruparel K, *et al.* (2011) Abnormal modulation of amygdala activity in schizophrenia in response to direct- and averted-gaze threat-related facial expressions. *American Journal of Psychiatry* **168**: 293–301.

Ragland JD, Laird AR, Ranganath C, *et al.* (2009) Prefrontal activation deficits during episodic memory in schizophrenia. *American Journal of Psychiatry* **166**: 863–874.

Rasetti R, Mattay VS, Wiedholz LM, *et al.* (2009) Evidence that altered amygdala activity in schizophrenia is related to clinical state and not genetic risk. *American Journal of Psychiatry* **166**: 216–225.

Roffman JL, Gollub RL, Calhoun VD, *et al.* (2008) MTHFR 677C→T genotype disrupts prefrontal funciton in schizophrenia through an interaction with COMT 158 VA → Met. *Proceedings of the National Academy of Sciences* **105**: 17573–17578.

Roth BL. K_i determinations, receptor binding profiles, agonist and/or antagonist functional data, HERG data, MDR1 data, etc. as appropriate was generously provided by the National Institute of Mental Health's Psychoactive Drug Screening Program, Contract # HHSN-271-2008-00025-C (NIMH PDSP). The NIMH PDSP is directed by Bryan L.Roth MD, PhD at the University of North Carolina at Chapel Hill and Project Officer Jamie Driscol at NIMH, Bethesda MD, USA. For experimental details please refer to the PDSP website http://pdsp.med.unc.edu.

Satterthwaite TD, Wolf DH, Loughead J, *et al.* (2010) Association of enhanced limbic response to threat with decreased cortical facial recognition memory response in schizophrenia. *American Journal of Psychiatry* **167**: 418–426.

Shahid M, Walker GB, Zorn SH, Wong EHF (2009) Asenapine: a novel psychopharmacologic agent with a unique human receptor signature. *Journal of Psychopharmacology* **23**: 65–73.

Singh J, Robb A, Vijapurkar U, Nuamah I, Hough D (2011) A randomized, double-blind study of paliperidone extended-release in treatment of acute schizophrenia in adolescents. *Biological Psychiatry* **70**: 1179–1187.

Stahl SM (2010) The serotonin-7 receptor as a novel therapeutic target. *Journal of Clinical Psychiatry* **71**: 1414–1415.

Stahl SM, Mignon L, Meyer JM (2009) What comes first: atypical antipsychotic or the metabolic syndrome? *Acta Psychiatrica Scandinavica* **119**: 171–179.

Tamminga CA, Stan AD, Wagner AD (2010) The hippocampal formation in schizophrenia. *American Journal of Psychiatry* **167**: 1178–1193.

Tan HY, Chen Q, Sust S, *et al.* (2007) Epistasis between catechol-O-methyltransferase and type II metabotropic glutamate receptor 3 genes on working memory brain function. *Proceedings of the National Academy of Sciences* **104**: 12536–12541.

Umbricht D, Yoo K, Youssef E, *et al.* (2010) Investigational glycine transporter type 1 (GlyT1) inhibitor RG1678: results of the proof-of-concept study for the treatment of negative symptoms in schizophrenia. Abstract from the American College of Neuropsychopharmacology (ACNP) 49th Annual Meeting, Miami Beach, Florida, December 5–9, 2010.

Ursu S, Kring AM, Gard MG, *et al.*(2011) Prefrontal cortical deficits and impaired cognition-emotion interactions in schizophrenia. *American Journal of Psychiatry* **168**: 276–285.

Wykes T, Huddy V, Cellard C, McGurk SR, Czobar P (2011) A meta-analysis of cognitive remediation for schizophrenia: methodology and effect sizes. *American Journal of Psychiatry* **168**: 472–485.

Chapters 6 (mood disorders), 7 (antidepressants), and 8 (mood stabilizers)

aan het Rot, M, Collins KA, Murrough JW, *et al.* (2010) Safety and efficacy of repeated-dose intravenous ketamine for treatment-resistant depression. *Biological Psychiatry* **67**: 139–145.

Alvarez E, Perez V, Dragheim M, Loft H, Artigas F (2012) A double-blind, randomized, placebo-controlled, active reference study of Lu AA21004 in patients with major depressive disorder. *International Journal of Neuropsychopharmacology* **15**: 589–600.

BALANCE investigators and collaborators; Geddes JR, Goodwin GM, Rendell J, *et al.* (2010) Lithium plus valproate combination therapy versus monotherapy for relapse prevention in bipolar I disorder (Balance): a randomized open-label trial. *Lancet* **375**: 385–395.

Bang-Andersen B, Ruhland T, Jorgensen M, *et al.* (2011) Discovery of 1-[2-(2,4-Dimethylphenylsulfanyl) phenyl] piperazine (LuAA21004): a novel multimodal compound for the treatment of major depressive disorder. *Journal of Medicinal Chemistry* **54**: 3206–3221.

Bergink V, Bouvy PF, Vervoort JSP, *et al.* (2012) Prevention of postpartum psychosis and mania in women at high risk. *American Journal of Psychiatry* **169**: 609–616.

Bogdan R, Williamson DE, an Hariri AR (2012) Mineralocorticoid receptor Iso/Val (rs5522) genotype moderates the association between previous childhood emotional neglect and amygdala reactivity. *American Journal of Psychiatry* **169**: 515–522.

Chiu CT, Chuan DM (2010) Molecular actions and therapeutic potential of lithium in preclinical and clinical studies of CNS disorders. *Pharmacology & Therapeutics* **128**: 281–304.

Chowdhury GMI, Behar KL, Cho W, *et al.* (2012) ^{1}H-[^{13}C]-nuclear magnetic resonance spectroscopy measures of ketamine's effect on amino acid neurotransmitter metabolism. *Biological Psychiatry* **71**: 1022–1025.

Cipriani A, Pretty H, Hawton K, Geddes JR (2005) Lithium in the prevention of suicidal behavior and all-cause mortality in patients with mood disorders: a systematic review of randomized trials. *American Journal of Psychiatry* **162**: 1805–1819.

DiazGranados N, Ibrahim LA, Brutsche NE, *et al.* (2010) Rapid resolution of suicidal ideation after a single infusion of an N-methyl-D-aspartate antagonist in patients with treatment-resistant depressive disorder. *Journal of Clinical Psychiatry* **71**: 1605–1611.

Duman RS, Voleti B (2012) Signaling pathways underlying the pathophysiology and treatment of depression: novel mechanisms for rapid-acting agents. *Trends in Neurosciences* **35**: 47–56.

Frodl T, Reinhold E, Koutsouleris N, *et al.* (2010) Childhood stress, serotonin transporter gene and brain structures in major depression. *Neuropsychopharmacology* **35**: 1383–1390.

Goldberg JF, Perlis RH, Bowden CL, *et al.* (2009) Manic symptoms during depressive episodes in 1,380 patients with bipolar disorder: findings from the STEP-BD. *American Journal of Psychiatry* **166**: 173–181.

Grady M, Stahl SM (2012) Practical guide for prescribing MAOI: debunking myths and removing barriers. *CNS Spectrums* **17**: 2–10.

Ibrahim L, DiazGranados N, Franco-Chaves J, *et al.* (2012) Course of improvement in depressive symptoms during a single intravenous infusion of ketamine vs add-on riluzole: results from a 4-week, double-blind, placebo-controlled study. *Neuropsychopharmacology* **37**: 1526–1533.

Leon AC, Solomon DA, Li C, *et al.* (2012) Antiepileptic drugs for bipolar disorder and the risk of suicidal behavior: a 30-year observational study. *American Journal of Psychiatry* **169**: 285–291.

Mork A, Pehrson A, Brennum LT, *et al.* (2012) Pharmacological effects of Lu AA21004: a novel multimodal compound for the treatment of major depressive disorder. *Journal of Pharmacology and Experimental Therapeutics* **340**: 666–675.

Pasquali L, Busceti CL, Fulceri F, Paparelli A, Fornai F (2010) Intracellular pathways underlying the effects of lithium. *Behavioral Pharmacology* **21**: 473–492.

Perlis RH, Ostacher MJ, Goldberg JF, *et al.* (2010) Transition to mania during treatment of bipolar depression. *Neuropsychopharmacology* **35**: 2545–2552.

Price JL, Drevets WC (2010) Neurocircuitry of mood disorders. *Neuropsychopharmacology* **35**: 192–216.

Price RB, Nock MK, Charney DS, Mathew SJ (2009) Effects of intravenous ketamine on explicit and implicit measures of suicidality in treatment-resistant depression. *Biological Psychiatry* **66**: 522–526.

Rao U, Chen LA, Bidesi AS, *et al.* (2010) Hippocampal changes associated with early-life adversity and vulnerability to depression. *Biological Psychiatry* **67**: 357–364.

Roiser JP, Elliott R, Sahakian BJ (2012) Cognitive mechanisms of treatment in depression. *Neuropsychopharmacology* **37**: 117–136.

Roy A, Gorodetsky E, Yuan Q, Goldman D, Enoch MA (2010) Interaction of FKBP5, a stress-related gene, with childhood trauma increases the risk for attempting suicide. *Neuropsychopharmacology* **35**: 1674–1683.

Salvadore G, Cornwell BR, Sambataro F, *et al.* (2010) Anterior cingulate desynchronization and functional connectivity with the amygdala during a working memory task predict rapid antidepressant response to ketamine. *Neuropsychopharmacology* **35**: 1415–1422.

Schwartz TL, Siddiqui US, Stahl SM (2011) Vilazodone: a brief pharmacologic and clinical review of the novel SPARI (serotonin partial agonist and reuptake inhibitor). *Therapeutic Advances in Psychopharmacology* **1**: 81–87.

Stahl SM (2010) Psychiatric stress testing: novel strategy for translational psychopharmacology. *Neuropsychopharmacology* **35**: 1413–1414.

Stahl SM, Fava M, Trivedi M, *et al.* (2010) Agomelatine in the treatment of major depressive disorder: an 8 week, multicenter, randomized, placebo-controlled trial. *Journal of Clinical Psychiatry* **71**: 616–626.

Undurraga J, Baldessarini RJ, Valenti M, *et al.* (2012) Bipolar depression: clinical correlates of receiving antidepressants. *Journal of Affective Disorders* **139**: 89–93.

Yatham LN, Liddle PF, Sossi V, *et al.* (2012) Positron emission tomography study of the effects of tryptophan depletion on brain serotonin$_2$ receptors in subjects recently remitted from major depression. *Archives of General Psychiatry* **69**: 601–609.

Zajecka J, Schatzberg A, Stahl SM, *et al.* (2010) Efficacy and safety of agomelatine in the treatment of major depressive disorder: a multicenter, randomized, double-blind, placebo-controlled trial. *Journal of Clinical Psychopharmacology* **30**: 135–144.

Zarate CA, Brutsche NE, Ibrahim L, *et al.* (2012) Replication of ketamine's antidepressant efficacy in bipolar depression: a randomized controlled add-on trial. *Biological Psychiatry* **71**: 939–946.

Chapter 9 (anxiety)

Anderson KC, Insel TR (2006) The promise of extinction research for the prevention and treatment of anxiety disorders. *Biological Psychiatry* **60**: 319–321.

Aupperle RL, Allard CB, Grimes EM, *et al.* (2012) Dorsolateral prefrontal cortex activation during emotional anticipation and neuropsychological performance in posttraumatic stress disorder. *Archives of General Psychiatry* **69**: 360–371.

Barad M, Gean PW, Lutz B (2006) The role of the amygdala in the extinction of conditioned fear. *Biological Psychiatry* **60**: 322–328.

Batelaan NM, Van Balkom AJLM, Stein DJ (2010) Evidence-based pharmacotherapy of panic disorder: an update. *International Journal of Neuropsychopharmacology* **15**: 403–415.

Bonne O, Vythilingam M, Inagaki M, *et al.* (2008) Reduced posterior hippocampal volume in posttraumatic stress disorder. *Journal of Clinical Psychiatry* **69**: 1087–1091.

De Kleine RA, Hendriks GJ, Kusters WJC, Broekman TG, van Minnen A (2012) A randomized placebo-controlled trial of D-cycloserine to enhance exposure therapy for posttraumatic stress disorder. *Biological Psychiatry* **71**: 962–968.

Hermans D, Craske MG, Mineka S, Lovibond PF (2006) Extinction in human fear conditioning. *Biological Psychiatry* **60**: 361–368.

Ipser JC, Stein DJ (2012) Evidence-based pharmacotherapy of post-traumatic stress disorder (PTSD). *International Journal of Neuropsychopharmacology* **15**: 825–840.

Jovanovic T, Ressler KJ (2010) How the neurocircuitry and genetics of fear inhibition may inform our understanding of PTSD. *American Journal of Psychiatry* **167**: 648–662.

Linnman C, Zeidan MA, Furtak SC, *et al.* (2012) Resting amygdala and medial prefrontal metabolism predicts functional activation of the fear extinction circuit. *American Journal of Psychiatry* **169**: 415–423.

Mercer KB, Orcutt HK, Quinn JF, *et al.* (2012) Acute and posttraumatic stress symptoms in a prospective gene X environment study of a university campus shooting. *Archives of General Psychiatry* **69**: 89–97.

Monk S, Nelson EE, McClure EB, *et al.* (2006) Ventrolateral prefrontal cortex activation and attentional bias in response to angry faces in adolescents with generalized anxiety disorder. *American Journal of Psychiatry* **163**: 1091–1097.

Myers KM, Carlezon WA (2012) D-cycloserine effects on extinction of conditioned responses to drug-related cues. *Biological Psychiatry* **71**: 947–955.

Onur OA, Schlaepfer TE, Kukolja J, I. (2010) The N-methyl-D-aspartate receptor co-agonist D-cycloserine facilitates declarative learning and hippocampal activity in humans. *Biological Psychiatry* **67**: 1205–1211.

Orr SP, Milad MR, Metzger LJ, *et al.* (2006) Effects of beta blockade, PTSD diagnosis, and explicit threat on the extinction and retention of an aversively conditioned response. *Biological Psychology* **732**: 262–271.

Otto MW, Basden SL, Leyro TM, McHugh K, Hofmann SG (2007) Clinical perspectives on the combination of D-cycloserine and cognitive behavioral therapy for the treatment of anxiety disorders. *CNS Spectrums* **12**: 51–56, 59–61.

Otto MW, Tolin DF, Simon NM, *et al.* (2010) Efficacy of D-cycloserine for enhancing response to cognitive-behavior therapy for panic disorder. *Biological Psychiatry* **67**: 365–370.

Raskind MA, Peskind ER, Hoff DJ, *et al.* (2007) A parallel group placebo controlled study of prazosin for trauma nightmares and sleep disturbance in combat veterans with post-traumatic stress disorder. *Biological Psychiatry* **61**: 928–934.

Rauch SL, Shin LM, Phelps EA (2006) Neurocircuitry models of posttraumatic stress disorder and extinction: human neuroimaging research – past, present and future. *Biological Psychiatry* **60**: 376–382.

Sandweiss DA, Slymen DJ, Leardmann CA, *et al.*; Millennium Cohort Study Team (2011) Preinjury psychiatric status, injury severity, and postdeployment posttraumatic stress disorder. *Archives of General Psychiatry* **68**: 496–504.

Sauve W, Stahl SM (2011) Psychopharmacological treatment.In Moore BA, Penk WE (eds.) *Treating PTSD in Military Personnel: a Clinical Handbook.* New York, NY: Guilford Press, pp. 155–172.

Shin LM, Bush G, Milad MR, *et al.* (2011) Exaggerated activation of dorsal anterior cingulate cortex during cognitive interference: a monozygotic twin study of posttraumatic stress disorder. *American Journal of Psychiatry* **168**: 979–985.

Stein MB, McAllister TW (2009) Exploring the convergence of posttraumatic stress disorder and mild traumatic brain injury. *American Journal of Psychiatry* **166**: 768–776.

Vaiva G, Ducrocq F, Jezequel K, Averland B, *et al.* (2003) Immediate treatment with propranolol decreases posttraumatic stress disorder two months after trauma. *Biological Psychiatry* **54**: 947–949.

van Zuiden M, Geuze E, Willemen HLDM, *et al.* (2011) Pre-existing high glucocorticoid receptor number predicting development of posttraumatic stress symptoms after military deployment. *American Journal of Psychiatry* **168**: 89–96.

Chapter 10 (pain)

Apkarian AV, Sosa Y, Sonty S, *et al.* (2004) Chronic back pain is associated with decreased prefrontal and thalamic gray matter density. *Journal of Neuroscience* 24: 10410–10415.

Bar KJ, Wagner G, Koschke M, *et al.* (2007) Increased prefrontal activation during pain perception in major depression. *Biological Psychiatry* 62: 1281–1287.

Benarroch EE (2007) Sodium channels and pain. *Neurology* 68: 233–236.

Brandt MR, Beyer CE, Stahl SM (2012) TRPV1 antagonists and chronic pain: beyond thermal perception. *Pharmaceuticals,* special issue "Emerging pain targets and therapy" 5: 114–132.

Davies A, Hendrich J, Van Minh AT, *et al.* (2007) Functional biology of the alpha 2 beta subunits of voltage gated calcium channels. *Trends in Pharmacological Sciences* 28: 220–228.

Dooley DJ, Taylor CP, Donevan S, Feltner D (2007) Ca^{2+} channel $\alpha_2\delta$ ligands: novel modulators of neurotransmission. *Trends in Pharmacological Sciences* 28: 75–82.

Farrar JT (2006) Ion channels as therapeutic targets in neuropathic pain. *Journal of Pain* 7 (1, Supplement 1).

Gracely RH, Petzke F, Wolf JM, Clauw DJ (2002) Functional magnetic resonance imaging evidence of augmented pain processing in fibromyalgia. *Arthritis and Rheumatism* 46: 1222–1343.

McLean SA, Williams DA, Stein PK, *et al.* (2006) Cerebrospinal fluid corticotropin-releasing factor concentration is associated with pain but not fatigue symptoms in patients with fibromyalgia. *Neuropsychopharmacology* 31: 2776–2782.

Miljanich GP (2004) Ziconotide: neuronal calcium channel blocker for treating severe chronic pain. *Current Medicinal Chemistry* 11: 3029–3040.

Nickel FT, Seifert F, Lanz S, Maihofner C (2012) Mechanisms of neuropathic pain. *European Neuropsychopharmacology* 22: 81–91.

Norman E, Potvin S, Gaumond I, *et al.* (2011) Pain inhibition is deficient in chronic widespread pain but normal in major depressive disorder. *Journal of Clinical Psychiatry* 72: 219–224.

Stahl SM (2009) Fibromyalgia: pathways and neurotransmitters. *Human Psychopharmacology* 24: S11–S17.

Wall PD, Melzack R (eds.) (1999) *Textbook of Pain*, 4th edn. London: Harcourt.

Williams DA, Gracely RH (2006) Functional magnetic resonance imaging findings in fibromyalgia. *Arthritis Research and Therapy* 8: 224–232.

Chapter 11 (sleep/wake)

Abadie P, Rioux P, Scatton B, *et al.* (1996) Central benzodiazepine receptor occupancy by zolpidem in the human brain as assessed by positron emission tomography. *Science* 295: 35–44.

Aloia MS, Arnedt JT, Davis JD, Riggs RL, Byrd D (2004) Neuropsychological sequelae of obstructive sleep apnea-hypopnea syndrome: a critical review. *Journal of the International Neuropsychological Society* 10: 772–785.

Bettica P, Squassante L, Groeger JA, *et al.* (2012) Differential effects of a dual orexin receptor antagonist (SB-649868) and zolpidem on sleep initiation and consolidation, SWS, REM sleep, and EEG power spectra in a model of situational insomnia. *Neuropsychopharmacology* 37: 1224–1233.

Cao M, Guilleminault C (2011) Hypocretin and its emerging role as a target for treatment of sleep disorders. *Current Neurology and Neuroscience Reports* 11: 227–234.

Cauter EV, Plat L, Scharf MB, *et al.* (1997) Simultaneous stimulation of slow-wave sleep and growth hormone secretion by gamma-hydroxybutyrate in normal young men. *Journal of Clinical Investigation* 100: 745–753.

Chahine LM, Chemali ZN (2006) Restless legs syndrome: a review. *CNS Spectrums* 11: 511–520.

Coleman PJ, Schreier JD, Cox CD, *et al.* (2012) Discovery of [(2R,5R)-5-{[(5-fluoropyridin-2-yl)oxy]methyl}-2-methylpiperidin-1-yl][5-methyl-2-(pyrimidin-2-yl) phenyl]methanone (MK-6096): a dual orexin receptor antagonist with potent sleep-promoting properties. *ChemMedChem* 7: 415–424.

Czeisler CA, Walsh JK, Roth T, *et al.* (2005) Modafinil for excessive sleepiness associated with shift-work sleep disorder. *New England Journal of Medicine* 353: 476–486.

Dawson GR, Collinson N, Atack JR (2005) Development of subtype selective $GABA_A$ modulators. *CNS Spectrums* 10: 21–27.

DiFabio R, Pellacani A, Faedo S, *et al.* (2011) Discovery process and pharmacological characterization of a novel dual orexin 1 and orexin 2 receptor antagonist useful for treatment of sleep disorders. *Bioorganic & Medicinal Chemistry Letters* 21: 5562–5567.

Dinges DF, Weaver TE (2003) Effects of modafinil on sustained attention performance and quality of life in OSA patients with residual sleepiness while being treated with CPAP. *Sleep Medicine* 4: 393–402.

Drover DR (2004) Comparative pharmacokinetics and pharmacodynamics of short-acting hypnosedatives: zaleplon, zolpidem and zopiclone. *Clinical Pharmacokinetics* 43: 227–238.

Durmer JS, Dinges DF (2005) Neurocognitive consequences of sleep deprivation. *Seminars in Neurology* 25: 117–129.

Ellis CM, Monk C, Simmons A, *et al.* (1999) Functional magnetic resonance imaging neuroactivation studies in normal subjects and subjects with the narcoleptic syndrome: actions of modafinil. *Journal of Sleep Research* **8**: 85–93.

Fava M, McCall WV, Krystal A, *et al.* (2006) Eszopiclone co-administered with fluoxetine in patients with insomnia coexisting with major depressive disorder. *Biological Psychiatry* **59**: 1052–1060.

Hart CL, Haney M, Vosburg SK, *et al.* (2006) Modafinil attenuates disruptions in cognitive performance during simulated night-shift work. *Neuropsychopharmacology* **31**: 1526–1536.

Hening W, Walters AS, Allen RP, *et al.* (2004) Impact, diagnosis and treatment of restless legs syndrome (RLS) in a primary care population: the REST (RLS Epidemiology, Symptoms, and Treatment) primary care study. *Sleep Medicine* **5**: 237–246.

Krystal AD, Walsh JK, Laska E, *et al.* (2003) Sustained efficacy of eszopiclone over 6 months of nightly treatment: results of a randomized, double-blind, placebo-controlled study in adults with chronic insomnia. *Sleep* **26**: 793–799.

Landrigan CP, Rothschild JM, Cronin JW, *et al.* (2004) Effect of reducing interns' work hours on serious medical errors in intensive care units. *New England Journal of Medicine* **351**: 1838–1848.

Madras BK, Xie Z, Lin Z, *et al.* (2006) Modafinil occupies dopamine and norepinephrine transporters in vivo and modulates the transporters and trace amine activity in vitro. *Journal of Pharmacology and Experimental Therapeutics* **319**: 561–569.

Makris AP, Rush CR, Frederich RC, Kelly TH (2004) Wake-promoting agents with different mechanisms of action: comparison of effects of modafinil and amphetamine on food intake and cardiovascular activity. *Appetite* **42**: 185–195.

Nofzinger EA, Buysse DJ, Germain A, *et al.* (2004) Functional neuroimaging evidence for hyperarousal in insomnia. *American Journal of Psychiatry* **161**: 2126–2129.

Nutt D, Stahl SM (2010) Searching for perfect sleep: the continuing evolution of GABA$_A$ receptor modulators as hypnotics. *Journal of Psychopharmacology* **24**: 1601–1612.

Sakurai T, Mieda M (2011) Connectomics of orexin-producing neurons: interface of systems of emotion, energy homeostasis and arousal. *Trends in Pharmacological Sciences* **32**: 451–462.

Saper CB, Lu J, Chou TC, Gooley J (2005) The hypothalamic integrator for circadian rhythms. *Trends in Neurosciences* **3**: 152–157.

Saper CB, Scammell TE, Lu J (2005) Hypothalamic regulation of sleep and circadian rhythms. *Nature* **437**: 1257–1263.

Scammell TE, Winrow CJ (2011) Orexin receptors: pharmacology and therapeutic opportunities. *Annual Review of Pharmacology and Toxicology* **51**: 243–266.

Schwartz JRL, Nelson MT, Schwartz ER, Hughes RJ (2004) Effects of modafinil on wakefulness and executive function in patients with narcolepsy experiencing late-day sleepiness. *Clinical Neuropharmacology* **27**: 74–79.

Steiner MA, Lecourt H, Strasser DS, Brisbare-Roch C, Jenck F (2011) Differential effects of the dual orexin receptor antagonist almorexant and the GABA$_A$-α1 receptor modulator zolpidem, alone or combined with ethanol, on motor performance in the rat. *Neuropsychopharmacology* **36**: 848–856.

Thomas RJ, Kwong K (2006) Modafinil activates cortical and subcortical sites in the sleep-deprived state. *Sleep* **29**: 1471–1481.

Thomas RJ, Rosen BR, Stern CE, Weiss JW, Kwong KK (2005) Functional imaging of working memory in obstructive sleep-disordered breathing. *Journal of Applied Physiology* **98**: 2226–2234.

U.S. Xyrem Multicenter Study Group (2003) A 12-month, open-label, multicenter extension trial of orally administered sodium oxybate for the treatment of narcolepsy. *Sleep* **26**: 31–35.

Willie JT, Chemelli RM, Sinton CM, *et al.* (2003) Distinct narcolepsy syndromes in *orexin recepter-2* and *orexin* null mice: molecular genetic dissection of non-rem and rem sleep regulatory processes. *Neuron* **38**: 715–730.

Winrow CJ, Gotter AL, Cox CD, *et al.* (2012) Pharmacological characterization of MK-6096 – a dual orexin receptor antagonist for insomnia. *Neuropharmacology* **62**: 978–987.

Wu JC, Gillin JC, Buchsbaum MS, *et al.* (2006) Frontal lobe metabolic decreases with sleep deprivation not totally reversed by recovery sleep. *Neuropsychopharmacology* **31**: 2783–2792.

Zeitzer JM, Morales-Villagran A, Maidment NT, *et al.* (2006) Extracellular adenosine in the human brain during sleep and sleep deprivation: an in vivo microdialysis study. *Sleep* **29**: 455–461.

Chapter 12 (attention deficit hyperactivity disorder)

Arnsten AFT (2006) Fundamentals of attention deficit/hyperactivity disorder: circuits and pathways. *Journal of Clinical Psychiatry* **67** (Suppl 8): 7–12.

Arnsten AFT (2006) Stimulants: therapeutic actions in ADHD. *Neuropsychopharmacology* **31**: 2376–2383.

Arnsten AFT (2009) Stress signaling pathways that impair prefrontal cortex structure and function. *Nature Reviews Neuroscience* 10: 410–422.

Arnsten AFT, Li BM (2005) Neurobiology of executive functions: catecholamine influences on prefrontal cortical functions. *Biological Psychiatry* 57: 1377–1384.

Avery RA, Franowicz JS, Phil M, *et al.* (2000) The alpha 2A adrenoceptor agonist, guanfacine, increases regional cerebral blood flow in dorsolateral prefrontal cortex of monkeys performing a spatial working memory task. *Neuropsychopharmacology* 23: 240–249.

Berridge CW, Devilbiss DM, Andrzejewski ME, *et al.* (2006) Methylphenidate preferentially increases catecholamine neurotransmission within the prefrontal cortex at low doses that enhance cognitive function. *Biological Psychiatry* 60; 1111–1120.

Berridge CW, Shumsky JS, Andrzejewski ME, *et al.* (2012) Differential sensitivity to psychostimulants across prefrontal cognitive tasks: differential involvement of noradrenergic α_1- and α_2-receptors. *Biological Psychiatry* 71: 467–473.

Biederman J (2004) Impact of comorbidity in adults with attention deficit/hyperactivity disorder. *Journal of Clinical Psychiatry* 65 (Suppl 3): 3–7.

Biederman J, Petty CR, Fried R, *et al.* (2007) Stability of executive function deficits into young adult years: a prospective longitudinal follow-up study of grown up males with ADHD. *Acta Psychiatrica Scandinavica* 116: 129–136.

Clerkin SM, Schulz KP, Halperin JM, *et al.* (2009) Guanfacine potentiates the activation of prefrontal cortex evoked by warning signals. *Biological Psychiatry* 66: 307–312.

Easton N, Shah YB, Marshall FH, Fone KC, Marsden CA (2006) Guanfacine produces differential effects in frontal cortex compared with striatum: assessed by phMRI BOLD contrast. *Psychopharmacology* 189: 369–385.

Faraone SV, Biederman J, Spencer T, *et al.* (2006) Diagnosing adult attention deficit hyperactivity disorder: are late onset and subthreshold diagnoses valid? *American Journal of Psychiatry* 163: 1720–1729.

Fusar-Poli P, Rubia K, Rossi G, Sartori G, Balottin U (2012) Striatal dopamine transporter alterations in ADHD: pathophysiology or adaptation to psychostimulants? A meta-analysis. *American Journal of Psychiatry* 169: 264–272.

Grady M, Stahl SM (2012) A horse of a different color: how formulation influences medication effects. *CNS Spectrums* 17: 63–69

Hannestad J, Gallezot JD, Planeta-Wilson B, *et al.* (2010) Clinically relevant doses of methylphenidate significantly occupy norepinephrine transporters in humans in vivo. *Biological Psychiatry* 68: 854–860.

Jakala P, Riekkinen M, Sirvio J, *et al.* (1999) Guanfacine, but not clonidine, improves planning and working memory performance in humans. *Neuropsychopharmacology* 20: 460–470.

Kessler RC, Adler L, Barkley R, *et al.* (2006) The prevalence and correlates of adult ADHD in the United States: results from the National Comorbidity Survey Replication. *American Journal of Psychiatry* 163: 716–723.

Kessler RC, Green JG, Adler LA, *et al.* (2010) Structure and diagnosis of adult attention-deficit/hyperactivity disorder. *Archives of General Psychiatry* 67: 1168–1178.

Kollins SH, McClernon JM, Fuemmeler BF (2005) Association between smoking and attention deficit/hyperactivity disorder symptoms in a population-based sample of young adults. *Archives of General Psychiatry* 62: 1142–1147.

Madras BK, Miller GM, Fischman AJ (2005) The dopamine transporter and attention deficit/hyperactivity disorder. *Biological Psychiatry* 57: 1397–1409.

Pingault JB, Tremblay RE, Vitaro F, *et al.* (2011) Childhood trajectories of inattention and hyperactivity and prediction of educational attainment in early adulthood: a 16-year longitudinal population-based study. *American Journal of Psychiatry* 168: 1164–1170.

Seidman LJ, Valera EM, Makris N, *et al.* (2006) Dorsolateral prefrontal and anterior cingulate cortex volumetric abnormalities in adults with attention-deficit/hyperactivity disorder identified by magnetic resonance imaging. *Biological Psychiatry* 60: 1071–1080.

Spencer TJ, Biederman J, Madras BK, *et al.* (2005) In vivo neuroreceptor imaging in attention deficit/hyperactivity disorder: a focus on the dopamine transporter. *Biological Psychiatry* 57: 1293–1300.

Spencer TJ, Bonab AA, Dougherty DD, *et al.* (2012) Understanding the central pharmacokinetics of spheroidal oral drug absorption system (SODAS) dexmethylphenidate: a positron emission tomography study of dopamine transporter receptor occupancy measured with C-11 altropane. *Journal of Clinical Psychiatry* 73: 346–352.

Stahl SM (2009) Norepinephrine and dopamine regulate signals and noise in the prefrontal cortex. *Journal of Clinical Psychiatry* 70: 617–618.

Stahl SM (2009) The prefrontal cortex is out of tune in attention-deficit/hyperactivity disorder. *Journal of Clinical Psychiatry* 70: 950–951.

Stahl SM (2010) Mechanism of action of stimulants in attention deficit/hyperactivity disorder. *Journal of Clinical Psychiatry* 71: 12–13.

Stahl SM (2010) Mechanism of action of α2A-adrenergic agonists in attention-deficit/hyperactivity disorder with or without oppositional symptoms. *Journal of Clinical Psychiatry* 71: 223–224.

Steere JC, Arnsten AFT (1997) The alpha 2A noradrenergic receptor agonist guanfacine improves visual object discrimination reversal performance in aged rhesus monkeys. *Behavioral Neuroscience* 111: 883–891.

Surman CBH, Biederman J, Spencer T, *et al.* (2011) Deficient emotional self regulation and adult attention deficit hyperactivity disorder: a family risk analysis. *American Journal of Psychiatry* 168: 617–623.

Swanson J, Baler RD, Volkow ND (2011) Understanding the effects of stimulant medications on cognition in individuals with attention-deficit hyperactivity disorder: a decade of progress. *Neuropsychopharmacology* 36: 207–226.

Turgay A, Goodman DW, Asherson P, *et al.*; for the ADHD Transition Phase Model Working Group (2012) Lifespan persistence of ADHD: the life transition model and its application. *Journal of Clinical Psychiatry* 73: 192–201.

Turner DC, Clark L, Dowson J, Robbins TW, Sahakian BJ (2004) Modafinil improves cognition and response inhibition in adult attention deficit/hyperactivity disorder. *Biological Psychiatry* 55: 1031–1040.

Turner DC, Robbins TW, Clark L, *et al.* (2003) Cognitive enhancing effects of modafinil in healthy volunteers. *Psychopharmacology* 165: 260–269.

Vaughan BS, March JS, Kratochvil CJ (2012) The evidence-based pharmacological treatment of pediatric ADHD. *International Journal of Neuropsychopharmacology* 15: 27–39.

Wang M, Ramos BP, Paspalas CD, *et al.* (2007) α2A-Adrenoceptors strengthen working memory networks by inhibiting cAMP-HCN channel signaling in prefrontal cortex. *Cell* 129: 397–410.

Wigal T, Brams M, Gasior M, *et al.*; 316 Study Group (2010) Randomized, double-blind, placebo-controlled, crossover study of the efficacy and safety of lisdexamfetamine dimesylate in adults with attention-deficit/hyperactivity disorder: novel findings using a simulated adult workplace environment design. *Behavioral and Brain Functions* 6: 34–48.

Wilens TE (2007) Lisdexamfetamine for ADHD. *Current Psychiatry* 6: 96–98, 105.

Yang L, Cao Q, Shuai L, *et al.* (2012) Comparative study of OROS-MPH and atomoxetine on executive function improvement in adhd: a randomized controlled trial. *International Journal of Neuropsychopharmacology* 15: 15–16.

Zang YF, Jin Z, Weng XC, *et al.* (2005) Functional MRI in attention deficit hyperactivity disorder: evidence for hypofrontality. *Brain and Development* 27: 544–550.

Zuvekas SH, Vitiello B (2012) Stimulant medication use in children: a 12-year perspective. *American Journal of Psychiatry* 169: 160–166.

Chapter 13 (dementia)

Albert MS, DeKosky ST, Dickson D, *et al.* (2011) The diagnosis of mild cognitive impairment due to Alzheimer's disease: recommendations from the National Institute on Aging and Alzheimer's Association Workgroup. *Alzheimer's & Dementia* 7: 270–279.

Alexopoulos GS (2003) Role of executive function in late life depression. *Journal of Clinical Psychiatry* 64 (Suppl 14): 18–23.

Bacher I, Rabin R, Woznica A, Sacvco KA, George TP (2010) Nicotinic receptor mechanisms in neuropsychiatric disorders: therapeutic implications. *Primary Psychiatry* 17: 35–41.

Ballard C, Ziabreva I, Perry R, *et al.* (2006) Differences in neuropathologic characteristics across the Lewy Cody dementia spectrum. *Neurology* 67: 1931–1934.

Barnes DE, Yaffe K, Byers AL, *et al.* (2012) Midlife vs late-life depressive symptoms and risk of dementia. *Archives of General Psychiatry* 69: 493–498.

Buccafusco JJ (2009) Emerging cognitive enhancing drugs. *Expert Opinion on Emerging Drugs* 14: 577–589.

Buchman AS, Boyle PA, Yu L, *et al.* (2012) Total daily physical activity and the risk of AD and cognitive decline in older adults. *Neurology* 78: 1323–1329.

Chetelat G, Villemagne VL, Villain N, *et al.* (2012) Accelerated cortical atrophy in cognitively normal elderly with high β-amyloid deposition. *Neurology* 78: 477–484.

Citron M (2004) β-Secretase inhibition for the treatment of Alzheimer's disease: promise and challenge. *Trends in Pharmacological Sciences* 25: 92–97.

Clark CM, Schneider JA, Bedell BJ, *et al.*; AV45-A07 study group (2011) Use of florbetapir-PET for imaging β-amyloid pathology. *JAMA* 305: 275–283.

Cummings JL (2011) Biomarkers in Alzheimer's disease drug development. *Alzheimer's & Dementia* 7: e13–e44.

Deutsch SI, Rosse RB, Deutsch LH (2006) Faulty regulation of tau phosphorylation by the reelin signal transduction pathway is a potential mechanism of pathogenesis and therapeutic target in Alzheimer's disease. *European Neuropsychopharmacology* 16: 547–551.

Dickerson BC, Stoub TR, Shah RC, *et al.* (2011) Alzheimer-signature MRI biomarker predicts AD dementia in cognitively normal adults. *Neurology* 76: 1395–1402.

Ercoli L, Siddarth P, Huang SC, *et al.* (2006) Perceived loss of memory ability and cerebral metabolic decline in persons with the apoplipoprotein E-IV genetic risk for Alzheimer disease. *Archives of General Psychiatry* 63: 442–448.

Ewers M, Sperling RA, Klunk WE, Weiner MW, Hampel H (2011) Neuroimaging markers for the prediction and early diagnosis of Alzheimer's disease dementia. *Trends in Neuroscience* 34: 430–442.

Fleisher AS, Chen K, Liu X, *et al.* (2011) Using positron emission tomography and florbetapir F 18 to image amyloid in patients with mild cognitive impairment or dementia due to Alzheimer disease. *Archives of Neurology* 68: 1404–1411.

Forster S, Grimmer, T, Miederer I, *et al.* (2012) Regional expansion of hypometabolism in Alzheimer's disease follows amyloid deposition with temporal delay. *Biological Psychiatry* 71: 792–797.

Frakey LL, Salloway S, Buelow M, Malloy P (2012) A randomized, double-blind, placebo-controlled trial of modafinil for the treatment of apathy in individuals with mild-to-moderate Alzheimer's disease. *Journal of Clinical Psychiatry* 73: 796–801.

Gomar JJ, Bobes-Bascaran MT, Conejero-Goldberg C, Davies P, Goldbert TE; Alzheimer's Disease Neuroimaging Initiative (2011) Utility of combinations of biomarkers, cognitive markers, and risk factors to predict conversion from mild cognitive impairment to Alzheimer disease in patients in the Alzheimer's Disease Neuroimaging Initiative. *Archives of General Psychiatry* 68: 961–969.

Grimmer T, Tholen S, Yousefi BH, *et al.* (2010) Progression of cerebral amyloid load is associated with the apolipoprotein E ε4 genotype in Alzheimer's disease. *Biological Psychiatry* 68: 879–884.

Grothe M, Heinsen H, Teipel SF (2012) Atrophy of the cholinergic basal forebrain over the adult age range and in early states of Alzheimer's disease. *Biological Psychiatry* 71: 805–813.

Hasselmo ME, Sarter M (2011) Nodes and models of forebrain cholinergic neuromodulation of cognition. *Neuropsychopharmacology* 36: 52–73.

Herrmann N, Chau SA, Kircanski I, Lanctot KL (2011) Current and emerging drug treatment options for Alzheimer's disease. *Drugs* 71: 2031–2065.

Huey ED, Putnam KT, Grafman J (2006) A systematic review of neurotransmitter deficits and treatments in frontotemporal dementia. *Neurology* 66: 17–22.

Jack CR, Albert MS, Knopman DS, *et al.* (2011) Introduction to the recommendations from the National Institute on Aging and the Alzheimer's Association workgroups on diagnostic guidelines for Alzheimer's disease. *Alzheimer's & Dementia* 7: 257–262.

Jack CR, Lowe VJ, Weigand SD, *et al.*; Alzheimer's Disease Neuroimaging Initiative (2009) Serial PIB and MRI in normal, mild cognitive impairment and Alzheimer's disease: implications for sequence of pathological events in Alzheimer's disease. *Brain* 132: 1355–1365.

Kales HC, Kim HM, Zivin K, *et al.* (2012) Risk of mortality among individual antipsychotics in patients with dementia. *American Journal of Psychiatry* 169: 71–79.

Lane RM, Potkin SG, Enz A (2006) Targeting acetylcholinesterase and butyrylcholinesterase in dementia. *International Journal of Neuropsychopharmacology* 9: 101–124.

Lee GJ, Lu PH, Hua X, *et al.*; Alzheimer's Disease Neuroimaging Initiative (2012) Depressive symptoms in mild cognitive impairment predict greater atrophy in Alzheimer's disease-related regions. *Biological Psychiatry* 71: 814–821.

Matsuzaki T, Sasaki K, Tanizaki Y, *et al.* (2010) Insulin resistance is associated with the pathology of Alzheimer disease. *Neurology* 75: 764–770.

McKhann GM, Knopman DS, Chertkow H, *et al.* (2011) The diagnosis of dementia due to Alzheimer's disease: recommendations from the National Institute on Aging and the Alzheimer's Association Workgroup. *Alzheimer's & Dementia* 7: 263–269.

Pomara N, Bruno D, Sarreal AS, *et al.* (2012) Lower CSF amyloid beta peptides and higher F-2 isoprostanes in cognitively intact elderly individuals with major depressive disorder. *American Journal of Psychiatry* 169: 523–530.

Purandare N, Burns A, Morris J, *et al.* (2012) Association of cerebral emboli with accelerated cognitive deterioration in Alzheimer's disease and vascular dementia. *American Journal of Psychiatry* 169: 300–308.

Rabinovici GD, Rosen HJ, Alkalay A, *et al.* (2011) Amyloid vs FDG-PET in the differential diagnosis of AD and FTLD. *Neurology* 77: 2034–2042.

Reisberg B, Doody R, Stöffler A, *et al.* (2003) Memantine in moderate-to-severe Alzheimer's disease. *New England Journal of Medicine* 348: 1333–1341.

Rodrigue KM, Kennedy KM, Devous MD, *et al.* (2012) B-amyloid burden in healthy aging. regional distribution and cognitive consequences. *Neurology* 78: 387–395.

Scheinin NM, Aalto S, Kaprio J, *et al.* (2011) Early detection of Alzheimer disease. *Neurology* 77: 453–460.

Schneider LS, Dagerman KS, Insel P (2005) Risk of death with atypical antipsychotic drug treatment for dementia. *JAMA* 294: 1935–1943.

Sink KM, Holden KF, Yaffe K (2005) Pharmacological treatment of neuropsychiatric symptoms of dementia. *JAMA* 293: 596–608.

Sperling RA, Aisen PS, Beckett LA, *et al.* (2011) Toward defining the preclinical stages of Alzheimer's disease: recommendations from the National Institute on Aging and the Alzheimer's Association Workgroup. *Alzheimer's & Dementia* 7: 280–292.

Tariot PN, Farlow MR, Grossberg GT, *et al.* (2004) Memantine treatment in patients with moderate to severe Alzheimer's disease already receiving donepezil. *JAMA* 291: 317–324.

Tartaglia MC, Rosen JH, Miller BL (2011) Neuroimaging in dementia. *Neurotherapeutics* **8**: 82–92.

Townsend M (2011) When will Alzheimer's disease be cured? A pharmaceutical persepctive. *Journal of Alzheimer's Disease* **24**: 43–52.

Valenzuela MJ, Matthews FE, Brayne C, *et al.*; Medical Research Council Cognitive Funciton and Ageing Study (2012) Multiple biological pathways link cognitive lifestyle to protection from dementia. *Biological Psychiatry* **71**: 783–791.

Vigen CLP, Mack WJ, Keefe RSE, *et al.* (2011) Cognitive effects of atypical antipsychotic medications in patients with Alzheimer's disease: outcomes from CATIE-AD. *American Journal of Psychiatry* **168**: 831–839.

Wagner M, Wolf S, Reischies FM, *et al.* (2012) Biomarker validation of a cued recall memory deficit in prodromal Alzheimer disease. *Neurology* **78**: 379–386.

Williams MM, Xiong C, Morris JC, Galvin JE (2006) Survival and mortality differences between dementia with Lewy bodies vs Alzheimer's disease. *Neurology* **67**: 1935–1941.

Wishart HA, Saykin AJ, McAllister TW, *et al.* (2006) Regional brain atrophy in cognitively intact adults with a single APOE ε4 allele. *Neurology* **67**: 1221–1224.

Wolk DA, Grachev ID, Buckley C, *et al.* (2011) Association between in vivo fluorine 18-labeled flutemetamol amyloid positron emission tomography imaging and in vivo cerebral cortical histopathology. *Archives of Neurology* **68**: 1398–1403.

Chapter 14 (disorders of reward, drug abuse, and their treatment)

Adan RAH, Vanderschuren LJMJ, la Fleur SE (2008) Anti-obesity drugs and neural circuits of feeding. *Trends in Pharmacological Sciences* **29**: 208–217.

Anton RF, O'Malley SS, Ciraulo DA, *et al.* (2006) Combined pharmacotherapies and behavioral interventions for alcohol dependence. The COMBINE study: a randomized controlled trial. *Journal of American Medical Association* **295**: 2003–2017.

Balodis IM, Kober H, Worhunsky PD, *et al.* (2012) Diminished frontostriatal activity during processing of monetary rewards and losses in pathological gambling. *Biological Psychiatry* **71**: 749–757.

Bauman MH, Ayestas MA, Partilla JS, *et al.* (2012) The designer methcathinone analogs, mephedrone and methylone, are substrates for monoamine transporters in brain tissue. *Neuropsychopharmacology* **37**: 1192–1203.

Berlin HA, Rolls ET, Iversen SD (2005) Borderline personality disorder, impulsivity, and the orbitofrontal cortex. *American Journal of Psychiatry* **162**: 2360–2373.

Bradberry CW (2002) Dose-dependent effect of ethanol on extracellular dopamine in mesolimbic striatum of awake rhesus monkeys: comparison with cocaine across individuals. *Psychopharmacology* **165**: 67–76.

Carhart-Harris RL, Erritzoe D, Williams T, *et al.* (2012) Neural correlates of the psychedelic state as determined by fMRI studies with psilocybin. *Proceedings of the National Academy of Sciences* **109**: 2138–2143.

Chamberlain SR, del Campo N, Dowson J, *et al.* (2007) Atomoxetine improved response inhibition in adults with attention deficit/hyperactivity disorder. *Biological Psychiatry* **62**: 977–984.

Chamberlain SR, Menzies L, Hampshire A, *et al.* (2008) Orbitofrontal dysfunction in patients with obsessive–compulsive disorder and their unaffected relatives. *Science* **321**: 421–422.

Chamberlain SR, Muller U, Blackwell AD, *et al.* (2006) Neurochemical modulation of response inhibition and probabilistic learning in humans. *Science* **311**: 861–863.

Chamberlain SR, Robbins TW, Winder-Rhodes S, *et al.* (2011) Translational approaches to frontostriatal dysfunction in attention-deficit/hyperactivity disorder using a computerized neuropsychological battery. *Biological Psychiatry* **69**: 1192–1203.

Clark L, Robbins TW, Ersche KD, Sahakian BJ (2006) Reflection impulsivity in current and former substance users. *Biological Psychiatry* **60**: 515–522.

Collins GT, Narasimhan D, Cunningham AR, *et al.* (2012) Long-lasting effects of a PEGylated mutant cocaine esterase (CocE) on the reinforcing and discriminative stimulus effects of cocaine in rats. *Neuropsychopharmacology* **37**: 1092–1103.

Crunelle CL, Miller ML, Booij J, van den Brink W (2010) The nicotinic acetylcholine receptor partial agonist varenicline and the treatment of drug dependence: a review. *European Neuropsychopharmacology* **20**: 69–79.

Culbertson CS, Bramen J, Cohen MS, *et al.* (2011) Effect of bupropion treatment on brain activation induced by cigarette-related cues in smokers. *Archives of General Psychiatry* **68**: 505–515.

Dahchour A, DeWitte P (2003) Effects of acamprosate on excitatory amino acids during multiple ethanol withdrawal periods. *Alcoholism: Clinical and Experimental Research* **3**: 465–470.

Dalley JW, Everitt BJ (2009) Dopamine receptors in the learning, memory and drug reward circuitry. *Seminars in Cell and Developmental Biology* **20**: 403–410.

Dalley JW, Everitt BJ, Robbins TW (2011) Impulsivity, compulsivity, and top-down cognitive control. *Neuron* **69**: 680–694.

Dalley JW, Mar AC, Economidou D, Robbins TW (2008) Neurobehavioral mechanisms of impulsivity: fronto-striatal systems and functional neurochemistry. *Pharmacology, Biochemistry and Behavior* **90**: 250–260.

DeWitte P (2004) Imbalance between neuroexcitatory and neuroinhibitory amino acids causes craving for ethanol. *Addictive Behaviors* **29**: 1325–1339.

DeWitte P, Littleton J, Parot P, Koob G (2005) Neuroprotective and abstinence-promoting effects of acamprosate: elucidating the mechanism of action. *CNS Drugs* **6**: 517–537.

DiIorio CR, Watkins TJ, Dietrich MS, *et al.* (2012) Evidence for chronically altered serotonin function in the cerebral cortex of female 3, 4-methylenedioxymethamphetamine polydrug users. *Archives of General Psychiatry* **69**: 399–409.

Erritzoe D, Frokjaer VG, Holst KK, *et al.* (2011) In vivo imaging of cerebral serotonin transporter and serotonin $_{2A}$ receptor binding in 3,4-methylenedioxymethamphetamine (MDMA or "ecstasy") and hallucinogen users. *Archives of General Psychiatry* **68**: 562–576.

Ersche KD, Bullmore ET, Craig KJ, *et al.* (2010) Influence of compulsivity of drug abuse on dopaminergic modulation of attentional bias in stimulant dependence. *Archives of General Psychiatry* **67**: 632–644.

Ersche KD, Jones PS, Williams GB, *et al.* (2012) Abnormal brain structure implicated in stimulant drug addiction. *Science* **335**: 601–604.

Ersche KD, Turton AJ, Pradhan S, Bullmore ET, Robbins TW (2010) Drug addiction endophenotypes: impulsive versus sensation-seeking personality traits. *Biological Psychiatry* **68**: 770–773.

Evins AE, Culhane MA, Alpert JE, *et al.* (2008) A controlled trial of bupropion added to nicotine patch and behavioral therapy for smoking cessation in adults with unipolar depressive disorders. *Journal of Clinical Psychopharmacology* **28**: 660–666.

Ferris MJ, Calipari ES, Mateo Y, *et al.* (2012) Cocaine self-administration produces pharmacodynamic tolerance: differential effects on the potency of dopamine transporter blockers, releasers, and methylphenidate: *Neuropsychopharmacology* **37**: 1708–1716.

Fineberg NA, Potenza MN, Chamberlain SR, *et al.* (2010) Probing compulsive and impulsive behaviors, from animal models to endophenotypes: a narrative review. *Neuropsyhcopharmacology* **35**: 591–604.

Flament MF, Bissada H, Spettigue W (2012) Evidence-based pharmacotherapy of eating disorders. *International Journal of Neuropsychopharmacology* **15**: 189–207.

Franklin T, Wang Z, Suh JJ, *et al.* (2011) Effects of varenicline on smoking cue-triggered neural and craving responses. *Archives of General Psychiatry* **68**: 516–526.

Gadde KM, Allison DB, Ryan DH, *et al.* (2011) Effects of low-dose, controlled-release, phentermine plus topiramate combination on weight and associated comorbidities in overweight and obese adults (CONQUER): a randomised, placebo-controlled, phase 3 trial. *Lancet* **377**: 1341–1352.

Gadde KM, Franciscy DM, Wagner HR, Krishnan KR (2003) Zonisamide for weight loss in obese adults. *JAMA* **289**: 1820–1825.

Gadde KM, Yonish GM, Foust MS, Wagner HR (2007) Combination therapy of zonisamide and bupropion for weight reduction in obese women: a preliminary, randomized, open-label study. *Journal of Clinical Psychiatry* **68**: 1226–1229.

Garbutt JC, Kranzler HR, O'Malley SS, *et al.* (2005) Efficacy and tolerability of long-acting injectable naltrexone for alcohol dependence. a randomized controlled trial. *Journal of American Medical Association* **293**; 1617–1625.

Gearhardt AN, Yokum S, Orr PT, *et al.* (2011) Neural correlates of food addiction. *Archives of General Psychiatry* **68**: 808–816.

Gillan CM, Papmeyer M, Morein-Zamir S, *et al.* (2011) Disruption in the balance between goal-directed behavior and habit learning in obsessive–compulsive disorder. *American Journal of Psychiatry* **168**: 719–726.

Grant JE, Kim SW, Hartman BK (2008) A double-blind, placebo-controlled study of the opiate antagonist naltrexone in the treatment of pathological gambling urges. *Journal of Clinical Psychiatry* **69**: 783–789.

Greenberg BD, Malone DA, Friehs GM, *et al.* (2006) Three year outcomes in deep brain stimulation for highly resistant obsessive–compulsive disorder. *Neuropsychopharmacology* **31**: 2384–2393.

Greenberg BD, Rauch SL, Haber SN (2010) Invasive circuitry-based neurotherapeutics: stereotactic ablation and deep brain stimulation for OCD. *Neuropsychopharmacology* **35**: 317–336.

Greenway FL, Whitehouse MJ, Guttadauria M, *et al.* (2008) Rational design of a combination medication for the treatment of obesity. *Obesity* **17**: 30–39.

Greeven A, van Balkom AJLM, van Rood YR, van Oppen P, Spinhoven P (2006) The boundary between hypochondriasis and obsessive–compulsive disorder: a cross-sectional study from the Netherlands. *Journal of Clinical Psychiatry* **67**: 1682–1689.

Haber SN, Knutson B (2010) The reward circuit: linking primate anatomy and human imaging. *Neuropsychopharmacology* **35**: 4–26.

Hart CL, Marvin CB, Silver R, Smith EE (2012) Is cognitive functioning impaired in methamphetamine users? A critical review. *Neuropsychopharmacology* **37**: 586–608.

Hay PJ, Claudino AM (2012) Clinical psychopharmacology of eating disorders: a research update. *International Journal of Neuropsychopharmacology* **15**: 209–222.

Heinz A, Reimold M, Wrase J, *et al.* (2005) Correlation of stable elevations in striatal μ-opioid receptor availability in detoxified alcoholic patients with alcohol craving: a positron emission tomography study using carbon 11-labeled carfentanil. *Archives of General Psychiatry* **62**: 57–64.

Higgins GA, Silenieks LB, Rossmann A, *et al.* (2012) The 5-HT$_{2C}$ receptor agonist lorcaserin reduces nicotine self-administration, discrimination, and reinstatement: relationship to feeding behavior and impulse control. *Neuropsychopharmacology* **37**: 1177–1191.

Jastreboff AM, Potenza MN, Lacadie C, *et al.* (2011) Body mass index, metabolic factors, and striatal activation during stressful and neutral-relaxing states: a fMRI study. *Neuropsychopharmacology* **36**: 627–637.

Jonkman S, Pelloux Y, Everitt BJ (2012) Drug intake is sufficient, but conditioning is not necessary for the emergence of compulsive cocaine seeking after extended self-administration. *Neuropsychopharmacology* **37**: 1612–1619.

Kiefer F, Jahn H, Tarnaske T, *et al.* (2003) Comparing and combining naltrexone and acamprosate in relapse prevention of alcoholism. *Archives of General Psychiatry* **60**: 92–99.

Kiefer F, Wiedemann K (2004) Combined therapy: what does acamprosate and naltrexone combination tell us? *Alcohol and Alcoholism* **39**: 542–547.

King DP, Paciga S, Pickering E, *et al.* (2012) Smoking cessation pharmacogenetics: analysis of varenicline and bupropion in placebo-controlled clinical trials. *Neuropsychopharmacology* **37**: 641–650.

King PJ (2005) The hypothalamus and obesity. *Current Drug Targets* **6**: 225–240.

Koob GF, Le Moal M (2008) Addiction and the brain antireward system. *Annual Review of Psychology* **59**: 29–53.

Koob GF, Volkow ND (2010) Neurocircuitry of addiction. *Neuropsychopharmacology* **35**: 217–238.

Kovacs FE, Knop T, Urbanski MJ, *et al.* (2012) Exogenous and endogenous cannabinoids suppress inhibitory neurotransmission in the human neocortex. *Neuropsychopharmacology* **37**: 1104–1114.

Kuczenski R, Segal DS (2005) Stimulant actions in rodents: implications for attention-deficit/hyperactivity disorder treatment and potential substance abuse. *Biological Psychiatry* **57**: 1391–1396.

Lawrence AJ, Luty J, Bogdan NA, Sahakian BJ, Clark L (2009) Impulsivity and response inhibition in alcohol dependence and problem gambling. *Psychopharmacology* **207**: 163–172.

Leyton M, Boileau I, Benkelfat C, *et al.* (2002) Amphetamine-induced increases in extracellular dopamine, drug wanting, and novelty seaking: a PET/[^{11}C]raclopride study in healthy men. *Neuropsychopharmacology* **27**: 1027–1035.

Lindsey KP, Wilcox KM, Votaw JR, *et al.* (2004) Effect of dopamine transporter inhibitors on cocaine self-administration in rhesus monkeys: relationship to transporter occupancy determined by positron emission tomography neuroimaging. *Journal of Pharmacology and Experimental Therapeutics* **309**: 959–969.

Little KY, Krolewski DM, Zhang L, Cassin BJ (2003) Loss of striatal vesicular monoamine transporter protein (VMAT2) in human cocaine users. *American Journal of Psychiatry* **160**: 47–55.

Lobo DSS, Kennedy JL (2006) The genetics of gambling and behavioral addictions. *CNS Spectr* **11**: 931–939.

Lodge DJ, Grace AA (2006) The hippocampus modulates dopamine neuron responsivity by regulating the intensity of phasic neuron activation. *Neuropsychopharmacology* **31**: 1356–1361.

Lotipour S, Mandelkern M, Alvarez-Estrada M, Brody AL (2012) A single administration of low-dose varenicline saturates α4β2* nicotinic acetylcholine receptors in the human brain. *Neuropsychopharmacology* **37**: 1738–1748.

Mandyam CD, Koob GF (2012) The addicted brain craves new neurons: putative role for adult-born progenitors in promoting recovery. *Trends in Neurosciences* **35**: 250–260.

Martinez D, Gil R, Slifstein M, *et al.* (2005) Alcohol dependence is associated with blunted dopamine transmission in the ventral striatum. *Biological Psychiatry* **58**: 779–786.

Martinez D, Narendran R, Foltin RW, *et al.* (2007) Amphetamine-induced dopamine release: markedly blunted in cocaine dependence and predictive of the choice to self-administer cocaine. *American Journal of Psychiatry* **164**: 622–629.

Mason BJ (2003) Acamprosate and naltrexone treatment for alcohol dependence: an evidence-based risk-benefits assessment. *European NeuroPsychopharmacology* **13**: 469–475.

Mason BJ (2005) Acamprosate in the treatment of alcohol dependence. *Expert Opinion on Pharmacotherapy* **6**: 2103–2115.

Mason BJ, Crean R, Goodell V, *et al.* (2012) A proof-of-concept randomized controlled study of gabapentin: effects on cannabis use, withdrawal and executive function deficits in cannabis-dependent adults. *Neuropsychopharmacology* **37**: 1689–1698.

Mason BJ, Goodman AM, Chabac S, Lehert P (2006) Effect of oral acamprosate on abstinence in patients with alcohol dependence in a double-blind, placebo-controlled trial: the role of patient motivation. *Journal of Psychiatric Research* **40**: 382–392.

McElroy SL, Hudson JI, Capece JA, *et al.* (2007) Topiramate for the treatment of binge eating disorder associated with obesity: a placebo-controlled study. *Biological Psychiatry* **61**: 1039–1048.

Menzies L, Chamberlain SR, Laird AR, *et al.* (2008) Integrating evidence from neuroimaging and neuropsychological studies of obsessive–compulsive disorder: the orbitofronto-striatal model revisited. *Neuroscience and Biobehavioral Reviews* **32**: 525–549.

Miedl SF, Peters J, Buchel C (2012) Altered neural reward representations in pathological gamblers revealed by delay and probability discounting. *Archives of General Psychiatry* **69**: 177–186.

Milad MR, Rauch SL (2012) Obsessive–compulsive disorder: beyond segregated cortico-striatal pathways. *Trends in Cognitive Sciences* **16**: 43–51.

Narendran R, Lopresti BJ, Martinez D, *et al.* (2012) In vivo evidence for low striatal vesicular monoamine transporter 2 (VMAT2) availability in cocaine abusers. *American Journal of Psychiatry* **169**: 55–63.

Nathan PJ, O'Neill BV, Mogg K, *et al.* (2012) The effects of the dopamine d_3 receptor antagonist GSK598809 on attentional bias to palatable food cues in overweight and obese subjects. *International Journal of Neuropsychopharmacology* **15**: 149–161.

Nestler EJ (2005) Is there a common molecular pathway for addiction? *Nature Neuroscience* **11**: 1445–1449.

Netzeband JG, Gruol DL (1995) Modulatory effects of acute ethanol on metabotropic glutamate responses in cultured purkinje neurons. *Brain Research* **688**: 105–113.

Overtoom CCE, Bekker EM, van der Molen MW, *et al.* (2009) Methylphenidate restores link between stop-signal sensory impact and successful stopping in adults with attention deficit/hyperactivity disorder. *Biological Psychiatry* **65**: 614–619.

Peng, XO, Xi ZX, Li X, *et al.* (2010) Is slow-onset long-acting monoamine transport blockade to cocaine as methadone is to heroin? implication for anti-addiction medications. *Neuropsychopharmacology* **35**: 2564–2578.

Petrakis IL, Poling J, Levinson C, *et al.*; VA New England VISN I MIRECC Study Group (2005) Naltrexone and disulfiram in patients with alcohol dependence and comorbid psychiatric disorders. *Biological Psychiatry* **57**: 1128–1137.

Pettinati HM, O'Brien CP, Rabinowitz AR, *et al.* (2006) The status of naltrexone in the treatment of alcohol dependence: specific effects on heavy drinking. *Journal of Clinical Psychopharmacology* **26**: 610–625.

Richter MA, de Jesus DR, Hoppenbrouwers S, *et al.* (2012) Evidence for cortical inhibitory and excitatory dysfunction in obsessive compulsive disorder. *Neuropsychopharmacology* **37**: 1144–1151.

Robbins TW, Gillan CM, Smith DG, de Wit S, Ersche KD (2012) Neurocognitive endophenotypes of impulsivity and compulsivity: towards dimensional psychiatry. *Trends Cogn Sci* **16**: 81–91.

Roozen HG, deWaart R, van der Windt DAW, *et al.* (2005) A systematic review of the effectiveness of naltrexone in the maintenance treatment of opioid and alcohol dependence. *European Neuropsychopharmacology* **16**: 311–323.

Salamone JD, Correa M, Mingote S, Weber SM (2002) Nucleus accumbens dopamine and the regulation of effort in food-seeking behavior: implications for studies of natural motivation, psychiatry, and drug abuse. *The Journal of Pharmacology and Experimental Therapeutics* **305**: 1–8

Schauer PR, Kashyap SR, Wolski K, *et al.* (2012) Bariatric surgery versus intensive medical therapy in obese patients with diabetes. *New England Journal of Medicine* **366**: 1567–1576.

Schneider S, Peters J, Bromberg U, *et al.*; IMAGEN Consortium (2012) Risk taking and the adolescent reward system: a potential common link to substance abuse. *American Journal of Psychiatry* **169**: 39–46.

Selzer J (2006) Buprenorphine: reflections of an addictions psychiatrist. *American Society of Clinical Psychopharmacology* **9**: 1466–1467.

Shaw P, Gilliam M, Liverpool M, *et al.* (2011) Cortical development in typically developing children with symptoms of hyperactivity and impulsivity: support for a dimensional view of attention deficit hyperactivity disorder. *American Journal of Psychiatry* **168**: 143–151.

Smith BM, Thomsen WJ, Grottick AJ (2006) The potential use of selective 5-HT$_{2C}$ agonists in treating obesity. *Expert Opinion on Investigational Drugs* **15**: 257–266.

Solinas M, Goldberg SR (2005) Motivational effects of cannabinoids and opioids on food reinforcement depend on simultaneous activation of cannabinoid and opioid systems. *Neuropsychopharmacology* **30**: 2035–2045.

Spencer TJ, Biederman J, Ciccone PE, *et al.* (2006) PET study examining pharmacokinetics, detection and likeability, and dopamine transporter receptor occupancy of short- and long-acting oral methylphenidate. *American Journal of Psychiatry* **163**: 387–395.

Steinberg MB, Greenhaus S, Schmelzer AC, *et al.* (2009) Triple-combination pharmacotherapy for medically ill smokers: a randomized trial. *Annals of Internal Medicine* **150**: 447–454.

Sugam JA, Day JJ, Wightman RM, Carelki RM (2012) Phasic nucleus accumbens dopamine encodes risk-based decision-making behavior. *Biological Psychiatry* **71**: 199–205.

Thomsen WJ, Grottick AJ, Menzaghi F, *et al.* (2008) Lorcaserin, a novel selective human 5-hydroxytryptamine$_{2C}$ agonist: in vitro and in vivo pharmacological characterization. *Journal of Pharmacology and Experimental Therapeutics* **325**: 577–587.

Tiihonen J, Krupitsky E, Verbitskaya E, *et al.* (2012) Naltrexone implant for the treatment of polydrug dependence: a randomized controlled trial. *American Journal of Psychiatry* **169**: 531–536.

Urban NBL, Girgis RR, Talbot PS, *et al.* (2012) Sustained recreational use of ecstasy is associated with altered pre and postsynaptic markers of serotonin transmission in neocortical areas: a PET study with [^{11}C]DASB and [^{11}C]MDL 100907. *Neuropsychopharmacology* **37**: 1465–1473.

Van de Giessen E, de Bruin K, la Fleur SE, van den Brink W, Booij J (2012) Triple monoamine inhibitor tesofensine decreases food intake, body weight, and striatal dopamine D2/D3 receptor availability in diet-induced obese rats. *European Neuropsychopharmacology* **22**: 290–299.

Van Holst RJ, Veltman DJ, Buchel C, van den Brink W, Goudriaan AE (2012) Distorted expectancy coding in problem gambling: is the addictive in the anticipation? *Biological Psychiatry* **71**: 741–748.

Volkow ND (2006) Stimulant medications: how to minimize their reinforcing effects? *American Journal of Psychiatry* **163**: 359–361.

Volkow ND, O'Brien CP (2007) Issues for DSM-V: should obesity be included as a brain disorder? *American Journal of Psychiatry* **164**: 708–710.

Volkow ND, Wang GJ, Fowler JS, *et al.* (2004) Evidence that methylphenidate enhances the saliency of a mathematical task by increasing dopamine in the human brain. *American Journal of Psychiatry* **161**: 1173–1180.

Volkow ND, Wang GJ, Fowler JS, Tomasi D, Telang F (2011) Addiction: beyond dopamine reward circuitry. *Proceedings of the National Academy of Sciences* **108**: 15037–15042.

Weathers JD, Stringaris AR, Deveney CM, *et al.* (2012) A development study of the neural circuitry mediating motor inhibition in bipolar disorder. *American Journal of Psychiatry* **169**: 633–641.

Wee S, Hicks MJ, De BP, *et al.* (2012) Novel cocaine vaccine linked to a disrupted adenovirus gene transfer vector blocks cocaine psychostimulant and reinforcing effects. *Neuropsychopharmacology* **37**: 1083–1091.

Wilding J, Van Gaal L, Rissanen A, Vercruysse F, Fitchet M (2004) A randomized double-blind placebo-controlled study of the long-term efficacy and safety of topiramate in the treatment of obese subjects. *International Journal of Obesity* **28**: 1399–1410.

Zack M, Poulos CX (2007) A D1 antagonist enhances the rewarding and priming effects of a gambling episode in pathological gamblers. *Neuropsychopharmacology* **32**: 1678–1686.

Index

THE STORY OF

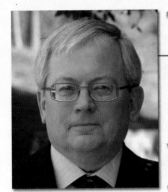

Stahl's Essential
Psychopharmacology

The Essential Psychopharmacology franchise began 17 years ago as a published offshoot of my lectures for mental health professionals.

I have always had to 'see' something before I could understand it, especially disease mechanisms and drug actions, and thus developed a compendium of figures and diagrams for my lectures. With my longterm illustrator Nancy Muntner, we gradually developed a 'visual language' for psychopharmacology with icons and figures that have become the signature feature of **Stahl's Essential Psychopharmacology**.

The original textbook – **Stahl's Essential Psychopharmacology**, the Fourth Edition of which you have in your hands now – explained how drugs work but not how to use them, so the **Prescriber's Guide** was created as a companion to the textbook. For this, in addition to our characteristic use of unique icons, we also included standard evidence based drug information. I also added 'tips and pearls' based on the art of psychopharmacology and derived as much from my experience in clinical practice as from the evidence.

More recently, we added two additional core educational resources. A **Case Studies** book, which is about living through the treatments that work, the treatments that fail, and the mistakes made along the journey – psychiatry in real life – and a **Self-Assessment Examination in Psychiatry** book with 150 questions and answers designed to help the reader to identify areas of competence or the need for further study.

Also available are the books in the **Stahl's Illustrated Series**, which evolved to answer the need for a distillation of focused therapeutic areas in a highly visual and easy to digest format in the size of a pocketbook.

More details of these publications appear in the following pages, and please remember that all of these resources are also available via your computer at **Stahl's Essential Psychopharmacology Online**.

four 'must-haves' Stahl's Essential Psychopharmacology

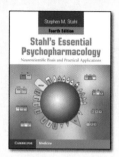

Stahl's Essential Psychopharmacology
Neuroscientific Basis and Practical Applications
Fourth Edition

- Long established as the preeminent source of education and information in its field

- Features the author's highly-praised writing style with clear, easy-to-follow illustrations

- Thoroughly updated and extensively revised for the fourth edition, taking account of advances in neurobiology and recent clinical developments to explain the concepts underlying the drug treatment of psychiatric disorders with a sleek new look and feel, larger page size, and two-column layout

- Indispensable for all professionals and students in mental health

978-1-107-68646-5 • Pbk • 616 pp • 2013   978-1-107-02598-1 • Hbk • 616 pp • 2013

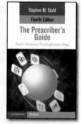

The Prescriber's Guide
Fourth Edition

Also available as an app! Visit the App Store for details!

- Completely revised and updated edition of the most widely-used prescribing guide specifically for psychopharmacology

- With new drug additions, and every drug entry revised and updated to take into account new regulations and uses

- Full color throughout, with information distilled into pragmatic formulary that gives all information that prescribers need to treat patients effectively

- Indexes by name, use, and class

978-0-521-17364-3 • Pbk • 712 pp • 2011

Available on the App Store

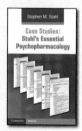

Case Studies

- Designed with the distinctive, user-friendly presentation that has been so popular in *Stahl's Essential Psychopharmacology* and *The Prescriber's Guide*

- Describes a wide-ranging and representative selection of clinical scenarios, making use of icons, questions/answers and tips

- Cases are followed through the complete clinical encounter, from start to resolution, acknowledging all the complications, issues, decisions, twists and turns along the way

- Psychiatry in real life!

978-0-521-18208-9 • Pbk • 408 pp • 2011

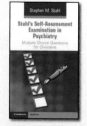

Stahl's Self-Assessment Examination in Psychiatry
Multiple Choice Questions for Clinicians

- Builds on Dr Stahl's exceptional ability to communicate complex principles and make them accessible

- Offers 150 self-assessment questions derived from Dr Stahl's Online Master Psychopharmacology Program, each followed by thorough explanation of correct and incorrect answer choices

- Ideal for those preparing for formal tests, including the American Board of Psychiatry and Neurology, and achieving CME and MoC credits towards ongoing ABPN re-accreditation

978-1-107-68159-0 • Pbk • 344 pp • 2012

Stahl's Illustrated Series

These books are designed to be fun. In full-color throughout, with illustrations in the style of the classic *Essential Psychopharmacology and Prescriber's Guide*, they provide a speedy way to learn or review specific concepts in psychopharmacology.

The visual learner will find that these books make psychopharmacology concepts easy to master, while the non-visual learner will enjoy a shortened text version of complex psychopharmacology concepts.

Within each book, each chapter builds on previous chapters, synthesizing information from basic biology and diagnostics to building treatment plans and dealing with complications and comorbidities. And, to help guide the reader toward more in-depth learning about particular concepts, each book ends with a Suggested Reading section.

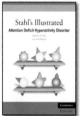

Stahl's Illustrated Attention Deficit Hyperactivity Disorder

978-0-521-13315-9
Pbk • 166 pp • 2009

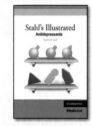

Stahl's Illustrated Antidepressants

978-0-521-75852-9
Pbk • 200 pp • 2009

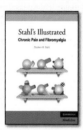

Stahl's Illustrated Chronic Pain and Fibromyalgia

978-0-521-13322-7
Pbk • 166 pp • 2009

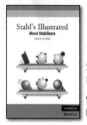

Stahl's Illustrated Mood Stabilizers

978-0-521-75849-9
Pbk • 176 pp • 2009

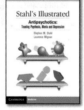

Stahl's Illustrated Antipsychotics: Treating Psychosis, Mania and Depression Second Edition

978-0-521-14905-1
Pbk • 166 pp • 2009

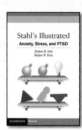

Stahl's Illustrated Anxiety, Stress, PTSD

978-0-521-15399-7
Pbk • 200 pp • 2010

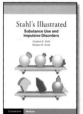

Stahl's Illustrated Substance Use and Impulsive Disorders

978-1-107-67453-0
Pbk • 183 pp • 2012

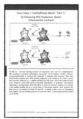

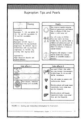

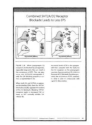

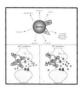

Also available

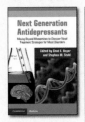

Next Generation Antidepressants
Moving Beyond Monoamines to Discover Novel Treatment Strategies for Mood Disorders

Chad E Beyer, PhD, MBA, University of Colorado School of Medicine, Aurora, USA, Dr Stephen M Stahl, MD, PhD, University of California, San Diego, USA

- Looks at the future of mood-disorder research in order to help build a better picture of the disease process and lead to new opportunities for patient stratification and treatment

- Essential reading for all those involved in psychopharmacologic drug development, and mental health clinicians seeking preview of discoveries soon to influence their practice

978-0-521-76058-4 • Hbk • 150 pp • 2010

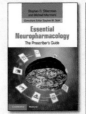

Also available as an app! Visit the App Store for details!

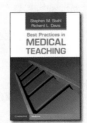
Available on the App Store

Essential Neuropharmacology
The Prescriber's Guide

Stephen D Silberstein, MD, Jefferson Medical College, Philadelphia, USA, Michael J Marmura, MD, Jefferson Medical College, Philadelphia, USA, Dr Stephen M Stahl, MD, PhD, University of California, San Diego, USA (Consultant Editor)

- Expertly reviews the most important medications used by neurologists in their practice

- Evidence is taken from recent clinical trials, which helps the reader relate the content to everyday clinical practice

- Detailed descriptions of each medication enable user to make quick and informed decisions with the confidence

978-0-521-13672-3 • Pbk • 420 pp • 2010

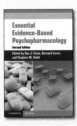

Essential Evidence-Based Psychopharmacology
Second Edition

Prof Dan Stein, University of Cape Town, South Africa, Dr Bernard Lerner, Hadassah-Hebrew University Medical Center, Israel, Dr Stephen M Stahl, MD, PhD, University of California, San Diego, USA

- Fully updated, this volume summarizes the wealth of new developments in the field of psychopharmacology and sets them within context of day-to-day clinical practice

- Organized according to the DSM-V listing and covering all major conditions, this book is invaluable to all practicing and training clinicians in a mental health or a less specialized environment

978-1-107-00795-6 • Pbk • 336 pp • 2012

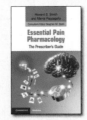

Best Practices in Medical Teaching

Dr. Stephen M Stahl, MD, PhD, University of California, San Diego, USA, Richard L Davis, Arbor Scientia, Carlsbad, USA

- Written by two of the leading experts in medical communication, this book illustrates the general principles of effective medical presentation by applying the principles of adult learning

- Features examples of how to design a successful lecture, along with chapter summary, progress check, and performance self-assessment test to ensure that concepts are understood

978-0-521-15176-4 • Pbk • 192 pp • 2011

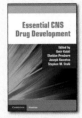

Essential CNS Drug Development

Amir Kalali, MD, University of California, San Diego, USA, Joseph Kwentus, MD, University of Mississippi, Jackson, USA, Sheldon Preskorn, MD, University of Kansas School of Medicine, Wichita, USA, Dr. Stephen M Stahl Stahl, MD, PhD, University of California, San Diego, USA

- Explains the complicated process of CNS drug development in an engaging fashion, covering drug development from pre-clinical research through all phases of clinical trials, to reporting to the regulatory authorities

- User-friendly format and style enable readers to find important information quickly and easily

- Unique resource for drug developers, investigators, academics and clinicians

978-0-521-76606-7 • Hbk • 218 pp • 2012

Essential Pain Pharmacology
The Prescriber's Guide

Howard S Smith, MD, Albany Medical Center, USA, Marco Pappagallo, MD, New York Medical Home for Chronic Pain, USA, Dr Stephen M Stahl, MD, University of California, San Diego, USA

- Clear and concise, this book presents most up-to-date and comprehensive array of agents available for prescribing

- A user-friendly must-have on the shelf of every physician

978-0-521-75910-6 • Pbk • 575 pp • 2012

Stahl's Essential Psychopharmacology Online

Now online, and more user-friendly than ever!

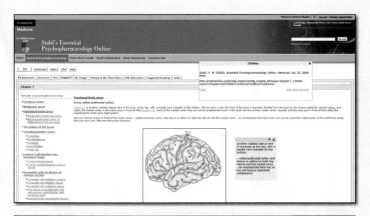

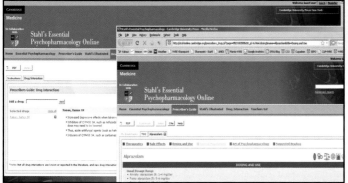

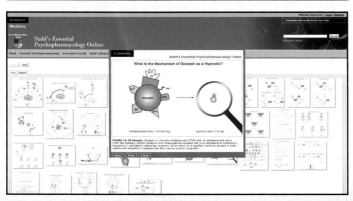

Features the **full text and all the illustrations** from the latest editions of *Stahl's Essential Psychopharmacology, The Prescriber's Guide*, the books currently available in the *Stahl's Illustrated Series*, and other books authored and co-authored by Dr Stahl, **all searchable on the same platform**.

- **Search drugs** by class, name, type, or use across all content, then **easily filter** your results

- Use **quick search** for easy use during patient appointments

- **Download illustrations and tables** for presentations and lectures

- **Cite, bookmark** or **take** notes at the click of a button

- **Link directly** to suggested readings

- **Use one-click access** to the Neuroscience Education Institute's **CME** portal

For more information including pricing, visit **www.stahlonline.org** and click on the 'Subscribe Today' button.

CNS
Spectrums
The Journal of the
Neuroscience Education Institute

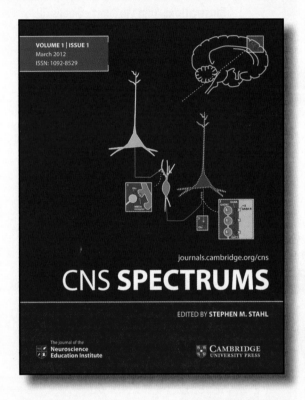

VOLUME 1 | ISSUE 1
March 2012
ISSN: 1092-8529

journals.cambridge.org/cns

CNS SPECTRUMS

EDITED BY **STEPHEN M. STAHL**

The journal of the
**Neuroscience
Education Institute**

CAMBRIDGE
UNIVERSITY PRESS

ISSN: 1092-8529
EISSN: 2165-6509

Editor: Stephen M. Stahl, University of California School of Medicine, San Diego, USA and Cambridge University, Cambridge, UK

Cambridge Journals announced the acquisition of *CNS Spectrums* in November 2011. The journal joined Cambridge University Press' established titles in Psychiatry and Psychopharmacology, and now forms an exciting parallel to *Stahl's Essential Psychopharmacology*.

CNS Spectrums was reconfigured and relaunched in 2012. Building upon its previous status, the new Editor-in-Chief, Dr. Stephen M. Stahl, has formed a new editorial board and developed the aims and scope of the journal to fully bridge the clinical information needs of psychiatrists and neurologists. As of 2013, *CNS Spectrums* publishes bimonthly.

For more information, please visit
journals.cambridge.org / cns

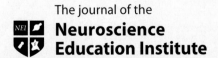

The journal of the
**Neuroscience
Education Institute**

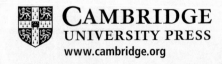

CAMBRIDGE
UNIVERSITY PRESS
www.cambridge.org